VALVULAR HEART DISEASE

THIRD EDITION

VALVULAR HEART DISEASE

THIRD EDITION

Edited by

Joseph S. Alpert, M.D.
Robert S. and Irene P. Flinn Professor of Medicine
Head, Department of Medicine
University of Arizona College of Medicine;
University Medical Center
Tucson, Arizona

James E. Dalen, M.D., M.P.H.
Vice President for Health Science
Dean, University of Arizona College of Medicine;
Cardiologist
University Medical Center
Tucson, Arizona

Shahbudin H. Rahimtoola, M.B., F.R.C.P., M.A.C.P., M.A.C.C.
George C. Griffith Distinguished Professor of Cardiology
Professor of Medicine
University of Southern California
Los Angeles, California

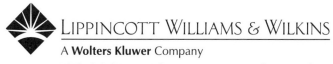

LIPPINCOTT WILLIAMS & WILKINS
A **Wolters Kluwer** Company
Philadelphia · Baltimore · New York · London
Buenos Aires · Hong Kong · Sydney · Tokyo

Acquisitions Editor: Ruth W. Weinberg
Developmental Editor: Anjou K. Dargar
Production Editor: Frank Aversa
Manufacturing Manager: Kevin Watt
Cover Designer: David Levy
Compositor: Lippincott Williams & Wilkins, Desktop Division
Printer: Maple Press

© 2000 by **LIPPINCOTT WILLIAMS & WILKINS**
227 East Washington Square
Philadelphia, PA 19106-3780 USA
LWW.com

Printed in the USA

Library of Congress Cataloging-in-Publication Data

Valvular heart disease / edited by Joseph S. Alpert, James E. Dalen, Shahbudin H. Rahimtoola. — 3rd ed.
    p. cm.
    Includes bibliographical references and index.
    ISBN 0-7817-2310-8
    1. Heart valves—Diseases. I. Alpert, Joseph S. II. Dalen, James E., 1932-
III. Rahimtoola, Shahbudin H.
    RC685.V2 V34 1999
    616.1'25—dc21
                                                                99-16809
                                                                CIP

10   9   8   7   6   5   4   3   2   1

*This book is dedicated to our mentors and colleagues
who are no longer alive but whose inspiration remains with us:
Lewis Dexter, Richard Gorlin, Niels A. Lassen,
Thomas W. Smith, and Jay M. Sullivan.*

Contents

Contributing Authors

Joseph S. Alpert, M.D.
Robert S. and Irene P. Flinn Professor of
 Medicine
Head, Department of Medicine
University of Arizona College of Medicine;
University Medical Center
1501 North Campbell Avenue
P. O. Box 245035
Tucson, Arizona 85724-5035

Robert O. Bonow, M.D.
Goldberg Distinguished Professor
Department of Medicine
Northwestern University Medical School;
Chief, Division of Cardiology
Northwestern Memorial Hospital
250 East Superior Street
Chicago, Illinois 60611-2950

Allen P. Burke, M.D.
Co-Chair and Staff Pathologist, A.F.I.P.
Department of Cardiovascular Pathology
Armed Forces Institute of Pathology
14th Street, Alaska Avenue, N.W.
Washington, D.C. 20306-6000

Blase A. Carabello, M.D.
Professor of Medicine
Department of Medicine
Main Baylor Plaza; Baylor College of Medicine;
Chief of Medical Service
VA Medical Center
VAMC 111, 2002 Holcombe Boulevard
Houston, Texas 77030

Antonio J. Chamoun, M.D.
Fellow, Division of Cardiology
University of Texas Medical Branch at Galveston
301 University Boulevard
5.106 John Sealy Annex
Galveston, Texas 77555-0553

Y. Chandrashekhar, M.D.
Assistant Professor of Medicine
Division of Cardiology
University of Minnesota School of Medicine
Minneapolis, Minnesota 55455

James E. Dalen, M.D., M.P.H.
Vice President for Health Sciences
Dean, University of Arizona College of
 Medicine;
Cardiologist
University Medical Center
1501 North Campbell Avenue
Tucson, Arizona 85724

Mark J. DiNubile, M.D.
Associate Professor of Medicine
University of Medicine and Dentistry of New
 Jersey,
Robert Wood Johnson Medical School;
Division of Infectious Diseases
Cooper Health System
Camden, New Jersey 08103

Gordon A. Ewy, M.D.
Professor and Chief of Medicine
Department of Medicine
University of Arizona College of Medicine;
Director, Diagnostic Cardiology
Arizona Health Sciences Center
1501 North Campbell Avenue
Tucson, Arizona 85724-5037

Andrew Farb, M.D.
Staff Cardiovascular Pathologist
Department of Cardiovascular Pathology
Armed Forces Institute of Pathology
14th Street, Alaska Avenue, N.W.
Washington, D.C. 20306-6000

Paul E. Fenster, M.D.
Associate Professor of Medicine
Department of Medicine
University of Arizona College of Medicine;
Director of Adult Echocardiography
University Medical Center
1501 North Campbell Avenue, Room 6404
Tucson, Arizona 85724-5037

Robert L. Frye, M.D.
Rose M. and Morris Eisenberg Professor of
  Medicine
Mayo Clinic
Rochester, Minnesota 55905

Joel M. Gore, M.D.
Professor of Medicine
University of Massachusetts Medical School;
Director, Division of Cardiovascular Medicine
University of Massachusetts Memorial Health
  Care
55 Lake Avenue, North
Worcester, Massachusetts 01655

Howard R. Horn, M.D.
The L. W. Diggs Alumni Professor of Medicine
and Chair of Excellence in Medical Education
Department of Medicine
The University of Tennessee, Memphis Health
  Science Center;
Senior Cardiologist
U.T. Bowld Hospital
951 Court Avenue, Room 754, Bowld
Memphis, Tennessee 38163

Gilbert E. Levinson, M.D. (deceased)
Professor of Medicine
University of Massachusetts Medical School;
Chief, Department of Medicine
St. Vincent's Hospital
Worcester, Massachusetts 01655

Karam C. Mounzer, M.D.
Assistant Professor of Clinical Medicine
Department of Internal Medicine/Infectious
  Disease
University of Medicine and Dentistry
  of New Jersey,
401 Haddon Avenue;
Attending, Department of Internal Medicine
Cooper Health System
1 Cooper Plaza
Camden, New Jersey 08103

**Jagat Narula, M.B., M.D., D.M., Ph.D.,
  F.A.C.C.**
Associate Professor of Medicine
Staff Physician
Director, Heart Failure and Transplant Center
Director, Center of Molecular Cardiology
MCP Hahnemann University School of Medicine
Broad & Vine, Mail Stop 115
Philadelphia, Pennsylvania 19102

Robert A. O'Rourke, M.D.
Charles Conrad Brown Distinguished Professor
  in Cardiovascular Disease
Department of Medicine/Cardiology
University of Texas Health Science Center
  at San Antonio
7703 Floyd Curl Drive;
Director of C.C.U.
Audie L. Murphy Veterans Hospital
7400 Merton Minter Boulevard
San Antonio, Texas 78284-7872

John A. Paraskos, M.D.
Professor of Medicine
Department of Medicine, Cardiology
University of Massachusetts Medical School;
Director of Cardiovascular Center
  and Ambulatory Cardiology Services
University of Massachusetts Memorial
  Health Care
55 Lake Avenue, North
Worcester, Massachusetts 01655

**Shahbudin H. Rahimtoola, M.B.,
  F.R.C.P., M.A.C.P., M.A.C.C.**
George C. Griffith Distinguished Professor of
  Cardiology
Professor of Medicine
University of Southern California
2025 Zonal Avenue
Los Angeles, California 90033

**Kodangudi B. Ramanathan, M.D.,
  M.R.C.P.**
Professor of Medicine
Department of Medicine/Cardiology
The University of Tennessee
951 Court Avenue, Room 353D
Memphis, Tennessee 38163;
Chief, Division of Cardiology
VA Medical Center
1030 Jefferson Street
Memphis, Tennessee 38104

P. Syamasundar Rao, M.D., F.A.C.C.
Professor of Pediatrics
Division of Pediatric Cardiology
St. Louis University School of Medicine;
Director, Center for Transcatheter Treatment
  of Heart Defects in Children
Cardinal Glennon Children's Hospital
1465 South Grand Boulevard
St. Louis, Missouri 63104-1095

Maurice Enriquez-Sarano, M.D.
Mayo Clinic
E16A
200 First Street, S.W.
Rochester, Minnesota 55905

Hartzell V. Schaff, M.D.
Stuart W. Harrington Professor of Surgery
Division of Cardiovascular Surgery
Mayo Clinic and Foundation
200 First Street, S.W.
Rochester, Minnesota 55905;
Consultant, Cardiovascular Surgery
Saint Mary's Hospital
1216 Second Street, S.W.
Rochester, Minnesota 55902

Paul D. Stein, M.D.
Professor of Medicine (Henry Ford)
Medical Director, Cardiac Wellness Center
Henry Ford Heart and Vascular Institute
6525 Second Avenue
Detroit, Michigan 48202

Abdul Jamil Tajik, M.D.
Thomas J. Watson, Jr., Professor of Medicine
    and Pediatrics
Department of Internal Medicine;
Chair, Division of Cardiovascular Diseases
Mayo Clinic
200 First Street, S.W.
Rochester, Minnesota 55905

Kathryn A. Taubert, Ph.D.
Associate Professor
Department of Physiology
University of Texas Southwestern Medical
    School
5323 Harry Hines Boulevard
Dallas, Texas 75235;
Senior Scientist
Department of Science and Medicine
American Heart Association
7272 Greenville Avenue
Dallas, Texas 75231-4596

Hoang M. Thai, M.D.
Assistant Professor of Clinical Medicine
University of Arizona College of Medicine
Veteran's Administration Medical Center, Section
    of Cardiology
1501 North Campbell Avenue
P.O. Box 245037
Tucson, Arizona 85724-5037

Renu Virmani, M.D.
Chair, Department of Cardiovascular Pathology
Armed Forces Institute of Pathology
14th Street, Alaska Avenue, N.W., Building 54,
    Room 2005
Washington, D.C. 20306-6000

Preface

Remarkable changes have occurred in the epidemiology, natural history, diagnostic evaluation, and therapy of patients with valvular heart disease during the last twenty-five years. Today, individuals with valvular heart disease can look forward to longer survival and better quality of life than was the case for earlier generations. When the first edition of this text was published in 1981, rheumatic heart disease was common. Today, adult cardiologists see fewer of these cases. On the other hand, degenerative valve diseases such as calcific, atherosclerotic aortic stenosis have become more frequent. Myxomatous degeneration of the mitral valve has also assumed a greater role among patients with valvular heart disease.

Catheter therapy for valvular stenosis had not been conceived in 1981 and hence was not mentioned in the first edition of *Valvular Heart Disease*. Today, catheter valvuloplasty is a commonly employed therapeutic intervention. Other new diagnostic or management strategies include anticoagulation for atrial fibrillation, transesophageal echocardiography, and vasodilator therapy for chronic valvular regurgitation, to mention a few of the many changes that have occurred.

The first two editions of *Valvular Heart Disease* were written primarily by faculty at the University of Massachusetts Medical School. In this third edition we have increased the number of editors with the edition of Dr. Rahimtoola, a Distinguished Professor of Cardiology at the University of Southern California, and we have sought to expand the scope of authors by including experts from around the country. This edition has undergone extensive editing and updating, and numerous figures and tables have been added throughout the text. However, we have retained our original intent: to offer the reader a complete, authoritative, and readable source of information concerning all forms of valvular heart disease. We believe that we have succeeded in reaching this goal.

Joseph S. Alpert
James E. Dalen
Shahbudin H. Rahimtoola

Acknowledgments

This book would not have been possible without the constant assistance of many individuals who offered advice, technical assistance, and continuing support. The editors thank the following individuals: Barbara Raney and Charlene Sass for superb technical assistance, Ruth Weinberg for sage advice, and Anjou Dargar for editorial excellence. Finally, we express our love and appreciation to our families, from whom precious hours were stolen in order to complete this book.

VALVULAR HEART DISEASE

THIRD EDITION

1

Pathogenesis and Pathology of Valvular Heart Disease

Andrew Farb, Renu Virmani, and Allen P. Burke

*Department of Cardiovascular Pathology, Armed Forces Institute of Pathology,
Washington, DC 20306*

Our current understanding of the pathogenesis of valvular heart disease rests on the pioneering pathologic studies by Jesse Edwards, Ariela Pomerance, and William C. Roberts. Their work led to the recognition that rheumatic scarring is not the only important cause of valve disease and underscored the significance of degenerative changes associated with advancing age. Barlow's studies of the mitral valve defined the entity of myxomatous degeneration, currently the most frequent cause of mitral valve insufficiency requiring surgical intervention. Increased longevity in patients has been accomplished through improvements in early detection and assessment of valvular heart disease by advances in cardiac imaging, especially echocardiography, along with the development of surgical techniques to replace native diseased valves. Many of these advances occurred in the 1960s and 1970s, and there has been further remarkable progress in the last two decades through better understanding of valvular and myocardial physiology, establishment of criteria for the optimal timing for surgical intervention,

and the recognition of improved outcomes via valve repair and other valve preserving surgical procedures rather than simple valve replacement.

CLASSIFICATION OF VALVULAR HEART DISEASE

Valvular heart disease may be classified by the underlying etiology and by the physiologic abnormality (Table 1-1); clearly, there will be overlap between these two schemes. In this chapter, our discussion of mitral valve pathology is presented based on underlying etiology. Because the physiologic abnormalities associated with aortic valve dysfunction are predominately responsible for the clinical presentation, we focus the section on aortic valve pathology based on the hemodynamic consequences of the valve lesion (i.e., stenosis or incompetence or both). Diseases of the tricuspid and pulmonary valves are discussed individually, and endocarditis is treated as a separate section. Finally, valve abnormalities occurring in the setting of systemic diseases are presented. Over the last several decades, the epidemiology of the most frequent causes of valvular heart disease has undergone dramatic changes concurrent with the reduction in rheumatic disease. These changes are presented as a function of patient age, a critical

The opinions or assertions contained herein are the private views of the authors and are not to be construed as official or reflecting the views of the Department of the Army, the Department of the Air Force, or the Department of Defense.

CHAPTER 1

TABLE 1-1. *Classification of valvular heart disease*

Mitral valve
  Congenital disorders: Parachute mitral valve, cleft mitral valve
  Myxomatous degeneration (mitral valve prolapse)
  Acute rheumatic fever and post-rheumatic scarring
  Mitral annular calcification
  Papillary muscle ischemia and infarction
  Mitral annular dilatation (dilated cardiomyopathy)
  Hypertrophic cardiomyopathy
Tricuspid valve
  Post-rheumatic scarring
  Tricuspid insufficiency secondary to annular dilatation (pulmonary hypertension)
  Ebstein's anomaly
  Myxomatous degeneration (tricuspid valve prolapse)
Aortic valve
  Aortic stenosis
    Congenial: unicuspid and bicuspid valves
    Degenerative tricuspid aortic stenosis
    Post-rheumatic scarring
  Aortic insufficiency
    Diseases of valve
      Congenital bicuspid valve
      Post-rheumatic scarring
      Myxomatous degeneration (aortic valve prolapse)
    Diseases of the aortic root
      Hypertension
      Marfan's syndrome
      Ehlers-Danlos syndrome
      Pseudoxanthoma elasticum
      Idiopathic aortic dilatation (annuloaortic ectasia)
      Aortic dissection
      Trauma
Pulmonary valve
  Congenital bicuspid valve
   Isolated pulmonic stenosis
   Tetralogy of Fallot
  Pulmonic insufficiency secondary to annular dilatation (pulmonary hypertension)
  Post-rheumatic scarring
Endocarditis
  Infective
  Noninfective
Valvular abnormalities in systemic disease
  Carcinoid heart disease
  Systemic lupus erythematosus
  Rheumatoid arthritis
  Seronegative spondyloarthropathy (HLA-B27 disease)
  Whipple's disease
  Hypereosinophilic syndrome

factor in the presentation of the various etiologies of valve disease.

ATRIOVENTRICULAR VALVES

Mitral Valve

Normal Anatomy of the Mitral Valve

The normal mitral valve consists of an anterior mitral leaflet connected by the commissures to the posterior mitral leaflet (Fig. 1-1A). The anterior mitral leaflet length (typically 1.5 to 2.5 cm [mean 2.0 cm]) is greater than the posterior leaflet (0.8 to 1.4 cm [mean 1.1 cm]), and the chordae tendineae arise at a 45-degree angle from the anterior leaflet on the ventricular surface. The mean width of the anterior leaflet is 3.3 ± 0.5 cm, and the mean posterior leaflet width is 4.8 ± 0.9 cm. The chordae insert into the anterolateral and the posterome-

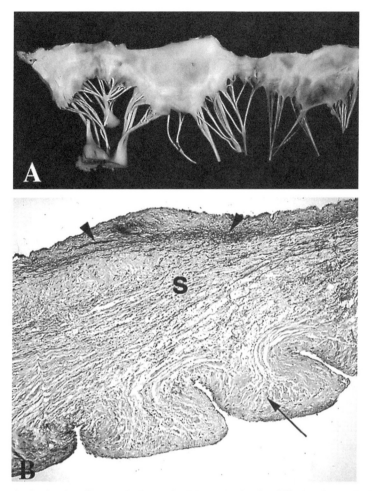

FIG. 1-1. Normal mitral valve. Gross photograph of the mitral valve **(A)** showing anterior and posterior leaflets. The anterior leaflet is larger and the chordae arise from the ventricular surface at a 45-degree angle. The anterior leaflet is separated from the posterior leaflet by the commissures and by fan-shaped branching commissural chordae. The posterior leaflet has three, often poorly defined, scallops, each with chordal attachments. A photomicrograph of a mitral valve leaflet **(B)** (Movat pentachrome stain) demonstrates the atrial surface rich in elastic fibers (*arrowheads*), proteoglycan-rich spongiosa (*S*) in the midportion, and dense collagenous tissue (*arrow*) that extends toward the ventricular surface of the leaflet.

dial papillary muscles. The commissural chordae branch and fan out from the papillary muscle, whereas the leaflet chordae are usually single and branch and fan out near their leaflet insertion sites. The chordae are usually thin and delicate, and their length varies from one sixth to one seventh the length of the left ventricle. The normal annular circumference is less than 10 cm, and the normal mitral valve orifice area is 4 to 6 cm^2.

The anterior mitral leaflet is in direct continuity with the posterior noncoronary cusp of the aortic valve. There is considerable variability in the sizes of the three scallops of the posterior leaflet. Similarly, variability exists in the papillary muscle heads and the extension of the muscle bundles into the chordae tendineae. Histologically (Fig. 1-1B), the mitral valve consists of three layers: the atrialis (a fibroelastic layer forming the atrial aspect of the leaflet), the spongiosa (delicate fibromyxomatous tissue rich in proteoglycans in the midportion of the valve), and the fibrosa (dense layer of collagen extending toward the ventricular surface and providing basic structural support) covered by thin fibroelastic tissue (ventricularis). The mitral annulus does not form a complete ring around the mitral valve. Instead, it is a C-shaped structure with the gap located at the anterior mitral leaflet.

Epidemiology and Etiology of Mitral Valve Disease

Before the 1960s, the predominant etiology of mitral valve disease in surgically excised mitral valves was rheumatic mitral stenosis (Tables 1-2 to 1-4); however, this finding has changed in the United States and in other industrialized nations in the last few decades as the incidence of untreated streptococcal infections and subsequent acute rheumatic fever has declined (1–3). Today, the most frequent cause of mitral valve disease leading to surgical intervention is mitral valve prolapse (4). Olson et al. (4) reported in 1987 gross pathologic observations in 712 patients who had undergone mitral valve replacement at various time points (1965, 1970, 1975, 1980, and 1985). Mitral stenosis was present in 452 valves; 99% were secondary to Postinflammatory disease, and 1% were secondary to congenital mitral stenosis. There were 262 cases of pure mitral incompetence, with mitral valve prolapse accounting for 38%, postinflammatory disease 31%, ischemic mitral regurgitation 11%, and idiopathic chordal rupture 4%. Notably, the number of rheumatic valves declined from 89% in 1965 to 51% in 1985. In a more recent study, Dare et al. (5) reported a similar incidence of rheumatic valves (49%, Table 1-4). The incidence of post-rheumatic disease among surgically excised mitral valves seen at our Institute from 1992 to 1996 was even less (35%).

TABLE 1-2. *Classification of mitral valve disease by functional abnormality, etiology, and mean age at presentation*

Functional abnormality	Diagnosis	Total (%)	Mean age (yr)
Mitral stenosis ± regurgitation	Postinflammatory disease (postrheumatic scarring)	25–40[a]	55
	Ergotamine-induced valve disease	<1	Adult
	Fenfluramine-phentermine	Unknown, Probably <1	Adult
	Mucopolysaccharidosis	<1	Childhood
	Congenital valve disease	<1	First decade of life
Mitral regurgitation	Mitral valve prolapse	15–30[a]	65
	Postinflammatory disease (postrheumatic scarring)	10	55
	Ischemic heart disease	4–8	70
	Endocarditis	2–5	50
	Carcinoid	<1	Adult
	Hypertrophic Cardiomyopathy	<1	Adult
	Postradiation therapy	<1	Young adult
	Congenital valve Disease	<1	Childhood
	Idiopathic chordal Rupture	<1	Adult

[a]The relative proportion of valve replacement for mitral valve prolapse has risen in recent years, with a concomitant drop in the proportion of valves removed for post-inflammatory valve disease.
From ref. 99, with permission.

TABLE 1-3. *Pathology of mitral regurgitation treated surgically as a function of patient age*

Diagnosis	Incidence (%)	
	Age < 60 yr	Age > 60 yr
Post-inflammatory disease	40	20
Mitral valve prolapse	33	45
Ischemic heart disease	5	18
Endocarditis	7	5
Other	15	12

From ref. 14, with permission.

The etiology of mitral valve disease can be classified as congenital or acquired (2). Congenital conditions of the mitral valve that may be corrected surgically include mitral valve prolapse, cleft mitral valve (almost always associated with primum atrial septal defect), parachute mitral valve (part of Shone's syndrome), and deformed mitral valve with direct leaflet attachment to papillary muscles without intervening chordae tendineae. Acquired diseases of the mitral valve include acute rheumatic fever and post-rheumatic scarring, infective endocarditis, mitral annular calcification, connective tissue disease, radiation heart disease, ergotamine-induced valvular disease (6), and the recently described valvular pathology associated with the use of the weight-reducing agents fenfluramine-phentermine (7). Other diseases that secondarily lead to mitral valve disease include coronary artery disease with papillary muscle dysfunction and cardiomyopathies (hypertrophic, dilated, and restrictive).

Mitral Valve Prolapse

The prevalence of mitral valve prolapse (myxomatous degeneration of the mitral valve, systolic click-murmur syndrome, Barlow's syndrome, billowing mitral cusp syndrome, floppy mitral valve syndrome, and redundant mitral valve) in the general population is 3% to 5%, is twice as frequent in women than in men, and is reported in all age groups (8). Most patients are asymptomatic. Symptomatic mitral regurgitation occurs in 10% to 15% of patients and is more common in men older than 50 years (9). Currently, mitral valve prolapse is the most common pathology seen in patients undergoing mitral valve surgery (8).

Pathologically, the spectrum of mitral valve prolapse ranges from mild to severe myxomatous changes (10) (Fig. 1-2). In mild forms, the posterior valve leaflet (especially the intermediate scallop) is involved and is longer than normal with myxomatous degeneration and mild prolapse into the left atrium. The mild form is usually seen as an incidental finding without clinical sequelae. In the more severe form of prolapse, all scallops of posterior leaflet are involved (with or without involvement of the anterior leaflet) and the degree of myxomatous change, valve thickening, and elongation is excessive (11,12). Chordal elongation is typically present (Fig. 1-2C), and extensive prolapse of the leaflets into the left atrium is seen. Further, chordal insertion on the ventricular leaflet surface is often haphazard and chaotic (Fig. 1-2D), such that there is poor leaflet structural support.

TABLE 1-4. *Pathology of surgically excised mitral valves from 1965 to 1996*

Etiology	Olson et al.[4] (1965)	Olson et al.[4] (1985)	Dare et al.[5] (1990)	AFIP (1992–1996)
Post-rheumatic	124 (89%)	43 (51%)	47 (49%)	47 (35%)
Myxomatous mitral valve	5 (4%)	21 (25%)	27 (29%)	57 (43%)
Papillary muscle ischemia	0	8 (10%)	7 (7%)	5 (4%)
Endocarditis	1	2 (2%)	5 (5%)	10 (8%)
Miscellaneous	10 (7%)	10 (12%)	9 (9%)	14 (11%)
Age (yr)[a]	47 (12–61)	61 (15–82)	61 (8–85)	56 (12–87)
Total	140	84	95	133

[a]Ranges in parentheses.
AFIP, Armed Forces Institute of Pathology.

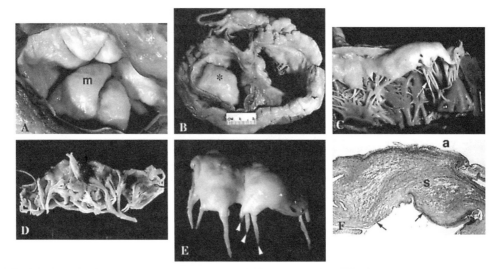

FIG. 1-2. Mitral valve prolapse. An atrial view of the mitral valve **(A)** shows marked anterior and posterior leaflet hooding and prolapse toward the left atrium. The middle scallop (*m*) of the posterior leaflet is maximally affected. Removal of both atria **(B)** exposes the mitral and tricuspid valves. There is severe prolapse of the middle scallop of the posterior mitral leaflet (*), without involvement of the other leaflets. The opened mitral valve (*C*) shows myxomatous degeneration of the prolapsed middle scallop of the posterior leaflet with chordal elongation (*arrow*). Surgically excised posterior leaflet **(D)** viewed from the ventricular surface demonstrates multiple haphazardly inserted chordae. One scallop excised in mitral valve repair **(E)** shows hooding and myxomatous degeneration with chordal rupture (*arrowhead*). Histologically **(F)**, the atrial surface (*a*) of a prolapsed mitral valve shows elastic fibers; the spongiosa (*s*) is expanded and disrupts the collagenous ventricular layer (*arrows*). (**E:** From Virmani R, Burke AP, Farb A. Pathology of valvular heart disease. In: Rahimtoola SH, ed. *Valvular Heart Disease.* Vol. XI. *Atlas of Heart Diseases.* St. Louis, MO: Mosby, 1997:1.11, with permission.)

The frequency of chordal rupture (Fig. 1-2E) has been reported to be present in 20% to 74% of surgically excised mitral valves. The prolapse is most severe when there are multiple ruptured chords (flail mitral valve). Annular calcification may be present and is frequent in patients with significant mitral regurgitation.

Histologically (Fig. 1-2F), the leaflet spongiosa in mitral valve prolapse is expanded, and there is focal disruption of the fibrosa by the proteoglycan-rich spongiosa. These pathologic changes are best appreciated when the valve is appropriately embedded and stained for proteoglycans by Movat stain or alcian blue stain.

Valve surgery is recommended in symptomatic patients with severe mitral regurgitation and in asymptomatic patients with severe re-gurgitation associated with left ventricular dilatation or dysfunction (13). In the past, the whole mitral valve, including chordae and papillary muscles, was removed. However, through better understanding of the important role played by the subleaflet valve apparatus in preserving left ventricular function and preventing left ventricular dilatation, it is now highly desirable to repair the valve, without valve replacement, by segmental valve resection (mitral valvuloplasty), with or without annuloplasty. When valve repair is performed, usually a portion of the posterior leaflet (which has maximal myxomatous degeneration) is resected. When valve repair is not feasible and valve replacement by a prosthetic valve is performed, the posterior leaflet and chordal attachments to the papillary muscle and mitral annulus are often left in place (4).

Cardiac complications of mitral valve prolapse (mitral regurgitation, need for valve surgery, and endocarditis) are associated with increased severity of the disease (i.e., increased leaflet thickness and length) (14). Although the incidence of sudden death in mitral valve prolapse in the absence of significant mitral regurgitation is low, it is not insignificant (14–19). In sudden death cases evaluated at autopsy, lengths of both the anterior and posterior leaflets and leaflet thickness are significantly greater than prolapse that occurs as an incidental finding (14,16). Additionally, subvalvular friction lesions caused by contact of chordae tendineae with the adjacent ventricular endocardium are more frequently observed in sudden death cases.

Acute and Chronic Rheumatic Mitral Valve Disease

The incidence of acute rheumatic fever has been in sharp decline in the United States. The reasons for this epidemiologic change is multifactorial and is related to a combination of improved socioeconomic conditions, a lower incidence of streptococcal infection, and the introduction of antibiotics. In the 1980s, there was an outbreak of acute rheumatic fever in several geographic locations. The two most important factors responsible for this rise in new cases were the significant increase in the number of immigrants entering the United States from parts of the world where acute rheumatic fever is still prevalent (Mexico, Asia, and Central and South America) and the appearance of new strains of streptococci that are particularly associated with acute rheumatic fever. The largest number of recent nonimmigrant cases of acute rheumatic fever were seen in Utah in 1985, and over 80% of the cases came from middle class families; carditis was present in 68% of cases (3).

Acute rheumatic carditis results from an altered immune response to group A hemolytic streptococcus infection and has been linked to histocompatability antigen HLA-B5 (20). The immune response is characterized by an excessive synthesis of antistreptococcal, antistreptolysin, anti-DNAase, and antihyaluronidase antibodies. Clinical signs and symptoms of rheumatic fever occur 2 to 6 weeks after the initial streptococcal pharyngitis, and the overall attack rate is less than 5% (21). The immunologic targets in the heart include: (1) glycoproteins; (2) the myocardial and smooth muscle cell sarcolemma, which cross-react with streptococcal membrane antigens; and (3) myocyte myosin, which shares antigens with streptococcal M protein.

The diagnosis of acute rheumatic fever is confirmed by serologic evidence of a preceding streptococcal infection with either two major Jones' criteria (carditis, polyarthritis, chorea, erythema marginatum, subcutaneous nodules) or one major and two minor Jones' criteria (fever, arthralgias, previous rheumatic fever or rheumatic heart disease, elevated erythrocyte sedimentation rate, positive C-reactive protein, or prolonged PR interval on electrocardiogram) (21–23). Clinically, a murmur may be absent unless there is severe mitral regurgitation and heart failure. Pathologically, small verrucous vegetations are present along the lines of valve closure. The mitral and the aortic valves are most commonly involved; rarely, the tricuspid and the pulmonic valves are involved.

Histologically, inflammation may be present in all three layers of the heart (pancarditis): endocarditis, myocarditis, and pericarditis. Aschoff bodies are seen within the myocardium (atria and papillary muscles in surgically removed tissue) and on the valve leaflets (24). The Aschoff nodule consists of focal fibrinoid necrosis, lymphocytes, macrophages, and plasma cells. Two types of macrophages may be seen in an Aschoff nodule: an Anitschkow's cell (also known as an Aschoff's cell, caterpillar cell, and owl-eyed cell) and a multinucleated Anitschkow's cell (Aschoff's giant cell). The Anitschkow's cells have round to oval nuclei and chromatin condensation at the nuclear periphery. In the center of the nucleus, chromatin strands connect the periphery of nucleus to the center with clearing in between. The most frequent location of Aschoff bodies is the endocardium of the atria and ventricles. In patients undergoing surgery for chronic post-rheumatic mitral scarring, the frequency of Aschoff nodules in excised atrial appendages and papillary muscles is 11% and 1%, respectively (24).

In chronic rheumatic mitral valve disease, a history of previous acute rheumatic fever is elicited in up to 50% of patients with mitral stenosis (4). Post-inflammatory scarring is presumed to be post-rheumatic in most cases, unless there is a history of some other non-rheumatic inflammatory disease. The latent period between acute rheumatic fever and chronic rheumatic valve disease is as long as 10 to 20 years, but an interval as short as 2 years has also been reported (22). Post-rheumatic valvular scarring is more prevalent in women, with a male-to-female ratio of approximately 0.4:1. Signs and symptoms of chronic valvular scarring typically appear in the third and fourth decades, and the age at which valvular surgery is usually performed is the fifth decade in the Western world. In contrast, in underdeveloped countries, severe post-rheumatic valve deformity may occur in adolescents. The risk of developing chronic valvular deformities is highest in patients with rheumatic carditis that results in congestive heart failure.

Rheumatic mitral stenosis is by far the most frequent clinical manifestation of chronic rheumatic heart disease; mixed mitral stenosis and regurgitation is not uncommon, and pure mitral regurgitation is rare. Roberts and Virmani (24) reviewed all patients who underwent valve surgery at the National Institutes of Health from 1964 to 1975. They reported that Aschoff nodules were present in the atrial appendages almost exclusively in patients with mitral stenosis with or without regurgitation and with or without other valve involvement; only one patient with pure mitral regurgitation had Aschoff nodules. Concurrent involvement of the aortic valve is common; involvement of the tricuspid and/or pulmonic valves is rare.

The valve area in mild mitral stenosis is less than 2 to 4 cm², moderate mitral stenosis 1 to 2 cm², and severe stenosis less than 1 cm². Signs and symptoms include dyspnea, congestive heart failure, arrhythmias (especially atrial fibrillation), and pulmonary hypertension. Increased symptoms correlate with valve areas of less than 1 cm². Valve surgery is indicated in symptomatic patients with severe stenosis and/or regurgitation (25). At surgery, the posterior leaflet and its chordal attachment to the papillary muscles are typically left intact, and the anterior leaflet is removed. Preservation of chordal structures is associated with improved cardiac function and reduced risk of postoperative left ventricular rupture or dilatation. The surgical specimen consists of either the entire mitral valve (Fig. 1-3) or anterior leaflet with or without portion of posterior leaflet. In autopsy cases of severe mitral stenosis, there is marked dilatation of the left atrium (Fig. 1-3) with or without right ventricular hypertrophy and right atrial dilatation. In patients with significant regurgitation, the findings are similar except that the left ventricular cavity is dilated, the extent of which depends on the severity of mitral incompetence (26). If there is concomitant aortic stenosis, the left ventricle will be hypertrophied and nondilated.

Post-rheumatic scarring results in fusion of parts of the mitral valve apparatus—commissures, leaflets, and/or chordae—leading to stenosis (Fig. 1-3). Commissural fusion alone is seen in 30%, fusion of leaflets alone in 15%, and fusion of the chordae alone in 10%; in the remainder, more than one valve structure is involved. Leaflet fibrosis occurs with or without calcification, which may be focally present at the fused commissures and ulcerate the leaflet surface. Thickening, fusion, and shortening of chordae results in the formation of a fibrous tunnel below the leaflets and give the classic "fish mouth" appearance of the severely stenotic mitral valve when viewed from the left ventricular aspect (Fig. 1-3A). Microscopically, the normal architecture of the valve is replaced by collagen with interspersed fibroblasts and focal neocapillary-formation. Varying degrees of chronic inflammatory cell infiltrates, consisting of lympho-

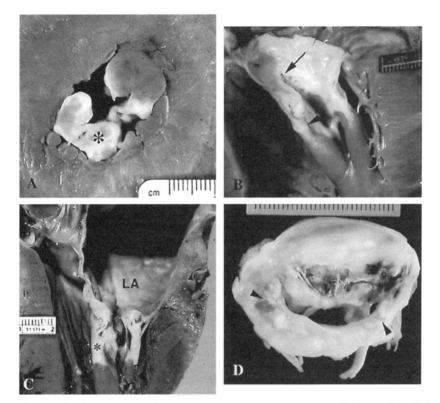

FIG. 1-3. Rheumatic mitral stenosis. Mitral valve as viewed from the ventricular surface **(A)** showing a markedly stenotic valve with chordae fusion and fibrosis (*). **B:** Commissural fusion *(arrow)* with leaflet fibrosis and severe chordal fusion *(arrowhead)* and shortening. Long axis view of the mitral valve **(C)** demonstrates marked chordal fusion (*), fibrosis, and shortening resulting in a stenotic orifice; secondary left atrial *(LA)* dilatation is present. Viewed from the atrial surface, a surgically excised mitral valve **(D)** shows commissural fusion, leaflet thickening, and focal calcification. (**B** and **C:** From Virmani R, Burke AP, Farb A. Pathology of valvular heart disease. In: Rahimtoola SH, ed. *Valvular Heart Disease.* Vol. XI. *Atlas of Heart Diseases.* St. Louis, MO: Mosby, 1997:1.9, with permission.)

cytes, plasma cells, and macrophages, are not uncommon. Aschoff nodules are only rarely described in the valve removed surgically but are more frequently seen in countries that have a high prevalence of rheumatic heart disease.

Aging Changes and Mitral Annular Calcification

The anterior and posterior leaflets at birth are translucent, gelatinous, and transmit light, but after the age of 20 they become opaque. By age 50, the mitral anterior leaflet is opaque and fibrotic and heavily infiltrated with lipids. The lines of closure on the anterior and posterior valve leaflets are thickened and nodular by the age of 70 years, and calcification is often focally present in the annulus. Mitral annular calcification is frequently seen in patients with Marfan's syndrome, mitral valve prolapse, and Hurler's syndrome. It is typically seen in renal failure patients on long-term dialysis with secondary hyperparathyroidism. In these patients, the calcification may be severe, extend into the valve leaflets and/or left atrium, and cause mitral stenosis. Hypertension and hyperlipidemia are also associated with annular calcification.

Annular calcification of the mitral valve is found at autopsy in 10% of individuals dying after the age of 50 years. In most cases, annu-

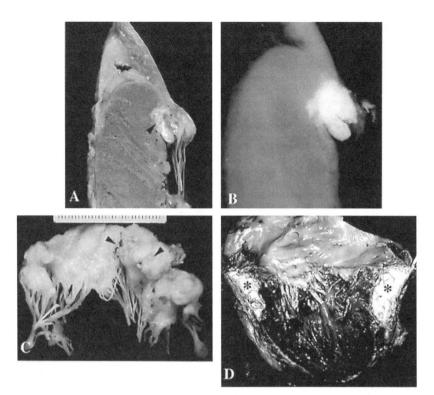

FIG. 1-4. Mitral annular calcification. Heavy calcification of the mitral annulus is present at the insertion of the posterior mitral leaflet (*arrowhead*: gross photo, **A**; corresponding radiograph, **B**). Surgically excised mitral valve from a 67-year-old man with end-stage renal disease with mitral stenosis secondary to extensive nodular annular calcification (**C**, *arrowheads*), most predominantly involving the posterior leaflet and extending into the body of the leaflets, with relative sparing of the valve margins and chordae. Heart from a 47-year-old man with end-stage renal disease and hypertension **(D)**. Note large masses of mitral annular calcification (*) that extends into the left ventricular wall. A semisolid chalky material fills the center of the areas of calcification. The left atrium is dilated (secondary to mitral regurgitation), and the mitral valve is focally fibrotic with thickening of the chordae tendineae. (**A:** From ref. 99, p. 46, with permission.)

lar calcification is of little significance; however, when severe, it may be responsible for mitral regurgitation. Women are more frequently affected than men. Over 50% of patients with severe mitral annular calcification have involvement of the aortic valve, but rarely does it lead to aortic stenosis.

Pathologically, the calcified annulus is located between the mitral valve cusp and the ventricular wall (Fig. 1-4, A and B). Calcification may range from mild, with focal small calcific deposits, to severe, with large calcific nodules involving the entire annulus projecting into the left ventricular cavity or as spurs that project into the left ventricular myocardium. The calcification involves more than one third of the annulus in 88% of patients, the posterior annulus alone in 10.5%, and the whole annulus in 1.5% (27). The calcification extends into the myocardium in 12% of the patients and into the papillary muscles in 4.5% (27). Rarely, severe annular calcification causes significant mitral stenosis that is treated with valve replacement (Fig. 1-4C). Occasionally, large calcified areas may become semisolid and necrotic (Fig. 1-4D) and may be confused with an annular abscess cavity on echocardiography.

Ischemic Mitral Regurgitation and Papillary Muscle Dysfunction

Mitral regurgitation of variable severity is seen in 30% of patients with coronary artery atherosclerosis who are being considered for coronary bypass surgery (28,29). In most cases, the regurgitation is mild; however, chronic severe regurgitation secondary to ischemic heart disease is associated with a poor prognosis. Ischemic mitral regurgitation is more common in men, reflecting the higher prevalence of the coronary disease in males. The mechanism of chronic ischemic mitral regurgitation involves papillary muscle dysfunction, mitral annular dilatation, or both. The most common myocardial finding is healed infarction of one or both papillary muscles (Fig. 1-5). Alternatively, acute severe mitral regurgitation results from infarction and rupture of a papillary muscle during acute myocardial infarction (Fig. 1-5).

The posterior papillary muscle has a single blood supply from posterior descending coronary artery and becomes infarcted more frequently than the anterolateral papillary muscle, which has a dual blood supply from the diagonal branches (from the left anterior descending coronary artery) and obtuse marginal branches from the left circumflex coronary artery. Although papillary muscle dysfunction is most frequently seen in the setting of coronary atherosclerosis, it can also result from shock, severe anemia, coronary

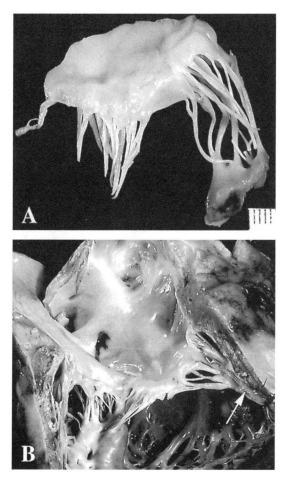

FIG. 1-5. Ischemic mitral valve disease. A 65-year-old man presented with an acute inferior myocardial infarction with acute mitral regurgitation secondary to the rupture of the posteromedial papillary muscle. The anterior mitral leaflet **(A)** with its ruptured and infarcted papillary muscle was excised. Chronic mitral regurgitation and congestive heart failure secondary to healed posterior wall myocardial infarction was present in this 60-year-old man **(B)**. Note scarred and thinned posterior papillary muscle (*arrow*) and left atrial dilatation.

arteritis, anomalous coronary arteries, abscess formation, congenital malposition of the papillary muscles, and infiltration of the papillary muscles by sarcoidosis, neoplasms, and amyloidosis. Annular dilatation, secondary to myocardial infarction or dilated cardiomyopathy, results in the alteration of the anatomic relationship between the papillary muscles and the chordae tendineae, resulting in mitral regurgitation.

Surgical treatment consists of resection of the entire valve or just the anterior mitral leaflet (28,29). Because the pathologic findings are in the papillary muscles, the valve leaflets and the chordae tendineae are usually unremarkable. In pathologic specimens that contain the papillary muscle, the muscle is thin and atrophic from scarring in chronic regurgitation. In papillary muscle rupture from acute ischemic injury, myocyte coagulation necrosis is evident, and platelets and fibrin are present along the ruptured muscle surface.

Tricuspid Valve Disease

Normal Anatomy of the Tricuspid Valve

The anatomy of the tricuspid valve is the most variable of all the four valves. The tricuspid valve normally measures 10 to 12.5 cm in circumference and usually consists of three leaflets: the anterior, septal, and the posterior leaflets, each separated from one another by commissures. However, the septal leaflet is highly variable and may often be rudimentary or absent without any clinical consequences (30). The septal leaflet forms a useful landmark, because just above its insertion in the right atrium lies the atrioventricular node and on its anterior-most insertion lies the membranous septum. The anterior leaflet is the largest; it is suspended across the anterior wall of the right ventricular cavity and separates the inflow portion of the right ventricle from the outflow. The chordae tendineae from the anterior and the posterior leaflets attach to a large single anterior papillary muscle that arises from the anterior free wall of the right ventricle and fuses with the moderator band. Several small posterior papillary muscles are attached to the posterior wall into which insert the chordae tendineae from the posterior and the septal leaflets. The septal papillary muscle is often rudimentary or even absent, and chordae from the septal and anterior leaflet insert either into the septal papillary muscle or directly into the ventricular septum.

Post-rheumatic (Post-inflammatory) Tricuspid Valve Disease

The overall incidence of post-rheumatic tricuspid valve disease is low. Of the 543 autopsy cases of rheumatic heart disease reported by Roberts and Virmani (24), functional tricuspid valve stenosis occurred in 8 cases (2%) and was seen only in the presence of mitral and aortic valve stenosis, with some degree of tricuspid valve involvement seen in 64 cases (12%). Although post-rheumatic scarring is the most frequent cause of pure tricuspid valve stenosis, rheumatic tricuspid stenosis is much less frequent than regurgitation. Of the 363 surgically excised tricuspid valves studied by Hauck et al. (31), post-rheumatic disease was observed in 194 (53%) and, of these, pure tricuspid valve stenosis was seen in 3% of cases, tricuspid stenosis and incompetence was observed in 41%, and tricuspid incompetence in 56%. All 194 cases with post-rheumatic tricuspid valve disease had mitral valve disease, 68% had combined mitral stenosis and incompetence, 26% had pure mitral stenosis, and 12% had pure mitral incompetence.

The pathologic features of rheumatic tricuspid disease consist of leaflet thickening and fusion of one or more commissures (Fig. 1-6). Chordal thickening and fusion are usually less severe than in the mitral valve. The extent of fibrosis and retraction of the leaflets, together with presence or absence of commissural fusion, determines whether the tricuspid valve will be incompetent, stenotic, or both. Commissural fusion is observed in all cases of pure tricuspid stenosis, 95% of cases with stenosis and regurgitation, and 51% of cases with pure tricuspid regurgitation. In contrast

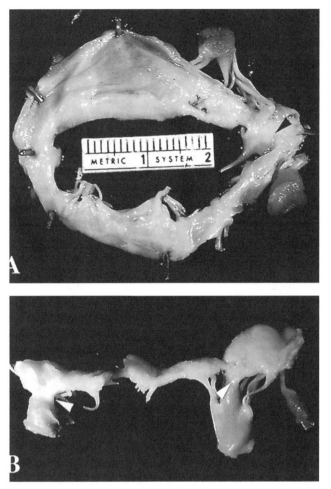

FIG. 1-6. Postrheumatic tricuspid valve scarring. Surgically removed tricuspid valve **(A)** from a patient who also underwent mitral and aortic valve replacement for mitral and aortic stenosis secondary to chronic rheumatic valvular disease. Note thickened, rolled, free margins of the valve leaflets and commissural fusion **(arrowhead)**. Diffuse tricuspid leaflet thickening with shortened, fused, and thickened chordae (*arrowheads*) is evident **(B)**.

to mitral stenosis, leaflet calcification is less common in rheumatic tricuspid valve disease.

Other uncommon causes of tricuspid valve stenosis include tricuspid atresia, right atrial tumors, Whipple's disease, methysergide therapy, infective endocarditis, and carcinoid heart disease.

Tricuspid Valve Insufficiency

Tricuspid valve insufficiency in adults most commonly occurs as a result of left ventricular failure (secondary to ischemic heart disease or any left-sided valve disease), cardiomyopathy, or primary lung disease. In these cases of secondary tricuspid insufficiency, tricuspid annular dilatation is present, but the tricuspid valve is structurally normal except for focal fibrous leaflet thickening. Intrinsic diseases of the tricuspid valve associated with tricuspid regurgitation include postrheumatic scarring, Ebstein's anomaly, infective endocarditis (32), valvular clefts as part of the atrioventricular canal defect, papillary muscle dysfunction secondary to infarction, trauma, endomyocardial fibrosis, hypereosinophilic syndrome, post-radiation (33), rheumatoid arthritis (34), and right ventricular pacemakers. In the surgical series of excised tricuspid valve by Hauck et al. (31), pure tricuspid incompetence was present in 269 (74%), and the underlying etiology was post-rheumatic in 109 (41%), Ebstein's anomaly in 38 (14%), congenital dysplasia or annular dilatation in 49 (18%), pulmonary venous hypertension in 56 (21%), infective endocarditis in 11 (4%), carcinoid syndrome in 2, trauma in 1, iatrogenic damage in 1, and indeterminate causes in 2.

Ebstein's Anomaly

Ebstein's anomaly of the heart is an uncommon congenital abnormality, accounting for less than 1% of congenital heart defects (35). The pathologic features of Ebstein's anomaly can be separated into anomalies of the valve and abnormalities of the right ventricle. Ebstein's anomaly consists of downward displacement of the tricuspid valve toward the right ventricle so that part of the right ventricle becomes a functional part of the right atrium (i.e., atrialization). Mild atrialization may be present in which the downward shift of the septal and posterior leaflets results in a relatively normal tricuspid valve orifice. Typically, there is mild valve incompetence, and occasionally, Ebstein's anomaly may go undetected into adulthood. In the most severe form, the septal leaflet is plastered to the septum, the posterior leaflet is plastered to the posterior ventricular wall, and the anterior leaflet is enlarged and abnormally attached to a muscular shelf that separates the inlet of the ventricle from the trabecular portion. The anterior leaflet may be large and "sail-like," and the valve cusps may not separate, forming a diaphragm with small peripheral openings and resulting in a stenotic orifice.

As a result of the downward displacement of the tricuspid valve, the right ventricle becomes divided into an atrialized chamber and a distal true ventricular chamber. The proximal right ventricular chamber may be larger or smaller than the distal chamber and its size depends on the extent of downward displacement of the tricuspid valve. The endocardium of the atrialized portion of the right ventricle is usually fibrotic, with poorly developed trabeculations. Often, there is aneurysmal dilatation of the fibrotic posterior wall, which may be devoid of myocytes. The distal chamber is located behind the anterior tricuspid valve leaflet. Right ventricular dilatation is present in 60% of cases.

Ebstein's anomaly may exist as an isolated finding but is frequently associated with a membranous ventricular septal defect. An atrial septal defect is common, and pulmonary stenosis or atresia may be present. Ebstein's anomaly is frequently associated with pulmonary atresia with an intact ventricular septum. In patients surviving beyond infancy, exercise intolerance, cyanosis resulting from right ventricular dysfunction, tricuspid valve insufficiency, and right-to-left shunting may be seen (36).

Myxomatous Degeneration of the Tricuspid Valve (Tricuspid Valve Prolapse)

The morphology of tricuspid valve prolapse is identical to that found in mitral valve prolapse. Grossly, there is ballooning and redundancy of leaflet tissue with variable attenuation of the chordae tendineae. Prolapse most commonly involves the anterior tricuspid valve leaflet, less frequently the septal leaflet, and rarely the posterior leaflet. Histologic findings are similar to those described in mitral valve prolapse.

The prevalence of tricuspid valve prolapse is estimated to be between 0.1% and 5.5% and is found in approximately 22% (range, 3% to 54%) of patients with mitral valve prolapse; isolated tricuspid valve prolapse is much less frequent (37). Tricuspid regurgitation is commonly seen in patients with tricuspid prolapse, is usually mild, and does not correlate with the severity of the prolapse. In surgically excised valves, it may be difficult to make the diagnosis of tricuspid valve prolapse, and therefore one may have to rely on clinical data and on the finding of enlarged tricuspid annulus. However, if the valve area were to be measured it would be much larger than that of a normal valve or in regurgitant tricuspid valves secondary to ischemic heart disease or pulmonary hypertension. In the series by Hauck et al. (31), tricuspid valve prolapse was not mentioned among the surgically excised tricuspid valves. Tricuspid valve prolapse may be a marker of more extensive organ involvement in patients with Marfan's syndrome. Additionally, tricuspid valve prolapse may identify a subset of patients with mitral valve prolapse who have a relatively worse prognosis than those in whom tricuspid valve is normal.

SEMILUNAR VALVES

Aortic Valve

Normal Anatomy of the Aortic Valve

The aortic valve consists of three semicircular cusps (left, right, and posterior [noncoronary] cusps) that attach to the aorta (Fig. 1-7A). The cusps and sinuses of Valsalva are generally equally sized, but mild asymmetry (more than 5% difference from the average cusp area) of two or all three cusps is common in otherwise normally functioning valves (38–40). The narrow space between each adjacent cusp where they attach to the aorta is referred to as a commissure (three per normal semilunar valve). The sinotubular junction, which separates the sinuses of Valsalva from the aorta, is formed by a line joining the three commissures (41). In the aortic valve, a linear relationship has been described relating increased cusp area and sinus of Valsalva volume with increased patient age, heart weight, and aortic area at the sinotubular junction (38). The line of closure of the semilunar valve is just below the free edge (Fig. 1-7B), the center of which contains a small nodule (noduli Arantii) from which a thin fibrous projection often emanates (Lambl's excrescence). Fenestrations in the valve cusps above the line of closure

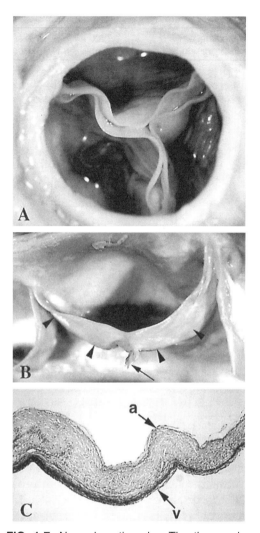

FIG. 1-7. Normal aortic valve. The three valve cusps **(A)** show complete coaptation with minor variability of the cusp sizes and three open (nonfused) commissures. An individual aortic valve cusp is shown **(B)**. The line of valve closures (*arrowheads*) is below the free edge, and a centrally place nodule of Arantii with Lambl's excrescence (*arrow*) is present. Histologically **(C)** (Movat pentachrome stain), the ventricular surface (*v*) has a dark-staining elastic layer, a loose connective tissue middle layer containing proteoglycans, and a dense collagenous layer that extends toward the aortic surface (*a*).

have no functional significance. Histologically (Fig. 1-7C), valve cusps consist of a fibroelastic layer on the ventricular surface (ventricularis), proteoglycan-rich connective tissue in the midportion, dense collagen extending toward the aortic surface, and a thin fibroelastic layer on the aortic surface (arterialis). The distal two thirds of the semilunar valve cusps are avascular (41).

Aortic Stenosis: Classification, Clinical Presentation, and Treatment

Diseases of the aortic valve resulting in stenosis may be categorized into congenital lesions (e.g., unicuspid or bicuspid valves), postinflammatory scarring (typically post-rheumatic), or degenerative changes (e.g., senile calcific aortic stenosis) (Table 1-5). The typical age at presentation generally correlates with underlying pathologic lesion (39). Most often, unicuspid aortic stenosis presents in childhood or adolescence and accounts for only 4% to 6% of aortic stenosis in adults. In contrast, in aortic stenosis secondary to congenital bicuspid valves, patients usually present in the fifth and sixth decades, and bicuspid aortic valves account for 50% of surgical valve replacements in adult patients less than 70 years old (42). Finally, in patients 70 or more years old, tricuspid degenerative aortic stenosis is responsible for nearly 50% of surgical valve replacements (42). With the aging of the general population and the decline in the incidence of rheumatic fever, the frequency of aortic valve surgery for calcific tricuspid aortic stenosis has increased concurrent with a decreased frequency of postinflammatory aortic valve scarring (43–45).

The normal aortic valve area is greater than 2.0 cm^2. Mild aortic stenosis is present at valve areas of 1.5 to 2.0 cm^2, moderate stenosis 0.8 to 1.5 cm^2, and severe stenosis less than 0.8 cm^2. The rate of progression from mild to severe stenosis is quite variable among individual patients (46). In serial cardiac catheterization studies, the presence and extent of aortic valve calcification on initial study was associated with a more rapid progression toward severe aortic stenosis (47). Despite hemodynamic evidence of severe aortic stenosis, patients may remain asymptomatic for years and require no specific therapy. However, the appearance of cardiac symptoms (syncope, cardiac angina, dyspnea, and/or heart failure) are associated with increased mortality from aortic stenosis and herald the need for valve replacement irrespective of the underlying valve morphology (48–50). Improvements in symptoms and survival after aortic valve replacement in symptomatic patients has been documented even in elderly individuals. There appears to be no role for prophylactic aortic valve replacement in asymptomatic patients with aortic stenosis (51). It is uncertain whether individuals undergoing coronary artery bypass surgery should have simultaneous aortic valve replacement if mild-to-moderate aortic stenosis is present (50). Patient subgroups at increased risk for aortic valve calcification leading to stenosis include those with disorders of calcium and phosphate metabolism (e.g., end-stage renal disease with dialysis treatment, primary hyperparathyroidism) and abnormalities of bone metabolism (e.g., Paget's disease) (46).

TABLE 1-5. *Surgical pathology of aortic stenosis*

Etiology	Mayo Clinic (1965)[55]	University of Minnesota (1979–1983)[44]	London (1976–1979)[43]	Mayo Clinic (1990)[45]	AFIP (1990–1997)
Bicuspid	49%	49%	56%	36%	30%
Post-rheumatic	33%	23%	24%	9%	13%
Degenerative	0%	28%	12%	51%	49%
Unicuspid	10%	1%	0%	0%	6%
Other	7%	0%	8%	2%	2%

AFIP, Armed Forces Institute of Pathology.

Morphology of Aortic Stenosis

Congenital Unicuspid Aortic Valve

There are two morphologic types of unicuspid aortic valves: a domed-shaped acommissural valve in which three aborted commissures (or raphes) are present or a unicommissural valve that has a slitlike opening (described as an "exclamation point" orifice) that reaches the aortic wall at one intact commissures with two raphes present (Fig. 1-8, A and B). Leaflet dysplasia is common, and calcification may or may not be severe, with the degree of calcification typically increasing after commissurotomy. Unicommissural unicuspid aortic valves account for 60% of aortic stenosis cases in patients less than 15 years old (52). Patients with congenital unicuspid valves are at increased risk for infective endocarditis.

Congenital Bicuspid Aortic Valve

Congenital bicuspid aortic valves are present in 1% to 2% of the general population (male-to-female ratio, 1.4–4:1) and are the most frequent cause of aortic stenosis in the 50- to 70-year-old age group. Aortic stenosis is the most common physiologic consequence of congenital bicuspid aortic valves, affecting nearly 80% of valves studied at autopsy (52). Post-inflammatory (post-rheumatic) scarring of a congenital bicuspid valve is associated with an earlier age of presentation for surgical intervention (53). Like patients with congenital unicuspid aortic valves, individuals with congenital bicuspid aortic valves are at increased risk for aortic dissection and infective endocarditis. The risk for endocarditis is less in stenotic bicuspid aortic valves compared with bicuspid valves with normal function or only mild dysfunction (54).

Most commonly, the congenitally bicuspid aortic valve has two leaflets of unequal size with the larger conjoint cusp located anteriorly within the aortic root (79% of excised stenotic bicuspid valves [55]) and the smaller cusp found posteriorly; less commonly, the right and noncoronary cusps are conjoint (Fig. 1-8C), and the rarest morphology is a conjoint left and noncoronary cusp (55–57). The size of the conjoint cusp is less than two times the size of the nonconjoint cusp. The conjoint cusp contains a median raphe (aborted third commissure) in approximately 75% of cases of excised valves (55). If not heavily calcified, the raphe is rich in elastic tissue. In most cases, the raphe does not reach the free edge of the conjoint cusp and demonstrates no separation into two cusp margins, which is best appreciated by viewing the valve from ventricular aspect. The raphe does not usually reach to the same level on its aortic insertion as the commissures of the other two cusps.

Variations of the raphe in congenitally bicuspid aortic valves include raphal ridges that reach the free margin of the cusp or partial separation of the raphe into cusp margins. These variants may cause problems in deciding whether a congenitally bicuspid valve is present versus an acquired bicuspid valve (e.g., postinflammatory fusion of one of the three commissures). In cases in which it is difficult to distinguish between a congenitally bicuspid valve and an acquired bicuspid valve, the median raphe or area of commissural fusion may be examined histologically. A raphe in a congenitally bicuspid valve is rich in elastic tissue; fused commissures secondary to postinflammatory scarring consist of nonelastic fibrous tissue. However, this difference is not particularly sensitive because marked raphal calcification may destroy the elastic tissue. Another bicuspid valve variant, accounting for 6% of surgically excised bicuspid aortic valves in one series (58), is a fenestrated raphe that consists of a fibrous strand that extends from the sinus wall to the free cusp edge. This morphology may be particularly difficult to distinguish by echocardiographic imaging (58). Occasionally, the bicuspid valve is composed of two cusps of equal size with no median raphe. Dystrophic calcification begins in the raphe, if present, and extends into the cusp tissue. In significant aortic stenosis secondary to a bicuspid aortic valve, calcification extends into the cusp tissue of the conjoint and nonconjoint cusps and calcific nodules may

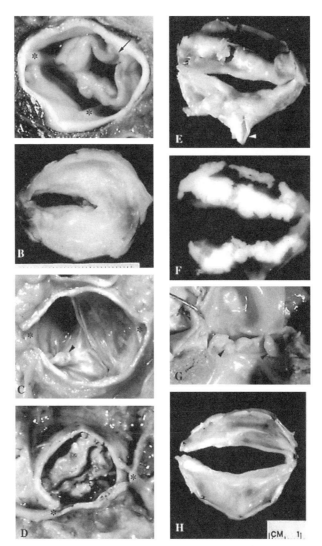

FIG. 1-8. Unicuspid and bicuspid aortic valve pathology. Stenotic unicuspid dysplastic aortic valve **(A)** from a 19-year-old woman who died suddenly while dancing. Note the eccentric valve orifice, single commissure (*arrow*), and thickened dysplastic leaflet with rudimentary raphae (*). Surgically excised stenotic congenital unicuspid, unicommissural aortic valve **(B)** with dysplastic leaflet, and eccentric valve orifice ("exclamation point"). A nonstenotic, functionally normal, mildly calcified congenitally bicuspid valve is shown **(C)**. A median raphe is present (*arrowhead*) in the right cusp, and the commissures are located anteriorly and posteriorly. Coronary arteries are indicated (*). The more typical location of the cusps and commissures in a congenital bicuspid stenotic aortic valve is demonstrated **(D)**. The commissures are placed right and left and both coronary arteries (*) arise from the anterior sinus. Severe cusp calcification is present, which obscures the raphe. Surgically excised stenotic congenitally bicuspid aortic valve (**E**, with corresponding radiograph **F**) with marked calcification and median raphe (*arrowhead*). A bicuspid dysplastic aortic valve in a child with congenital aortic stenosis is shown **(G)** consisting of two thickened and gelatinous cusps (*arrowheads*). Pure aortic insufficiency with a bicuspid valve is presented **(H)**. Note the increased annular circumference, nonspecific cusp fibrosis, most pronounced near the line of valve closure, and absence of valve calcification. (**A:** From Virmani R, Burke AP, Farb A. *Valvular Heart Disease*. Vol. XI. *Atlas of Heart Diseases*. St. Louis, MO: Mosby, 1997:1.3, with permission. **B:** From ref. 99, p. 53, with permission.)

ulcerate the cusp surface (Fig. 1-8, D through F). When young individuals present with cardiac symptoms secondary to a congenital bicuspid valve, the cusps are typically thickened and dysplastic (Fig. 1-8G).

Degenerative Calcific Tricuspid Aortic Valve

Degenerative tricuspid aortic stenosis is more common in men (male-to-female ratio, 1.6:1) and is the most frequent indication for isolated aortic valve replacement. In stenotic tricuspid aortic valves, calcification occurs most prominently in the base of the cusps on the aortic aspect and extends superiorly to-

ward the midportion of the cusp with sparing of the free margin (closing edge) (Fig. 1-9, A through C). Typically, nodular calcific deposits are superimposed on a fibrotic cusp (59); conversely, in congenital bicuspid valve stenosis, calcification occurs diffusely within the cusp spongiosa (59). Commissural fusion is rare in tricuspid aortic valve stenosis unless there has been a concomitant associated inflammatory or infectious disorder.

The pathogenesis of calcification of tricuspid aortic valves and risk factors for the development of aortic stenosis are uncertain. Mild asymmetry has been suggested as a possible factor in the etiology of acquired

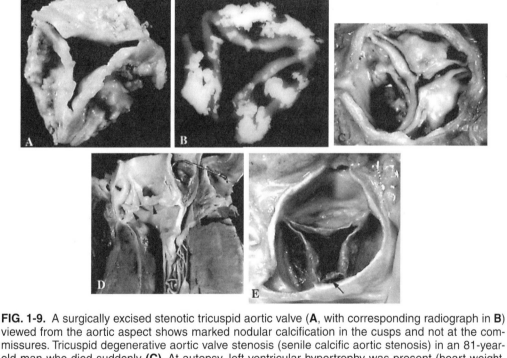

FIG. 1-9. A surgically excised stenotic tricuspid aortic valve (**A**, with corresponding radiograph in **B**) viewed from the aortic aspect shows marked nodular calcification in the cusps and not at the commissures. Tricuspid degenerative aortic valve stenosis (senile calcific aortic stenosis) in an 81-year-old man who died suddenly **(C)**. At autopsy, left ventricular hypertrophy was present (heart weight, 675 g). Large nodular calcific deposits are present on the aortic surface of the valve cusps extending in the sinuses of Valsalva; the free edges of the valve cusps are relatively spared. Chronic aortic regurgitation secondary to aortic valve prolapse is shown **(D)**. There is fibromyxomatous thickening of the aortic valve cusps that prolapse toward the left ventricular outflow tract (*arrowheads*), and a endocardial jet lesion of chronic aortic insufficiency is present (*) on the interventricular septum. An incidental quadricuspid aortic valve was found at autopsy in a 53-year-old woman **(E)**. The four cusps are dissimilar in size; the right and the left sinuses are normal, and the posterior sinus contains two cusps with a smaller left posterior cusp (*arrow*). (**E:** From Virmani R, Burke AP, Farb A. Pathology of valvular heart disease. In: Rahimtoola SH, ed. *Valvular Heart Disease.* Vol. XI. *Atlas of Heart Diseases.* St. Louis, MO: Mosby, 1997:1.3, with permission.)

tricuspid aortic stenosis (39,40); however, the high prevalence of differences in cusp size (more than 50% in individuals) makes it unlikely that isolated cusp asymmetry is sufficient to account for severe stenosis in most cases. An association between coronary atherosclerosis (with its epidemiologic risk factors) and tricuspid valve aortic stenosis has been observed. In patients older than age 40 years having aortic valve replacement, the presence of at least three of four of the following factors—age older than 65 years, total serum cholesterol more than 200 mg/dL, body mass index greater than 29 kg/m², and coronary atherosclerosis—was associated with a low probability (10% to 29%) of a *congenitally* abnormal (unicuspid or bicuspid) aortic valve; in contrast, patients lacking three or four of these clinical variables have a high probability for a congenitally abnormal aortic valve (60). In other studies, increasing age, smoking, hypertension, height, increased lipoprotein(a), and increased low-density lipoprotein levels have been associated with an increased prevalence of aortic valvular sclerosis (61–63). Increased rates of concurrent coronary bypass surgery in patients with tricuspid aortic valve stenosis compared with bicuspid aortic valve stenosis suggest that risk factors for the development of coronary artery atherosclerotic plaques may play a role in the pathogenesis of cusp calcification (64). Histologic studies of early aortic lesions in mildly thickened tricuspid aortic valves demonstrate subendothelial thickening, intra- and extracellular neutral lipids, fine mineralization, and basement membrane disruption (65). Immunohistochemical stains showed that these early lesions contain an inflammatory infiltrate composed of macrophages (foam and non-foam cell), scattered T lymphocytes, and rare smooth muscle cells (65). A similar, albeit more advanced, lesion was observed in clinically stenotic aortic valves (65). Of the lymphocytes infiltrating excised stenotic valves, T-helper cells were most frequently observed in the vicinity of calcific deposits and the endothelium expressed receptors for inter-

leukin-2 (66). These data suggest that an active inflammatory process, and not solely age-related degenerative change, may be involved in etiology of tricuspid aortic stenosis. Relatively less diastolic pressure loads imparted on the coronary cusps (left and right) compared with the noncoronary cups due to the presence of the coronary ostia may be an explanation of the increased incidence of degenerative changes in the noncoronary cusp (67).

Post-inflammatory Aortic Stenosis

Post-inflammatory aortic stenosis is presumed to be post-rheumatic, but less than 50% of patients have a history of rheumatic fever (55). Chronic post-inflammatory pathologic changes may occur in bicuspid or tricuspid aortic valves and occur with equal frequency in men and women. Commissural fusion is the most important diagnostic feature of postinflammatory aortic stenosis. Fusion of one, two, or all three commissures may be present (Fig. 1-10, A and B). Fusion of only one commissure results in an acquired bicuspid valve morphology (Fig. 1-10C), and fusion of all three commissures produces a dome-shaped valve. Commissures may be completely fused from the aortic wall to the free edge or only partially fused near the aortic wall insertion and remain separate at the free edge. The severity of stenosis increases as the number of fused commissures increases (55). The valve cusps themselves are diffusely fibrotically thickened. Variable degrees of cusp calcification may occur beginning in the fused commissures and extending into the cusp body (in contrast to congenital bicuspid valves in which calcification occurs in the cusps themselves and largely spares the commissures). Histologically, the fused commissure consists of fibrous connective tissue without elastic tissue. The valve cusps are fibrotic and contain foci of calcification, vascularization (small thick-walled vessels), myxomatous change, and chronic inflammation. Aschoff nodules are rare but may be seen with a recent history of acute rheumatic fever.

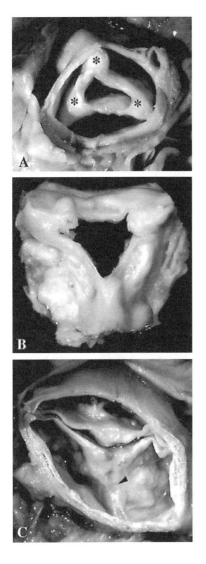

FIG. 1-10. Postrheumatic aortic valve disease. A 44-year-old man with known heart disease was found dead. At autopsy, he had an enlarged heart with severe mitral stenosis and aortic stenosis **(A)**. Note fusion of all three aortic valve commissures (*), thickening and fibrosis of all three aortic leaflets, and no calcification. A surgically excised aortic valve **(B)** in a 50-year-old woman with mitral and aortic stenosis. All three commissures are fused, and cusp fibrosis and calcification are evident with calcification present both in the commissures and leaflets. An acquired bicuspid stenotic aortic valve **(C)** was found in this 65-year-old man who died while awaiting valve replacement. The anterior commissure is fused (*arrowhead*), and this commissure is at the same level as and equidistant from the other two nonfused commissures. (**C**: From Virmani R, Burke AP, Farb A. Pathology of valvular heart disease. In: Rahimtoola SH, ed. *Valvular Heart Disease*. Vol. XI. *Atlas of Heart Diseases*. St. Louis, MO: Mosby, 1997:1.5, with permission.)

Nonvalvular Aortic Stenosis

Congenital supravalvular and subvalvular aortic stenoses are unusual etiologies for aortic stenosis (Fig. 1-11). Dysplasia and thickening of the aortic valve cusps may be present. Supravalvular aortic stenosis may occur as part of the Williams' syndrome or as an isolated finding. Subvalvular stenosis may be caused by a discrete fibrous membrane or tunnel-like narrowing of the left ventricular outflow tract. A discussion of hypertrophic cardiomyopathy with asymmetric hypertrophy causing subaortic stenosis is beyond the scope of this chapter.

Aortic Insufficiency

Aortic insufficiency may be due to lesions in the aortic valve cusps themselves or in the ascending aorta, resulting in the failure of valve cusps to close effectively (Table 1-6). Disease of the ascending aorta is now the most common cause of pure aortic insufficiency (68). Post-inflammatory scarring as an etiology of aortic insufficiency has declined

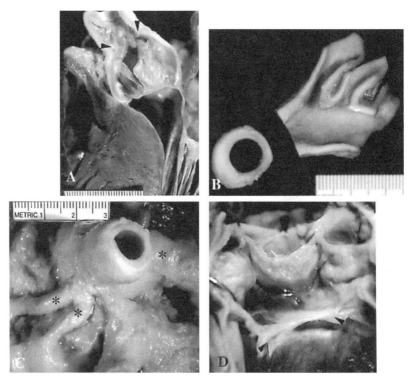

FIG. 1-11. Supravalvular and subvalvular aortic stenosis. Supravalvular aortic stenosis **(A, B, and C)** was found at autopsy in this 35-year-old man. Note the markedly thickened and narrowed aorta beginning at and extending above the sinotubular junction **(A,** *arrowheads*). The aortic valve cusps are also thickened. The thickening extends into the aortic arch **(B)**, and the epicardial coronary arteries are thickened, dysplastic, and dilated **(C,** *). Subaortic stenosis may occur either from a localized fibrous ridge or, less commonly, from a longer diffuse fibrous tunnel. Note a discreet fibrous ridge **(D,** *arrowheads*) underlying the aortic valve in a 15-year-old boy who died suddenly. The valve has three dysplastic valve cusps. **(D:** From Virmani R, Burke AP, Farb A. Pathology of valvular heart disease. In: Rahimtoola SH, ed. *Valvular Heart Disease.* Vol. XI. *Atlas of Heart Diseases.* St. Louis, MO: Mosby, 1997:1.3, with permission.)

in incidence as the frequency of acute rheumatic fever has declined (68). Aortic root dilatation is more common in men; postinflammatory disease is more common in women. In older individuals (60 to 80 years old), dilatation of the aorta is most often idiopathic or related to systemic hypertension, whereas in younger persons (20 to 40 years old), Marfan's syndrome and congenital heart disease are more frequently seen.

TABLE 1-6. *Surgical pathology of aortic regurgitation*

Etiology	Mayo Clinic (1965)[68]	London (1980)[43]	Mayo Clinic (1990)[45]	AFIP (1990–1997)
Postrheumatic	47%	26%	14%	15%
Aortic dilatation and/or degenerative valve changes[a]	19%	31%	50%	53%
Bicuspid	17%	26%	14%	19%
Endocarditis	4%	11%	1%	10%
Other	13%	6%	21%	3%

[a]Degenerative valve changes refers to tricuspid aortic valves with cusp fibrosis or myxomatous degeneration. AFIP, Armed Forces Institute of Pathology.

Clinical Presentation of Aortic Regurgitation

Clinically, chronic severe regurgitation may be well tolerated for many years without associated symptoms. Surgical intervention for chronic aortic regurgitation is indicated for patients with symptoms of left-sided heart failure (dyspnea, orthopnea, and fatigue) or objective evidence of left ventricular dysfunction or dilatation (50). In contrast to chronic regurgitation, acute severe aortic regurgitation (most commonly caused by infectious endocarditis, aortic dissection, or trauma) is typically extremely poorly tolerated, may precipitate acute cardiovascular collapse, and often requires urgent surgery.

Pathology of Aortic Regurgitation

With respect to etiology, intrinsic abnormalities of the aortic cusps leading to chronic aortic insufficiency are diverse and include congenital cusp lesions (e.g., congenital bicuspid aortic valve), post-inflammatory (post-rheumatic) scarring, myxomatous degeneration, infectious disease (endocarditis), connective tissue disease, and acquired cusp deformity secondary to nonvalvular congenital heart disease. For example, in membranous ventricular septal defect, prolapse of the right aortic cusp into the left ventricular outflow tract may occur, rendering the valve incompetent. Case reports of aortic valve repair or replacement have been published for Behçet's syndrome, hypereosinophilic syndrome, mucopolysaccharidoses (Hunter-Hurler phenotype), amyloidosis, and post-methysergide therapy.

When clinically important, congenital bicuspid aortic valves are most often stenotic; however, bicuspid valves account for 7% to 20% of cases of pure chronic aortic insufficiency (Fig. 1-8H) and may be increasing in incidence (68,69). The valve consists of two aortic unequally sized cusps, and a median raphe is frequently present in the conjoint (larger) cusp. An indentation of the conjoint cusp of congenitally bicuspid valves was a frequent finding (43% of cases) in one surgical series (70). An uncommon variant is a raphal cord that extends from the sinus wall to the free edge that produces cusp retraction. Regurgitant bicuspid valve cusps show varying degrees of fibrous thickening and rolled edges, and prolapse of the valve cusp(s) toward the left ventricle may be present (71,72). There is an increased incidence of structural abnormalities of the aortic root (cystic medial change) in patients with congenitally bicuspid aortic valves so that regurgitation may be primarily caused by aortic root dilatation rather than lesions in the valve cusps themselves. In one surgical series of pure aortic regurgitation, there was a 31% incidence of aortic root dilatation among bicuspid aortic valves (68). Superimposed infective endocarditis is a common cause of aortic regurgitation in nonstenotic bicuspid aortic valves (73,74).

A definitive history of rheumatic fever is uncommon (less than 10% of cases) in apparent post-inflammatory cusp scarring, leading to chronic aortic regurgitation. Diffuse fibrosis of valve cusps results in contracture and shortening, and calcification is typically mild or absent. If significant commissural fusion is present, the hemodynamic lesion is likely to be mixed stenotic and regurgitant.

Myxomatous aortic valves may be seen in Marfan's syndrome, in myxomatous degeneration of the mitral valve (mitral valve prolapse), or as an isolated aortic valve finding (75). In one study of surgically excised aortic valves for severe regurgitation, 13 of 55 patients (24%) had myxomatous degeneration in the absence of Marfan's syndrome; 85% were males and 77% had systemic hypertension (76). Pathologically, the aortic valve cusps are thickened by myxomatous tissue and may be redundant (Fig. 1-9D). Histologically, the spongiosa of the valve cusp is expanded by proteoglycans and occupies more than 50% of the cusp, resulting in discontinuity of the zona fibrosa. The etiology of the valvular myxomatous degeneration is not known but may involve an abnormality of collagen synthesis. It has been suggested that fibrotic, nonredundant, and retracted cusps may represent a later stage of myxomatous degeneration of the aortic valve (77). Miscellaneous causes of aortic regurgitation include a quadricuspid valve (Fig. 1-9E) and large noninfected fenestrations (78). Rarely, no etiology for aortic insufficiency is found.

In acute aortic insufficiency secondary to aortic dissection, the dissecting hematoma extending to commissural attachments or into the valve cusps results in cuspal malalignment. Of 189 cases of noniatrogenic aortic dissection, congenital aortic valve lesions were present in 16 (8.5%) patients (14 with bicuspid valves and 2 with unicuspid valves), all of whom had an intimal tear in the ascending aorta (79). In traumatic laceration of the proximal aorta, there may be avulsion of the cuspal attachment to the sinus of Valsalva wall.

A detailed discussion of the various causes of proximal aortic dilatation that may result in aortic insufficiency is beyond the scope of this chapter. Causes of ascending aortic dilatation that can produce severe aortic insufficiency include hypertension, aortic dissection, annuloaortic ectasia, traumatic aortic laceration, Marfan's syndrome, Ehlers-Danlos syndrome, oteogenesis imperfecta, pseudoxanthoma elasticum, and aortitis. Most cases of dilatation of the aorta (74% to 90%) are idiopathic (annuloaortic ectasia). Pathologically, valve cusps may be thin and stretched or fibrotically thickened. The cusp free edges may be rolled secondary to chronic severe regurgitation. Occasionally, foci of chronic inflammation may be encountered in the valve cusps as part of the accompanying aortitis.

Combined Aortic Stenosis and Regurgitation

Combined significant aortic stenosis and aortic regurgitation is a common indication for valve replacement, accounting for approximately 25% to 30% of aortic valve surgery cases. The age range at time of surgery is 40 to 80 years with a male-to-female ratio of 1.5:1. Symptoms and signs are similar to those of aortic stenosis or regurgitation. Postinflammatory disease is the most common etiology (approximately 70% of cases) and is assumed to be post-rheumatic; however, a definitive history of rheumatic fever is rare. Congenital bicuspid valves account for 25%

of cases, and the remaining cases are caused by miscellaneous conditions (congenital unicuspid valve, infectious endocarditis, and congenitally dysplastic tricuspid aortic valve). Aortic valve damage secondary to external beam radiation requiring valve surgery has been reported (80).

Pathologically, valvular stenosis is produced by leaflet calcification, fibrosis, and commissural fusion that restricts cusp excursion. The degree of calcification is generally less extensive than in pure aortic stenosis. Regurgitation is produced by leaflet fibrosis and retraction that prevents closing edges to align in diastole. One, two, or all three commissures may be fused.

Pulmonary Valve

Normal Anatomy of the Pulmonary Valve

The pulmonary valve consists of three semicircular cusps (left, right, and anterior cusps) and three commissures, and its annulus is approximately 1.5 cm above the level of the aortic annulus (41). Except for the absence of coronary ostia, the pulmonary valve is similar in structure to the aortic valve (41).

Pathology of the Pulmonary Valve

Congenital pulmonary valve disease may be an isolated finding (e.g., congenital pulmonary artery stenosis) or may occur in association with other congenital cardiac anomalies (e.g., tetrology of Fallot and ventricular septal defect). When present, pulmonic stenosis is most frequently a congenital lesion and as an isolated cardiac abnormality is typically associated with survival into adulthood (81,82). Morphologically, the stenotic pulmonic valve may have three normally placed commissures with dysplastic cusps, two cusps and two commissures (bicuspid valve), one cusp and one commissure (unicuspid, unicommissural valve), or one cusp and no commissure (unicuspid, acommissural valve) (Fig. 1-12A) (78–80). Valve cusps are thickened to a variable degree involving the entire length of the cusp (83). Histologically, there is increased cusp myxo-

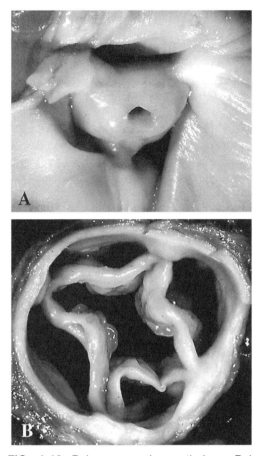

FIG. 1-12. Pulmonary valve pathology. Pulmonary stenosis may occur as an isolated congenital anomaly, and the stenosis is either valvular or both valvular and infundibular. The stenotic unicuspid acommissural pulmonary valve **(A)** is from a neonate; a dome- or funnel-shaped fibromyxomatous pulmonary valve with three raphal ridges was present. This quadricuspid pulmonary valve with mild dysplasia **(B)** was found in a 12-year-old girl with tunnel subaortic stenosis. Quadricuspid pulmonary valves are more frequently encountered than quadricuspid aortic valves and are usually an incidental finding. (**A and B:** From Virmani R, Burke AP, Farb A. Pathology of valvular heart disease. In: Rahimtoola SH, ed. *Valvular Heart Disease.* Vol. XI. *Atlas of Heart Diseases.* St. Louis, MO: Mosby, 1997:1.19–1.20, with permission.)

matous tissue with occasional increased cusp collagen and elastic tissue (83). Currently, congenital pulmonic stenosis is most often treated with percutaneous balloon valvuloplasty (84,85). Surgical removal of the pulmonic valve is most frequently performed for tetrology of Fallot (86); the valve is typically bicuspid and is associated with a hypoplastic annulus (37). Pulmonic stenosis may also be encountered in carcinoid heart disease (see below), and post-rheumatic valve scarring resulting in commissural fusion rarely causes significant valvular stenosis.

Similar to aortic regurgitation in which aortic root dilatation is the most common etiology, pulmonic regurgitation is most frequently caused by pulmonary trunk dilatation secondary to pulmonary hypertension (of any etiology), idiopathic pulmonary trunk dilatation, or Marfan's syndrome (41). Less common etiologies of pulmonic regurgitation include pulmonary valve carcinoid plaques, post-rheumatic scarring, endocarditis (86), trauma, congenitally absent or dysplastic leaflets, or surgical treatment of right ventricular and pulmonic valve congenital heart disease (87).

Quadricuspid pulmonary valve is the most frequent congenital pulmonary valve anomaly seen at autopsy (Fig. 1-12B) but is most often an incidental finding without clinical physiologic consequences (37).

ENDOCARDITIS

Infective Endocarditis

Infective endocarditis is defined by microbial infection of the valve endocardial surface often accompanied by destruction of underlying valvular structures. The median age of patients with infective endocarditis has increased from approximately 30 to 40 years from the preantibiotic era to 45 to 65 years in the last few decades. The incidence of infective endocarditis increases after the age of 30 years, increasing to greater than 15 to 30 cases per 100,000 person-years (88). Infective endocarditis is more frequent in men, with a male-to-female ratio varying from 1.6:2.5 to 1.

Approximately 55% to 75% of infective native valve endocarditis cases occur in the setting underlying valve abnormalities (89, 90) (Table 1-7). In adults, the underlying valve disease in native valve infective endocarditis is mitral valve prolapse in 29%, degenerative calcified valve disease in 21%, bicuspid aortic valve or other congenital abnormalities in 13%, and post-rheumatic scarring in 6%. Infective endocarditis is seen in normal valves in 31%, and many of these patients have underlying noncardiac conditions that predisposes to intravascular infection such as intravenous drug abuse, immunosuppressive therapy, alcoholic abuse, and colon carcinoma. Because of the reduction in rheumatic heart disease, other predisposing conditions such as mitral valve prolapse, nosocomial endocarditis in the elderly, and endocarditis in intravenous drug abusers have become relatively more common.

The microbiologic agents causing endocarditis have also changed because of the alterations in the underlying conditions that predispose to endocarditis and the increasing age of the population (90). *Staphylococcus aureus* is the most frequent cause of endocarditis in intravenous drug abusers, and gram-negative bacilli and *Candida* species are not uncommon in these individuals. *Streptococcus bovis* endocarditis is associated with colon carcinoma. *Streptococcus pneumoniae* endocarditis may be seen in alcoholics and pneumococcal sepsis. Gram-negative organisms are encountered in vegetations in diabetics and fungi in patients receiving immunosuppressive therapy (91–93). *Streptococcus viridans* remains a common organism in subacute cases of infective endocarditis and in post-rheumatic valve disease (94).

The pathogenesis of infective endocarditis initially involves formation of a sterile thrombus on an abnormal valve endocardial surface, followed by colonization, reproduction of microorganisms, and invasion of the valve tissue (95). Transient bacteremia is frequently seen in dental extraction, periodontal surgery, and oropharyngeal, gastrointestinal, urologic, or gynecologic invasive diagnostic or surgical procedures (96). Vegetations in infective endocarditis are more often on the left-sided valves.

TABLE 1-7. *Predisposing conditions and microorganism in native valve infectious endocarditis as a function of patient age*

	Children (%)		Adults (%)	
	Neonates	2 mo to 15 yr	15–60 yr	>60 yr
Predisposing condition				
RVD	—	2–10	25–30	8
CHD	28	75–90[a]	10–20	2
MVP	—	5–15	10–30	10
DVD	—	—	Rare	30
IVDA	—	—	15–35	10
Other	—	—	10–15	10
Normal	72[b]	2–5	25–45	25–40
Microbiology				
Streptococci	15–20	40–50	45–65	30–45
Enterococci	—	4	5–8	15
S. aureus	40–50	25	30–40	25–30
Coagulase-negative staphylococci	10	5	3–5	5–8
GNB	10	5	4–8	5
Fungi	10	1	1	Rare
Polymicrobial	4	—	1	Rare
Other	—	—	1	2
Culture negative	4	0–15	3–10	5

CHD, congenital heart disease; DVD, degenerative valve disease; GNB, gram-negative bacteria (frequently *Haemophilus* species, *Actinobacillus actinomycetemitans, Cardiobacterium hominis*); IVD, intravenous drug abuse; MVP, mitral valve prolapse; RVD, rheumatic valve disease.
[a]Fifty percent of cases follow surgery and may involve implanted devices and foreign material.
[b]Often tricuspid valve infective endocarditis.
From ref. 94, with permission.

The aortic valve (39% to 46%) is slightly more frequently involved than the mitral valve (30% to 35%), and combined aortic and mitral valve lesions (18% to 24%) are not uncommon. Infective endocarditis is more likely to occur in the setting of underlying valvular regurgitation rather than stenosis because of increased pressure and flow in regurgitant lesions that augment endocardial damage. Endocarditis involving the right-sided valves is less frequent (9% to 11%) compared with the aortic and mitral valves but is particularly common in intravenous drug abuse secondary to repeated injections of a nonsterile material; the tricuspid valve is more frequently affected than the pulmonic valve. Right-sided endocarditis is also associated with pulmonary artery catheterization, but most vegetations are sterile.

Presenting cardiac signs and symptoms of infective endocarditis include valvular regurgitation murmurs, congestive heart failure secondary to severe regurgitation, infectious pericarditis, heart block, and myocardial infarction secondary to coronary embolization; valvular stenosis secondary to bulky vegetations are rare. Noncardiac signs and symptoms include fever, anemia, musculoskeletal pain, glomerulonephritis, peripheral arterial embolization, and septic shock. Valve surgery for acute infective endocarditis is indicated for significant heart failure, valve annular abscess, heart block, major organ embolization, and persistent bacteremia. At surgery, a portion of the vegetation should be sent for organism identification and antibiotic sensitivity testing. Special stains for bacteria, Brown and Hopps and Brown and Brenn tissue Gram stains, are helpful in identifying microorganisms. Brown and Brenn stain is superior for gram-positive organisms that upon death may not stain with Brown and Hopps stain. Gomori methenamine silver or periodic acid–Schiff staining for fungi should be performed to identify fungi.

We recently reported 13 cases of sudden death secondary to infectious endocarditis in intravenous drug users seen between 1992 and 1994 at the Office of the Chief Medical Examiner in Maryland, which corresponds to a yearly incidence of infective endocarditis-related sudden unexpected death of 12 per 100,000. By comparison, in a prospective 5-year study conducted in Sweden (97), the yearly clinical incidence of endocarditis among intravenous drug users was 111 per 100,000. Therefore, by combining these two population studies, one can estimate that intravenous drug users are about nine times more likely to acquire endocarditis than they are likely to die suddenly with endocarditis (11% mortality). Comparable figures among non-drug users are a 3.8 per 100,000 yearly risk of acquiring endocarditis and a 0.04 per 100,000 yearly risk of dying with endocarditis (98), indicating a 95-fold increased risk of acquiring infective endocarditis than dying of infective endocarditis (1% mortality rate). In our study, infective endocarditis in intravenous drug users was much more likely to occur in native valves compared with non-drug users (88% vs. 25%, $p = 0.004$). Tricuspid valve endocarditis is three times more common than aortic valve endocarditis in intravenous drug abusers admitted to the hospital with staphylococcal septicemia. In lethal cases, left-sided endocarditis is more common than right-sided endocarditis. Healed endocarditis is more common in right-sided valves than in left-sided valves (67% vs. 8%).

The characteristic lesion of endocarditis consists of a mass or vegetation composed of platelets and fibrin containing colonies of microorganisms (Fig. 1-13, A through F). Grossly infective vegetations are pink, red, or yellow and change to gray-yellow brown as they organize. Vegetations initially develop at the line of valve closure and are most often on the atrial surface of the atrioventricular valves and on the ventricular surface of the semilunar valves. Vegetations may be associated with valve leaflet erosion or perforations or rupture of chordae tendineae. Spread of infection from the closing edge of one valve to its opposite side results in "kissing lesions." Infectious endocarditis usually leads to valvular regurgitation; rarely, valve stenosis occurs secondary to bulky vegetations. Weakening of the leaflet due to surface erosion may result in the formation of a leaflet aneurysm that bulges into the left atrium from the mitral

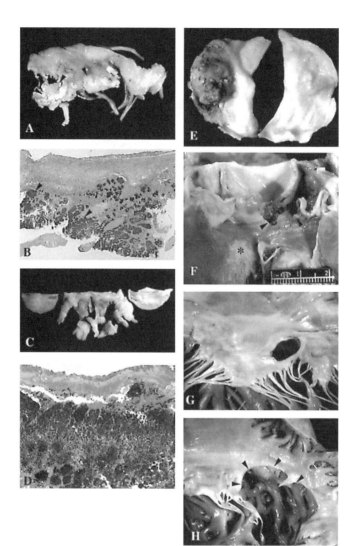

FIG. 1-13. Infective endocarditis. A 52-year-old man with mitral regurgitation, low-grade fever, and a mitral valve vegetation demonstrated on echocardiography underwent valve replacement. The excised mitral valve **(A)** demonstrated prolapse, ruptured chordae tendineae, and infective endocarditis characterized by bulky vegetations (*arrowheads*) that partially destroyed the valve leaflet. Histologically **(B)** (hematoxylin and eosin stain), the vegetation on the valve surface consisted of fibrin containing bacterial colonies (*arrowheads*) and interspersed acute inflammatory cells. **C:** Excised aortic valve from a 35-year-old intravenous drug user presented with acute aortic regurgitation and congestive heart failure. A large vegetation has resulted in multiple perforation of the middle aortic valve cusp. Silver methamine staining of the valve **(D)** revealed numerous microorganism colonies consistent with candida. A large infective vegetation secondary to *S. aureus* resulted in destruction of one cusp of a congenitally bicuspid aortic valve **(E)**. Subacute infectious endocarditis resulted in severe aortic regurgitation and sudden death in this 40-year-old man **(F)**. The left aortic valve cusp is perforated (*arrowheads*), and the adjacent sinus of Valsalva is dilated. The vegetations are small and organizing, and the chronicity of the aortic regurgitation is indicated by the endocardial thickening (*). Chronic mitral regurgitation secondary to healed mitral valve infective endocarditis is shown **(G)**. The valve leaflet surrounding the perforation is thickened. The chordae tendineae are intact, and the remainder of the underlying valve is unremarkable. Healed tricuspid valve endocarditis **(H)** from a 48-year-old intravenous drug user with chronic severe right-sided heart failure secondary to tricuspid regurgitation. A large portion of the anterior and septal leaflets are missing (*arrowheads*), and the margins of the remaining leaflets are mildly thickened.

valve and into the left ventricle from the aortic valve. Valve regurgitation may acutely worsen if there is perforation of the aneurysm (99). Histologically, the acute vegetation consists of platelets, fibrin, neutrophils, and microorganisms. Typically, there is associated acute and chronic inflammation.

Organizing healing vegetations contain varying degrees of chronic inflammatory cells, including lymphocytes, macrophages, plasma cells, and giant cells; neutrophils may be absent or scant in number. In healed lesions (Fig. 1-13, G and H), there may be focal leaflet thickening (which is most marked in the area of previous vegetation), calcification, or leaflet perforation. The area surrounding the perforation is thickened, and in an aneurysm, the valve surrounding the lesion is attenuated. Large friable vegetations are particularly prone to embolization. Clinically apparent emboli are seen in 15% to 35% of cases of infective endocarditis (94,100), and the incidence of emboli in autopsy series is substantially higher (45% to 65%) (101).

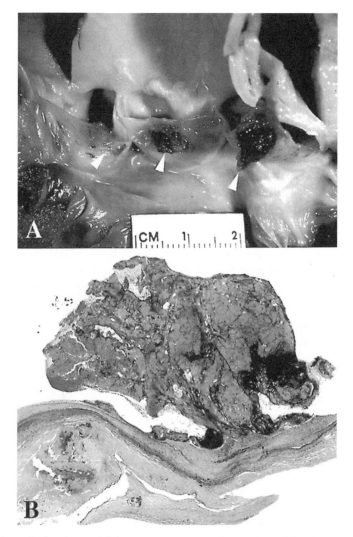

FIG. 1-14. A: Marantic (nonbacterial thrombotic) aortic valve endocarditis characterized by vegetations of varying sizes near the lines of closure on all three cusps (*arrowheads*). **B:** Histologically, marantic vegetations consist of fibrin-rich hypocellular thrombi attached to the valve surface in the absence of destruction of the underlying normal valve.

Noninfectious Endocarditis (Marantic Endocarditis, Nonbacterial Thrombotic Endocarditis)

Noninfectious endocarditis most frequently occurs in the setting of an underlying malignancy, chronic inflammatory disease, disseminated intravascular coagulation, uremia, burns, and intracardiac catheters. At autopsy, noninfectious endocarditis is reported in 1.3% of patients. Although seen at all ages, these vegetations are more common with increasing age. The etiology of these valvular vegetations is unknown but may involve platelet and fibrin deposition on valves that have endothelial injury in the setting of a hypercoagulable state (e.g., lupus anticoagulant, antiphospholipid antibodies [102], underlying adenocarcinoma, disseminated intravascular coagulation) or trauma (intracardiac catheter related). In the left heart, aortic valve involvement is more common than the mitral valve. The tricuspid and the pulmonic valve vegetations may occur secondary to central venous catheter-induced endocardial trauma. Even in patients with nonterminal illness, surgery is rarely performed unless there is significant embolization.

The vegetations may be small or large and are gray-pink, friable, soft or firm masses along the line of valve closure on the atrial surface of the atrioventricular valves and on the ventricular surface of the semilunar valves (Fig. 1-14A). Histologically, marantic vegetations are composed of platelet fibrin deposits with scant inflammatory cells (Fig. 1-14B). Most importantly, there is no associated valve ulceration or perforation, the underlying valve is almost always unremarkable, and no microorganisms are present.

VALVULAR ABNORMALITIES IN SYSTEMIC DISEASE

Carcinoid Heart Disease

Carcinoid heart disease occurs in 20% to 50% of patients with carcinoid syndrome (flushing, telengiectasias, diarrhea, and bronchoconstriction) secondary to a metastatic carcinoid tumor (103). The pathogenesis of carcinoid plaques is unknown but may be related to endothelial injury from vasoactive agents produced by the carcinoid tumor; circulating plasma serotonin levels (104) and urinary 5-hydroxyindoleacetic acid (105) are higher in patients with carcinoid heart disease compared with those with carcinoid tumors but no cardiac involvement. Carcinoid heart disease is an important cause of morbidity and mortality (103,106), is associated with a mean survival of 1 to 2 years (105,106), and may be treated with valve replacement or palliative valvotomy in selected cases (103,107, 108). In the Mayo Clinic series of 363 surgically excised tricuspid valves, 5 valves were removed because of carcinoid syndrome. Valve replacement in patients older than age 60 years is associated with a high postoperative mortality rate (109).

Tricuspid valve carcinoid plaques occur with equal frequency to pulmonic valve plaques (Fig. 1-15, A to C). On the tricuspid valve, accumulation of carcinoid plaques deposited on the valve surface results in tricuspid regurgitation with or without stenosis (103). Pure tricuspid valve stenosis secondary to carcinoid valve disease is rare. On the pulmonary valve, carcinoid plaques most often cause pulmonic stenosis, with pulmonic regurgitation being less common. The histology of carcinoid valve plaques consists of smooth muscle cells within a proteoglycan matrix that are deposited on the normal valvular endothelium. These plaques on the ventricular endocardial surface of the tricuspid valve result in leaflet and chordal thickening.

Recently, valve lesions similar to those seen in the carcinoid syndrome have been identified in patients taking the weight-reducing agents fenfluramine and phentermine (7,110). Connolly et al. (7) found apparently new valvular heart disease in 24 women who had been treated with these agents in combination for approximately 1 year. Valve abnormalities were severe enough to require surgery in five patients. Pathologic evaluation of excised valve demonstrated plaques consisting of smooth muscle cells in a connective tissue matrix encasing otherwise unremark-

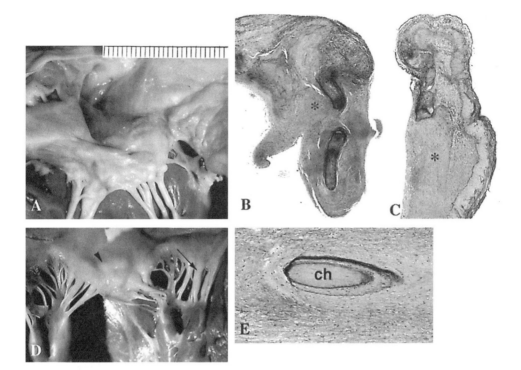

FIG. 1-15. Carcinoid and fenfluramine-phentermine–associated valve disease. The opened right atrium and tricuspid valve **(A)** show markedly thickened valve leaflets with chordae thickening and fusion. Clinically, the patient had mild tricuspid stenosis and regurgitation in the setting of a small bowel carcinoid tumor with liver metastasis. Grossly, the thickened and fibrotic tricuspid valve resembles postrheumatic scarring; however, histologically **(B)**, the underlying valve structure is well preserved, but the atrial and ventricular surfaces of the valve are surrounded by carcinoid plaque consisting of smooth muscle cells in a proteoglycan matrix (*, staining of proteoglycans by Movat pentachrome stain). Combined stenosis and regurgitation resulted from carcinoid plaque on the arterial surface of the pulmonary valve cusp (**C**, *). Lesions similar to those associated with the carcinoid syndrome have been described in patients treated methysergide and ergotamine treatment and most recently in patients receiving the weight-reducing agents fenfluramine-phentermine. Mitral valve leaflet and chordal thickening in a 48-year-old woman treated with fenfluramine-phentermine for over 1 year is shown **(D)**. Smooth muscle cells in a proteoglycan matrix surrounding a mitral valve chord (*ch*) is shown **(E)**.

able valve structures (Fig. 1-15, D and E), identical to the pathology of carcinoid or ergotamine heart disease (7).

Systemic Lupus Erythematosus

Cardiac involvement in systemic lupus erythematosus (SLE) includes pericarditis, myocarditis, endocardial and valvular lesions, and conduction system abnormalities. First described by Libman and Sacks in 1924, valvular lesions are present at autopsy in 50% of SLE cases and are clinically insignificant in most cases.

Antiphospholipid antibodies associated with SLE were first noted in 1985 (111). In most cases, antiphospholipid antibodies occur in the setting of SLE, but antiphospholipid antibodies in the absence of SLE are increasingly recognized. The antiphospholipid syndrome is defined by the presence of antiphospholipid antibodies, arterial and venous thrombosis, recurrent pregnancy loss, and thrombocytopenia. One third of patients with primary antiphospholipid syndrome have valvular involvement. The frequency of valve lesions is higher in SLE patients with antiphospholipid antibodies compared with those in which antiphospholipid antibodies are absent (48% vs. 21%, respectively) (112). Antiphospholipid antibodies determined by ELISA with the negatively charged phospholipid cardiolipin are called anticardiolipin antibodies (aCLs) (102). In SLE patients with antiphospholipid antibodies, the highest aCLs levels (more than 100 units) are seen in more than 50% of patients with valvular abnormalities; moderate aCL levels are present in 37% with valvular defects, and 14% of those with valve defects had no elevation of aCLs (113). Other factors associated with valvulopathy include increasing age, increased duration of SLE or antiphospholipid syndrome, and a history of arterial thrombosis. In patients with antiphospholipid antibodies, valve lesions are often associated with thromboembolic events (114). Patients with embolic events are more likely to have elevated aCLs than those without elevated levels, and those with embolic events are typically younger than those without (115).

Since the introduction of two-dimensional echocardiography, 35% of SLE patients have been shown to have valvulopathy; valve thickening in the midportion or the base of the posterior mitral leaflet is the most common echo finding (112). The most common hemodynamic valvular abnormality in SLE is mitral regurgitation, which occurs in 22% to 26% of all patients with SLE and antiphospholipid antibodies. Aortic regurgitation is less common, occurring in 6% to 10%. Stenosis of the mitral or aortic valve is rare as is right-sided valvular disease. Superimposed infective endocarditis in patients with valve lesions is uncommon (116).

Pathologically, valve lesions in SLE (Libman-Sacks endocarditis) are pinhead, warty, sessile, fibrinous vegetations, 3 to 4 mm in size, located predominantly near the valve tips (Fig. 1-16A) on the ventricular surface of the mitral valve, may be adherent to chordae, and variably extend onto the atrial valve sur-

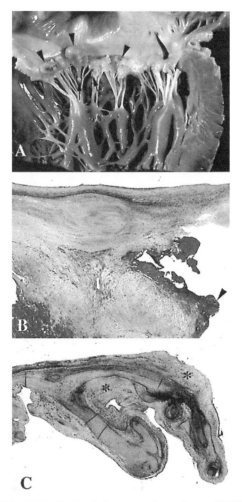

FIG. 1-16. Systemic lupus erythematosus (SLE). A 21-year-old women with SLE diagnosed 2 years antemortem developed systemic hypertension and renal failure. At autopsy **(A)**, Libman-Sacks verrucous vegetations (*arrowheads*) were evident on the anterior and posterior mitral valve leaflets with smaller chordal vegetations present (arrows). Histologically **(B)**, the mitral valve was fibrotic, and an organizing fibrinous vegetation (*arrowhead*) was present on the undersurface of the valve in this field (Movat pentachrome stain). A histologic section of the posterior mitral leaflet from a 42-year-old woman with a long history of SLE treated with immunosuppressive therapy demonstrates healed Libman-Sacks endocarditis characterized by fibrosis (*) on the atrial and ventricular surfaces of the valve (**C**, Movat pentachrome stain). (**C:** From Virmani R, Burke AP, Farb A. Pathology of valvular heart disease. In: Rahimtoola SH, ed. *Valvular Heart Disease.* Vol. XI. *Atlas of Heart Diseases.* St. Louis, MO: Mosby, 1997:1.14, with permission.)

face (117). On the aortic valve, Libman-Sacks vegetations are most commonly found near the commissures. The vegetations are firmly attached to the valve surface. Similar vegetations have been described in patients with the antiphospholipid syndrome. Histologically (Fig. 1-16B), the vegetations are characterized by the presence of fibrin at varying stages of organization, neovascularization, and mononuclear cell infiltrates. Before the advent of steroid treatment, more extensive inflammation was present associated with focal necrosis and hematoxylin bodies, the tissue counterpart to lupus erythematosus cells (118,119). Healed lesions of Libman-Sacks endocarditis consist of fibrous plaques with or without focal calcification (120). When the lesions are extensive, there is typically marked fibrosis (Fig. 1-16C), thickening, scarring, and retraction of the valve that leads to valvular regurgitation (120). However, surgery for valve abnormalities in SLE is rarely performed.

How antiphospholipid antibodies induce valvular damage is unknown, but it has been postulated that they promote thrombosis on the injured valve endothelium. Several biologic effects of antiphospholipid antibodies have been shown *in vitro* that may be responsible for the increased endothelial cell procoagulant activity: increased production of platelet activating factor, increased tissue factor activity, and inhibition of plasminogen activator release (121). However, the precise mechanisms that initiate valve damage *in vivo* have not been identified. Immunohistochemical studies have shown valvular immunoglobulin deposits with complement colocalization. Further, valves with immunoglobulin present have also been shown to stain positively for aCLs (122). Thus, it would appear that antiphospholipid antibodies play an important role in the pathogenesis of cardiac valve lesions.

Rheumatoid Arthritis

Although fibrinous pericarditis is the most frequent cardiac manifestation of rheumatoid arthritis, the classic cardiac lesion is the rheumatoid nodule that may involve the myocardium, endocardium, and valves (123). Involvement of the heart by rheumatoid granulomas at autopsy in patients with rheumatoid arthritis is 1% to 5%.

In a study of 214 patients with rheumatoid arthritis followed for 18 years, valvular disease was found during follow-up in 6 (3%), and the most frequent site of involvement was the mitral valve followed by aortic valve and rarely the tricuspid valve (124). At autopsy, rheumatoid nodules may be present in any of the four cardiac valves (34). Valve involvement by rheumatoid nodules does not usually lead to valvular dysfunction, but when present, valvular regurgitation is more common than stenosis. The frequency of clinical valve involvement correlates with the duration of the disease (125).

Pathologically, rheumatoid nodules are located at the base of the valve near its annular attachment in the center of the valve leaflet. The nodules have a central area of necrosis with surrounding palisading histiocytes, giant cells, extensive lymphocyte infiltration, and a variable number of plasma cells. At the site of the nodule, the valve appears grossly thickened. At the valve annulus, the nodules may bulge into the ventricular cavity. Rupture of a valvular rheumatoid nodule has been reported (126). The acute lesions may heal, resulting in valve sclerosis and scarring with chronic inflammation, but rheumatoid nodules may no longer be present. Fibrous scarring and retraction of the leaflets may result in further valve incompetence.

Seronegative Spondyloarthopathies (HLA-B27–associated Heart Disease)

The seronegative spondyloarthopathies (ankylosing spondylitis, Reiter's syndrome, and psoriatic arthritis) are associated with HLA-B27 histocompatability antigen and occasionally involve the aortic root and aortic valve cusps to produce significant chronic aortic regurgitation. The valve cusps are scarred and fibrotically thickened, particularly in their basal portion, which results in cusp retraction, inward rolling of valve cusp free edges, and foci of chronic inflammation (127). The aortitis of ankylosing spondylitis may extend below the aortic valve and produce a subaortic fibrous ridge (128). The prevalence of aortic regurgitation in ankylosing spondylitis ranges from 2% to 10% (127,129) of affected patients and increases with age, disease duration, and presence of peripheral arthritis (128,130). Mitral valve involvement is secondary to aortic valve abnormalities; the base of the mitral valve shows a hump or a ridge from fibrosis and inflammation extending from the aortic valve (127). Functionally, the mitral valve is competent unless there is severe dilatation of the left ventricle and mitral annulus secondary to aortic regurgitation. Conduction abnormalities are well documented in patients with ankylosing spondylitis.

In one study, the prevalence of aortic regurgitation in 164 patients with Reiter's disease was 2.8% (131). In patients undergoing aortic valve surgery for relapsing polychondritis, aortic root dilatation is responsible for significant aortic regurgitation in nearly 80% of cases with aortic valve pathology (fibrosis of valve cusps with elastic tissue loss and cystic degeneration) in the absence of aortic root dilatation, which was responsible for the remaining 20% (132). The aortic valve annulus is dilated and there is fibrosis and retraction of the aortic valve leaflets, resulting in valve incompetence.

Whipple's Disease

Valvular involvement in Whipple's disease is usually overshadowed by the intestinal symptoms. Endocarditis in Whipple's disease is characterized by infiltration of the valve by macrophages, interspersed acute inflammatory cells, and valve surface vegetations, usually resulting in valvular regurgitation (133). Healing of the acute lesions may result in commissural fusion and resultant valve stenosis (134). The causative organism of Whipple's disease has recently been identified as a gram-positive actinomycete (*Tropheryma whippeli*) (135).

Hypereosinophilic Syndrome (Loeffler's Endocarditis)

The hypereosinophilic syndrome is characterized by chronic eosinophilia of more than 1,500 eosinophils/mm^2 for at least 6 months or at the time of death, thromboembolic phenomena, and generalized arteritis. The cause of hypereosinophilia is idiopathic in most cases; occasionally, it may be secondary to leukemia, parasitic infestation, allergic or hypersensitivity reaction, or neoplasms such as Hodgkin's disease. The hypereosinophilic syndrome typically occurs in middle-aged men (in the fourth decade) but has been reported in all ages. Cardiac involvement, typically involving both ventricles, is seen in at least 75% of cases, and cardiac dysfunction is responsible for the high rates of morbidity and mortality. In the acute phase, the heart may be enlarged, and there are eosinophil-rich mural thrombi on the endocardium of the ventricular apex, ventricular inflow, and on the ventricular surface of the atrioventricular valves (Fig. 1-17A). A portion of the posterior mitral and the tricuspid valve leaflets may be adherent to the underlying ventricular wall, resulting in regurgitation (Fig. 1-17B). Small intramuscular arteries may contain thrombi, and eosinophilic myocarditis may be evident depending on the stage of the disease. Upon degranulation of the eosinophils, Charcot-Leiden crystals with surrounding giant cells and macrophages may be seen. In the late phase of the disease, the endocardium is markedly thickened, extending from the apex to the papillary muscles; neither eosinophils nor myocarditis may be present. The disease at this late phase is indistinguishable from endocardial fibrosis (Davies disease), a disease common in tropical and subtropical Africa, especially Uganda and Nigeria, and also reported in Brazil, Colombia, and Sri Lanka.

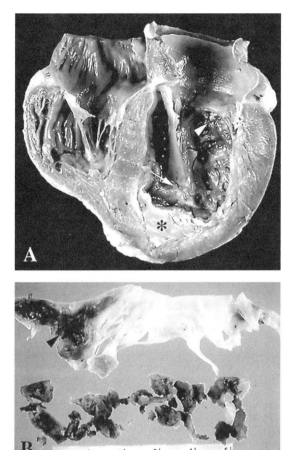

FIG. 1-17. Hypereosinophilic syndrome. The heart **(A)** from a 9-year-old boy with eosinophilic leukemia of 9-months duration shows biventricular dilatation and hypertrophy (four-chamber view). Note the organizing mural thrombus at the apex of the left ventricle (*), enveloping the posteromedial papillary muscle (*arrow*), and extending up and inferior to the posterior mitral valve leaflet (*arrowhead*). Endocardial fibrosis is present in the right ventricular apex extending into the papillary muscle. A surgically removed mitral valve and multiple fragments of endocardial thrombus **(B)** from a patient with hypereosinophilic syndrome shows attached focally organizing thrombus on the ventricular surface of the leaflet (*arrowhead*). **(A:** From Virmani R, Burke AP, Farb A. Pathology of valvular heart disease. In: Rahimtoola SH, ed. *Valvular Heart Disease.* Vol. XI. *Atlas of Heart Diseases.* St. Louis, MO: Mosby, 1997:1.15, with permission.)

MISCELLANEOUS LESIONS

Valve papillary fibroelastoma (136) and valve myxoma are rare causes of systemic emboli. Now rare, tertiary syphilis can result in proximal aortic root dilatation and aortic cusp scarring, resulting in significant aortic regurgitation.

REFERENCES

1. Rose AG. Etiology of valvular heart disease. *Curr Opin Cardiol* 1996;11:98–113.
2. Hanson T, Edwards B, Edwards JE. Pathology of surgically excised mitral valves. *Arch Pathol Lab Med* 1985;109:823–828.
3. Feldman T. Rheumatic heart disease. *Curr Opin Cardiol* 1996;11:126–130.
4. Olson LJ, Subramanian R, Ackermann DM, Orszulak TA, Edwards WD. Surgical pathology of the mitral valve: a study of 712 cases spanning 21 years. *Mayo Clin Proc* 1987;62:22–34.
5. Dare AJ, Harrity PJ, Tazelaar HD, Edwards WD, Mullany CJ. Evaluation of surgically excised mitral valves: revised recommendations based on changing operative procedures in the 1990s. *Hum Pathol* 1993;24: 1286–1293.
6. Hendrikx M, Van Dorpe J, Flameng W, Daenen W. Aortic and mitral valve disease induced by ergotamine therapy for migraine: a case report and review of the literature. *J Heart Valve Dis* 1996;5:235–237.
7. Connolly HM, Crary JL, McGoon MD, et al. Valvular heart disease associated with fenfluramine-phentermine. *N Engl J Med* 1997;337:581–588.
8. Chesler E, Gornick CC. Maladies attributed to myxomatous mitral valve. *Circulation* 1991;83:328–332.
9. Perloff JK, Child JS. Clinical and epidemiologic issues in mitral valve prolapse: overview and perspective. *Am Heart J* 1987;113:1324–1332.
10. Virmani R, Atkinson JB, Byrd BF 3d, Robinowitz M, Forman MB. Abnormal chordal insertion: a cause of mitral valve prolapse. *Am Heart J* 1987;113: 851–858.

11. Becker AE, De Wit AP. Mitral valve apparatus. A spectrum of normality relevant to mitral valve prolapse. *Br Heart J* 1979;42:680–689.

12. Baker PB, Bansal G, Boudoulas H, Kolibash AJ, Kilman J, Wooley CF. Floppy mitral valve chordae tendineae: histopathologic alterations. *Hum Pathol* 1988;19:507–512.

13. Enriquez-Sarano M, Orszulak TA, Schaff HV, Abel MD, Tajik AJ, Frye RL. Mitral regurgitation: a new clinical perspective. *Mayo Clin Proc* 1997;72:1034–1043.

14. Duren DR, Becker AE, Dunning AJ. Long-term follow-up of idiopathic mitral valve prolapse in 300 patients: a prospective study. *J Am Coll Cardiol* 1988;11:42–47.

15. Dollar AL, Roberts WC. Morphologic comparison of patients with mitral valve prolapse who died suddenly with patients who died from severe valvular dysfunction or other conditions. *J Am Coll Cardiol* 1991;17:921–931.

16. Farb A, Tang AL, Atkinson JB, McCarthy WF, Virmani R. Comparison of cardiac findings in patients with mitral valve prolapse who die suddenly to those who have congestive heart failure from mitral regurgitation and to those with fatal noncardiac conditions. *Am J Cardiol* 1992;70:234–239.

17. Pocock WA, Bosman CK, Chesler E, Barlow JB, Edwards JE. Sudden death in primary mitral valve prolapse. *Am Heart J* 1984;107:378–382.

18. Kligfield P, Levy D, Devereux RB, Savage DD. Arrhythmias and sudden death in mitral valve prolapse. *Am Heart J* 1987;113:1298–1307.

19. Morales AR, Romanelli R, Boucek RJ, Tate LG, Alvarez RT, Davis JT. Myxoid heart disease: an assessment of extravalvular cardiac pathology in severe mitral valve prolapse. *Hum Pathol* 1992;23:129–137.

20. Bronze MS, Dale JB. The reemergence of serious group A streptococcal infections and acute rheumatic fever. *Am J Med Sci* 1996;311:41–54.

21. Shiffman RN. Guideline maintenance and revision. 50 years of the Jones criteria for diagnosis of rheumatic fever. *Arch Pediatr Adolesc Med* 1995;149:727–732.

22. Stollerman GH. Rheumatic fever. *Lancet* 1997;349:935–942.

23. Markowitz M, Gerber MA. The Jones criteria for guidance in the diagnosis of rheumatic fever. Another perspective [editorial; comment]. *Arch Pediatr Adolesc Med* 1995;149:725–726.

24. Roberts WC, Virmani R. Aschoff bodies at necropsy in valvular heart disease. *Circulation* 1977;57:803–807.

25. Carabello BA. Indications for valve surgery in asymptomatic patients with aortic and mitral stenosis. *Chest* 1995;108:1678–1682.

26. Hutchison SJ, Tak T, Mummaneni M, et al. Morphological characteristics of the regurgitant rheumatic mitral valve. *Can J Cardiol* 1995;11:765–769.

27. Carpentier AF, Pellerin M, Fuzellier JF, Relland JY. Extensive calcification of the mitral valve anulus: pathology and surgical management. *J Thorac Cardiovasc Surg* 1996;111:718–729.

28. Czer LS, Maurer G, Trento A, et al. Comparative efficacy of ring and suture annuloplasty for ischemic mitral regurgitation. *Circulation* 1992;86:II46–II52.

29. David TE, Bos J, Rakowski H. Mitral valve repair by replacement of chordae tendineae with polytetrafluoroethylene sutures. *J Thorac Cardiovasc Surg* 1991;101:495–501.

30. Davies MJ. The tricuspid valve. In: Davies MJ, ed. *Pathology of Cardiac Valves*. London: Butterworths, 1980:124–131.

31. Hauck AJ, Freeman DP, Ackermann DM, Danielson GK, Edwards WD. Surgical pathology of the tricuspid valve: a study of 363 cases spanning 25 years. *Mayo Clin Proc* 1988;63:851–863.

32. Burke AP, Kalra P, Li L, Smialek J, Virmani R. Infectious endocarditis and sudden unexpected death: incidence and morphology of lesions in intravenous addicts and non-drug abusers. *J Heart Valve Dis* 1997;6:198–203.

33. Knight CJ, Sutton GC. Complete heart block and severe tricuspid regurgitation after radiotherapy. Case report and review of the literature. *Chest* 1995;108:1748–1751.

34. Roberts WC. Cardiac valvular lesions in rheumatoid arthritis. *Arch Intern Med* 1968;122:141–146.

35. Anderson KR, Lie JT. Pathologic anatomy of Ebstein's anomaly of the heart revisited. *Am J Cardiol* 1978;41:739–745.

36. Giuliani ER, Fuster V, Brandenburg RO, Mair DD. Ebstein's anomaly: the clinical features and natural history of Ebstein's anomaly of the tricuspid valve. *Mayo Clin Proc* 1979;54:163–173.

37. Farb A, Burke AP, Virmani R. Anatomy and pathology of the right ventricle (including acquired tricuspid and pulmonic valve disease). *Cardiol Clin* 1992;10:1–21.

38. Silver MA, Roberts WC. Detailed anatomy of the normally functioning aortic valve in hearts of normal and increased weight. *Am J Cardiol* 1985;55:454–461.

39. Roberts WC. The structure of the aortic valve in clinically isolated aortic stenosis. An autopsy study of 162 patients over 15 years of age. *Circulation* 1970;42:91–97.

40. Vollebergh FEMG, Becker AE. Minor congenital variations of cusp size in tricuspid aortic valves. Possible link with isolated aortic stenosis. *Br Heart J* 1977;39:1006–1011.

41. Waller BF. Morphological aspects of valvular heart disease. Part 1. *Curr Prob Cardiol* 1984;9:1–65.

42. Passik CS, Ackerman DM, Pluth JR, Edwards WD. Temporal changes in the causes of aortic stenosis: A surgical pathologic study of 646 cases. *Mayo Clin Proc* 1987;62:119–123.

43. Davies MJ. *Pathology of Cardiac Valves*. London: Butterworths, 1980:18–58.

44. Peterson MD, Roach RM, Edwards JE. Types of aortic stenosis in surgically removed valves. *Arch Pathol Lab Med* 1985;109:829–832.

45. Dare AJ, Veinot JP, Edwards WD, Tazelaar HD, Schaff HV. New observations on the etiology of aortic valve disease: A surgical pathologic study of 236 cases from 1990. *Hum Pathol* 1993;24:1330–1338.

46. Faggiano P, Aurigemma GP, Rusconi C, Gaasch WH. Progression of valvular aortic stenosis in adults: literature review and clinical implications. *Am Heart J* 1996;132:408–417.

47. Davies SW, Gershlick AH, Balcon R. Progression of aortic stenosis: A long-term retrospective study. *Eur Heart J* 1991;12:10–14.

48. Ross JJ, Braunwald E. Aortic stenosis. *Circulation* 1968;38[Suppl V]:V61–V67.

49. O'Keefe JHJ, Vlietstra RE, Bailey KR, Holmes DRJ. Natural history of candidates for balloon aortic valvuloplasty. *Mayo Clin Proc* 1987;62:986–991.

50. Carabello BA, Crawford FA Jr. Valvular heart disease. *N Engl J Med* 1997;337:32–41.

51. Pellika PA, Nishimura RA, Bailey KR, Tajik JA. The natural history of adults with asymptomatic, hemodynamically significant aortic stenosis. *J Am Coll Cardiol* 1990;15:1012–1017.

52. Roberts WC. Morphologic aspects of cardiac valve dysfunction. *Am Heart J* 1992;123:1610–1632.

53. Sadee AS, Becker AE, Verheul JA. The congenital bicuspid aortic valve with post-inflammatory disease—a neglected pathological diagnosis of clinical relevance. *Eur Heart J* 1994;15:503–506.

54. Arnett EN, Roberts WC. Acute infective endocarditis: a clinicopathologic analysis of 137 patients. *Curr Probl Cardiol* 1976;1:1–76.

55. Subramanian R, Olson LJ, Edwards WD. Surgical pathology of pure aortic stenosis: a study of 374 cases. *Mayo Clin Proc* 1984;59:683–690.

56. Moore GW, Hutchins GM, Brito JC, Kang H. Congenital malformations of the semilunar valves. *Hum Pathol* 1980;11:367–372.

57. Lerer PK, Edwards WD. Coronary arterial anatomy in bicuspid aortic valve: Necropsy study of 100 hearts. *Br Heart J* 1981;45:142–147.

58. Walley VM, Antecol DH, Kyrollos AG, Chan KL. Congenitally bicuspid aortic valves: study of a variant with fenestrated raphe. *Can J Cardiol* 1994;10:535–542.

59. Isner JM, Chokshi SK, DeFranco A, Braimen J, Slovenkai GA. Contrasting histoarchitecture of calcified leaflets from stenotic bicuspid versus stenotic tricuspid aortic valves. *J Am Coll Cardiol* 1990;15:1104–1108.

60. Mautner GC, Mautner SL, Cannon RO, Hunsberger SA, Roberts WC. Clinical factors useful in predicting aortic valve structure in patients > 40 years of age with isolated valvular aortic stenosis. *Am J Cardiol* 1993;72:194–198.

61. Nistal JF, Garcia-Martinez V, Fernandez MD, Hurle A, Hurle JM, Revuelta JM. Age-dependent dystrophic calcification of the aortic valve leaflets in normal subjects. *J Heart Valve Dis* 1994;3:37–40.

62. Stewart BF, Siscovick D, Lind BK, et al. Clinical factors associated with calcific aortic valve disease. Cardiovascular Health Study. *J Am Coll Cardiol* 1997;29:630–634.

63. Gotoh T, Kuroda T, Yamasawa M, et al. Correlation between lipoprotein(a) and aortic valve sclerosis assessed by echocardiography (the JMS Cardiac Echo and Cohort Study). *Am J Cardiol* 1995;76:928–932.

64. Davies MJ, Treasure T, Parker DJ. Demographic characteristics of patients undergoing aortic valve replacement for stenosis: relation to valve morphology. *Heart* 1996;75:174–178.

65. Otto CM, Kuusisto J, Reichenbach DD, Gown AM, O'Brien KD. Characterization of the early lesion of "degenerative" valvular aortic stenosis. Histological and immunohistochemical studies. *Circulation* 1994;90:844–853.

66. Olsson M, Dalsgaard CJ, Haegerstrand A, Rosenqvist M, Ryden L, Nilsson J. Accumulation of T lymphocytes and expression of interleukin-2 receptors in non-rheumatic stenotic aortic valves. *J Am Coll Cardiol* 1994;23:1162–1170.

67. Young ST, Lin SL. A possible relation between pressure loading and thickened leaflets of the aortic valve: a model simulation. *Med Eng Phys* 1994;16:465–469.

68. Olson LJ, Subramanian R, Edwards WD. Surgical pathology of pure aortic regurgitation: a study of 225 cases. *Mayo Clin Proc* 1984;59:835–841.

69. Roberts WC, Morrow AG, McIntosh CL, Jones M, Epstein SE. Congenitally bicuspid aortic valve causing severe, pure aortic regurgitation without superimposed infective endocarditis. Analysis of 13 patients requiring aortic valve replacement. *Am J Cardiol* 1980;47:206–209.

70. Sadee AS, Becker AE, Verheul HA, Bouma B, Hoedemaker G. Aortic valve regurgitation and the congenitally bicuspid aortic valve: a clinico-pathological correlation. *Br Heart J* 1992;67:439–441.

71. Stewart WJ, King ME, Gillam LD, Guyer DE, Weyman AE. Prevalence of aortic valve prolapse with bicuspid aortic valve and its relation to aortic regurgitation: a cross-sectional echocardiographic study. *Am J Cardiol* 1984;54:1277–1282.

72. Mills P, Leech G, Davies M, Leatham A. The natural history of a non-stenotic bicuspid aortic valve. *Br Heart J* 1978;40:951–957.

73. Turri M, Thiene G, Bortolotti U, Milano A, Mazzucco A, Gallucci V. Surgical pathology of aortic valve disease. A study based on 602 specimens. *Eur J Cardiothorac Surg* 1990;4:556–560.

74. Roberts WC. The congenitally bicuspid aortic valve. A study of 85 autopsy cases. *Am J Cardiol* 1960;23:72–83.

75. McKay R, Yacoub MH. Clinical and pathological findings in patients with "floppy" valves treated surgically. *Circulation* 1973;48[Suppl I]:III63–III73.

76. Allen WM, Matloff JM, Fishbein MC. Myxoid degeneration of the aortic valve and isolated severe aortic regurgitation. *Am J Cardiol* 1985;55:439–444.

77. Lakier JB, Copans H, Rosman HS, et al. Idiopathic degeneration of the aortic valve: a common cause of isolated aortic regurgitation. *J Am Coll Cardiol* 1985;5:347–351.

78. Kaplan J, Farb A, Carliner NH, Virmani R. Large aortic valve fenestrations producing chronic aortic regurgitation. *Am Heart J* 1991;122:1475–1477.

79. Roberts CS, Roberts WC. Dissection of the aorta associated with congenital malformation of the aortic valve. *J Am Coll Cardiol* 1991;17:712–716.

80. Beckman DJ, Bandy M, Evans M. Extensive radiation injury of the aortic valve, ascending aorta, left main coronary artery and right ventricle. *Cardiovasc Surg* 1994;2:117–118.

81. Kaplan S, Adolf RJ. Pulmonic valve stenosis in adults. *Cardiovasc Clin* 1979;10:327–339.

82. Waller BF, Howard J, Fess S. Pathology of pulmonic valve stenosis and pure regurgitation. *Clin Cardiol* 1995;18:45–50.

83. Gikonyo BM, Lucas RV, Edwards JE. Anatomic features of congenital pulmonary valvar stenosis. *Pediatr Cardiol* 1987;8:109–116.

84. Sherman W, Hershman R, Alexopoulos D, et al. Pulmonic balloon valvuloplasty in adults. *Am Heart J* 1990;119:186–190.

85. Marantz PM, Huhta JC, Mullins CE, et al. Results of

balloon valvuloplasty in typical and dyplastic pulmonary valve stenosis: Doppler echocardiographic follow-up. *J Am Coll Cardiol* 1988;12:476–479.

86. Altrichter PM, Olson LJ, Edwards WD, Puga FJ, Danielson GK. Surgical pathology of the pulmonary valve: a study of 116 cases spanning 15 years. *Mayo Clin Proc* 1989;64:1352–1360.

87. Braunwald E. Valvular heart disease. In: Braunwald E, ed. *Heart Disease: A Textbook of Cardiovascular Medicine*. Philadelphia: W.B. Saunders, 1997:1007–1076.

88. King JW, Nguyen VQ, Conrad SA. Results of a prospective statewide reporting system for infective endocarditis. *Am J Med Sci* 1988;295:517–527.

89. Watanakunakorn C, Burkert T. Infective endocarditis at a large community teaching hospital, 1980–1990. A review of 210 episodes. *Medicine (Baltimore)* 1993; 72:90–102.

90. McKinsey DS, Ratts TE, Bisno AL. Underlying cardiac lesions in adults with infective endocarditis. The changing spectrum. *Am J Med* 1987;82:681–688.

91. Terpenning MS, Buggy BP, Kauffman CA. Infective endocarditis: clinical features in young and elderly patients. *Am J Med* 1987;83:626–634.

92. MacMahon SW, Roberts JK, Kramer-Fox R, Zucker DM, Roberts RB, Devereux RB. Mitral valve prolapse and infective endocarditis. *Am Heart J* 1987;113: 1291–1298.

93. Danchin N, Voiriot P, Briancon S, et al. Mitral valve prolapse as a risk factor for infective endocarditis. *Lancet* 1989;1:743–745.

94. Karchmer AW. Infective endocarditis. In: Braunwald E, ed. *Heart Disease: A Textbook of Cardiovascular Medicine*. Philadelphia: W.B. Saunders, 1997: 1077–1104.

95. Baddour LM, Christensen GD, Lowrance JH, Simpson WA. Pathogenesis of experimental endocarditis. *Rev Infect Dis* 1989;11:452–463.

96. Durack DT. Current issues in prevention of infective endocarditis. *Am J Med* 1985;78:149–156.

97. Cherubin CE, Sapira JD. The medical complications of drug addiction and the medical assessment of the intravenous drug user: 25 years later. *Ann Intern Med* 1993;119:1017–1028.

98. Hogevik H, Olaison L, Andersson R, Lindberg J, Alestig K. Epidemiologic aspects of infective endocarditis in an urban population. A 5-year prospective study. *Medicine (Baltimore)* 1995;74:324–339.

99. Virmani R, Burke AP, Farb A. *Atlas of Cardiovascular Pathology.* Philadelphia: W.B. Saunders, 1996:64–68.

100. Mansur AJ, Grinberg M, da Luz PL, Bellotti G. The complications of infective endocarditis. A reappraisal in the 1980s. *Arch Intern Med* 1992;152:2428–2432.

101. Nakayama DK, O'Neill JA Jr, Wagner H, Cooper A, Dean RH. Management of vascular complications of bacterial endocarditis. *J Pediatr Surg* 1986;21: 636–639.

102. Hojnik M, George J, Ziporen L, Shoenfeld Y. Heart valve involvement (Libman-Sacks endocarditis) in the antiphospholipid syndrome. *Circulation* 1996;93: 1579–1587.

103. Moyssakis IE, Rallidis LS, Guida GF, Nihoyannopoulos PI. Incidence and evolution of carcinoid syndrome in the heart. *J Heart Valve Dis* 1997;6:625–630.

104. Robiolio PA, Rigolin VH, Wilson JS, et al. Carcinoid heart disease. Correlation of high serotonin levels with valvular abnormalities detected by cardiac catheterization and echocardiography. *Circulation* 1995;92: 790–795.

105. Himelman RB, Schiller NB. Clinical and echocardiographic comparison of patients with the carcinoid syndrome with and without carcinoid heart disease. *Am J Cardiol* 1989;63:347–352.

106. Connolly HM, Nishimura RA, Smith HC, et al. Outcome of cardiac surgery for carcinoid heart disease. *J Am Coll Cardiol* 1995;25:410–416.

107. Defraigne JO, Jerusalem O, Soyeur D, Jacquet N, Limet R. Successful tricuspid valve replacement and pulmonary valvulotomy for carcinoid heart disease. *Acta Chir Belg* 1996;96:170–176.

108. Konstantinov IE, Peterffy A. Tricuspid and pulmonary valve replacement in carcinoid heart disease: two case reports and a review of the literature. *J Heart Valve Dis* 1997;6:193–197.

109. Robiolio PA, Rigolin VH, Harrison JK, et al. Predictors of outcome of tricuspid valve replacement in carcinoid heart disease. *Am J Cardiol* 1995;75:485–488.

110. Cannistra LB, Davis SM, Bauman AG. Valvular heart disease associated with dexfenfluramine [letter]. *N Engl J Med* 1997;337:636.

111. D'Alton JG, Preston DN, Bormanis J, Green MS, Kraag GR. Multiple transient ischemic attacks, lupus anticoagulant and verrucous endocarditis. *Stroke* 1985;16:512–514.

112. Nesher G, Ilany J, Rosenmann D, Abraham AS. Valvular dysfunction in antiphospholipid syndrome: prevalence, clinical features, and treatment. *Semin Arthritis Rheum* 1997;27:27–35.

113. Nihoyannopoulos P, Gomez PM, Joshi J, Loizou S, Walport MJ, Oakley CM. Cardiac abnormalities in systemic lupus erythematosus: association with raised anticardiolipin antibodies. *Circulation* 1990;82: 369–375.

114. Leung WH, Wong KL, Lau CP, Wong CK, Liu HW. Association between antiphospholipid antibodies and cardiac abnormalities in patients with systemic lupus erythematosus. *Am J Med* 1990;89:411–419.

115. Barbut D, Borer JS, Gharavi A, et al. Prevalence of anticardiolipin antibody in isolated mitral or aortic regurgitation, or both, and possible relation to cerebral ischemic events. *Am J Cardiol* 1992;70:901–905.

116. Lehmen TJA, Palmeri ST, Hastings C, Klippel JH, Plotz PH. Bacterial endocarditis complicating systemic lupus erythematosus. *J Rheumatol* 1983;10: 655–658.

117. Libman E, Sacks B. A hitherto undescribed form of valvular and mural endocarditis. *Arch Intern Med* 1924;33:701–737.

118. Bulkley BH, Roberts WC. The heart in systemic lupus erythematosus and the changes induced in it by corticosteroid therapy: a study of 36 necropsy patients. *Am J Med* 1975;58:243–264.

119. Mandell BF. Cardiovascular involvement in systemic lupus erythematosus. *Semin Arthritis Rheum* 1987;17: 126–141.

120. Galve E, Candell-Riera J, Pigrau C, Permanyer-Miralda G, Garcia-Del-Castillo H, Soler-Soler J. Prevalence, morphologic types, and evolution of cardiac valvular disease in systemic lupus erythematosus. *N Engl J Med* 1988;319:817–823.

121. Kornberg A, Blank M, Kaufman S, Shoenfeld Y. In-

duction of tissue factor-like activity in monocytes by anti-cardiolipin antibodies. *J Immunol* 1994;153: 1328–1332.

122. Ziporen L, Goldberg I, Arad M, et al. Libman-Sacks endocarditis in the antiphospholipid syndrome: immunopathologic findings in deformed heart valves. *Lupus* 1996;5:196–205.

123. Sokoloff L. Cardiac involvement in rheumatoid arthritis and allied disorders: current concepts. *Mod Conc Cardiovasc Dis* 1964;33:847–850.

124. Nemchinov EN, Kanevskaia MZ, Chichasova NV, Telepneva LM, Krel AA. Heart defects in rheumatoid arthritis patients. The results of a multiyear prospective clinico-echocardiographic study. *Ter Arkh* 1994;66: 33–38.

125. MacDonald WJ Jr, Crawford MH, Klippel JH, Zvaifler NJ, O'Rourke RA. Echocardiographic assessment of cardiac structure and function in patients with rheumatoid arthritis. *Am J Med* 1977;63:890–896.

126. Howell A, Say J, Hedworth-Whitty R. Rupture of the sinus of Valsalva due to severe rheumatoid heart disease. *Br Heart J* 1972;34:537–540.

127. Bergfeldt L. HLA-B27-associated cardiac disease. *Ann Intern Med* 1997;127:621–629.

128. O'Neil TW, Brersnihan B. The heart in ankylosing spondylitis. *Ann Rheum Dis* 1992;51:705–706.

129. Kinsella TD, Johnson LG, Sutherland IR. Cardiovascular manifestations of ankylosing spondylitis. *Can Med Assoc J* 1974;111:1309–1311.

130. Graham DC, Smyth HA. The carditis and aortitis of ankylosing spondylitis. *Bull Rheum Dis* 1958;9: 171–174.

131. Good AE. Reiter's disease: a review with special attention to cardiovascular and neurologic sequelae. *Semin Arthritis Rheum* 1974;3:263–286.

132. Lang-Lazdunski L, Hvass U, Paillole C, Pansard Y, Langlois J. Cardiac valve replacement in relapsing polychondritis. A review. *J Heart Valve Dis* 1995;4:227–235.

133. McAllister HA Jr, Fenoglio JJ Jr. Cardiac involvement in Whipple's disease. *Circulation* 1975;52:152–156.

134. Rose AG. Mitral stenosis in Whipple's disease. *Thorax* 1978;33:500–503.

135. Relman DA, Schmidt TM, MacDermott RP, Falkow S. Identification of the uncultured bacillus of Whipple's disease. *N Engl J Med* 1992;327:293–301.

136. Ragni T, Grande AM, Cappuccio G, et al. Embolizing fibroelastoma of the aortic valve. *Cardiovasc Surg* 1994;2:639–641.

2

Rheumatic Fever

Y. Chandrashekhar and Jagat Narula

Division of Cardiology, University of Minnesota School of Medicine, Minneapolis, Minnesota 55455;
Center of Molecular Cardiology, MCP Hahnemann University School of Medicine,
Philadelphia, Pennsylvania 19102

Acute rheumatic fever (RF), a noninfectious delayed complication of streptococcal sore throat due to group A β-hemolytic streptococcus (GABHS) (1,2), is an enigmatic disease that has ravaged humankind since the industrial revolution (3). Although the disease has been largely controlled in the industrialized nations (4,5), which were devastated by it in the early and middle part of this century (6,7), it continues to surface intermittently even in the most developed countries (8,9). It still is a major problem in the developing world. Given the inexplicable nature of the rise and fall, RF constitutes a major challenge to health care providers. Interestingly, group A streptococcal infection, the only species that cause acute RF, carrier rates have remained unabated (10). RF and the threat of residual heart disease make it imperative that we recognize and manage acute episodes of disease effectively.

HISTORY

The historical evidence of RF is clouded because RF is a multisystemic disease, wherein the clinical manifestations come at varying intervals in its natural history. Therefore, the definitive diagnosis had to await the institution of a set of diagnostic criteria (11). Even so, the evolution of the thought process in this field is a fascinating story. The earliest descriptions of RF are relatively recent, except for one probable description of what might be rheumatic heart disease (RHD) in the Hippocratic era (12), and involve the pioneers of modern medicine (13). There are no descriptions of this disease in the early recorded history or from anatomic studies on cadavers or mummies. The crowded and poor working conditions fostered by the industrial revolution probably contributed to the spread of virulent streptococcal infections and RF. It is interesting to note that similar crowded conditions in army barracks during World War II were associated with ravaging epidemics of RF (6). The disease, as expected, was a puzzle to early clinicians. Each manifestation of the disease was described separately (14,15) and put together only in the 1700s (15,16). Finally, the diagnostic criteria were established in 1944 by T. Duckett Jones (11) at a time when RF devastated many nations (6,17). The strength of these criteria is attested by the fact that they have hardly changed since their inception (18).

Early RF literature is full of reports where children were cloistered in sanatoria for much of their childhood. These patients were subjected to a regular medical supervisory regimen consisting of periodic throat cultures, blood sampling, and clinical assessments, all meant to detect and prevent streptococcal infection (19). Visitation by relatives was limited to a few hours and a couple of times of a month. In some places, visitors were cultured and screened lest they infect the wards of the sanitoria (20). These measures, which today seem like penal servitude, were all that the medical profession could offer to the patients of RF. Even as late as World War II, a high proportion of adults were afflicted with RHD, and this was the single most common cause of draft rejection in the United States armed forces (21). All this changed dramatically when sulfonamides were shown to prevent streptococcal infections (22,23) and prevent first attacks of RF (24), and this initiated the concept of long-term prophylaxis (25). The mid-1940s also saw the introduction of penicillin to prevent RF (26). A large number of studies followed with the largest contributions coming from the Irvington House Sanatoria in New York (27–34). The American Heart Association (AHA) recognized the importance of preventing RF and regularly contributed authoritative position statements on secondary prophylaxis (35). The World Health Organization (WHO) has contributed at a global level by providing knowledge, finances, and guidelines for secondary prophylaxis in many developing nations and has stressed the role of secondary prevention.

EPIDEMIOLOGY OF RHEUMATIC FEVER AND HEART DISEASE

Magnitude of Problem and Projections

RF is a major cardiovascular health problem in many nations of the world (1,36). Although traditionally considered to be a disease associated with poverty and overcrowding, RF continues to persist, even among the middle class populace, who have excellent access to medical care in the first world nations (8,9). After an unexplained fall in the incidence of RF in the United States and Europe (4,5), the disease has shown outbreaks in some of these countries in an equally unexplained way (9,37). Developing nations never had the privilege of seeing a reduction in RF (36–38). More tragically, RF commonly affects the young (39–40) and adversely affects national productivity.

The incidence and prevalence of RF worldwide are enormous (41,41a). The prevalence of RF and RHD is highly variable, with the highest rates in the middle eastern and sub-Saharan African regions (41). The total burden of RF is enormous. For instance, it is estimated that 3.2 million patients had RHD in India in 1991, and at least two thirds of these were young children (42). Data on the secular trends in RF in developing countries are inadequate (43). It appears, however, that the number of patients with RF and RHD in these countries is not decreasing (1,36,41). In contrast, the annual incidence of RF in developed nations is less than 5 per million and prevalence of RHD is less than 50 per million (44). These rates represent a sharp decline from the levels seen 30 to 40 years ago, when the numbers were similar to that now seen in underdeveloped countries. The causes for this reduction are unclear and may be related to better socioeconomic status and reduced crowding (44) because the decline antedated the discovery of penicillin (45). In addition, a change in the virulence of streptococci (10) and better medical care have contributed significantly. The recent resurgence of RF in 24 states (46) in the United States, predominantly affecting white middle class families, underscores the fact that we know very little about the cyclic rise and fall of RF.

Agent, Host, and Environmental Factors

Only GABHS throat infections (47,48) strong enough to induce an immunologic response (49,50) are capable of triggering an episode of RF. GABHS are found in a fair number of asymptomatic subjects (1) and form a ready reservoir for transmission to susceptible individuals. The number of streptococcal infections and sore throats worldwide has not changed appreciably since the early part of this century (10), even during the decline of RF in the developed world. Whereas 0.3% of patients develop RF after a streptococcal throat, 3% develop it during epidemics of streptococcal pharyngitis and an even larger number develop it if they have had a previous episode of RF (Fig. 2-1) (1,35).

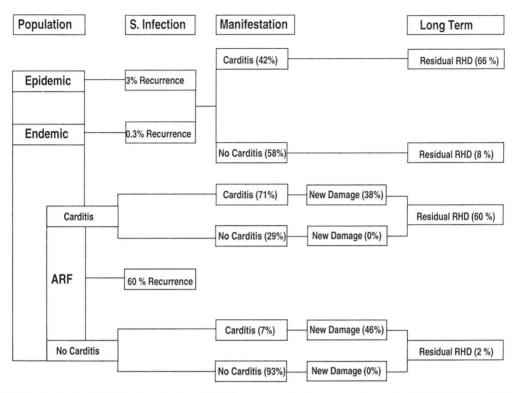

FIG. 2–1. Natural history of acute rheumatic fever compiled from a number of published studies (42). Presence of an epidemic and previous carditis are important determinants of prognosis in acute rheumatic fever.

There is evidence that the strain of the bacteria and its virulence (rheumatogenicity) also influences the attack rate for RF (10,51). Symptomatic throat infections are most often associated with RF, but more than one third of the infections that trigger RF are asymptomatic (47). Recent epidemics in the United States show an even higher incidence of asymptomatic streptococcal infection in first attacks of RF (8). Not all infections, even those associated with an immune response, result in a recurrence, suggesting that important host factors might exist. Thus, homozygotic twins have higher concordance for RF than heterozygotes (52), a higher risk is seen in some ethnic races (53–55), and genetic markers may identify individuals at higher risk for developing RF (56–58). Finally, environmental factors like crowding, poverty, health education, and access to medical care continue to influence the development of RF.

Social and Economic Burden

RHD is one of the most common causes of cardiovascular mortality and morbidity in the world (1,36,38,40). It accounts for 35% to 40% of cardiovascular admissions to hospitals in developing countries, with the major proportion of their patients undergoing cardiac surgery (1,59). RF is more aggressive in the young, especially in the developing world (36,39,60), and is the most common cause of mortality of young in these nations (36). RF and RHD therefore impose a significant burden on the total health budget in these countries, which can ill afford it in face of numerous other health problems. As an example, in India, which apart from being a developing nation has good epidemiologic data on RF, the prevalence of RF/RHD among school children is 2 to 11 per 1,000, with a mean of 6 per 1,000 (61). The adult rates are uncertain, with published figures between 123 and 200 per 100,000 population (40). With a population of over 850 million, which increases annually at the rate of over 1.9% a year, the monetary costs of this disease are phenomenal in a poor country where a number of other health-related conditions compete for the meager health budget. India allocates a mere 2% of their gross national product, compared with 5% to 10% in the developed world. There are far fewer tertiary-level centers to treat this extraordinary RHD burden, and a number of patients die awaiting surgical intervention. The costs of supportive medical therapy, loss of productive years, and human misery are incalculable. This is a familiar story in most developing countries (62). Disturbing data are available even from richer nations like South Africa and New Zealand (63–65). The cost of treating RF/RHD in 1 year was over 5 to 9 million dollars in New Zealand (64). Of the 3.6 million dollars spent in Auckland alone, chronic RHD accounted for 71% of the expense, whereas preventive efforts received 13% of the allocation (65). Similarly, between 1982 and 1987, South Africa spent 206 million SA Rands on valve surgery alone in patients with RF (66).

PATHOGENESIS

The exact mechanism by which GABHS initiates RF is unclear. Similarly, it is unknown as to why only throat infections and not skin or other streptococcal infections convert to RF (48). One reason why RF proves to be such an enigma is the lack of an animal model (67). A number of theories have been proposed at various times (68). RF was earlier believed to be the result of direct injury mediated by streptococci (69) or its toxins (70). The more plausible explanation suggests that RF is an immune- (cellular and antibody) mediated injury (71–74). The current understanding proposes that rheumatogenic streptococci contain multiple antigenic determinants (75–81) that mimic (in part) normal human tissue antigens (67,73,82,83); these antigens are recognized as foreign by the susceptible host (57,58,84,85) and result in a hyperactive immune response (both humoral and cellular) (67,71,84). In addition, there is a breakdown of immunologic tolerance, which allows autoreactive immune-mediated injury (67,82, 83).

A number of streptococcal antigens have been implicated in triggering aberrant immune response in RF. Group A polysaccharide has an N-acetyl glucosamine moiety that cross-reacts with antibodies to the heart valve tissue (75), and patients with significant valvular heart disease have an excess of such cross-reactive antibodies (74,79). Antibodies to the streptococcal peptidoglycan complexes have been implicated in rheumatic arthritis (81). The streptococcal M protein (78,86) has homology with the cardiac contractile proteins, including myosin and tropomyosin, and structural proteins like keratin, laminin, and vimentin, which are common in the cardiac interstitium (87). These M protein epitopes trigger heart cross-reactive antibodies (86,88). They can also act as a superantigen and lead to a more widespread immune response (89). In addition, myosin cross-reactivity has also been demonstrated for a streptococcal membrane component (80,90). A number of problems exist with a humoral theory of genesis in RF. Myocyte necrosis is not a prominent feature of rheumatic carditis (91). It is unclear how the heart reactive antibodies, which react with antigens normally sequestered intracellularly by intact membranes, mediate cardiac damage. Cross-reactive antibodies are also seen in patients without evidence of RF and persist for long periods of time (92). Cellular immunity instead may contribute significantly to the pathogenesis of RF. There is a significant T-cell infiltration in the valvular tissue and synovium (91). Membrane antigens from group A streptococci can stimulate T cells cytotoxic for cardiac but not skeletal muscle cells (93,94). More recently, it has been shown that T cells isolated from valve tissue of patients with RHD respond to streptococcal M5 protein sequence stretches and are cross-reactive with cardiac myosin (86,95).

Immune responses, both humoral (79,84) and cellular (96,97), are more vigorous in patients with RF compared with the normal population. Two streptococcal antigens, the pepsin generated fraction of M protein (89) and a streptococcal pyrogenic exotoxin (98), are believed to behave as superantigens. These antigens do not bind to antigen binding clefts in T or B cells and can amplify an immune response (99) by clonal expansion of T and B cells, release of cytokines (100), and adhesion molecules (101), which could help localize immune responses to certain tissues. Finally, superantigenic stimulation may help T cells respond to antigens like M proteins, which they might not in absence of such stimulation (102).

Because only a small proportion of patients infected with streptococci develop RF (1,6,10,19,32,34,103), it is conceivable that host factors are important in determining susceptibility to RF (84). Identifying individuals with a high likelihood of developing RF might be useful in targeting prophylactic efforts. A previous attack of RF identifies a subgroup with increased susceptibility to a recurrence (6,103). Similarly, an increased risk in families with a history of RF (104) and the higher concordance rate in homozygous twins compared with heterozygous twins suggests a role for familial susceptibility in addition to the environmental factors (52). Certain races, like the Samoans in Hawaii (53) and the aboriginal Maori races in New Zealand (54), have increased susceptibility to RF. There is an association, albeit sometimes confusing, between RF and RHD and human leukocyte antigen (HLA) subgroups; RF risk has been associated with increased prevalence of HLA-DR4 in the United States (84,105) and Saudi Arabia (85) and with increased prevalence of DR3 and DQw2 in India (56,106). However, DR2 has an increased prevalence in the African American population in the United States, whereas it seems to be protective in Indians (56). Some other markers, such as a B-cell alloantigen D8/17, have showed a strong association with susceptibility to RF (57,58), sug-gesting it may be possible to identify susceptible groups prospectively in the future.

PATHOLOGIC CHARACTERISTICS OF CARDIAC INVOLVEMENT

RF is considered a multisystem connective tissue disease and is characterized by inflammatory, either exudative or fibrotic, lesions in a number of systems, including the heart, joints, and the subcutaneous tissue (107). The Aschoff granuloma is the pathologic hallmark of RF (108). It consists of a central area of fibrinoid necrosis surrounded by cells of histiocytic-macrophagic origin (Anitschkow cells) that show a typical "owl eye-shaped" nucleus. These cells are usually found in the subendocardial or perivascular regions (109), in the myocardium, and sometimes in the pericardium. A number of features at gross and microscopic examination of surgically excised tissue have been defined to correlate with rheumatic activity (110–112). These include fibrinous pericarditis with epicardial involvement; pinhead vegetations on valve leaflets with edema or hemorrhage in the leaflet tissue; and microscopic findings, including fibrinoid necrosis in the valve leaflet, cellular infiltrates, and neovascularization of valves.

There is surprisingly little histopathologic damage to the myocardium, even in patients with florid clinical carditis and heart failure (91,113,114). Myocyte necrosis is uncommon, and the cellular infiltrate is confined to the interstitium. The conduction system also shows little pathology even in the presence of clinical conduction defects (115). The valves show the brunt of pathologic damage. Macroscopically, valves are dull and thickened, unlike the smooth pliable normal appearance, and show small verrucous vegetations on the atrial surface of the mitral valve, the chords, and the ventricular surface of the aortic valve. These are composed of fibrin and are the equivalent of the changes seen on echocardiography (116). The valves are significantly inflamed and edematous and demonstrate extensive pallisading mononuclear infiltration. Aschoff bodies are occasionally seen. There is granulation tissue and fibrous scarring in the late stages of the disease. The valves involved in order of frequency are the mitral, aortic, tricuspid, and pulmonary (2,107,108). The endocardium of the left ventricle often shows inflammation and contains Aschoff bodies. A scar in the left atrium, the McCallum's patch, probably reflects a regurgitant jet lesion (107) rather than rheumatic inflammation. Older literature described a vasculitis with areas of fibrinoid necrosis in the aorta and in muscular myocardial vessels (117). The pathologic features observed in endomyocardial biopsies in RF patients are not of significant diagnostic value (91). Aschoff bodies are seen in 30% to 40% of patients with proven or suspected carditis and have not been noted in patients without carditis.

CLINICAL FEATURES

Joint Symptoms

Arthritis is a major manifestation of RF and frequently is the symptom that brings the patient to clinical attention (118,119). Arthritis occurs in more than two thirds of patients (119–121) and may be the sole manifestation in older patients with RF. Large joints of the extremity are usually involved, although smaller joints including those in the hand and feet may occasionally be inflamed (2,120, 121). Hips and the spine or axial joints are rarely affected. The joints are hot, tender, and often show symptoms disproportionate to the physical findings (2). The joints are inflamed at various intervals, each cycle lasts several days, and this gives a migratory character to joint pains. Monoarticular arthritis is uncommon (122). Joint aspirates usually show more than 10,000 leukocytes/mm^3. Arthritis resolves in most patients within 3 to 4 weeks and does not result in any permanent damage. A condition called Jaccoud's arthritis, which involves small joints and causes deformities, was thought to be due to RF, but this has never been proved (123).

Arthralgia is joint pain without objective signs of inflammation and is common in rheumatic recurrences (2,124) and in patients with RHD in developing countries (125–127). Arthralgia, being so nonspecific, is not accepted as a major criteria for the diagnosis of RF (1,18), but clinicians in the developing world have suggested that they see arthralgia more often than arthritis. Therefore, it may be acceptable to consider diagnosis of RF in a patient with known RHD on the basis of migratory polyarthalgia. However, it is important to note that even in the developing world, first attacks of RF are more often associated with arthritis rather than arthralgias (128).

Some forms of polyarthritis after pharyngitis may be a poststreptococcal reactive phenomenon. Poststreptococcal arthropathy is an unclear entity that develops shortly after streptococcal infection. Adults are often affected, and the condition is characterized by recurrent, severe, prolonged polyarthritis that is not very responsive to nonsteroidal anti-inflammatory drugs. It is not clearly associated with other manifestations of RF, but some patients end up with residual heart disease (129,130). It has been suggested that these patients are given prophylaxis similar to patients with RF. However, there are little data to provide any definite recommendations concerning prophylaxis.

Cardiac Involvement

Although RF is a systemic disease with multiorgan involvement, none of its manifestations, except for carditis, leave behind significant residua. Therefore, carditis is predominantly responsible for the morbidity and mortality associated with acute RF (40), and preventing acute rheumatic carditis reduces cardiac sequelae (45). Studies on the frequency of cardiac involvement in RF (131) have severe limitations. Most are hospital-based data and do not differentiate recurrences from first attacks of RF (131); this artificially inflates the prevalence of carditis. It is therefore not surprising that cardiac involvement has been reported to occur from nearly one third to almost 99% of cases in various series and in 33% to 46% of cases in prospective series (8,119,120,128). Clinical carditis was seen in 72% of patients in the recent resurgence of RF in the United States (8), reminiscent of that seen in the early part of this century (132), possibly due to more virulent strains of streptococci (such as M types 5 and 18). Echocardiography further clouds the data on the incidence of carditis in acute RF. Echocardiography is inherently more sensitive in detecting subclinical valvular regurgitation and would increase the incidence of carditis in acute RF. In the Utah series, clinical carditis was seen in 72% of patients, whereas echocardiography-detected carditis was seen in 91% (8). It is important to note that most of this increase was in the detection of mild mitral regurgitation (MR), which usually heals (133), and by itself is unlikely to influence prognosis significantly if recurrences are effectively prevented.

Acute rheumatic carditis can present in a number of ways, including subclinical cardiac involvement; indolent, subacute, acute, or even fulminant congestive heart failure; mitral or aortic regurgitation of varying severity, pericarditis, and conduction disturbances. Younger patients often present with insidious onset carditis, whereas joint involvement is common in older patients (2). The advent of penicillin and a change in rheumatogenecity of the streptococcus have made carditis milder than before. Carditic episodes, which are somewhat uncommon in the older adult, often present with unexplained worsening of congestive heart failure. There is a curious association in the way RF often presents. Patients who have significant arthritis less commonly have severe carditis (118,119). The joint discomfort often forces patients to seek medical attention sooner and more often than patients with carditis, which is often asymptomatic or mildly symptomatic initially. This is unfortunate because the former in general have good prognosis, whereas the latter, with ominous consequences, may be missed.

Clinical Recognition of Carditis

Rheumatic carditis is an early manifestation; almost 80% of patients who develop carditis do so within the first 2 weeks of the onset of RF (118,134). Rheumatic carditis is a pancarditis (135) involving the pericardium, the myocardium, and the endocardium. Although both pericardial and myocardial involvement can contribute to the clinical picture of an acute attack of RF, it is important to emphasize that valvular involvement is responsible for the unfavorable prognosis. Second, rheumatic carditis cannot be easily diagnosed without valvular involvement. One general schema for the diagnosis of acute rheumatic carditis is shown in Table 2-1.

TABLE 2-1. *Simplified schema for the diagnosis of acute rheumatic carditis[a]*

Criteria	First attacks	Recurrences
Valvulitis	New onset	Change in murmur
	Apical systolic murmur	New onset murmur
	Carey coombs murmur	
	Aortic regurgitation murmur	
	Evanescent murmurs	Evanescent murmurs
Myocarditis	Unexplained cardiomegaly	Worsening cardiomegaly
	Unexplained CHF/gallop sounds	Worsening CHF
Pericarditis	Pericardial rubs	Pericardial rubs
	Unexplained pericardial effusion	Pericardial effusion
Miscellaneous methods	Conduction disturbances or unexplained tachycardia[b]	
	Echocardiographic imaging[c]	
	Nuclear imaging	
	Morphologic evidence at surgery	
	Histologic evidence at biopsy or pathology	

[a]Needs supportive evidence for the presence of acute rheumatic fever using Jones criteria. In patients with known rheumatic heart disease, acute rheumatic fever can be diagnosed with minor criteria *along with* evidence for antecedent streptococcal infection.
[b]These would be considered soft criteria.
[c]Significance of these methods is controversial.
CHF, Congestive heart failure.
From ref. 91, with permission.

Endocarditis

Pathologic studies reveal that endocardial inflammation most commonly afflicts the mitral and aortic valves, and for practical purposes the clinical diagnosis of rheumatic endocarditis depends on the presence of mitral and/or aortic valve regurgitation murmurs. It is also clear that we may miss lesser degrees of endocardial inflammation because the diagnosis has been traditionally based on the auscultatory documentation of regurgitant murmurs. Mitral valve disease is seen in 70% to 75% of the patients, whereas mitral plus aortic valve disease occurs in an additional 20% to 25%; isolated aortic valve disease is uncommon and is found in 5% to 8% of patients. Pathologic studies report tricuspid valve involvement in 30% to 50% of patients, but clinical tricuspid valve involvement is rare in the first attack of RF (135). The pulmonary valve involvement is almost never recognized clinically and is equally rare pathologically.

The most common evidence of carditis is a blowing pansystolic MR murmur. It is usually grades II to IV, radiates to the axilla, and sometimes is associated with an apical, low-pitched, short, mid-diastolic rumble without a presystolic accentuation (Carey Coombs murmur). MR is commonly of mild-to-moderate severity in acute RF but may be severe occasionally. The severity of MR is of prognostic significance; mild MR often resolves without residua if recurrent attacks are effectively prevented and greater severity of mitral valvular involvement portends occurrence of chronic valvular heart disease (Fig. 2-2). Aortic valve regurgitation in acute rheumatic carditis is usually mild to moderate. Valvular stenosis does not occur in acute rheumatic carditis; valve stenosis is evidence for chronic RHD, often in patients with multiple previous attacks of rheumatic carditis.

Echocardiography has clarified the mechanism of valve regurgitation in RF (116). MR is due to a combination of active inflamma-

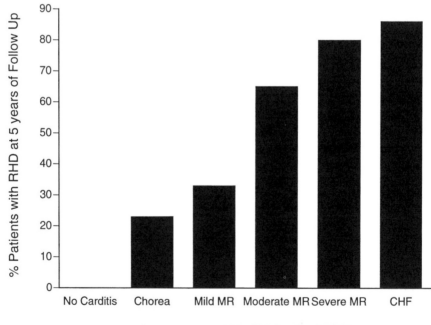

FIG. 2-2. Initial presentation of RF and likelihood of development of RHD on follow-up.

tory valvulitis, valve prolapse, annular dysfunction or dilatation, and ventricular enlargement. Patients with mild-to-moderate MR show left ventricular dilatation with mild or no annular dilatation and less commonly mitral valve prolapse (116). In patients with more severe degrees of MR, especially in those coming to surgery during carditis, marked annular dilatation, chordal elongation, and anterior mitral leaflet prolapse are commonly seen (110,136). The Aschoff nodules have a predilection for valve rings (137), and this may account for annular dysfunction and dilatation. Rarely, the stretched chordae may rupture, resulting in flail leaflets and severe acute regurgitation (138). Most patients with acute RF and carditis have mild-to-moderate MR that frequently disappears on follow-up (118,119,133,134). It is therefore likely that a functional mechanism rather than structural alterations in the valve or annulus may be operative in the pathogenesis of the more milder forms of MR. Valvulitis and rheumatic involvement of the aortic ring causes aortic regurgitation, sometimes with aortic valve prolapse.

Myocarditis

Myocarditis is often indicated by the presence of a soft first sound, gallop sounds, cardiomegaly, and/or congestive cardiac failure. New onset cardiomegaly or a recent change in cardiac size (especially if it improves once the carditis resolves) is suggestive of myocarditis, more so in the absence of a significant pericardial effusion. Congestive heart failure in patients with rheumatic carditis has been traditionally believed to be due to severe myocardial inflammation (113,139). A number of observations available today indicate that myocyte damage is not the primary cause of congestive failure in RF. There is so little myocardial damage in patients dying from acute RF that it is difficult to explain why the patient died (140). Myocardial biopsies in patients with active rheumatic carditis do not show significant evidence of myocyte damage (91). The left ventricular systolic function and myocardial contractility are normal in patients with rheumatic carditis and congestive failure (116,139). Although the assessment of pure myocardial contractility is difficult in the presence of MR, the observation that congestive failure does not occur in the absence of hemodynamically significant valvular lesions and the rapid clinical improvement after mitral valve replacement during active carditis are strong evidence against myocarditis per se as the cause of congestive failure (139,140). It is now generally believed that congestive heart failure in patients with acute rheumatic carditis is caused by severe MR.

Pericarditis

Clinical rheumatic pericarditis occurs in 6% to 15% of patients during the acute stage of RF, and the presence of a pericardial friction rub in this setting is evidence for rheumatic carditis. The rub can be evanescent and may be confused with a murmur. Rheumatic pericarditis is always associated with findings of valvular involvement, although a pericardial rub can, at times, mask the presence of underlying valvular murmurs. If there are no valvulitis-related murmurs after the friction rub has resolved, one can safely conclude that the pericarditis was non-rheumatic (2). Rheumatic pericarditis is often associated with a serosanguinous or hemorrhagic effusion that usually resolves without residua; rare reports have described the occurrence of pericardial tamponade (141) or pericardial constriction (142). It has been suggested that the presence of pericarditis indicates severe carditis (2).

Inapparent (Silent) Carditis

Several observations suggest that at times active rheumatic carditis may be clinically silent or not suspected. Patients with chorea and no clinical evidence for carditis develop mitral stenosis on follow-up, suggesting multiple subclinical attacks of carditis (143). Furthermore, histopathologic evidence for active carditis has been reported in the absence of clinical evidence for carditis (111,112,114). Endomyocardial biopsies in patients with RHD and unexplained congestive failure with raised antistreptolysin O (ASO) titers have shown histologic evidence of active rheumatic carditis in 40% of patients (91), supporting the contention that active rheumatic carditis is present in the absence of other features. Marcus et al. (112) showed that a number of patients without clinical or even gross morphologic evidence had carditis at histology. These data reinforce that our clinical ability to diagnose carditis is limited at best. More recently, echocardiography (MR or visualization of valvular nodules [116]) has been proposed for identifying subclinical carditis in patients with acute RF who do not have audible murmurs (8,144–148) and is discussed below in the section on diagnosis.

Neurologic Manifestation

Chorea (the term originally used by Paracelsus to describe the fanatic frenzied movements of a group of patients, labeled religious fanatics in a trance), a series of involuntary movements commonly involving the face and extremities with emotional lability, is an uncommon and mysterious major manifestation of acute RF. It also bears the colorful name of St. Vitus' dance in honor of the treatment of chorea in those days—a pilgrimage to the shrine of St. Vitus (the success of these treatments may have depended on the self-limiting nature of the chorea irrespective of the interventions, a fact still not changed today). As known to Osler, it commonly affects children between the ages 7 and 14 years, is rarely seen in adults, is more common in females, and is often associated with carditis and subcutaneous nodules (2).

Chorea is usually a late manifestation and appears several weeks after an acute attack of RF, at a time when other manifestations have disappeared, and patients often do not fulfill the Jones' criteria (143). The onset is usually gradual. The patient appears increasingly nervous, is dysarthric, makes grimacing gestures, has difficulty in writing, and shows characteristic purposeless movements of the arms and legs. These involuntary movements are increased by effort or excitement, are absent during sleep, and may be associated with muscular weakness. The pathogenesis of chorea remains unclear (149). Sydenham's chorea is usually a self-limited condition and recovers without residua. Mild cases may subside within a few weeks, although relapses are not uncommon. There is a high incidence of chronic RHD in patients with chorea, and these patients are therefore considered a high-risk group for secondary prophylaxis strategies (42).

Skin Manifestations

Subcutaneous nodules, a late manifestation of RF, occur in 1% to 21% of patients (150), and the presence of subcutaneous nodules usually suggests underlying carditis. The nodules are firm and painless, 0.5 to 3.0 cm, and are usually on bony prominence or vertebral spinous processes and on extensor tendons. They usually appear in crops and disappear within 8 to 12 weeks in most patients.

Similar to subcutaneous nodules, erythema marginatum is usually indicative of underlying carditis. Erythema marginatum, unlike subcutaneous nodules, however, can be an early or a late manifestation and can be present in the absence of features to indicate active RF (2). It occurs in less than 10% to 15% of patients, is present on the trunk and proximal extremities as a serpigenous macular nonpruritic rash, and is often very evanescent.

Other Features

A number of other signs and symptoms seen in patients with acute RF and in view of their nonspecific nature are called minor manifestations for diagnostic purposes. These include fever, prolonged PR interval, and elevated acute-phase reactants (Table 2-2).

TABLE 2-2. *The Jones' criteria for diagnosis of acute rheumatic fever*

Major criteria	Minor criteria
Carditis	Previous rheumatic fever or rheumatic heart disease
Polyarthritis	Arthralgia
Chorea	Fever
Subcutaneous nodules	ESR
Erythema marginatum	Positive C-reactive protein
	Leukocytosis
	Prolonged PR interval

Needs two major criteria or one major plus two minor criteria for diagnosis. Needs supportive evidence for recent streptococcal infection for all diagnosis. Chorea, indolent carditis, and poststreptococcal arthritis may not fulfill the Jones' criteria at the time of diagnosis.

DIAGNOSIS AND LABORATORY INVESTIGATIONS

The Jones' criteria are universally used for the diagnosis of RF (Table 2-2). The Jones' criteria have been classified in major and minor manifestations of the disease. At least two major or one major and two minor criteria in the presence of evidence for a recent streptococcal throat infection are needed for the diagnosis of RF. The division into major and minor criteria imply the diagnostic import of each parameter rather than any pathophysiologic significance. The Jones' criteria were introduced in 1944 (11) and have been periodically revised. These criteria have the endorsement of both the AHA and WHO (1,35) and serve to reduce misdiagnosis of RF. Several manifestations of Jones' criteria need to be discussed. Joint manifestations have been divided in (objective) arthritis and (subjective) arthralgia and are respectively considered as major and minor manifestations. There have been concerns that arthralgias are more common than frank arthritis in developing countries. It has been argued therefore that arthralgia should be used as a major criterion. This is not well accepted because arthralgias are nonspecific and could reduce the specificity of the Jones' criteria. Other data suggest that arthritis is more common during first attacks (124,128), unlike the situation in recurrent attacks, even in developing countries. Because the recent Jones' criteria update is applicable only for diagnosing first attacks, the AHA or WHO have kept arthralgia a minor criteria. It is accepted, however, that arthralgias may be important for the diagnosis of RF in patients with recurrent attacks, especially in those with RHD (1).

The second contested issue is the prerequisite of documenting a recent streptococcal infection for the diagnosis of RF. It has been argued that lack of appropriate facilities in developing countries makes it difficult to meet this parameter. The need for evidence of streptococcal infection makes the criteria highly specific. In several studies (1,3,5, 112), the sensitivity and specificity of Jones' criteria were 77% and 97%, respectively, when compared with histologic proof of rheumatic activity. One last group where the diagnosis of RF can be made without completely fulfilling the Jones' criteria is patients with what is termed "indolent carditis" (1). It needs to be emphasized that some patients in developing countries, especially young children, present with vague symptoms with features insufficient to suggest RF. Physical examination identifies RHD often with congestive heart failure (91). Acute-phase reactants are elevated consistent with an active inflammatory state, whereas ASO titer may elevated. These patients pose a difficult problem and are often considered to have acute RF; a WHO study group (1) considered this a valid diagnostic group and has exempted them the stringent requirements of the Jones' criteria.

Evidence for Streptococcal Throat Infection

Although one can use clinical, microbiologic, or even streptococcal antigen tests as evidence of streptococcal throat infection, none of these differentiate a carrier state from active infection. Moreover, because RF is a postinfectious complication, occurring some time after the infective episode, microbiologic evidence is usually very limited. Thus, the evidence for recent streptococcal infection as needed by the Jones' criteria is usually obtained using the antistreptococcal antibody tests (1,35). Although these tests have little value in the diagnosis or treatment of acute streptococcal pharyngitis, elevated or rising antistreptococcal antibody titers provide reliable confirmation of a recent GABHS infection of sufficient severity to elicit an immune response. Because only the latter are associated with RF (47–50), measuring the immune response to GABHS is a very useful test to establish recent streptococcal infection. The most commonly used antibody assays are ASO and antideoxyribonuclease B (anti-DNase B), although other tests, including antibodies to hyaluronidase, streptokinase, and nicotinamide adenine dinulceotidase, are also available (151).

The antibody response to these streptococcal antigens is seen in the first month and remains detectable at a plateau level up to 3 to 6 months after the infection (152). The antibodies become undetectable in the next 6 to 12 months. ASO test results are determined by an agglutination test (153) or a hemolytic inhibition test. Healthy people have some detectable ASO titer from previous minor streptococcal infections. In adults and in preschool children, the ASO titers are usually less than 85 Todd units/mL, whereas school-aged children can have ASO titers up to 170 Todd units/mL. Local normal levels need to be determined for each laboratory; if these are not available, an ASO greater than 240 units in adults or greater than 330 units in children is used for diagnosis (151). The best diagnostic specificity is obtained by demonstrating an interval increase in ASO in two paired serial samples (154), but this may delay the diagnosis. Increased ASO titers are seen in within 7 to 10 days, and because levels persist for some time, they are usually elevated (in 80%) during acute RF. An anti-DNase B test can be done if ASO is nondiagnostic because ASO titers rise and fall more rapidly than anti-DNase B, which remain elevated for several months after even uncomplicated streptococcal infections. Taking antibiotics or corticosteroids may influence the levels; liver disease or bacterial contamination of samples can falsely elevate ASO (155) but not anti-DNase B, which is falsely elevated in hemorrhagic pancreatitis (151). A rapid slide agglutination test that looks at antibodies against several (five) streptococcal antigens, the Streptozyme test, was thought to improve the detection of streptococcal infection (1,35). However, this test needs to be studied further before full acceptance.

Role for Echocardiography

Use of echocardiography for the diagnosis of rheumatic carditis remains a very controversial issue at present (42), and the inclusion of echocardiographic evidence of valvulitis has been repeatedly proposed for inclusion in Jones' criteria as a major manifestation. As mentioned above, the Jones' criteria were established to reduce inaccurate diagnosis of RF and were codified before the advent of modern diagnostic techniques. Clinically detectable valvular regurgitation (usually mitral and occasionally aortic) is the hallmark of acute carditis, and the clinical theory dictated that carditis could not be reliably diagnosed in absence of clinical signs of valve regurgitation. Moreover, the degree of MR or aortic regurgitation has been shown to be a very important prognostic factor (42,118,119). Previous studies done in an era where cardiac auscultation was a much practiced art showed that not all mitral or aortic murmurs were efficiently detected by clinical examination (42,103,118,119), and thus the incidence of carditis was different in various studies (131) and led to diametrically opposite conclusions on the risk of RHD after RF. Recent surveys have shown that clinical auscultation is a dying art, especially in countries with declining RF (156,157), and less than one third of the medicine programs in the United States teach auscultation in a structured way. The accuracy of medicine residents in detecting significant MR (the most important sign for acute carditis) is less than 40% to 50% (156,157). Skill levels do not change significantly with increasing periods of clinical training (156) and do not exceed those of a third-year medical student (157). Even cardiology fellows have a median diagnostic accuracy of only 22% (157). Skill levels have decreased since the 1960s (158). Physicians in training are aware of their deficiencies; internal medicine and cardiology fellows rated their clinical auscultation skills at a mean score of 2.5 out of a possible 5 (157). This might lead to a significant underdetection of carditis in RF.

Echocardiography consistently demonstrates valve regurgitation not detectable with clinical examination (8,144,145,148,159,160), allows the visualization of valve structure, and rules out other causes of valve dysfunction. It is therefore reasonable to suggest that echocardiography (which is like using an excellent clinician) should be incorporated into the diagnostic criteria for RF (148).

Does Echocardiography Perform Superiorly in the Diagnosis of Rheumatic Carditis?

In the Utah epidemic (8), echocardiography detected carditis in many patients who did not show cardiac involvement clinically; of the 74 patients with RF, Doppler detected carditis in 19% of subjects when there was no clinical evidence of cardiac involvement. In another report from the same group (160), asymptomatic cardiac involvement was detected in 47% of RF patients presenting with polyarthritis. Folger and colleagues (144,159) also found significant valvular involvement (with color flow Doppler) in patients with acute RF, polyarthritis, and no evidence of clinical carditis. In a study from New Zealand,

Abernathy et al. (145) found Doppler evidence of valvular involvement in 100% of patients with rheumatic carditis compared with a 79% clinical valvular involvement. They also found valve involvement in 13% of patients with RF and no clinical evidence of carditis, 30% of patients with possible RF, and none in febrile control subjects. However, all extra patients with carditis detected by echo-Doppler were also detected clinically in the next 2 weeks. Thus, in this study, echocardiography allowed earlier diagnosis but was not ultimately superior. Echocardiography also shows a high incidence of subclinical carditis in patients with chorea. In the Salt Lake study (8), chorea was the presenting feature in 31% of patients; among the 11 patients with chorea and no clinical carditis, Doppler revealed MR in 9 (82%). Patients with chorea frequently develop residual heart disease later in life, suggesting that a high proportion of subjects had carditis in the initial attack, even if not clinically detected; in one study, 22% of patients with pure chorea developed residual heart disease on long-term follow-up (118,119). Echocardiography may predict that subgroup destined to develop RHD in later life. A carefully done, large study from India, however, did not find evidence of Doppler regurgitation in patients without clinical carditis (116). It is important to note that 28% had trivial MR, and this needs to be carefully excluded from being considered as carditis (116).

How Specific Is Echocardiography?

Trivial to mild valvular regurgitation is quite common in the normal population (146), to the extent of 38% to 45% for MR and 15% to 77% for tricuspid regurgitation (TR) (161). Use of color Doppler can further overestimate the prevalence of physiologic regurgitation. Such transient valvular abnormalities may be even more common in populations with suspected RF who are febrile and have a hyperdynamic state. Physiologic regurgitation needs to be differentiated from organic rheumatic valvular dysfunction to avoid overdiagnosis of carditis in RF. A number of studies have well described the characteristics of benign murmurs (162,163). A holosystolic jet of MR, visible in two echocardiography planes and extending well beyond the valve leaflets, is usually accepted as evidence of carditis even in the absence of audible murmurs (144,145,148). In the absence of a gold standard for the diagnosis of carditis, diagnostic accuracy of these echocardiography findings cannot be easily evaluated. In the study from New Zealand, although control subjects had normal echocardiograms, Doppler abnormalities were also seen in two of three patients who did not end up with confirmed RF (145). Moreover, one patient in the carditis group had pulmonary regurgitation, an uncommon lesion in RF. One approach may be to see the way echocardiographic findings behave on serial follow-up (144). Persistent abnormalities, involvement of multiple valves, and disease progression may help the specificity of abnormal echocardiographic findings but involves a delay in diagnosis. More recently, echocardiography has been used to visualize nodular structures on inflamed valves (116); these appear to be the echocardiographic counterpart of nodular excrescences seen at pathology and have been proposed as a marker to identify carditis in patients with acute RF without audible murmurs. Transesophageal echocardiography is likely to show these nodules more clearly. The utility of diagnosis of valve nodules needs to be validated prospectively.

What Clinical Subgroups Are Best Detected by Echocardiography?

It is important to note that echocardiography is more sensitive than clinical examination in detecting only patients with very mild MR (116). Many milder forms of carditis resolve with good prophylaxis (42,103,118,119, 133,134,164–180), and it is not certain if this additional detection of "mild nonclinical carditis" is of prognostic significance. It should be remembered that the added ability of echocardiography would be inversely pro-

portional to the degree of clinical skills. In the Irvington house studies, a number of patients with established heart disease were found to have been misdiagnosed as having no cardiac involvement in previous episodes (103,118, 119). A concerted effort by experienced clinicians led to better recognition of carditis in the initial attack and thus better prediction of who would develop residual heart disease. A recent study has found that even experienced clinicians can occassionally miss moderate lesions and miss some abnormalities in patients with multivalvular involvement (145). Echocardiography may also be useful in detecting clinically silent carditis in some high-risk groups, like chorea or poststreptococcal reactive arthritis. Some studies have indeed suggested that echocardiography could pick up carditis in the group presenting with RF and noncardiac manifestations (144,159), but another study did not find such a benefit (116). Preexisting RHD would obscure the ability of echocardiography to detect subclinical carditis unless there is a florid interval change in echocardiographic findings. This would presuppose that a previous echocardiographic study is available, a situation unlikely in countries with the greatest problem of RF. Finally, RF is much more aggressive in developing countries where a large proportion of patients present with florid MR (116), and because patients are rarely seen in the first attacks, echocardiography may have a lesser role in detecting subclinical carditis.

Is Detecting "Echo-detectable" Carditis of Clinical Benefit?

An important role for echocardiography may be to detect the group that does not show cardiac involvement even with echocardiography during an attack of RF. In a prospective study, Vasan et al. (116) reported that patients without carditis on echocardiogram did not develop valve regurgitation on follow-up. One can possibly ensure such patients of a benign prognosis and may allow early discontinuation of secondary prophylaxis. There is a tremendous need for correct diagnosis of rheumatic carditis, and echocardiography will significantly improve our ability to do so. However, some questions need to be answered before accepting echocardiography as a primary modality of diagnosis in RF.

What will it mean in practical terms? Echocardiography is unlikely to modify the acute management of RF because present day treatment is not dependent on the presence or absence of carditis, especially if it is subclinical. What will it mean for secondary prevention and prognostication? All data showing low incidence of residual heart disease in patients without carditis have been from clinical studies (17,103,118,119,166,168,169,171–174,178, 179). If it is correct to assume that echocardiography will be predominantly useful in detecting subclinical carditis (116), a number of patients with "echocardiography-detectable" carditis would have been included in the low-risk group in previous studies, and this group probably did not suffer adversely by the misclassification. Most of the milder forms of rheumatic carditis naturally resolve (118,119, 166,168,169,178,179). It is not certain if the additional detection of "nonclinical" carditis is of prognostic significance. One limited study has shown that echocardiography-detectable carditis is not so benign. Folger et al. (144) found that four of six patients with Doppler evidence of valve involvement continued to have it 18 to 36 months later. However, one of these patients had a normal valve on follow-up and then redeveloped an abnormality, suggesting inadequate penicillin prophylaxis and recurrent RF. Similarly, it is not clear if detecting "subclinical" carditis will influence long-term strategies for prophylaxis. Some patients without clinical carditis in an index attack do develop carditis and cardiac damage in later attacks (42). It is possible that this occurs in patients with carditis too mild for clinical detection in index attack. Echocardiography might identify this subset and may thus aid prophylaxis. There is no clear evidence for this scenario as yet, and it needs clinical confirmation. A large echocardiographic report failed to demonstrate an incremental diagnostic utility of the echocardiogram in patients

with acute RF (116), and the AHA and others currently do not favor the diagnosis of carditis based on Doppler echocardiography in absence of clinical criteria to support the diagnosis (18,147).

What Is the Likely Place for Echocardiography in the Jones' Criteria?

Echocardiography is likely to get better and more widespread in the future, and such a powerful diagnostic tool cannot be denied a place in the management of any cardiovascular disorder. One way to optimize its role in RF is to include this modality in the Jones' criteria with multiple clear caveats. It is likely to have the most useful role in countries with widespread access to health care and with low RF burden; less than 115 cases were seen in the United States in 1994, and RF is no longer a reportable disease (165). Patients are more likely to be seen during first attacks of RF, and the additional cost and workload imposed by routine echocardiography is small and likely to be outweighed by its advantages. There is a significant prognostic implication of finding a normal heart or finding unrelated causes of cardiac murmurs in this population. In addition, with suboptimal auscultation skills (156,157), an echocardiogram will quickly resolve whether absence of a clinically detectable murmur is in fact truly so. This will protect patients with clinical carditis from being misclassified as patients with a more benign prognosis and prevent them from a more relaxed and inappropriate secondary prophylaxis regimen. Even if echocardiography inappropriately overdetects subclinical carditis, given the good medical follow-up in these countries, serial echocardiographic studies will resolve the significance of such valve dysfunction. If most resolve as expected, it has not changed anything adversely for the patients. There is a trend toward abbreviated periods of prophylaxis in the developed world. Even so, the period is sufficiently long to protect patients while the significance of subclinical carditis is being resolved. Moreover, this might help increase motivation for adequate prophylaxis for the necessary period. Detecting subclinical carditis and even mislabeling some patients with RF as having carditis for a short period of time until their clinical situation is resolved does not seem to adversely influence their well-being.

On the other hand, the clinical situation is quite different in the developing world (1,2,36,39,40,42). The incidence of RF and the prevalence of RHD is very high, whereas access to medical care is limited. The disease is more aggressive and needs more prolonged and aggressive prophylaxis. First attacks are rarely witnessed, and many patients present with recurrences and are likely to have established heart disease. Nonrheumatic causes of valvular murmur are proportionately less common given the wide prevalence of RHD. Physical examination is the most often used mode of diagnosis. In one study from India, clinical examination accurately detected patients with and without cardiac involvement, and echocardiography did not add to this ability (116). Echocardiographic facilities are not widely available, and tertiary care centers are far away from most of the rural population. Finally, the cost and additional workload imposed with the universal use of echocardiography in RF episodes will need to be worked out. The echocardiography experience in patients on anorectic drugs is a logical comparison. Detecting echocardiography-detectable carditis in this population is very costly and probably does not change the management strategies very much because the initial period of prophylaxis is no different in patients with and without carditis (21 years or 5 years since last attack). In this population, the presence of RHD is a reason for lifelong prophylaxis (1,35,42). If an echocardiogram needs to be done, doing it at the time of discontinuing prophylaxis might make more sense than during each attack of RF. Therefore, echocardiography cannot be recommended as a routine modality for investigation of RF as yet in these countries. Of course, the role of echocardiography in detecting and managing established RHD is unquestioned in any population.

MANAGEMENT

Risk Stratification in Rheumatic Fever

Risk stratification in RF has been the subject of many studies (Fig. 2-1). The following factors appear to be important in prognostication.

1. Number of RF recurrences. Many studies have shown that recurrences of RF are harmful (25,27,32,115,119,132,166–171,173–175) and constitute the most potent prognostic factor; recurrences increase cardiovascular mortality (132,176,177), increase residual heart disease (118,171–173), and may be responsible for the aggressive nature of the disease in the tropics. In historical studies, patients with multiple attacks of RF ended up with increased prevalence of heart disease (118,132,172). In fact, some types of lesions like mitral stenosis occurred only in those with multiple recurrences (174).

2. Presence of carditis in first attacks. One of the most important prognostic factor in RF is the detection of carditis in an acute episode of RF. Apart from its immediate adverse impact during the episode, carditis is an unfavorable long-term prognostic factor. The data from studies where both the initial and subsequent attacks were witnessed or evaluated (44,103,119,171,172) reveal that patients with recurrences eventually develop greater cardiac damage, not because cardiac damage occurred in later episodes but because patients with cardiac damage in the first attack were more prone to recurrent attacks. This has led to the belief that the first attack separates the RF population into two distinct subsets; those with cardiac involvement in the first attack are the ones likely to sustain recurrent attacks in future. This group also has more cardiac involvement in each subsequent attack leading to severe RHD. Feinstein and Stern (171) studied 105 recurrences in 79 patients on prophylaxis in the Irvington house cohort. Patients with carditis in the initial attack suffered frequent cardiac involvement in subsequent attacks, regardless of the degree of carditis in the previous episode. About half of this group developed new cardiac damage

during the subsequent recurrence. Similarly, the cardiac status in an attack was predictive of cardiac involvement in later attacks; not only did those with RHD have more cardiac involvement in secondary attacks, they also manifested more severe cardiac dysfunction in each later episode. Because cardiac damage, especially of the milder form, heals after an attack (166,178), cardiac status after an episode of RF is, however, not as good a discriminator between those destined for good versus poor prognosis. It is thus clear that recurrences are harmful in patients who have cardiac involvement in initial episodes.

The other group of patients identifiable in the first attack are those who escape cardiac involvement in the initial attacks. This group has fewer recurrences in their lifetime and each recurrence rarely involves the heart and, most importantly, rarely causes cardiac damage (17, 118,166,168,169,171–174,178). Thus, recurrences are benign in this population except for the noncardiac morbidity associated with the acute attack of RF.

3. Fidelity of secondary prophylaxis. Another important prognostic factor is the fidelity with secondary prophylaxis. Secondary prophylaxis not only prevents recurrences and reduces new cardiac damage, it also helps facilitate resolution of previous damage. In the often quoted study of Tompkins et al. (178), MR disappeared in over 70% of patients on regular prophylaxis. Although there was no control group, this benign course was not observed in the few patients not on prophylaxis. Majeed et al. (179) studied the course of cardiac involvement in patients presenting with the first attack of RF. Patients were analyzed by evaluating the incidence of residual heart disease at 5 years with respect to secondary prophylaxis. Although they could not demonstrate a significant difference in the residual heart disease between the two groups of subjects (good vs. poor prophylaxis) in the whole population, there was a significant influence of prophylaxis in patients with carditis during the initial attack. Among the patients with carditis, the greatest difference was seen in patients with mild carditis. Not surprisingly,

prophylaxis did not seem to reduce the incidence of residual heart disease in the patients with severe carditis to start with. The incidence of heart disease was low in the noncarditic group irrespective of prophylaxis. A reduction in the number of RF recurrences with chemoprophylaxis has translated into a reduction in mortality due to RHD (176), a reduction in prevalence of residual heart disease (118,166,168,169,178,180), and a greater likelihood of resolution of cardiac damage sustained during the first attack (118,166,178, 180).

4. Type of streptococcal prevalence in the community. There is increasing evidence that only some of the streptococci can precipitate RF, even in patients not on prophylaxis (19, 181,182). This suggests that some as yet unclear characteristic of the bacterium influences the occurrence of RF. Bacterial strains with increased mucoid capsules and those with higher M protein load appear to be particularly virulent (10). Some strains, such as M types 3, 5, 6, 14, 18, 19, and 24, are frequently found to be responsible for large epidemics (10), whereas others (M types 2, 4, 12, and 28) do not cause significant RF even during epidemics of streptococcal sore throat (19,183). Bacterial strains have shown unexplained changes in virulence over years (10, 184,185). Such a change is thought to account for the sudden unexpected resurgence of RF in the United States (186). Similarly, strains that were common during the widespread epidemics in the past are now being, for reasons unknown, isolated less frequently, and this might account for a reduction in RF.

5. Age of the patient and duration since last attack. The risk of recurrence is highest in the first year after an index attack of RF and decreases with time from the last attack (34,50,103,132,187). Similarly, the risk decreases with increasing age of the patient, and very few recurrences are seen in adults beyond ages 35 to 40 years. However, there remains a finite amount of risk in all patients with RF, perhaps forever. In the study by Bland and Jones (132), in the preprophylaxis era, the risk of recurrence remained small but

significant even up to 20 years after an attack of RF. Patients with more than one episode of RF have higher recurrence rates in some studies (25,103,188). As noted by Spagnuolo et al. (34), the risk of recurrent RF is greatly increased if more than one risk factor is present together.

Treatment of the Acute Episode

Therapy for acute RF has been a source of great disappointment; medical management of RF has not changed since the mid-1950s. It is also unfortunate that current medical therapy only modifies the symptomatic aspects of the disease and has not been shown to significantly change the natural history of the disease. Thus, none of the medical strategies reduce or even modify the occurrence of chronic RHD.

The treatment of an acute episode should initially involve eradication of any persistent GABHS using any accepted antibiotic regimen (see below). This is important to reduce infectivity and to reduce relapses. Anti-inflamatory agents, such as aspirin, have been used for controlling arthritis and the indices of systemic inflammation like erythrocyte sedimentation rate or C-reactive protein. In fact, the diagnosis of RF is questioned if high-dose salicylates do not significantly resolve joint pain and inflammation within 48 hours. Relatively high doses are needed, up to 8 to 10 g/day (100 mg/kg/day) for a period of 3 to 4 weeks (an arbitrary period based on the average duration of inflammation in the untreated patients from the earlier studies). These doses may be associated with significant gastric and other side effects that may reduce compliance, especially once the acute symptoms have resolved. In some patients, clinical rebounds are seen after discontinuation of salicylates and a gradual taper is beneficial. There are no data that salicylates or any other anti-inflamatory drugs modify the natural history of the disease, apart from modifying the acute symptomatic components of the disease (1,2).

Corticosteroids in rheumatic carditis have been used (189) almost since their discovery. Because RF is considered to be due to aberrant immune responses to the streptococcal antigens, the anti-inflammatory and immunosuppressive effects of steroids make them a logical choice. Almost all reports show that steroids rapidly resolve the toxic state, reduce inflammation (134), may reduce the incidence of new murmurs (190), help murmurs disappear faster (191), and help resolution of pericardial effusions (118,119). There is some evidence that steroids may be life saving in severe carditis (122). From 1950 to 1980, almost 135 reports, including 11 randomized trials, evaluated the role of steroids and compared them with salicylates in the treatment of RF. None of the major trials were able to show a significant effect of steroids in modifying the natural history of RF or reducing the prevalence of residual heart disease. There was no significant benefit of steroids over salicylates in most patients. However, most investigators believed that steroids controlled acute symptoms faster (192,193) and might have helped to resolve mitral murmurs (194). A recent meta-analysis on the treatment of rheumatic carditis again could not distinctly demonstrate any significant differences in reducing residual heart disease (assessed as the prevalence of a mitral murmur 1 year after RF) (195). However, the studies were very old, used varying methodology and entry criteria, allowed a significant number of patients to cross over to the steroid group, did not have sufficient power in some cases (193,195), and did not include a sufficient number of patients with severe carditis, the group in which the most significant benefit is expected. Moreover, the results were influenced predominantly by one of the negative trials, and the meta-analysis itself had a large degree of uncertainty. Thus, this question is not fully resolved in the literature.

A short course of steroids is commonly used in patients with severe carditis, based on its anti-inflamatory benefits described above. Prednisone 1 to 2 mg/kg/day is used for a period of 4 weeks with a tapering schedule once the acute symptoms resolve (after the first 2 weeks). There are no definitive end points for discontinuing anti-inflammatory therapy in

RF. A general measure is absence of clinical symptoms and signs of rheumatic activity in addition to normalization of acute phase reactants, usually the erythrocyte sedimentation rate. Too rapid a reduction can be accompanied by a rebound. The steroid taper period should also be covered with good doses of salicylates to prevent a relapse. If congestive heart failure continues to persist despite steroid therapy, surgical repair of mechanical lesions should be considered promptly instead of prolonged trials with high-dose steroids.

Surgical Therapy in the Acute Episode

It has been traditionally believed that surgical therapy is contraindicated in patients with acute RF given the profound inflammatory state. Some studies have showed that surgery, although feasible, is associated with increased mortality (196,197). The only major advance in treatment of acute carditis has been the recognition that patients can be operated in the acute stages of rheumatic carditis with gratifying results and valve repair or replacement in patients with severe congestive heart failure could be life saving. Surgery quickly reverses the prolonged course of congestive heart failure in patients with acute carditis and should be considered early in the course of refractory disease. It is important to realize that congestive heart failure during an acute episode is most often due to severe MR except in patients with long-standing RHD. Because mitral valve repair is often possible in the former situation, the threshold for recommending surgery should be appropriately low when operating for pure MR (110,112,198). If the patient is not responding adequately to medical treatment, the treatment of choice is valve surgery (112,140,198). Valve repair (annuloplasty), correction of valve prolapse, or mitral valve replacement can be done with less than 5% mortality. Essop et al. (140) reported 32 cases of mitral or mitral plus aortic valve replacement during active carditis. There was no mortality, and surgery was associated with rapid and remarkable improvement, including reduction in left ventricular dimensions. However, a series

with a much longer follow-up showed that acute rheumatic carditis does adversely influence the outcome of mitral valve repair (198). Skoularigis et al. (198) studied 254 patients (aged 6 to 52 years) with pure rheumatic regurgitation and heart failure (96% New York Heart Association grades III and IV), one third of whom showed acute rheumatic activity. Patients were followed for 60 ± 35 months after surgery. Acute and long-term (5-year) mortality was about 2.6% and 15%, respectively, primarily due to valve-related causes. A high incidence of valve failure occurred that necessitated reoperation (27%); presence of acute carditis was the strongest predictor of reoperation, and this was not influenced by strict penicillin prophylaxis. Indeed, among patients undergoing reoperation, a high proportion of patients having early reoperation showed rheumatic activity (47%) compared with those having late reoperations (24%). Thus, mitral valve repair may be inappropriate in patients whose valves look macroscopically inflamed at the time of surgery.

Strategies for the Prevention of Rheumatic Fever

Streptococcus remains an enigma in many ways, and little is known about the mechanism by which it causes RF and RHD. Fortunately, this has not been a significant impediment to successful prophylaxis. A number of preventive strategies have been developed. Primordial prevention involves measures to prevent the occurrence of a GABHS sore throat. Primary prophylaxis involves the effective recognition and treatment of GABHS sore throats and in turn prevents the development of RF (1,35). Secondary prophylaxis is the prevention of streptococcal sore throats in patients with previous episodes of RF and thereby prevents recurrent cardiac damage (1,35).

Primordial, Primary, and Secondary Prevention

Streptococcal pharyngitis is the only precipitating cause of RF. Primordial preventive efforts to reduce streptococcal infections are not feasible at present. Efforts to completely eradicate streptococci, as was done with the smallpox virus, are not feasible. Although measures to reduce exposure to streptococci may help, it is unlikely that dramatic socioeconomic changes would occur in the near future in most third world countries to achieve this. Even if they did occur, there is no certainty of effectiveness given the resurgence of RF in the developed world (8,9). Thus, immediate efforts in any primordial prophylactic program would have to be directed toward the host, reducing streptococcal infections through chemoprophylaxis or a vaccine and identifying host susceptibility. The latter is not widely feasible at present, but trials are in progress (199,200). Mass chemoprophylaxis (primordial or primary) can work in some high-risk situations (201,202) and has been used successfully even in some third world countries (192). However, it is excessively wasteful, cannot be applied easily on a daily long-term basis, and some data show that it has a poor efficacy unless carefully targeted (203). Attempts have been made to identify susceptible individuals using genetic markers with some success (57,58). Even though this would reduce the burden of primary prophylaxis by targeting only high-risk individuals, this has not yet been shown to be feasible. Although primary prevention is theoretically the best way to prevent cardiac damage, RF is often precipitated by subclinical streptococcal infections (8,19,47). It is therefore not possible for the physician to intervene effectively at this stage. Additionally, there are significant problems with the early detection of streptococcal sore throats (delay in seeking medical help, delay in diagnosis, differentiating carriers from active infection, etc.) that might limit the efficacy of primary prevention. Furthermore, none of the regimens are 100% effective, and RF recurrence can occur even when a symptomatic infection is optimally treated (35). Unlike solitary benzathene penicillin shots, other regimens for treating streptococcal sore throat need good compliance to complete a 10-day course, especially once symptoms resolve after the first few days. Finally, all programs compete for a limited amount of health care money, and primary prophylaxis is not the most cost-effective way (204), especially in third world countries. At the other end of the spectrum, there is no adequate treatment for an established attack of RF (195). Thus, secondary prevention—preventing recurrent RF episodes in patients with a prior history of RF—would be an appropriate strategy. Secondary prophylaxis is associated with the most satisfying outcome (205). It has been shown to be effective in a number of studies. The population targeted is at a higher risk of cardiac damage and has increased proclivity for recurrences. They are more easily identified, form a smaller proportion of the population than that for primary prophylaxis, and may be more motivated to follow medical advice. They are more likely to be under medical supervision, and a significant proportion can discontinue prophylaxis after a period of time (42,205).

Primary Preventive Strategies

Primary prevention of RF is the detection and treatment of streptococcal sore throat and requires eradication of GABHS from the throat.

Detection of Streptococcal Sore Throat

Acute pharyngitis is more often caused by viruses and other bacteria than by streptococci (35), and the clinical ability to differentiate between these causes in limited at best (206,207). Streptococcal sore throat often presents acutely with fever (101°F or more); painful deglutition; and may be associated with headache, abdominal pain, nausea, and vomiting, especially in children. Clinical signs include tonsillopharyngeal erythema with or without exudate and anterior cervical lymphadenitis. None of these findings are, however, specific for streptococcal infections. Hoarseness, runny nose, conjunctivitis cough, and diarrhea do not occur with streptococcal pharyngitis. Studies that have compared the accuracy of clinical judgment with throat cultures have shown that physicians identify 50% to 75% of GABHS cases correctly (206,207). Physicians also incorrectly label 20% to 40% of all those with a negative throat culture as having GABHS (206,207). A Canadian group of family physicians reported that using four criteria—tonsillar exudate, swollen anterior cervical nodes, a history of a fever of more than 38°C, and lack of a cough—could be used to stratify the risk of streptococcal throats with a sensitivity of 82% but a specificity of only 42% (207). Throat cultures (vigorous swabbing of both tonsils and the posterior pharynx) are needed for accurate diagnosis of streptococcal throat infections and are nearly always positive in the untreated patient with streptococcal throats. Unfortunately, the culture does not distinguish between acute infection and streptococcal carrier state and may need an antibody test in addition. However, a negative culture has a very high value; antibiotic therapy can be withheld in patients with sore throat if the throat culture is negative after incubation for 48 hours. In an effort to speed up the detection of streptococcal sore throats, a number of tests rely on the ability to detect streptococcal antigens. Most of these tests have a highly specificity but have a very low sensitivity, which makes a negative test worthless. Moreover, similar to the throat culture, a positive test does not differentiate between active infection and a carrier state and cannot by itself determine treatment. Newer tests are being developed that may have increased sensitivity, but further evaluations are needed before recommendations can be made for their clinical use. Thus, most clinicians rely on a high or rising levels of a streptococcal antibody test to generate evidence for a presumed recent streptococcal infection.

Treatment Protocols

No single regimen is completely effective in eradicating GABHS from the pharynx, and the choice of the drug regimen depends on the known clinical efficacy, ease of administration, cost, and side effects (Table 2-3). No

TABLE 2-3. *Prevention of rheumatic fever*

Agent	Dose	Mode	Duration
Primary prevention (treatment of streptococcal tonsillopharyngitis)[a]			
Benzathine penicillin G		i.m.	Once
<27 kg (60 lb)	0.6 MU		
>27 kg (60 lb)	1.2 MU		
Penicillin V		p.o.	10 days
Children	250 mg b.i.d./t.i.d.		
Adolescents and adults	500 mg b.i.d./t.i.d.		
With penicillin allergy			
Erythromycin (maximum 1 g/d)		p.o.	10 days
Estolate	20–40 mg/kg/d		
Ethylsuccinate	40 mg/kg/d		
Secondary prevention			
Benzathine penicillin G[b]	1.2 MU	i.m.	Every 4 wk[c]
Penicillin V[d]	250 mg b.i.d.	p.o.	Daily
Sulfadiazine[e]		p.o.	Daily
<27 kg (60 lb)	500 mg		
>27 kg (60 lb)	1,000 mg		
With penicillin and sulfa allergy			
Erythromycin	250 mg b.i.d.	p.o.	Daily

[a]Drugs not useful in primary prevention: sulfonamides, trimethoprim, tetracyclines, and chloramphenicol.
[b]Use drug at room temperature and with procaine penicillin to reduce pain. From Dajani A et al. *Pediatrics* 1995;96:758–764, with permission.
[c]Consider three weekly in high-risk situations including third world countries.
[d]May interfere with oral contraception.
[e]Avoid in pregnancy; more effective than penicillin and better choice if tolerated.

regimen has been found to be superior to penicillin in terms of cost or efficacy. Expert recommendations call for starting the drug after the results of the throat culture are available (1,35,208), although many practitioners do not wait for the culture results (209). This may not be appropriate because only a small fraction of sore throats are caused by streptococci and the delay in getting the throat culture results does not increase the risk of RF (210). Azithromycin (500 mg/day on the first day, 250 mg/day for 4 days) is an acceptable alternative in penicillin-allergic patients, although erythromycin-resistant GABHS has been described (211). Oral cephalosporins may be more effective than penicillins but are not yet approved by the U.S. Food and Drug Administration. The efficacy of treatment is usually determined clinically, and follow-up cultures are rarely used but may be useful in patients with a history of RF. Treatment failures should be treated with a different drug than one used in the previous regimen. Chronic GABHS carriers (asymptomatic patients without a positive immune response) do not need repeated efforts at eradication because they pose little threat to themselves or to others.

Strategies for Secondary Prophylaxis

Rationale

RF follows a different natural history in patients who have sustained previous attacks of RF compared with those without such history (19,118,167), and this strongly influences prophylaxis strategy (Fig. 2-1). RF is a recurrent disease (25,132,167,172,187). Patients with carditis in previous attacks have more recurrence per streptococcal infection (19,30, 32,34,47,50) than those without previous carditis, and those with preexisting RHD have the highest risk of recurrence (103,166,167). The risk of recurrence per infection may range up to 40% to 60% (19,103,167) in younger patients who have RHD with cardiac enlargement. Also, permanent cardiac damage is worse with recurrences, and the cumulative effects of all recurrences are responsible for the poor prognosis in RHD (1,25,118,171). However, recurrent episodes are not necessarily associated with additional cardiac damage in all patients. This is true especially in those patients with no cardiac involvement to begin with (169,171–174,179). Cardiac damage due to multiple recurrences can be most easily demonstrated in patients with the mildest initial cardiac involvement. Finally, recurrent RF can be prevented by preventing GABHS infections. A reduction in the number of RF recurrences with chemoprophylaxis has translated into a reduction in mortality due to RHD (176), a reduction in prevalence of residual heart disease (118,166,168,169,178,180), and greater healing of cardiac damage sustained during the first attack (118,166,178,180). Not surprisingly, secondary prophylaxis has also changed the natural history of RF in many studies (42,169,179).

Candidates for Prophylaxis and Length of Prophylaxis

Continuous prophylaxis (Table 2-4) should be considered for patients with well-documented histories of RF or chorea, with or without evidence of RHD. It should be initiated as soon as acute RF or RHD is diagnosed and should start with an antibiotic course to eradicate any GABHS in the throat. Streptococcal infections occurring in family members of patients with current or previous RF should be treated promptly to reduce the chance of recurrent throat infections.

The duration of prophylaxis depends on the potential risk of repeated streptococcal throat infections and the risk of a recurrence of RF with each such episode (1,35,42). Physicians must consider each individual situation when determining the appropriate duration of prophylaxis. The two main factors in making this decision are the presence of carditis in the RF episodes and the probability of acquiring streptococcal sore throat. The chance of RF is increased with a history of carditis or residual heart disease, multiple previous attacks, and younger age, whereas

TABLE 2-4. *Duration of secondary rheumatic fever prophylaxis[a]*

Category	Risk of recurrent streptococcal infections[b]		
	High	Not high	
		<40 yr	>40 yr[c]
RHD	Lifelong	Until 40 yr[c]	None[c]
Hx carditis and no RHD[d]	Until age 40 yr[c]	Until age 21 yr[c] or 10 yr since last attack[e]	None[f]
ARF and no carditis	Until age 21 yr[c] or 10 yr from last attack	Until age 21 yr[f] or 5 yr since last attack[e]	None[f]

[a]Each case is judged individually after considering the clinical situation and patient wishes.
[b]Modify prophylaxis in epidemic situations, especially if virulent streptococci reemerge.
[c]Should be at least 10 yr since last attack and should not have history of multiple attacks.
[d]Use echo if possible to prove or disprove RHD.
[e]Whichever is longer in duration.
[f]Should be at least 5 yr since last attack and should not have history of multiple attacks.
RHD, residual rheumatic heart disease of any severity; patients from developing countries, with large ARF burden, should be considered at high risk for recurrent streptococcal infections; ARF, acute rheumatic fever.

the risk decreases with increasing interval since the last attack. Streptococcal infections are more common in children, adolescents, parents of young children, teachers, health personnel in contact with children, persons living in closed quarters (like military recruits), and in poor, crowded neighborhoods. The AHA committee's recommendations are given in Table 2-4 with some modifications. The need for prophylaxis should be reassessed periodically. In all situations, the decision to discontinue prophylaxis should be made after discussing potential risks and benefits with the patient and after careful consideration of the risk factor profile.

Antibiotics for Secondary Prophylaxis

An intramuscular injection of benzathine penicillin G (0.6 to 1.2 million units depending on age and weight) every 4 weeks is the regimen of choice. The advantages of benzathine penicillin G include the need for just one injection each month and its unchallenged efficacy (1,35,42). On the other hand, the injection is somewhat painful, which can reduce compliance (42). There is preliminary evidence that a 3-week regimen (212-214) or even a 2-week regimen (215) of benzathine penicillin G is more efficacious in the developing countries with high RF loads. Another

study suggested the use of a higher dose—1.8 million units every 4 weeks (216). This needs to be further validated, however, and the effects of more frequent dosing must be balanced with the costs and possible loss of compliance. The use of penicillin levels has been suggested to allow a more pharmacologically optimum regimen (42), but there is significant controversy. Pain is a significant side effect with benzathine penicillin, and the use of local anesthesia along with the injection does not seem to help. Procaine penicillin injected along with benzathine penicillin is somewhat better tolerated. Severe allergic reactions are seen occasionally, but there are only a few well-documented reports of fatalities (217). The fear of this drug is worse than its risks. Recently, an international study prospectively evaluated the risks associated with benzathine penicillin in 1,790 patients over 2,736 patient-years of follow-up (218). Patients were chosen from 11 countries and were given benzathine penicillin made by 12 different manufacturers. A total of 32,430 injections were administered; 3.2% of patients showed allergic reactions and anaphylaxis occurred in 0.2%. One patient died (0.05%). This patient had received 24 injections previously without problems. Rheumatic recurrences occurred in 11.5% of patients without prophylaxis compared with 0.45% in those complying with the

TABLE 2-5. *Effect of secondary prophylaxis on recurrent rates in the Irvington House Studies*

| Category | Penicillin | | Sulfa | |
	Benzathine	Oral	Oral	Historical control[a]
Streptococcal infections	6.1	20.7	24	32
True infections	4.3	18.5	17.7	
Good prophylaxis	6.3	6.2	16.0	
ARF recurrences	0.4	5.5	2.8	15
Good prophylaxis	0.4	2.6	3.2	
Recurrence infection[b]	5.9	25.7	11.6	
Recurrence/true infection	8.3	28.7	15.7	48
Good prophylaxis	6.0	16	20	

All in terms of 100 patient-years. True infections exclude carriers.
[a]From Kuttner AG et al. *J Clin Invest* 1943;22:77–85.
[b]Per 100 infections.
From ref. 28, with permission.

regimen. There was no increase in the risk of reactions with longer duration of prophylaxis. These risks are no greater than those in patients not having RF (1 to 4/10,000 injections). The risk is lower in children less than 12 years old, and mortality is primarily seen in patients with severe heart disease. Skin testing is not universally mandated but may help in reducing the risk. Thus, benzathine is essentially safe, and the fear of reactions should not be an important consideration in choosing the method of prophylaxis. There is some limited evidence that penicillin might interfere with oral contraception (219). This might need to be discussed with patients using this form of contraception.

Oral agents are more appropriate for patients at a lower risk for RF recurrence, and some physicians might advise oral prophylaxis in highly compliant young adults who have not had a rheumatic recurrence in the last few years. Successful oral prophylaxis needs significant patient adherence, which might be difficult in patients without any discomfort; however, even with excellent compliance as seen in randomized trials, oral prophylaxis is inferior (Table 2-5) to monthly benzathene penicillin prophylaxis (32). Oral sulfa is superior to oral penicillin but may not be tolerated as well (1,35,42). It is important to note that sulfonamides do not eradicate streptococci from the throat even though they

can effectively prevent streptococcal sore throat and RF. Sulfonamide are associated with rashes and hematologic toxicity. The latter is seen in the initial few months of therapy. Sulfonamide prophylaxis is contraindicated in pregnancy due to the risk of kernicterus in the newborn (220). There are no published data about the use of other penicillins, macrolides, or cephalosporins for the secondary prevention of RF.

Subacute Bacterial Endocarditis and Rheumatic Fever Prophylaxis

Subacute bacterial endocarditis (SBE) is a significant problem in patients with RHD. There is no evidence that the incidence of SBE is declining in patients with RHD (1). Although it is known that penicillin-resistant organisms can colonize the individual receiving penicillin (221), there is no evidence that rheumatic individuals on secondary prophylaxis are at increased risk of SBE with penicillin-resistant organisms (222). Prophylaxis of SBE is often confused with that for RF. It should be emphasized that the doses used in prophylaxis for RF are very much inadequate as far as prophylaxis for SBE is concerned. Further, gram-negative bacteria may need coverage in a number of instances, and this is not achieved with the drugs used for RF.

Pregnancy and Postcardiac Surgery and Rheumatic Fever Prophylaxis

Prophylaxis needs to be continued during pregnancy and in the postcardiac surgical period. RHD occurs at a younger age in developing countries, and it is not uncommon to find young pregnant patients with florid RHD. Prophylaxis needs to be continued during pregnancy in these patients, but sulfonamides are contraindicated (220). Penicillin is safe, and the injectable form should be offered wherever possible. Patients need to continue prophylaxis after cardiac surgery, including valve replacement, because RF can recur in this population with involvement of other valves (223) or precipitate congestive heart failure.

STREPTOCOCCAL VACCINE

Probably the most effective way to reduce the global RF burden would be the development of an economic, safe, and effective antistreptococcal vaccine (224). This is not yet totally feasible, although vaccines are in various stages of trial. Two concepts have been used to make this possible. The streptococcal M protein has long been known to be an important determinant of streptococcal virulence (225). M proteins are type specific to each strain, and antibodies to M proteins effectively confer immunity to that strain. Dale et al. (226) showed distinct segments in the M protein structure with different functionality, including sites for toxic, cross-reactive, and immunizing epitopes. They identified the N-terminal sequence that is devoid of the more proximal human tissue homologous antigens. Also, this segment is not pyrogenic and toxic to humans. This segment induces protective immune response when injected in humans and may constitute an important vaccine (226,227). However, the N-terminal also contains the variable segment of the type-specific determinants, and such vaccines need to be multicomponent to contain all putative strains that could cause RF in each community (224). Moreover, with changes in the streptococcal strain in each community, induction of new strains by trade and travel and the possibility that bacteria can change the hypervariable region sequences to produce new antigenic epitopes or even exchange antigenic epitopes among themselves further complicates the issue (228,229). This variability has been shown to be related to changes in genes coding for the M protein (*emm* gene) and results in loss of susceptibility to opsonizing antibodies (228). Finally, a number of bacteria are not M typeable, especially those reported from Thailand and Australia (230), and this might pose a problem in vaccine efficacy. Since 1987, a number of improvements have been made in the vaccine. One of the current vaccines includes an octavalent antigenic peptide (231). In the other vaccine, recombinant streptococcal protein fragments are linked to *Escherichia coli* labile toxin that, apart from being a hapten, is likely to prevent mucosal colonization due to the formation of IgA antibodies (232).

The other method of vaccine development has used the cell wall end of the M protein (233). Previous work had shown that antibodies to the conserved C-terminal were not opsonizing but did reduce mucosal colonization (234,235), which would in turn reduce streptococcal infections. Contradictory studies have shown antibodies to the C-terminal conserved epitope have opsonizing capacity as well (236). The advantage of this approach would be that this region is relatively conserved (227) through streptococcal strains, and opsonizing antibodies to it would be useful against multiple strains. It has been found to induce T cells reactive against myosin (237) and could entail potential risk. Further work is in progress to obtain the B-cell–specific epitopes of this peptide. An effective streptococcal vaccine is likely to be available in the near future.

AGENDA FOR THE FUTURE

RF remains a major preventable disease of this century. Effectively managing streptococcal sore throat and preventing recurrent carditis through aggressive prophylaxis is still a major goal in preventing this disease. However, the success rates for this approach have been variable and quite dismal in most nations of the world.

The role of echocardiography in the diagnosis of carditis in RF is a matter of debate, and more studies will clarify its role. Given the insensitivity of our ability to detect murmurs on auscultation, an additional tool to detect cardiac involvement would be immensely useful. However, the utility of detecting subclinical valve dysfunction, especially in an era of declining incidence of RF, is unclear given the fact that most patients with milder forms of clinically detectable carditis resolve without residua when recurrences are prevented. This area needs immediate attention; we need an accurate way of differentiating normal from abnormal valvular regurgitation to limit labeling people with a diagnosis of RF unnecessarily. Any recommendation in this regard should keep in mind that most RF burden is in developing countries with very stringent health budgets and lack of widespread availability of experienced echocardiographers. The beneficial implications of an echocardiogram should far outweigh its disadvantages for it to be universally acceptable.

It is unfortunate that even though we have been successful in preventing recurrences of RF, we are not as yet able to effectively modulate the course and natural history of acute rheumatic carditis after an acute episode has occured. Anti-inflammatory therapy in its present form is a largely symptomatic treatment. There are no data on the use of newer immunosuppressive protocols to modify the course of rheumatic carditis, and this could be an area of great potential. Carditis in RF is very different from the more well-known forms of myocarditis in that there is little myocyte necrosis. The cause of congestive heart failure is clearly mechanical valve problems, which respond well to surgery. Surgery in the form of mitral valve repair or replacement can be done at low risk with gratifying results and should be considered early in the course of severe refractory carditis with mitral or, less commonly, aortic regurgitation.

Finally, acute RF remains a common and enigmatic problem worldwide and needs to be evaluated in a global perspective. Although socioeconomic factors are probably playing a major role in its occurrence in the third world today, the lack of a detailed knowledge of how and why streptococci cause RF is a major limitation in preventing this disease globally. In the absence of a likelihood of great social change in the world, an effective antistreptococcal vaccine is needed to favorably alter the epidemiology of RF.

REFERENCES

1. WHO Study Group. Rheumatic fever and rheumatic heart disease. WHO Technical Report Series No. 764. Geneva: World Health Organization, 1988.
2. Massell BF, Narula J. Rheumatic fever and rheumatic carditis. In: Braunwald E, ed. *The Atlas of Heart Diseases.* Current Medicine: Philadelphia, 1994:10.1–10.20.
3. English PC. Emergence of rheumatic fever in the nineteenth century. *Milbank Q* 1989;67[Suppl 1]:33–49.
4. Land MA, Bisno AL. Acute rheumatic fever: a vanishing disease in suburbia. *JAMA* 1983;249:895–898.
5. Gordis L. The virtual disappearance of rheumatic fever in the United States: lessons in the rise and fall of disease. *Circulation* 1985;72:1155–1162.
6. Rammelkamp CH, Denny FW, Wannamaker LW. Studies on the epidemiology of rheumatic fever in the armed services. In: Thomas L, ed. *Rheumatic Fever.* Minneapolis: University of Minnesota Press, 1952: 72–89.
7. Bland EF. Rheumatic fever. The way it was. *Circulation* 1987;76:1190–1195.
8. Veasy LG, Wiedmeier SE, Orsmond GS, et al. Resurgence of acute rheumatic fever in the intermountain area of the United States. *N Engl J Med* 1987;316: 421–427.
9. Bisno AL. The resurgence of acute rheumatic fever in the United States. *Annu Rev Med* 1990;41:319–329.
10. Stollerman GH. Rheumatogenic group A streptococci and the return of rheumatic fever. *Adv Intern Med* 1990;35:1–25.
11. Jones TD. Diagnosis of rheumatic fever. *J Am Med Assoc* 1944;126:481–484.
12. Adams F. *The genuine works of Hippocrates.* New York: Wood, 1886.
13. Taranta A. No contemptible distemper. A history of rheumatic fever and its idea. In: Narula J, Virmani R, Tandon R, Reddy KS, eds. *Rheumatic Fever.* Washington, DC: AFIP Press 1999;1–4.
14. Bright R. *Reports of Medical Cases, Selected with a View of Illustrating the Symptoms and Cure of Diseases by a Reference to Morbid Anatomy.* Vol. 1. London: Longman, 1832.

15. Wells WC. On rheumatism of the heart. *Trans Soc Improv Med Chir Knowl* 1812;3:373–424.
16. Cheadle WB. The various manifestations of the rheumatic state as exemplified in childhood and early life. *Lancet* 1889;1:812–817.
17. Findlay L. *The Rheumatic Infection in Childhood.* London: E Arnold, 1931.
18. Special Writing Group of the Committee on Rheumatic Fever, Endocarditis and Kawasaki Disease of the Council of Cardiovascular Disease in the Young of the American Heart Association. Guidelines for the diagnosis of rheumatic fever: Jones criteria 1992 update. *JAMA* 1992;268:2069–2073.
19. Kuttner AG, Krumwiede E. Observations on the effect of streptococcal upper respiratory infections on rheumatic children: a three-year study. *J Clin Invest* 1941;20:273–287.
20. Stroud WD. The clinical importance of the infections of the respiratory tract in rheumatic fever. Abstract of discussion. *J Am Med Assoc* 1939;113:902.
21. Rowntree LG, McGill KM, Folk OH. Health of selective service registrants. *J Am Med Assoc* 1942;118:1223–1227.
22. Coburn AF, Moore LV. The prophylactic use of sulfanilamide in streptococcal respiratory infections with especial reference to rheumatic fever. *J Clin Invest* 1939;18:147–155.
23. Thomas CB, France RA. Preliminary report of the prophylactic use of sulfanilamide in patients susceptible to rheumatic fever. *Bull Johns Hopkins Hosp* 1939;64:67–77.
24. Holbrook WP. The Army Air Force's rheumatic fever control program. *J Am Med Assoc* 1944;126:84–87.
25. Hansen AE. Rheumatic recrudesences: diagnosis and prevention. *J Pediatr* 1946;28:296–308.
26. Burke PJ. Penicillin prophylaxis in acute rheumatism. *Lancet* 1947;1:255–256.
27. Feinstein AR, Spagnuolo M. Mimetic features of rheumatic fever recurrences. *N Engl J Med* 1960;262:533–540.
28. Wood HF, Feinstein AR, Taranta A, et al. Rheumatic fever in children and adolescents: a long-term epidemiologic study of subsequent prophylaxis, streptococcal infections, and clinical sequelae. Ill. Comparative effectiveness of three prophylaxis regimens in preventing streptococcal infections and rheumatic recurrences. *Ann Intern Med* 1964;60[Suppl 5]:31–46.
29. Feinstein AR, Wood HF, Spagnuolo M, Taranta A, Tursky E, Kleinberg E. Oral prophylaxis of recurrent rheumatic fever. sulfadiazine vs a double dose penicillin. *J Am Med Assoc* 1964;188:489–492.
30. Johnson EE, Stollerman GH, Grossman BJ. Rheumatic recurrences in patients not receiving continuous prophylaxis. *J Am Med Assoc* 1964;190:407–413.
31. Feinstein AR, Spagnuolo M, Jonas S, et al. Prophylaxis of recurrent rheumatic fever. Ineffectiveness of intermittent "therapeutic" oral penicillin. *J Am Med Assoc* 1965;191:451–454.
32. Taranta A. Factors influencing recurrent rheumatic fever. *Annu Rev Med* 1967;18:159–172.
33. Feinstein AR, Spagnuolo M, Jonas S, et al. Prophylaxis of recurrent rheumatic fever. Therapeutic-continuous oral penicillin vs. monthly injections. *J Am Med Assoc* 1968;206:565–568.
34. Spagnuolo M, Pasternack B, Taranta A. The risk of rheumatic recurrences after streptococcal infections. Prospective study of clinical and social factors. *N Engl J Med* 1971;285:641–647.
35. Dajani AS, Bisno AL, Chung KJ, et al. Prevention of rheumatic fever: a statement for health professionals by the Committee on Rheumatic Fever, Endocarditis, and Kawasaki Disease of the Council on Cardiovascular Disease in the Young, the American Heart Association. *Circulation* 1988;78:1082–1086.
36. Aggarwal BL. Rheumatic heart disease unabated in developing countries. *Lancet* 1981;2:909–910.
37. Kaplan EL, Hill HR. Return of rheumatic fever: consequences, implications, and needs. *J Pediatr* 1987;111:244–246.
38. Markowitz M. Observations on the epidemiology and preventability of rheumatic fever in developing countries. *Clin Ther* 1981;4:240–251.
39. Roy SB, Bhatia ML, Lazaro EJ et al. Juvenile mitral stenosis in India. *Lancet* 1963;2:1193–1196.
40. Padmavati S. Rheumatic fever and rheumatic heart disease in developing countries. *Bull WHO* 1978;56:543–550.
41. Murray CJ, Lopez AD. *Global Health Statistics: A Compendium of Incidence, Prevalence and Mortality Estimates for over 200 Conditions. Global Burden of Disease and Injury Series*. Vol. II. Cambridge: Harvard School of Public Health, 1996:132–140.
41a. Vijaikumar M, Narula J, Reddy KS, Kaplan EL. Incidence of rheumatic fever and prevalence of rheumatic heart disease in India. *Int J Cardiol* 199;43:221–228.
42. Chandrashekhar Y. Secondary prevention. Theory, practice and analysis of available trials. In: Narula J, Virmani R, Tandon R, Reddy KS, eds. *Rheumatic Fever*. Washington, DC: AFIP Press 1999;399–442.
43. Quinn RW. Comprehensive review of morbidity and mortality trends for rheumatic fever, streptococcal disease and scarlet fever: the decline of rheumatic fever. *Rev Infect Dis* 1989;11:928–953.
44. Michaud C, Trejo-Gutierrez J, Cruz C, Pearson T. Rheumatic heart disease. In: Jamison DT, ed. *Disease Control Priorities in Developing Countries: A Summary*. Washington, DC: World Bank, 1993:221–232.
45. Massell BF, Chute CG, Walker AM, Kuriand GS. Penicillin and the marked decrease in morbidity and mortality from rheumatic fever in the United States. *N Engl J Med* 1988;318:280–286.
46. Kavey RE, Kaplan EL. Resurgence of acute rheumatic fever [letter]. *Pediatrics* 1989;84:585–586.
47. Feinstein AR, Spagnuolo M, Taranta A, Tursky E, Kleinberg E. Rheumatic fever in children and adolescents. A long-term epidemiologic study of subsequent prophylaxis, streptococcal infections, and clinical sequelae. VI. Clinical features of streptococcal infection and rheumatic recurrences. *Ann Intern Med* 1964;60[Suppl 5]:68–86.
48. Wannamaker LW. The chains that link the heart to the throat. *Circulation* 1973;48:9–18.
49. Stollerman GH, Lewis AJ, Schultz L, et al. Relationship of immune response to group A streptococci to the course of acute, chronic and recurrent rheumatic fever. *Am J Med* 1956;20:163–169.
50. Taranta A, Wood HF, Feinstein AR, Simpson R, Kleinberg E. Rheumatic fever in children and adolescents. A

long-term epidemiologic study of subsequent prophylaxis, streptococcal infections, and clinical sequelae. IV. Relation of the rheumatic fever recurrence rate per streptococcal infection to the titer, of streptococcal antibodies. *Ann Intern Med* 1964;60[Suppl 5]:47–57.

51. Bisno AL. The concept of rheumatogenic and non rheumatogenic group A streptococci. In: Read SE, Zabriskie JB, eds. *Streptococcal Diseases and the Immune Response*. New York: Academic Press, 1980: 789–803.

52. DiSciascio G, Taranta A. Rheumatic fever in children. *Am Heart J* 1980;99:635–658.

53. Chun LT, Reddy V, Rhoads GG. Occurrance and prevention of rhuematic fever among ethnic groups of Hawaii. *Am J Dis Child* 1984;138:476–478.

54. Wannamaker LW. Changes and changing concepts in the biology of group A streptococci and in the epidemiology of streptococcal infections. *Rev Infect Dis* 1979;1:967–975.

55. Ferguson GW, Schultz JM, Bisno AL. The epidemiology of acute rheumatic fever in a multiethnic, multiracial urban community: the Miami-Dade County experience. *J Infect Dis* 1991;164:72–75.

56. Taneja V, Mehra NK, Reddy KS, et al. HLA-DR/DQ and reactivity to B cell alloantigen D8/17 in Indian patients with rheumatic heart disease. *Circulation* 1989; 80:335–340.

57. Khanna AK, Buskirk DR, Williams RC Jr, et al. Presence of a non-HLA B cell antigen in rheumatic fever patients and their families as defined by a monoclonal antibody. *J Clin Invest* 1989;83:1710–1716.

58. Patarroyo ME, Winchester RJ, Vejerano A, et al. Association of a B cell alloantigen with susceptibility to rheumatic fever. *Nature* 1979;278:173–174.

59. Krishnaswami S, Joseph G, Richard J. Demands on tertiary care for cardiovascular diseases in India. Analysis of data for 1960–89. *Bull WHO* 1991;69: 325–330.

60. Chesler E, Levin S, du Plessis L, Freiman I, Rigers M, Joffe N. The pattern of rheumatic heart disease in the urbanised Bantu of Johannesburg. *S Afr Med J* 1966; 40:899–904.

61. Mathur KS, Wahal PK. Epidemiology of rheumatic heart disease—a study of 29,922 school children. *Indian Heart J* 1982;34:367–371.

62. Schwankhaus JD. Preventing rheumatic heart disease in developing countries. *Ann Intern Med* 1994;121:77.

63. McLaren MJ, Hawkins DM, Koornhof HJ, et al. Epidemiology of rheumatic heart disease in black school children of Soweto, Johannesburg. *Br Med J* 1975;3: 474–478.

64. Neutze JM. Rheumatic fever and rheumatic heart disease in the Eastern Pacific region. *N Z Med J* 1988; 101:404–406.

65. North DA, Heynes RA, Lennnon DR, Neutze J. Analysis of costs of acute rheumatic fever and rheumatic heart disease in Auckland. *N Z Med J* 1993;106: 400–403.

66. Donald PR, Van der Merwe PL. Secondary prophylaxis of group A beta hemolytic streptococcal throat infections. *S Afr Med J* 1989;75:248–249.

67. Zabriskie JB. Rheumatic fever: interplay between host, genetics and the microbe. *Circulation* 1985;71: 1077–1086.

68. McCarty M. Theories of pathogenesis of streptococcal complications. In: Wannamaker LW, Matsen JM, eds. *Streptococci and Streptococcal Diseases*. New York: Academic Press, 1972:517–526.

69. Thompson S, Innes J. Hemolytic streptococci in the cardiac lesions of acute rheumatism. *Br Med J* 1940;2: 733–736.

70. Hirschhorn K, Schreibman RR, Verbo S, Grushkin RH. The action of streptolysin S on peripheral leukocytes of normal subjects and patients with acute rheumatic fever. *Proc Natl Acad Sci USA* 1964;52: 1151–1157.

71. Kaplan MH, Meyeserian M, Kushner I. Immunologic cross reaction between group A streptococcal cells and human heart tissue. *Lancet* 1962;1:706–710.

72. Kaplan MH, Suchy ML. Immunologic relation of streptococcal and tissue antigens. II. Cross reaction of antisera to mammalian heart tissue to the cell wall constituents of cetain strains of group A streptococci. *J Exp Med* 1964;119:643–650.

73. Kaplan MH, Svec KH. Immunologic relation of streptococcal and tissue antigens. III. Presence in human sera of streptococcal antibody cross reactive with heart tissue. Association with streptococcal infection, rheumatic fever, and glomerulonephritis. *J Exp Med* 1964;119:651–666.

74. Dudding BA, Ayoub EM. Persistance of streptococcal group A antibody in patients with rheumatic valvular disease. *J Exp Med* 1968;128:1081–1098.

75. Goldstein I, Halpern B, Robert L. Immunological relationship between streptococcus A polysaccharide and the structural glucoproteins of heart valve. *Nature* 1967;213:44–47.

76. Dale JB, Beachey EH. Protective determinant of streptococcal M protein shared with sarcolemmal membrane protein of human heart. *J Exp Med* 1982;156: 1165–1176.

77. Dale JB, Beachey EH. Epitopes of streptococcal M protein shared with cardiac myosin. *J Exp Med* 1985; 162:583–591.

78. Bessen D, Jones KF, Fischetti VA. Evidence for two distinct classes of streptococcal M protein and their relationship to rheumatic fever. *J Exp Med* 1989;169: 269–283.

79. Ayoub EM, Dudding BA. Streptococcal group A carbohydrate antibody in rheumatic and non rheumatic bacterial endocarditis. *J Lab Clin Med* 1970;76: 322–332.

80. Barnett A, Cunningham MW. A new heart cross reactive antigen in streptococcus pyogenes is not M protein. *J Infect Dis* 1990;162:875–882.

81. Fox A, Brown RR, Anderle SS, et al. Arthropathic properties related to the molecular weight of peptidoglycan-polysaccharide polymers of streptococcal cell walls. *Infect Immun* 1982;35:1003–1010.

82. Stollerman GH. Rheumatogenic streptococci and autoimmunity. *Clin Immunol Immunopathol* 1991;61: 131–142.

83. Zabriskie JB. Mimetic relationships between group A streptococci andmammalian tissues. *Adv Immunol* 1967;7:147–188.

84. Ayoub EM. The search for host determinants of susceptibility to rheumatic fever: the missing link. *Circulation* 1984;69:197–201.

85. Rajapakse CN, Halim K, Al-Orainay I, Al-Nozha M, AlAska AK. A genetic marker for rheumatic heart disease. *Br Heart J* 1987;58:659–662.

86. Cunningham MW, McCormack JM, Fenderson PG, Ho MK, Beachey EH, Dale JB. Human and murine antibodies cross reactive with streptococcal M protein and myosin recognise the sequence GLN-LYS-SER-LYS-GLN in M protein. *J Immunol* 1989;143: 2677–2683.

87. Manjula BN, Trus BL, Fischetti VA. Presence of two distinct regions in the coiled coil structure of the streptococcal Pep M5 protein: relationship to mammalian coiled coil proteins and implications to its biological properties. *Proc Natl Acad Sci USA* 1985;82: 1064–1068.

88. Sarjent SJ, Beachey EH, Corbett CE, Dale JB. Sequence of protective epitopes of streptococcal M proteins shared with cardiac sarcolemmal membranes. *J Immunol* 1987;139:1285–1290.

89. Tomai MA, Kotb M, Majumdar G, Beachey EH. Superantigenicity of streptococcal M protein. *J Exp Med* 1990;172:359–362.

90. van de Rijn I, Zabriskie JB, McCarty M,. Group A streptococcal antigens cross reactive with myocardium. Purification of heart reactive antibody and isolation and characterisation of the streptococcal antigen. *J Exp Med* 1977;146:579–599.

91. Narula J, Chopra P, Talwar KK, et al. Does endomyocardial biopsy aid in the diagnosis of active rheumatic carditis? *Circulation* 1993;88:2198–2205.

92. Zabriskie JB, Hsu KC, Seegal BC. Heart reactive antibody associated with rheumatic fever: characterisation and diagnostic significance. *Clin Exp Immunol* 1970; 7:147–159.

93. Yand LC, Soprey PR, Wittner MK, Fox EN. Streptococcal induced cell mediated immune destruction of cardiac myofibres in vitro. *J Exp Med* 1977;146: 344–360.

94. Hutto J, Ayoub EM. Cytotoxicity of lymphocytes from patients with rhuemtic carditis to cardiac cells in vitro. In: Zabriskie JB, Read SE, eds. *Streptococcal Disease and the Immune Response.* New York: Academic Press, 1980:733–738.

95. Guilherme L, Cuhna-Neto E, Coehlo V, et al. Human heart infiltrating T cell clones from rheumatic heart disease recognise both streptococcal and cardiac proteins. *Circulation* 1995;92:415–420.

96. Read SE, Reid HF, Fischetti V, et al. Serial studies on the cellular immune response to streptococcal antigens in acute and convalescent rheumatic fever patients in Trinidad. *J Clin Immunol* 1986;6:433–441.

97. Sapru RP, Ganguly NK, Sharma S, Chandani RE, Gupta AK. Cellular reaction to group A beta hemolytic streptococcal membrane antigen and its relation to complement levels in patients with rheumatic heart disease. *Br Med J* 1977;2:422–424.

98. Abe J, Forrester J, Nakahara T, Lafferty JA, Kotzin DL, Leung DY. Selective stimulation of human T cells with streptococcal erthrogenic toxins A and B. *J Immunol* 1991;146:3747–3750.

99. Scherer MT, Ignatowicz L, Winslow GM, Kappler JW, Marrack P. Superantigens: bacterial and viral proteins that manipulate the immune system. *Annu Rev Cell Biol* 1993;9:101–128.

100. Hackett SP, Stevens DL. Streptococcal toxic shock syndrome: synthesis of tumour necrosis factor and interleukin 1 by monocytes stimulated with pyrogenic exotoxin A and streptolysin O. *J Infect Dis* 1992;165: 879–885.

101. Tomaya-Sorimachi N, Miyake K, Miyasaka M. Activation of CD44 induces ICAM-1/LFA-1 independent Ca^{2+}, Mg^{2+} independent adhesion pathway in lymphocyte endothelial cell interaction. *Eur J Immunol* 1993; 23:439–446.

102. Kotb M. Post streptococcal autoimmune sequelae: a link between infection and autoimmunity. In: Dalgleish AG, Albertini A, Paoletti R, eds. *The Impact of Biotechnology on Autoimmunity.* Boston: Kluwer Academic Publishers, 1994.

103. Taranta A, Kleinberg E, Feinstein AR, et al. Rheumatic fever in children and adolescents. A long-term epidemiologic study of subsequent prophylaxis, streptococcal infections, and clinical sequelae. V. Relation of the rheumatic fever recurrence rate per streptococcal infection to preexisting clinical features of the patients. *Ann Intern Med* 1964;60[Suppl 5]:58–67.

104. Pickles WN. A rheumatic family. *Lancet* 1943;2:241.

105. Anastasiou-Nana MI, Anderson JL, Carlquist LF, Nanas JN. HLA-DR typing and lymphocyte subset evaluation in rheumatic heart disease: a search for immune response factors. *Am Heart J* 1986;112:992–997.

106. Jhinghan B, Mehra NK, Reddy KS, Taneja V, Vaidya MC, Bhatia ML. HLA, blood groups and secretor status in patients with established rheumatic fever and rheumatic heart disease. *Tissue Antigens* 1986;27: 172–178.

107. Silver MD. Blood flow obstruction related to tricuspid, pulmonary and mitral valves. In: Silver MD, ed. *Cardiovascular Pathology*, 2nd ed. New York: Churchill Livingstone, 1991:944–960.

108. Baggenstoss AH, Titus JL. Rheumatic and collagen disorders of the heart. In Gould SE, ed. *Pathology of the Heart and Blood Vessels*, 3rd Edition. Springfield, IL: Charles C Thomas, 1968:649–722.

109. Virmani R, Roberts WC. Aschoff bodies in operatively excised atrial appendages and in papillary muscles. Frequency and clinical significance. *Circulation* 1977; 55:559–563.

110. Kinsley RH, Girdwood RW, Milner S. Surgical treatment during the acute phase of rheumatic carditis. In: Nyhus LM, ed. *Surgery Annual.* East Norwalk, CT: Appleton-Century-Crofts, 1981:299–323.

111. Edwards WD, Peterson K, Edwards JE. Active valvulitis associated with chronic rheumatic disease and active myocarditis. *Circulation* 1978;57:181–185.

112. Marcus RH, Sareli P, Pocock WA, Barlow JB. The spectrum of severe rheumatic valve disease in a developing country. Correlation among clinical presentation, surgical pathologic findings and hemodynamic sequalae. *Ann Intern Med* 1994;120:177–183.

113. Veasy GL. Myocardial dysfunction in active rheumatic carditis. *J Am Coll Cardiol* 1994;24:578.

114. Klibanoff E, Frieden J, Spagnuolo M, Feinstein AR. Rheumatic activity: a clinicopathologic correlation. *JAMA* 1966;195:895–900.

115. Gross G, Fried BM. Lesions in the atrioventricular conduction system occurring in rheumatic fever. *Am J Pathol* 1936;12:31–43.

116. Vasan R, Shrivastava S, Vijaya Kumar K, Narang R, Lister BC, Narula J. Echocardiographic evaluation of patients with acute rheumatic fever and rheumatic carditis. *Circulation* 1996;94:73–82.

117. Gross L, Kugel MA, Epstein EZ. Lesions of the coronary arteries and their branches in rheumatic fever. *Am J Pathol* 1935;11:253–279.

118. Feinstein AR, Stern EK, Spagnuolo M. The prognosis of acute rheumatic fever. *Am Heart J* 1964;68:817–834.

119. Feinstein AR, Spagnuolo M. The clinical pattern of acute rheumatic fever. a reappraisal. *Medicine (Baltimore)* 1962;41:279–305.

120. Sanyal SK, Thapar MK, Ahmed AH, et al. The initial attack of rheumatic fever during childhood in North India: a prospective study of the clinical profile. *Circulation* 1974;49:7–12.

121. Aggarwal BL, Aggarwal R. Rheumatic fever: clinical profile of the initial attack in India. *Bull WHO* 1986;64:573–578.

122. Amigo MC, Martinez-Levin M, Reyes PA. Acute rheumatic fever. *Rheum Clin North Am* 1993;19:333–350.

123. Gupta MS, Mehta L, Malhotra S, Malhotra KC. Jaccoud's arthritis. *J Assoc Physicians India* 1990;38:947–948.

124. Markowitz M. Evolution and critique of changes in the Jones criteria for the diagnosis of rheumatic fever. *N Z Med J* 1988;101:392–394.

125. Okuni M. Problems in clinical application of revised Jones criteria for rheumatic fever. *Jpn Heart J* 1971;12:436–441.

126. Battacharya S, Tandon R. The diagnosis of rheumatic fever. Evaluation of Jones criteria. *Int J Cardiol* 1986;12:285–294.

127. Pamavati S, Gupta V. Reappraisal of Jones criteria: the Indian experience. *N Z Med J* 1988;101:391–392.

128. Majeed HA, Khan N, Dabbagh M, et al. Acute rheumatic fever during childhood in Kuwait. The mild nature of the initial attack. *Ann Trop Pediatr* 1981;1:13–20.

129. Fink CW. The role of the streptococcus in post-streptococcal reactive arthritis and childhood polyarteritis nodosa. *J Rheumatol* 1991;29:14–20.

130. Deighton C. Beta hemolytic streptococci and reactive arthritis in adults. *Ann Rheum Dis* 1993;52:475–482.

131. Kothari SS, Chandrashekhar Y, Tandon RK. Rheumatic carditis. In: Narula J, Virmani R, Tandon R, Reddy KS, eds. *Rheumatic Fever.* Washington, DC: AFIP Press 199;257–270.

132. Bland EF, Jones TD. Rheumatic fever and rheumatic heart disease. A 20-year report on 1,000 patients followed since childhood. *Circulation* 1951;4:836–843.

133. Stollerman GH. Rheumatic carditis. *Lancet* 1995;346:390–391.

134. Massell BF, Fyler DC, Roy SB. The clinical picture of rheumatic fever. Diagnosis, immediate prognosis, course and therapeutic implications. *Am J Cardiol* 1958;1:436–449.

135. Kinare SG. Chronic valvular heart disease. *Ann Indian Acad Med Sci* 1972;8:48–51.

136. Marcus RH, Sareli P, Pocock WA, et al. Functional anatomy of severe mitral regurgitation in active rheumatic carditis. *Am J Cardiol* 1989;63;577–584.

137. Gross L, Friedberg CK. Lesions of cardiac valve rings in rheumatic fever. *Am J Pathol* 1936;12:469–493.

138. de Moor MM, Lachman PI, Human DG. Rupture of tendinous chords during acute rheumatic carditis in young children. *Int J Cardiol* 1986;12:353–357.

139. Essop MR, Wisenbaugh T, Sareli P. Evidence against a myocardial factor as the cause of left ventricular dilation in active rheumatic carditis. *J Am Coll Cardiol* 1993;22:826–829.

140. Edwards BS, Edwards JE. Congestive heart failure in rheumatic carditis: valvular or myocardial origin. *J Am Coll Cardiol* 1993;22:830–831.

141. Tan AT, Mah PK, Chia BL. Cardiac tamponade in acute rheumatic carditis. *Ann Rheum Dis* 1983;42:699–701.

142. Przybojewski JZ. Rheumatic constrictive pericarditis. A case report and review of the literature. *S Afr Med J* 1981;59:682–686.

143. Bland EF. Chorea as a manifestation of rheumatic fever. A long term perspective. *Trans Am Clin Climatol Assoc* 1961;73:209–213.

144. Folger GM, Hajar R, Robida A, Hajjar HS. Occurrence of valvar heart disease in acute rheumatic fever without evident carditis: color-flow Doppler identification. *Br Heart J* 1992;67:434–439.

145. Abernathy M, Bass N, Sharpe N, et al. Doppler echocardiography and the early diagnosis of carditis in acute rheumatic fever. *Aust N Z J Med* 1994;24:530–535.

146. Brand A, Dollberg S, Keren A. The prevalence of valvular regurgitation in children with structurally normal hearts: a color Doppler echocardiographic study. *Am Heart J* 1992;123:177–180.

147. Veasy LG. Echocardiography for the diagnosis of rheumatic fever. *JAMA* 1993;269:2084.

148. Wilson NJ, Neutze JM. Echocardiographic diagnosis of subclinical carditis in acute rheumatic fever. *Int J Cardiol* 1995;50:1–6.

149. Husby G, van de Rijn I, Zabriskie JB, et al. Antibodies reacting with cytoplasm of subthalamic and caudate nuclei neurons in chorea and acute rheumatic fever. *J Exp Med* 1976;144:1094–1110.

150. Behera M. Subcutaneous nodules in acute rheumatic fever. An analysis of age old dictums. *Indian Heart J* 1993;45:463–467.

151. Burdash NM, Teti G, Hund P. Streptococcal antibody tests in rheumatic fever. *Ann Clin Lab Sci* 1986;16:163–170.

152. Ayoub EM, Wannamaker LW. Evaluation of the streptococcal DNase B and DPNase antibody tests in acute rheumatic fever and glomerulonephritis. *Pediatrics* 1962;29:527–538.

153. Curtis GD, Kraak WA, Mitchell RG. Comparison of latex and hemolysin tests for determination of anti streptolysin O antibodies. *J Clin Pathol* 1988;41:1331–1333.

154. Stollerman GH, Markowitz M, Taranta A, Wannamaker LW, Whittermore R. Jones criteria (revised) for guidance in the diagnosis of rheumatic fever. *Circulation* 1965;32:664–668.

155. Watson KC, Kerr EJC. Partial characterisation of an inhibitor of streptolysin O produced by bacteria growth in serum. *J Med Microbiol* 1975;8:465–476.

156. St. Clair EW, Oddone EZ, Waugh RA, Corey GR, Feussner JR. Assessing housestaff diagnostic skills us-

ing a cardiology patient simulator. *Ann Intern Med* 1992;117:751–756.

157. Mangione S, Nieman L, Gracely E, Kaye D. The teaching and practice of cardiac auscultation during internal medicine and cardiology training. *Ann Intern Med* 1993;119:47–54.

158. Butterworth JS, Reppert EH. Auscultatory acumen in the general medical population. *J Am Med Assoc* 1960; 174:32–34.

159. Folger GM Jr, Hajar R. Doppler echocardiographic findings of mitral and aortic valvular regurgitation in children manifesting only rheumatic arthritis. *Am J Cardiol* 1989;63:1278–1280.

160. Veasy LG, Tani LY, Hill HR. Persistence of acute rheumatic fever in the intermountain area of the United States. *J Pediatr* 1994;125:673–674.

161. Yoshida K, Yoshikawa J, Shakuro M, et al. Color Doppler evaluation of valvular regurgitation in normal subjects. *Circulation* 1988;78:840–847.

162. Berger M, Hecht SR, Van Tosh A, Lingam U. Pulsed and continuos wave Doppler echocardiographic assessment of valvular regurgitation in normal subjects. *J Am Coll Cardiol* 1989;13:1540–1545.

163. Sahn DJ, Maciel BC. Physiological valvular regurgitation: Doppler echocardiography and potential for iatrogenic heart disease. *Circulation* 1988;78:1075–1077.

164. Mason T, Fisher M, Kujala G. Acute rheumatic fever in West Virginia. Not just a disease of children. *Arch Intern Med* 1991;151:133–136.

165. Anonymous. Summary of notifiable diseases—1994. *MMWR Morb Mortal Wkly Rep* 1993;43:53.

166. United Kingdom and United States Joint Report on Rheumatic Heart Disease. The natural history of rheumatic fever and rheumatic heart disease. Ten-year report of a cooperative clinical trial of ACTH, cortisone, and aspirin. *Circulation* 1965;32:457–476.

167. Massell BF. Factors in the pathogenesis of rheumatic fever recurrences. A study of streptococcal infections and rheumatic fever. *J Maine Med Assoc* 1962;53: 88–93.

168. Sanyal SL, Berry AM, Duggal S, et al. Sequelae of the initial attack of acute rheumatic fever in children from North India: a prospective 5-year follow-up study. *Circulation* 1982;65:375–379.

169. Majeed HA, Bhatnagar S, Yousof AM, Khuffash F, Yusuf AR. Acute rheumatic fever and the evolution of rheumatic heart disease: a prospective 12 year follow up report. *J Clin Epidemiol* 1992;45:871–875.

170. Kuttner AG, Mayer FE. Carditis during second attacks of rheumatic fever. Its incidence in patients without clinical evidence of cardiac involvement in their initial rheumatic episode. *N Engl J Med* 1963;268:1259–1261.

171. Feinstein AR, Stern EK. Clinical effects of recurrent attacks of acute rheumatic fever: a prospective epidemiologic study of 105 episodes. *J Chronic Dis* 1967; 20:13–27.

172. Feinstein AR, Wood HF, Spagnuolo M, et al. Rheumatic fever in children and adolescents. VII. Cardiac changes and sequelae. *Ann Intern Med* 1964; 60[Suppl 5]:87–123.

173. Majeed HA, Shaltout A, Yousof AM. Recurrences of acute rheumatic fever: a prospective study of 79 episodes. *Am J Dis Child* 1984;138:341–345.

174. Thomas GT. Five year follow up on patients with

rheumatic fever treated by bed rest, steroids or salicylates. *Br Med J* 1961;1:1635–1639.

175. Adatto IJ, Poske RM, Ponget JM, Pilz CG, Montgomery MM. Rheumatic fever in the adult. *JAMA* 1965;194:1043–1048.

176. Lue HC et al. Clinical and epidemiological features of rheumatic fever and rheumatic heart disease in Taiwan and the Far East. *Indian Heart J* 1983;35:139–146.

177. Taranta A. Should adults with rheumatic heart disease be kept on continuous prophylaxis. *Am J Cardiol* 1966; 18;627–629.

178. Tompkins DG, et al. Long term prognosis of rheumatic fever patients receiving regular intramuscular benzathine penicillin. *Circulation* 1972;45:543–551.

179. Majeed HA, Yousof AM, Khuffash FA, Yusuf AR, Farwana S, Khan N. The natural history of acute rheumatic fever in Kuwait: a prospective six year follow-up report. *J Chronic Dis* 1986;39:361–369.

180. United Kingdom and United States Joint Report on Rheumatic Heart Disease. The evolution of rheumatic heart disease in children. Five-year report of a cooperative clinical trial of ACTH, cortisone, and aspirin. *Circulation* 1960;22:503–515.

181. Bisno AL, Pearce IA, Stollerman GH. Streptococcal infections that fail to cause recurrences of rheumatic fever. *J Infect Dis* 1977;136:278–285.

182. Saslaw MS, Streitfeld MM. Group A beta hemolytic streptococci and rheumatic fever in Miami, Florida. 1. Bacteriologic observations from October 1954 through May 1955. *Dis Chest* 1959;35:175–193.

183. Berrios X, del Campo E, Guzman B, Bisno AL. Discontinuing rheumatic fever prophylaxis in selected adolescents and young adults: a prospective study. *Ann Intern Med* 1993;118:401–406.

184. Kaplan EL, Johnson DR, Cleary PP. Group A streptococcal serotypes isolated from patients and sibling contacts during the resurgence of rheumatic fever in the United States in the mid-1980s. *J Infect Dis* 1989; 159:101–103.

185. Schwartz B, Facklam RR, Breiman RF. Changing epidemiology of group A streptococcal infection in the USA. *Lancet* 1990;336:1167–1171.

186. Johnson DR, Stevens DL, Kaplan EL. Epidemiologics analysis of group A streptococcal serotypes associated with severe systemic infections, rheumatic fever, or uncomplicated pharyngitis. *J Infect Dis* 1992;166: 374–382.

187. Stollerman GH. The use of antibiotics for the prevention of rheumatic fever. *Am J Med* 1954;17:757–767.

188. Stollerman GH. Factors determining the attack rate of rheumatic fever. *JAMA* 1961;77:823–828.

189. Hench PS, Slocumb CH, Barnes AR, Smith HL, Polly HF, Kendall EC. The effects of adrenal cortical hormone (compound E) on the acute phase of rheumatic fever. *Mayo Clin Proc* 1949;25:277–297.

190. Rothman PE. Treatment of rheumatic carditis. A critical review. *Clin Pediatr* 1965;4:619–625.

191. Markowitz M, Kuttner AG. Treatment of acute rheumatic fever. *Am J Dis Child* 1962;104:137–144.

192. Combined Rheumatic Fever Study Group. A comparison of short term intensive prednisone and acetyl salicylic acid therapy in the treatment of acute rheumatic fever. *N Engl J Med* 1965;272:63–70.

193. Stolzer BL, Houser HB, Clark EJ. Therapeutic agents

in rheumatic carditis. *Arch Intern Med* 1955;95: 677–688.

194. Dorfman A, Gross JL, Lorincz AE. The treatment of acute rheumatic fever. *Pediatrics* 1961;27:692–706.

195. Albert DA, Harel L, Karrison T. The treatment of rheumatic carditis. A review and meta analysis. *Medicine (Baltimore)* 1995;74:1–12.

196. Duran CMG, Gometza B, De Vol EB. Valve repair in rheumatic mitral disease. *Circulation* 1991;84[Suppl III]:III-125–III-132.

197. Lewis BS, Geft IL, Milo S, Gotsman MS. Echocardiography and valve replacement in the critically ill patients with acute rheumatic carditis. *Ann Thoracic Surg* 1978;27:529–535.

198. Skoularigis J, Sinovich V, Joubert G, Sareli P. Evaluation of the long term results of mitral valve repair in 254 young patients with rheumatic mitral regurgitation. *Circulation* 1994;90[Pt II]:II-167–II-174.

199. Kehoe MA. Group A streptococcal antigens and vaccine potential. *Vaccine* 1991;9:797–806.

200. Prusakorn S, Currie B, Brandt E, et al. Towards a vaccine for rheumatic fever. Identification of conserved target epitope on M protein of group A streptococci. *Lancet* 1994;344:639–642.

201. Schneider WF, Chapman S, Schule VB, Krause RM, Krupier RC. Prevention of streptococcal pharyngitis among military personnel and their dependents by mass prophylaxis. *N Engl J Med* 1964;270: 1205–1212.

202. Arguedas A, Mohs E. Prevention of rheumatic fever in Costa Rica. *J Pediatr* 1992;121:569–572.

203. Chun LT, Reddy DV, Yamamoto LG. Rheumatic fever in children and adolescents in Hawaii. *Pediatrics* 1987;79:549–552.

204. Michaud C, Ramohan R, Narula J. Cost effectiveness analysis of intervention strategies for reduction of the burden of rheumatic fever. In: Narula J, Virmani R, Reddy KS, Tandon R, eds. *Rheumatic Fever.* Washington, DC: AFIP Press 1999;485–498.

205. Strasser T. Cost-effective control of rheumatic fever in the community. *Health Policy* 1985;5:159–164.

206. Kljakovic M. Sore throat presentation and management in general practice. *N Z Med J* 1993;106:381–383.

207. Krober MS, Bass JW, Michels GN. Streptococcal pharyngitis. Placebo-controlled double-blind evaluation of clinical response to penicillin therapy. *JAMA* 1985;253:1271–1274.

208. Canadian Pediatric Society. Group A streptococcus: a re-emergent pathogen. Infectious Diseases and Immunization Committee. *CMAJ* 1993;148:1909–1911.

209. Cochi SL. Management of pharyngitis in an era of declining rheumatic fever. 86th Ross Conference of Pediatric Research. Columbus, Ohio: Ross Laboratories 1984;51–59.

210. Catanzaro FJ, Stetson CA, Morris AJ, et al. Symposium on rheumatic fever and rheumatic heart disease. *Am J Med* 1954;17:749–756.

211. Seppala H, Nissinen A, Jarvinen H, et al. Resistance to erythromycin in group A streptococci. *N Engl J Med* 1992;326:292–297.

212. Lue HC, Wu MH, Hsieh KH, et al. Rheumatic fever recurrences: controlled study of 3-week versus 4-week benzathine penicillin prevention program. *J Pediatr* 1986;108:299–304.

213. Leu HC, Wu MH, Wang JK, Wu FF, Wu YN. Long term outcome of patients with rheumatic fever receiving benzathine penicillin G prophylaxis every three weeks versus every four weeks. *J Pediatr* 1994;125: 812–816.

214. Padmavati S, Gupta V, Prakash K, Sharma KB. Penicillin for rheumatic fever prophylaxis: 3-weekly or 4-weekly schedule. *J Assoc Physicians India* 1987;35: 753–755.

215. Kassem AS, Madkor AA, Massoud BZ, Zaher SR. Benzathine prophylaxis for rheumatic fever. 2 weekly versus 4 weekly regimens. *Indian J Pediatr* 1992;59: 741–748.

216. Currie BJ, Burt T, Kaplan EL. Penicillin concentrations after increased doses of benzathine penicillin G for prevention of secondary rheumatic fever. *Antimicrob Agents Chemother* 1994;38:1203–1204.

217. Weiss ME, Adkinson NF. Immune hypersensitive reactions to penicillin and related antibiotics. *Clin Allergy* 1988;18:515–540.

218. International Rheumatic Fever Study Group. Allergic reactions to long-term benzathine penicillin prophylaxis for rheumatic fever. *Lancet* 1991;337: 1308–1310.

219. WHO Principle Investigators. WHO Program for the prevention of rheumatic fever and rheumatic heart disease in 16 developing countries. Report from the phase 1 study. *Bull WHO* 1992;70:213–218.

220. Baskin CG, Law S, Wenger NK. Sulfadiazine rheumatic fever prophylaxis during pregnancy: does it increase the risk of kernicterus in the newborn. *Cardiology* 1980;65:220–225.

221. Naiman RA, Barrow JG. Penicillin resistant bacteria in the mouths and throats of children receiving continuous prophylaxis against rheumatic fever. *Ann Intern Med* 1963;58:768–772.

222. Doyle EF, Spagnuolo M, Taranta A, et al. The risk of bacterial endocarditis during anti-rheumatic prophylaxis. *J Am Med Assoc* 1967;201:807–812.

223. Hodes RM. Recurrence of rheumatic fever after valve replacement. *Cardiology* 1989;76:465–468.

224. Stollerman GH. Changing streptococci and prospects for global eradication of rheumatic fever. *Perspect Biol Med* 1997;40:165–189.

225. Lancefield RC. Specific relationship of cell composition to biological activity of hemolytic streptococci. *Harvey Lectures* 1941;35:251.

226. Dale JB, Seyter JM, Beachey EH. Type specific immunogenicity of a chemically synthesized peptide fragment of a type 5 streptococcal M protein. *J Exp Med* 1983;158:1727–1732.

227. Jones KF, Manjula BN, Johnston KH, Hollingshed SK, Scott JR, Fischetti VA. Location of variable and conserved epitopes among the multiple serotypes of streptococcal M protein. *J Exp Med* 1985;161:623–628.

228. Jones KF, Hollingshed SK, Scott JR, Fischetti VA. Spontaneous M6 protein size mutants of group A streptococci display variation in antigenic and opsonogenic epitopes. *Proc Natl Acad Sci USA* 1988;85: 8271–8275.

229. Bessen DE, Hollingshed SK. Allelic polymorphism of emm loci provides evidence for horizontal gene spread in group A streptococci. *Proc Natl Acad Sci USA* 1994: 91:3280–3284.

230. Hartas J, Goodfellow AM, Currie B, SriprakasH KS. Characterisation of group A streptococcal isolates

from tropical Australia with high prevalence of rheumatic fever: probing for signature sequences to identify members of the family of serotype 5. *Microbiol Pathol* 1995;18:345–354.

231. Dale JB, Simmons M, Chiang EC, Chiang EY. Recombitant octavalent group A streptococcal vaccine. *Vaccine* 1996;14:944–948.

232. Dale JB, Chiang EC. Intranasal immunization with recombitant group A streptococcal M protein fragment fused to the B subunit of E ColI labile toxin protects mice against systemic challenge infections. *J Infect Dis* 1995;171:1038–1041.

233. Bessen D, Fischetti VA. Synthetic peptide vaccine against mucosal colonisation by group A streptococci: protection against a heterologous M serotype which shared C repeat region epitopes. *J Immunol* 1990;145: 1251–1256.

234. Jones KF, Fischetti VA. The importance of the location of the antibody binding on the M6 protein for opsonisation and phagocytosis of group A M6 streptococci. *J Exp Med* 1988;167:1114–1123.

235. Bronze MS, Courtney HS, Dale JB. Epitopes of a group A streptococcal M protein that evoke cross protective local immune responses. *J Immunol* 1992;148: 888–893.

236. Bessen D, Fischetti VA. Influence of intranasal immunisation with synthetic peptides corresponding to conserved epitopes of M protein on mucosal colonisation by group A streptococci. *Infect Immun* 1988;56: 2666–2672.

237. Pruksakorn S, Currie BJ, Brandt E, et al. Identification of T cell autoepitopes that cross react with the C terminal segment of the M protein of the group A streptococci. *Int Immunol* 1994;6:1235–1244.

3

Mitral Stenosis

James E. Dalen and Paul E. Fenster

Department of Medicine, University of Arizona College of Medicine, Tucson, Arizona 85724

Mitral stenosis is the prototype of rheumatic heart disease. The mitral valve is the valve most frequently damaged by rheumatic carditis. In the classic study of Bland and Jones (1), 1,000 children treated for acute rheumatic fever at the House of the Good Samaritan in Boston were followed for 20 years. At the end of 20 years, 301 (30%) had died; 91% of these were cardiac deaths, mostly from severe carditis. Of the 699 patients alive 20 years later (average age, 28), 315 (45%) had evidence of rheumatic heart disease; the mitral valve was involved in all but 27 cases. Twenty years after the diagnosis of acute rheumatic fever, only 38% of the patients were alive and without evidence of rheumatic heart disease.

For all intents and purposes, one can assume that mitral stenosis in an adult is due to rheumatic heart disease. This is true even though about one half of patients with mitral stenosis do not give a history of acute rheumatic fever or chorea. The other rare causes of mitral stenosis include congenital mitral stenosis, mitral annular calcification, rheumatoid arthritis, and infective endocarditis.

THE NORMAL MITRAL VALVE

The normal mitral valve has been well described by Roberts and Perloff (2). The larger anterior leaflet does not have a true anulus and is continuous with the wall of the ascending aorta. The posterior leaflet is attached to and is part of the mural endocardium of the left atrium. The two mitral leaflets are attached by 120 chordae to the two papillary muscles. Each leaflet is attached by chordae to both papillary muscles (2). The mitral valve is in essence funnel-shaped (Fig. 3-1), with the apex within the left ventricle.

PATHOLOGIC FEATURES

The initial insult of rheumatic carditis involves the mitral leaflets, causing tiny translucent nodules along the line of closure of the leaflets (3). At this point, even though significant obstruction of the mitral valve is not present, one may hear a diastolic rumble (the Carey Coombs murmur) or a blowing systolic murmur at the apex (1). These murmurs are particularly likely to be heard when carditis has caused significant cardiac enlargement and tend to disappear as carditis resolves and heart size returns to normal (1). It takes decades from the onset of rheumatic carditis until significant symptomatic obstruction of the mitral valve occurs. In Wood's series (4), the latency period from acute rheumatic fever (average age, 12) until the onset of cardiac symptoms due to mitral stenosis (average age, 31) was 19 years.

The explanation for the long latency period is not clear. Smoldering rheumatic carditis has been suggested in the past; however, the hypothesis of Selzer and Cohn (3) seems more plausible. They suggested that the initial valvulitis (at the time of rheumatic carditis)

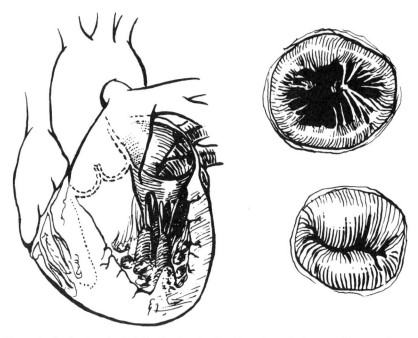

FIG. 3-1. Normal mitral valve. **Left:** Mitral valve *in situ*. Note funnel shape, with apex formed by papillary muscles. **Right:** Mitral valve shown from the left atrium during diastole (*top*) and systole (*bottom*).

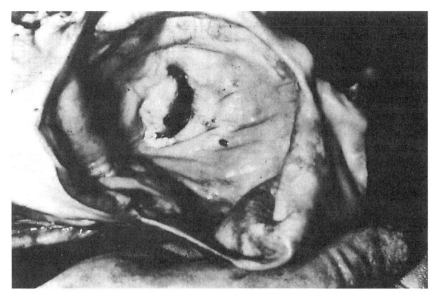

FIG. 3-2. Stenotic mitral valve as seen from the left atrium.

causes an abnormal flow pattern across the valve leaflets that eventually leads to thickening, fibrosis, and possible calcification of the valve cusps. This hypothesis is consistent with current concepts of the mechanism by which a nonobstructive congenital bicuspid aortic valve evolves (without smoldering carditis) into calcific aortic stenosis over a period of decades. It should be noted that this latency period is considerably shortened in certain third world nations such as India, the Philippines, and Kenya. In these countries, symptomatic mitral stenosis often occurs before age 20 (3,5,6). Attacks of rheumatic carditis are assumed to be more severe and/or more frequent in these countries.

When mitral stenosis is symptomatic, the anatomic features consist of thickened mitral cusps with or without calcific deposits, fusion of the valve commissures, and shortening and fusion of the chordae tendineae (2) (Fig. 3-2). Although the major obstruction to diastolic flow from the left atrium to the left ventricle in patients with mitral stenosis is usually due to fusion of the commissures, it may be below the valve itself, secondary to fusion of the chordae.

MEASUREMENT OF MITRAL VALVE OBSTRUCTION

The cross-sectional area of the normal mitral valve is 4 cm^2. There is no detectable pressure gradient across the normal mitral valve, even with increased flow as with exercise. The pioneering work of Gorlin and Gorlin in 1951 (7) made it possible to calculate the effective mitral valve area (MVA) at cardiac catheterization in patients with varying degrees of mitral stenosis. Their studies and applications of basic hydraulic formulas indicated that if one can measure the flow across the mitral valve and the simultaneous pressure gradient across the valve (i.e., left atrial mean diastolic pressure minus left ventricular mean diastolic pressure), one can calculate the MVA in square centimeters.

Mitral valve flow is measured by dividing cardiac output (mL/min) by the product of heart rate (beats/min) and the diastolic filling period per beat in seconds. The resultant calculated mitral valve flow is therefore expressed as mL flow/s diastole. The normal mitral valve flow is approximately 150 mL/s diastole (8). When cardiac output increases, mitral valve flow increases. If heart rate increases, the seconds of diastole per beat decreases because tachycardia shortens diastole more than systole; therefore, tachycardia increases mitral valve flow.

Left atrial mean diastolic pressure (LA$_{DM}$) may be measured directly by means of transseptal catheterization of the left atrium, or it can be measured by accurate measurement of pulmonary capillary wedge pressure (9). The resultant formula for MVA is therefore

$$\text{MVA (cm}^2) = \frac{\text{cardiac output (mL/min)}}{38 \, (\text{La}_{DM} - \text{LV}_{DM}) \times \text{heart rate} \times \text{diastolic filling period}}$$

or

$$\text{MVA} = \frac{\text{mitral valve flow (mL/s diastolic)}}{38 \, (\text{LA}_{DM} - \text{LV}_{DM})}$$

The number 38 is a constant based on certain assumptions. These assumptions have proved to be appropriate in that calculated MVA correlates well with MVA as measured at operation and with MVA as measured by cross-sectional echocardiography (10,11).

Pitfalls in the calculation of MVA by the Gorlin and Gorlin formula are as follows:

1. Conventional means of measuring cardiac output only measure forward flow; therefore, if mitral regurgitation is present, true mitral valve flow, which includes the regurgitant flow, is underestimated. In the presence of mitral regurgitation, therefore, calculated MVA is underestimated.
2. For the calculations to be accurate, the measurements of cardiac output, heart rate, diastolic filling period, and the pressure gradient must be simultaneous (12).
3. If the wedge pressure is to be used as a measure of left atrial pressure, the

catheter position must be confirmed by withdrawing a blood sample and showing that it is fully saturated (9). Confirmation of the wedge pressure by inspection of the contour of the pressure tracing, coupled with fluoroscopic evidence that the catheter is in a distal position, is not adequate.

By quantifying the degree of mitral valve obstruction, the measured MVA helps to explain the pathophysiology features of mitral stenosis.

The prime symptoms of mitral stenosis are caused by pulmonary venous hypertension. Pulmonary venous pressure is the same as pulmonary capillary pressure. As shown in Fig. 3-3, if one knows two of three variables, namely, MVA, mitral valve gradient, or mitral valve flow, one can easily predict the third variable. Thus, if a patient has a fixed MVA and mitral valve flow is increased (e.g., due to increased cardiac output), the gradient across the obstructed mitral valve will increase. The

symptoms of pulmonary venous hypertension will appear. In the presence of tight mitral stenosis (i.e., MVA $\leq$ 1.0 cm^2), the mitral valve gradient at rest, with normal mitral valve flow, will be sufficient to cause symptomatic pulmonary venous hypertension.

SYMPTOMS AND COMPLICATIONS

Pulmonary Venous Hypertension

Dyspnea, Orthopnea, and Paroxysmal Nocturnal Dyspnea

As pulmonary venous pressure increases, fluid is driven out of the pulmonary capillaries. This transudate decreases the compliance of the lungs and increases the work of breathing. The resultant symptom is dyspnea. One can see that with exercise this process is accelerated; thus, dyspnea increases on exertion. The supine position increases pulmonary venous pressure, leading to the symptoms of orthopnea and paroxysmal nocturnal dyspnea.

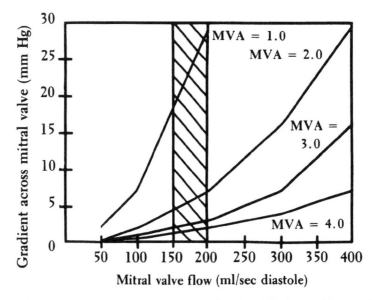

FIG. 3-3. The gradient across mitral valves of various sizes is plotted according to mitral valve flow. Note that when mitral valve flow is in the normal range (150 to 200 mL/s diastole), the gradient across a mitral valve with an area of 3.0 cm^2 is approximately 2 mm Hg. When the MVA is 2.0 cm^2, the gradient is 4 to 6 mm Hg. With an MVA of 1.0 cm^2, the gradient with normal mitral valve flow is 18 to 28 mm Hg.

Acute Pulmonary Edema

If pulmonary capillary pressure exceeds the tissue oncotic pressure of approximately 25 mm Hg and if the lymphatics are unable to decompress the resultant transudated fluid, acute pulmonary edema develops. Pulmonary edema may occur gradually and may be preceded by orthopnea and paroxysmal nocturnal dyspnea in a patient with tight mitral stenosis, or it may occur suddenly. Indeed, it can be one of the first overt signs of mitral stenosis. The sudden appearance of acute pulmonary edema can occur in patients with noncritical mitral stenosis (i.e., MVA ≥ 1.4 cm^2) if conditions occur that cause an abrupt increase in mitral valve flow. Such conditions include the following:

1. The onset of atrial fibrillation (AF) with a rapid ventricular response. This increases mitral valve flow by shortening the duration of diastole per beat.
2. Intercurrent conditions that increase cardiac output (e.g., thyrotoxicosis, pneumonia, and surgery, particularly if complicated by fluid overload, tachycardia, and fever) may increase mitral valve flow, causing the wedge pressure to reach pulmonary edema levels.
3. Pregnancy is one of the most common precipitants of pulmonary edema in patients with noncritical mitral stenosis. Pregnancy increases mitral valve flow by increasing cardiac output, heart rate, and the central blood volume. These effects are maximal at 25 to 27 weeks of gestation (13). Because more than two thirds of patients with mitral stenosis are women, such patients commonly give a history of the symptoms of pulmonary venous hypertension (often including pulmonary edema) during pregnancy. If the patient has noncritical mitral stenosis, these symptoms will abate postpartum, and symptoms of pulmonary venous hypertension may not reappear for several years, when the degree of mitral valve obstruction has become critical.

Hemoptysis

Wood (4) pointed out at least five causes of hemoptysis in patients with mitral stenosis. The most severe is sudden unexpected profuse hemorrhage of bright red blood (pulmonary apoplexy). This almost certainly results from a sudden increase in pulmonary venous pressure, and it may be one of the first signs of mitral stenosis. Such hemoptysis can be massive, requiring emergency surgery (3). Profuse hemoptysis of this type is an indication for mitral valve surgery. The other potential causes of hemoptysis in patients with mitral stenosis are

1. Blood-streaked sputum associated with attacks of dyspnea;
2. Blood-streaked sputum in association with attacks of bronchitis;
3. Pink frothy sputum accompanying acute pulmonary edema;
4. Hemoptysis due to pulmonary embolism inducing pulmonary infarction. In this circumstance, one should expect to find other evidence of pulmonary infarction such as infiltrate by x-ray and pleuritic pain (14).

"Winter Bronchitis"

Many clinicians believe that patients with mitral stenosis are prone to the development of attacks of bronchitis, particularly in the winter. Wood (4) reported winter bronchitis in 28% of 150 patients with mitral stenosis sufficiently severe to warrant surgical relief. Their average preoperative left atrial pressure was 23 mm Hg, indicating significant pulmonary venous hypertension. Spencer (15) pointed out that any condition that causes chronic passive congestion of the lung can cause chronic bronchial hyperemia. Such hyperemia causes hypersecretion of serous glands, leading to excessive bronchial mucus production. Mitral stenosis, as one of the common causes of chronic passive congestion of the lungs, may lead to the symptoms of bronchitis.

Pulmonary Vascular Disease

As mitral valve obstruction increases, left atrial, pulmonary venous, and wedge pressures increase. An increase in wedge pressure causes an obligatory increase in the pulmonary artery (PA) mean pressure if blood is to flow across the pulmonary bed. The average gradient across the pulmonary bed (i.e., PA mean minus left atrial mean pressure) is 10 to 12 mm Hg. If left atrial mean pressure increased to 20 mm Hg, PA mean pressure would be expected to increase to about 30 mm Hg. In this circumstance, the patient has pulmonary hypertension in that the normal PA mean pressure is 12 ± 2 mm Hg (16). The pulmonary hypertension, however, is entirely passive. That is, the observed pulmonary hypertension is completely explained by the increase in left atrial pressure.

Most patients with mitral stenosis have passive pulmonary hypertension (Fig. 3-4); however, in some patients, PA pressure rises out of proportion to the increase in wedge pressure (Fig. 3-5). In this circumstance, the gradient across the pulmonary bed may be even greater than the obstruction across the narrowed mitral valve. Such patients have pulmonary vascular disease or "reactive pulmonary hypertension." It would appear that pulmonary vascular disease is in some way related to the magnitude of the increase in pulmonary venous pressure (and thus in wedge pressure).

As shown in Fig. 3-6, reactive pulmonary hypertension is rare unless mitral stenosis is sufficiently severe to cause a pulmonary capillary pressure at rest of 20 to 25 mm Hg or more. Reactive pulmonary hypertension, however, does not occur in all patients who have grossly elevated wedge pressures. Some patients with severe left atrial hypertension continue to have a normal PA to left atrial gradient (i.e., they do not have reactive pulmonary hypertension) (Fig. 3-6). The reason reactive pulmonary hypertension develops in some patients with severe mitral stenosis (as reflected by severe left atrial hypertension) and not in others remains a mystery. One might assume that its incidence is due to the duration of left atrial hypertension; however, when we compared the PA–left atrial gradient to the duration of symptoms in 100 patients with pure mitral stenosis, we found no correlation (16). Reactive pulmonary hypertension

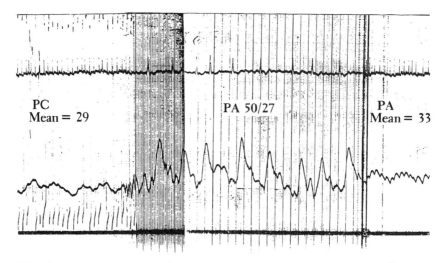

FIG. 3-4. Right heart pressures in a patient with tight mitral stenosis (MVA = 0.8 cm²). The mean pulmonary capillary wedge pressure is 29 mm Hg; the mean pulmonary artery pressure is 33 mm Hg. The gradient across the pulmonary bed is therefore only 4 mm Hg, indicating that the pulmonary hypertension is entirely passive.

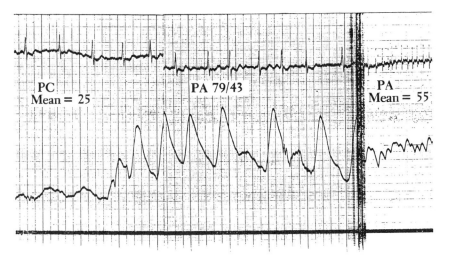

FIG. 3-5. Right heart pressures in a patient with tight mitral stenosis (MVA = 0.5 cm²), complicated by reactive pulmonary hypertension. Note that the gradient across the pulmonary bed (pulmonary artery mean pressure minus pulmonary capillary mean pressure) is grossly elevated at 30 mm Hg.

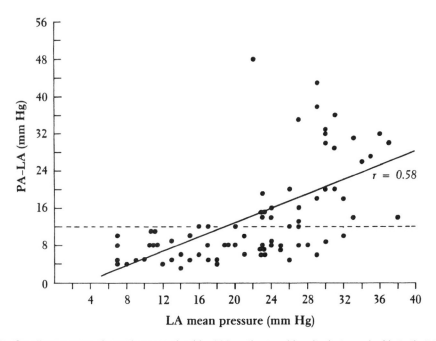

FIG. 3-6. Gradient across the pulmonary bed in 100 patients with mitral stenosis. Note that the gradient across the pulmonary bed remains normal; thus, reactive pulmonary hypertension does not occur, unless the left atrial mean pressure is at least 20 mm Hg. Also note that the pulmonary artery to left atrial gradient remains normal in some patients even when left atrial pressure is grossly elevated.

developed quickly in some patients with se-vere mitral stenosis. Others had symptoms of mitral stenosis for years without the development of reactive pulmonary hypertension.

A variety of theories and hypotheses for the cause of reactive pulmonary hypertension in patients with mitral stenosis has been presented and reviewed by Jordan (17):

1. Wood (18) proposed pulmonary vasoconstriction as the cause. He noted, however, that it did not occur in all patients with severe mitral stenosis and concluded that just what determines this vasoconstrictive response is unknown.
2. Doyle et al. (19) suggested that the pressure increase in the pulmonary veins of the lower lobes (where it is maximal in mitral stenosis) produces reflex arterial constriction.
3. Heath and Harris (20) extended this hypothesis to state that increased PA pressure causes reflex pulmonary arteriolar vasoconstriction; this causes a further increase in PA pressure, which causes further pulmonary vasoconstriction.
4. Welch et al. (21) attributed pulmonary vascular disease to obliteration of the pulmonary capillary bed by alveolar fibrosis. However, this hypothesis is inconsistent with the reversibility of pulmonary hypertension after successful surgical relief of mitral valve obstruction (22–24).
5. Jordan's (17) hypothesis is that increased pulmonary venous pressure causes fluid to pass into the alveolar walls, particularly in the lower lobes. Much of the fluid is removed by the lymphatics; however, residual fluid causes thickening and eventually fibrosis of the alveolar walls. Such fibrosis causes hypoventilation of the lower lobes, with resultant hypoxemia in the lower lobe pulmonary veins. The hypoxemia is sensed by chemoreceptors in the pulmonary veins, causing pulmonary arterial vasoconstriction in the region supplying these alveoli; as a result lower lobe perfusion decreases. The process eventually involves the middle and upper lung fields.

Most of these theories invoke pulmonary vasoconstriction. These theories are consistent with the decrease in PA pressure and pulmonary vascular resistance that occurs within days of surgery (23,25). None of these theories, however, explains why reactive pulmonary hypertension occurs in some patients with severe mitral stenosis but not in others. This is analogous to the situation of patients with secundum atrial septal defect: Severe pulmonary hypertension develops in some patients with atrial septal defect at an early age (third or fourth decade), whereas others may survive for decades without pulmonary hypertension (26).

Sequelae of Reactive Pulmonary Hypertension

The primary burden of reactive pulmonary hypertension (which may reach systemic levels) must be borne by the right ventricle. Right ventricular hypertension can be detected by electrocardiography (ECG) and physical examination and can be measured by Doppler echocardiography, if tricuspid regurgitation is present. The size of the right ventricle and the pulmonary arteries increases, as noted on the roentgenogram. The early work of Gorlin et al. (27) demonstrated that as pulmonary vascular disease (as measured by pulmonary vascular resistance) increases, right ventricular stroke volume decreases, with a resultant decrease in cardiac output. Others have also reported that cardiac output is decreased in patients with reactive pulmonary hypertension (pulmonary vascular disease) (3,18). Some have speculated that the decrease in cardiac output associated with pulmonary vascular disease has a protective effect, that is, it prevents or lessens the probability of pulmonary edema (12,18). Other observations have cast doubt on the concept that pulmonary vascular disease has such a protective effect (3,28).

Most patients with mitral stenosis complicated by reactive pulmonary hypertension are incapacitated and are class IV by New York Heart Association (NYHA) standards (class V by the authors' classification) (Table 3-1).

TABLE 3-1. *Stages of mitral stenosis*

Class	MVA (cm^2)	Symptoms
1. Minimal	>2.5	None
2. Mild	1.4–2.5	Dyspnea with exertion
3. Moderate	1.0–1.4	Dyspnea, orthopnea, paroxysmal nocturnal dyspnea, ±pulmonary edema
4. Severe	<1.0	Resting dyspnea; disabled (NYHA class IV); bed-chair
5. Reactive pulmonary hypertension	<1.0	As in severe disease, plus fatigue and right ventricular failure

MVA, mitral valve area; NYHA, New York Heart Association.

Eventually, the right ventricle may dilate and fail in response to severe pulmonary hypertension. Functional tricuspid regurgitation may occur, and the resultant murmur may be confused with the murmur of mitral regurgitation. With the advent of right ventricular failure, the neck veins distend, and hepatomegaly and peripheral edema appear. With longstanding right ventricular failure, ascites, cardiac cirrhosis, and cardiac cachexia may appear.

An unusual complication of severe pulmonary hypertension secondary to mitral stenosis is hoarseness resulting from paralysis of the left recurrent laryngeal nerve. This paralysis is due to compression of the nerve between the enlarged tense left PA and the aorta at the ligamentum arteriosum. By 1966, 142 such cases had been reported (29). Of eight such patients who survived surgical therapy, six recovered vocal cord function.

Other Complications

Atrial Fibrillation

AF is one of the most common complications of mitral stenosis. It may occur as paroxysmal episodes or as a sustained arrhythmia. In the former case, the patient may give a history of palpitations. In the latter case (persistent AF), it may cause the patient to seek medical attention because of symptoms of pulmonary venous hypertension.

The impact of AF on the patient with mitral stenosis depends almost entirely on the ventricular rate (30). As heart rate increases, the seconds of diastole per beat decrease; there-

fore, mitral valve flow (mL/s diastole) increases. In the presence of mitral stenosis, increased mitral valve flow causes increased left atrial and pulmonary venous pressure. The loss of atrial contraction per se has minimal impact on the patient with significant mitral stenosis (31). Unlike the situation in normal patients, atrial contraction does not cause an increase in flow across an obstructed mitral valve. This is reflected as a loss of the A wave in the M-mode echocardiogram of mitral stenosis patients who are in normal sinus rhythm.

Contrary to prior belief, the size of the fibrillatory waves in lead V_1 is unrelated to the size of the left atrium or even to the cause of AF. Coarse AF, which has large fibrillatory waves in V_1, does not correlate well with the presence or absence of mitral valve disease or with the size of the left atrium as detected by echocardiogram (32,33).

In most series of patients with mitral stenosis, the incidence of AF is about 40%; however, the incidence is clearly related to age, according to Deverall et al. (34) (Table 3-2). Echocardiographic studies by Henry et al. (35) showed a close correlation between left atrial size and AF. When the left atrium was smaller than 40 mm,

TABLE 3-2. *Age and AF in mitral stenosis*

Age when first seen (yr)	Number	% in AF
11–20	10	0
21–30	55	17
31–40	88	45
41–50	101	60
Over 51	44	80

AF, atrial fibrillation.
From ref. 34, with permission.

only 3 of 117 patients had AF; however, when the left atrium was larger than 40 mm, 80 of 148 patients (54%) had AF.

The most important impact of AF on the patient with mitral stenosis is that it greatly increases the probability of systemic embolism. The presence of AF in a patient with mitral valve disease is a clear indication for long-term anticoagulation (goal international normalized ratio (INR), 2.5; range, 2.0 to 3.0).

Systemic Embolism

Systemic emboli occur in patients with mitral stenosis because of the formation of clots within the left atrium, especially within the left atrial appendage. Systemic embolism appears to be unrelated to the severity of mitral stenosis. It may be the first symptom of mitral stenosis in a previously asymptomatic patient with mild mitral stenosis. A particularly tragic fact is that cerebral emboli are particularly common, accounting for 60% to 70% of episodes of systemic embolism in several reports (3,34). The exact incidence of systemic embolism in patients with mitral stenosis is difficult to assess. Some emboli may cause transient symptoms and go undetected.

Ellis and Harken (36) reported that in 1,500 consecutive patients undergoing mitral valvuloplasty, 18% had a definite history of systemic embolism before surgery. Deverall et al. (34) reported that 16% of 298 patients being evaluated for mitral stenosis had a history of systemic embolism.

Emboli are often fatal in patients with mitral stenosis. In a 10-year follow-up of 250 patients with unoperated mitral stenosis, Rowe et al. (37) found that 19% of 110 deaths in the first 10 years of follow-up were due to arterial embolism. In the follow-up series of Olesen (38), 22% of all deaths in patients with mitral stenosis were due to thromboembolism.

The two factors most closely associated with systemic embolism in patients with mitral stenosis are age and the presence of AF. The size of the left atrium is relevant in that as it enlarges it increases the probability of AF (39). In the classic series of Coulshed et al.

(40), 737 patients with predominant mitral stenosis were followed. Of 248 patients 35 years old or less (with normal sinus rhythm or AF), the incidence of embolization was 9%. Of 489 patients over 35, the incidence was 24%. Deverall et al. (34) found that the incidence of systemic emboli correlates better with years since initial rheumatic activity than with chronologic age per se.

As previously noted, the other major factor affecting the occurrence of systemic embolism is the presence of AF. Nearly all observers reported that most mitral stenosis patients who have systemic emboli are in AF. The relative impact of age and AF is somewhat hard to unravel, because the incidence of AF in patients with mitral stenosis increases with age. Coulshed et al. (40), however, showed that the presence of AF increases the probability of systemic embolism in young patients and in older patients with mitral stenosis (Table 3-3). Bannister (41) followed 105 patients with mitral stenosis who were not operated on because they were asymptomatic (class I) or had trivial symptoms (class II) for an average of 4.5 years. Systemic embolism occurred in 22 patients (21%) and was fatal in 5. Emboli were closely associated with the presence of AF and with age. More than half of these patients with mild mitral stenosis who were over age 40 and who had AF had systemic embolism during the short follow-up period of 4.5 years.

These data should make it clear that patients with mitral stenosis who are in AF or have a history of systemic embolism require long-term anticoagulation with warfarin at a dose sufficient to prolong the INR to 2.5 (range, 2.0

TABLE 3-3. *Incidence of systemic embolism in 737 patients with mitral stenosis*

Age (yr)	Rhythm	Number	% with emboli
≤35	Normal sinus rhythm	197	5
>35	Normal sinus rhythm	195	11
≤35	AF	51	27
>35	AF	294	32

AF, atrial fibrillation.
From ref. 40, with permission.

to 3.0) (42). Anticoagulation should be considered in patients in sinus rhythm who are aged 35 or older. Mitral valve disease is one of the diseases most commonly predisposing to systemic embolism and should be sought in all patients who present with systemic embolism.

Infective Endocarditis

Although the mitral valve is frequently affected by infective endocarditis, endocarditis is relatively uncommon in isolated mitral stenosis (3,43,44).

In the 10-year follow-up of medically treated mitral stenosis (in the preantibiotic era) by Rowe et al. (37), 5% of all deaths were due to endocarditis. In Olesen's series (38), at the end of an average 11 years of follow-up, 8% of all deaths were due to infections. Endocarditis is more frequent when mitral stenosis is complicated by mitral regurgitation or aortic regurgitation (3). Even though the reported incidence of infective endocarditis in patients with isolated mitral stenosis is less than with some other forms of valvular heart disease, antibiotic prophylaxis is clearly indicated. When endocarditis does occur in patients with mitral stenosis, it may cause mitral regurgitation or, rarely, it may increase the degree of stenosis (45). The complications of mitral stenosis are summarized in Table 3-4.

PRESENTATION

AF, systemic embolism, hemoptysis, or infective endocarditis may occur at any point in the course of mitral stenosis; however, symptoms related to pulmonary venous hypertension are closely related to the MVA, as shown in Table 3-1. Note in Table 3-1 that symptoms related to pulmonary venous hypertension do not occur unless the MVA is less than 2.5 cm^2. Also note that with a valve area of 1.4 to 2.5 cm^2, a very significant increase in mitral valve flow would have to occur before pulmonary venous pressure would rise high enough to cause dyspnea. Dyspnea, therefore, occurs only with exertion in patients with MVAs of 1.4 to 2.5 cm^2. Patients in class III (MVA 1.0 to 1.4 cm^2) have symptoms with ordinary activity; that is, with near normal mitral valve flow, the gradient across the obstructed valve causes the symptoms of pulmonary venous hypertension.

Patients in class IV have symptoms at rest. They correspond to NYHA class IV patients (i.e., they usually lead a bed-chair existence). As noted, in some class IV patients (i.e., patients with resting wedge pressure of 25 mm Hg or more), reactive pulmonary hypertension and right ventricular failure may develop. These patients are cardiac invalids and are classified here as class V.

TABLE 3-4. *Complications of mitral stenosis*

Unrelated to severity of mitral stenosis
  AF
  Systemic embolism
  Infective endocarditis
Related severity of mitral stenosis (as reflected by pulmonary venous pressure)
  Dyspnea
  Orthopnea, paroxysmal nocturnal dyspnea
  Pulmonary edema
  Hemoptysis (pulmonary apoplexy)
  "Winter bronchitis"
Related to reactive pulmonary hypertension (always preceded by severe mitral stenosis)
  Decreased exercise tolerance, fatigue
  Right ventricular failure
    Edema, hepatomegaly, with or without ascites
    Cardiac cirrhosis
    Cardiac cachexia
  Hoarseness (due to paralyzed left recurrent laryngeal nerve)

AF, atrial fibrillation.

DIAGNOSIS

Physical Findings

Although there are multiple clues to the presence of mitral stenosis by physical examination (Table 3-5), they often are subtle and are likely to be overlooked during a routine physical examination of an asymptomatic patient. The diagnosis of mitral stenosis is often first suspected when it causes one of the complications noted in Table 3-4. Once the diagnosis of mitral stenosis has been suspected, a careful physical examination usually confirms it.

By palpation, the point of maximal impulse is normal or small. A prominent point of maximal impulse is a clue to associated disease involving the left ventricle (e.g., mitral regurgitation, aortic valve disease, or systemic hypertension). A diastolic thrill might be felt at the apex; in this circumstance, one can expect to hear a very loud diastolic rumble. A parasternal lift is usually present if mitral stenosis is complicated by significant pulmonary hypertension.

A loud first heart sound (S_1) associated with closure of the diseased mitral valve is an important finding and may in fact be the first auscultatory finding to emerge in patients with mitral stenosis (46). A loud S_1 in the presence of AF should always alert the clinician to search for other evidence of mitral stenosis. A soft S_1 in patients with significant

mitral stenosis may be due to calcification of the mitral valve, associated mitral regurgitation, or aortic insufficiency. A third heart sound (S_3) is rarely heard in significant mitral stenosis because rapid filling of the left ventricle is prevented by the stenotic mitral valve.

A classic finding in mitral stenosis is the presence of an opening snap (OS). The OS may occur from 0.03 to 0.1 seconds after the second heart sound (S_2). As the severity of mitral stenosis increases and left atrial pressure rises, the mitral valve opens earlier and the S_2–OS interval decreases (47). An S_2–OS interval less than 0.08 seconds usually means tight mitral stenosis. An absent OS in significant mitral stenosis may be caused by calcification of the mitral valve.

The most diagnostic finding in patients with mitral stenosis is the presence of a diastolic rumble. This is best heard with the bell of the stethoscope lightly applied to the chest, with the patient in the left lateral position. One must explore the area between the apex and the lower left sternal border because the murmur may only be audible over a very small area of the precordium. In the early stages of mitral stenosis, the diastolic rumble is confined to mid-diastole. To hear the murmur, it may be necessary to listen to the patient after he or she has exercised. As the stenotic process progresses, the murmur extends to the S_1, often with presystolic accentuation (48,49). The presystolic component of the diastolic murmur (Fig. 3-7) is very important in that its presence makes it very unlikely that the patient has associated significant mitral regurgitation. In the past, it was taught that the crescendo presystolic murmur or mitral stenosis disappears when AF develops; however, Criley and Hermer (50) clearly documented that in AF, after short RR intervals, a definite crescendo presystolic murmur may occur and may be documented by phonocardiogram. With increasing severity, the diastolic rumble may occupy all of diastole.

It should be reemphasized that the classic diastolic rumble of mitral stenosis is easily missed. In our experience, the most sensitive auscultatory clue to the presence of mitral

TABLE 3-5. *Physical findings in mitral stenosis*

Palpation
  Point of maximal impulse is normal or decreased
  Right ventricular heave is present if patient has
    pulmonary hypertension
  Apical diastolic thrill may be present
Auscultation
  Loud S_1
  Opening snap
  Diastolic rumble, near apex
    Mid-diastolic
    Presystolic
    Pandiastolic
  Variably present
    Loud P_2
    Murmur of mitral regurgitation
    Murmur of tricuspid regurgitation

stenosis is the triple cadence of a loud S_1, normal S_2, and then the OS. This is easily appreciated, even with the diaphragm of the stethoscope. When this distinctive triple cadence is heard, a careful search with the bell usually reveals the classic diastolic rumble.

The presence of a pansystolic murmur at the apex could be caused by associated mitral regurgitation or by tricuspid regurgitation. If the systolic murmur is due to mitral regurgitation, it often radiates to the axilla and may be accompanied by an S_3 gallop. As noted, in the presence of mitral regurgitation, the S_1 is soft, and the presystolic component of the mitral stenosis murmur may be lost. With associated mitral regurgitation, the point of maximal impulse may be hyperkinetic. If the systolic murmur is due to tricuspid regurgitation, it may be loudest at the lower left sternal edge, increasing with inspiration. Tricuspid regurgitation in association with mitral stenosis is usually functional, that is, secondary to

pulmonary and therefore right ventricular hypertension. In the presence of tricuspid regurgitation therefore, one would expect to find a parasternal lift and signs of right ventricular hypertrophy by ECG.

A decrescendo diastolic blowing murmur may be heard along the left sternal border. In the past, this had been considered to be the Graham-Steele murmur of pulmonic insufficiency (secondary to pulmonary hypertension). Aortography demonstrates that the most common cause of a blowing diastolic murmur along the left sternal border in patients with mitral stenosis is associated aortic regurgitation. As noted by Bland and Jones (1), rheumatic carditis very frequently involves the aortic and the mitral valve.

A loud pulmonic component of S_2 (P_2) is suggestive but not diagnostic of pulmonary hypertension. A parasternal heave is far more specific for pulmonary hypertension in patients with mitral stenosis.

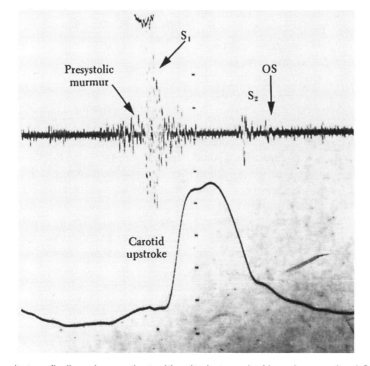

FIG. 3-7. Auscultatory findings in a patient with mitral stenosis. Note the very loud S_1, the opening snap, and the presystolic murmur that occurs just before the carotid upstroke.

Additional extracardiac physical findings depend on whether pulmonary hypertension is present and is sufficiently severe to have caused right ventricular failure. With right ventricular failure, the neck veins are distended and the liver is enlarged and often tender to palpation. Peripheral edema is usually present. With chronic right ventricular failure, ascites and cardiac cirrhosis with mild jaundice may occur.

"Mitral facies" is sometimes noted in severe mitral stenosis with low cardiac output and peripheral vasoconstriction. In addition to peripheral cyanosis, the lips and face may be cyanotic (4,46). Despite the cyanosis, there may be a malar flush or florid countenance as described by Levine (46). Sokolow and McIlroy (51) attribute the malar flush to dilated veins in the cheeks. All agree that these findings are limited to patients who have far-advanced mitral stenosis with a low cardiac output.

Electrocardiographic Findings

As mentioned earlier, nearly half of patients presenting with mitral stenosis have AF, and the incidence of AF increases with age. The size of the fibrillatory waves in lead V_1 (i.e., coarse vs. fine fibrillation) is unrelated to left atrial size and does not help to determine the cause of AF (32,33).

Patients still in normal sinus rhythm usually have signs of P mitrale. The most consistent sign of P mitrale is a widened P wave in lead II that may be notched, bifid, or have a flat top (Fig. 3-8). The terminal portion of the P wave in lead V_1 is usually negative in patients with left atrial enlargement. The latter finding is not specific for mitral valve disease and can occur in left ventricular failure from any cause. P pulmonale may develop in the presence of severe pulmonary hypertension.

Right ventricular hypertrophy is highly suggestive of pulmonary hypertension as is right axis deviation (8). Right ventricular hypertrophy in patients with mitral stenosis is ominous. Because the mortality without surgery is high, right ventricular hypertrophy

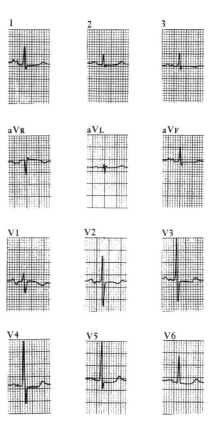

FIG. 3-8. P mitrale in a patient with mitral stenosis. Note the wide-notched P waves, particularly in leads II and III.

is considered by most clinicians to be an indication for surgical correction of mitral stenosis. If the patient has signs of significant pulmonary hypertension by physical examination or chest roentgenography but does not show evidence of right ventricular hypertrophy by ECG, one should look for another lesion causing left ventricular hypertrophy (e.g., mitral regurgitation, aortic valve disease, systemic hypertension). Overt left ventricular hypertrophy or combined ventricular hypertrophy also should alert the clinician to look for additional cardiac lesions.

Roentgenographic Findings

The most frequent roentgenographic findings in mitral stenosis are shown in Table 3-6.

TABLE 3-6. *Roentgenographic findings in mitral stenosis*

Left atrial enlargement
Redistribution of venous and arterial flow to upper lobes
Calcification of mitral valve
Kerley B lines
Enlarged pulmonary artery
Enlarged right ventricle

Left Atrial Enlargement

Left atrial enlargement is one of the earliest signs of mitral stenosis; however, its presentation may be subtle and limited to enlargement of the left atrial appendage, causing a straightening of the left heart border (Fig. 3-9). In more advanced cases, the left atrium is recognized as a double density on the posteroanterior film. Left atrial size by roentgenography is best quantified by a lateral view with barium in the esophagus. In this circumstance, isolated mitral stenosis with an enlarged left atrium causes posterior deviation of the esophagus. With significant left atrial enlargement, the left main stem bronchus may be elevated. Extreme left atrial enlargement, when the right heart border approaches or touches the right chest wall, is not seen in mitral stenosis. In ten such cases reported by DeSanctis et al. (52), all ten patients had significant mitral regurgitation. It is of interest that four patients reported slight to moderate dysphagia. Plaschkes et al. (53) reported that of 18 patients with a giant left atrium, all 18 had significant mitral regurgitation.

Redistribution of Blood Flow

Redistribution of blood flow to the upper lobes is characteristic of mitral stenosis (Fig. 3-10). This correlates best with the degree of mitral valve obstruction when it involves the venous and arterial circulation (54).

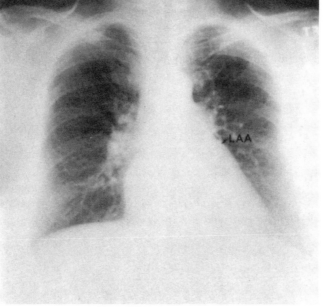

FIG. 3-9. Posteroanterior chest roentgenogram of a patient with mitral stenosis. Note the straightening of the left heart border due to enlargement of the left atrial appendage (*LAA*).

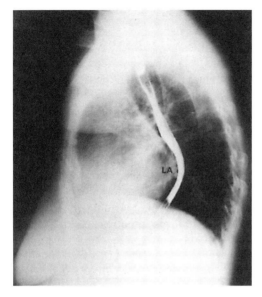

FIG. 3-10. Lateral chest roentgenogram during barium swallow in a patient with mitral stenosis. Note the discrete posterior deviation of the barium-filled esophagus due to the enlarged left atrium (*LA*). (This is the same patient as in Fig. 3-9.)

rior to the left ventricular endocardium (57,58). Studies using Doppler echocardiography have shown that MAC may cause mitral regurgitation or, even less commonly, mitral stenosis in patients without rheumatic heart disease (59). The presence of functional mitral stenosis at cardiac catheterization in six patients with MAC was reported by Osterberger et al. (60). Five of these patients underwent surgery; none had abnormalities of the mitral valve leaflets or chordae tendineae. None of the six patients had an OS or a diastolic rumble. In addition to causing mitral regurgitation or stenosis, MAC may lead to calcification of the aortic valve, conduction disturbances, and, rarely, endocarditis (58,61, 62).

The cause of MAC is unknown. It is generally believed to be a noninflammatory exaggeration of the normal aging changes (63). It may also be seen in younger patients with Marfan's or Hurler's syndrome and in patients with disorders of calcium metabolism (64, 65).

Calcification of Mitral Valve

Calcification of the mitral valve is an important finding in mitral stenosis. It helps determine whether surgical correction should be balloon valvuloplasty or valve replacement. Mitral valve calcification may be noted by plain film (posteroanterior and lateral) but is more reliably detected by fluoroscopy. In one study, the predictive accuracy of fluoroscopic detection of mitral valve calcification (compared with operative assessment) was 91% (55).

Mitral valve calcification should be distinguished from calcification of the mitral anulus, which is common in elderly patients, particularly in women. It has been reported in 8.5% to 10.0% of adult autopsies and in 43% of women over age 90 at autopsy (56). Mitral anular calcification (MAC) may be recognized by roentgenography but is most accurately detected by echocardiography by which it appears as a dense band of echoes posterior to the mitral valve moving parallel and ante-

Calcification of the Left Atrial Wall

Calcification within the left atrial wall is an uncommon complication of chronic rheumatic heart disease. It was noted in 26 of 1,826 patients with mitral valve disease studied at the University of Minnesota (66). Its main importance is that it is frequently associated with systemic embolism and left atrial thrombus (67).

Kerley B Lines

The presence of Kerley B lines is an important finding in patients with mitral stenosis. These are fine parallel densities in the peripheral lung fields that are perpendicular to a pleural surface and are most frequently seen in the costophrenic sulci. The lines are due to thickened interlobular septa and signify pulmonary venous hypertension. In a correlative study by Chen et al. (54), the mean left atrial pressure in mitral stenosis patients with multiple distinct Kerley B lines was 24 mm Hg.

Other studies have shown that Kerley B lines are associated with increased extravascular lung water in patients with mitral stenosis (68). These lines may persist after correction of mitral stenosis due to chronic scarring or hemosiderin deposition.

Pulmonary Artery and Right Ventricular Enlargement

Enlargement of the PA and right ventricle in patients with mitral stenosis is associated with pulmonary hypertension. Moore et al. (69) found a strong correlation ($R = 0.89$) between the size of the main PA and mean PA pressure. Chen et al. (54) reported that the best estimate of mean PA pressure is the diameter of the right PA at its widest point distal to the right middle lobe artery.

Echocardiographic Findings

The recognition of the ultrasound pattern of rheumatic mitral stenosis by M-mode echocardiography was the first clinical application of echocardiography. The subsequent development of two-dimensional imaging facilitated visualization of the abnormal valve anatomy, and the development of Doppler measurement of flow velocities facilitated the accurate noninvasive measurement of the mean valve gradient and calculation of valve area. Echo-Doppler techniques may also reveal the presence of mitral insufficiency and any associated involvement of the aortic and tricuspid valves. Echocardiography helps select patients for balloon valvuloplasty by predicting the likelihood of procedural success. Transesophageal echocardiography shows valve anatomy in greater detail and may be used to identify thrombus in the left atrium or left atrial appendage.

In 1957, Edler and Gustafson (70) reported that the closure rate of the anterior leaflet of the mitral valve measured by M-mode echocardiography (termed the E-F slope) is decreased in mitral stenosis (Fig. 3-11). They also reported that the E-F slope increases after successful mitral commissurotomy. It was

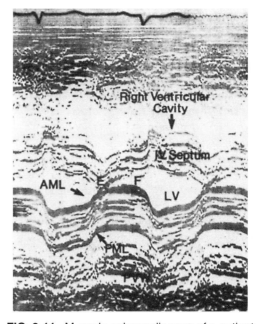

FIG. 3-11. M-mode echocardiogram of a patient with mitral stenosis. Note the decreased E-F slope, absent A wave, and thickened leaflets. The posterior mitral leaflet (*PML*) moves in an anterior direction with the anterior mitral leaflet (*AML*) during diastole. *IV*, interventricular; *LV*, left ventricle; *PVW*, posterior ventricular wall.

amply confirmed in the subsequent two decades that the E-F slope is decreased in patients with mitral stenosis. The E-F slope is simply a reflection of the rate of diastolic filling of the left ventricle (71). Any condition that decreases the rate of filling of the left ventricle may decrease the E-F slope. Although a decreased E-F slope is almost always present in severe mitral stenosis, it is not diagnostic of mitral stenosis.

The specificity of the diagnosis of mitral stenosis by M-mode echocardiography is greatly improved by visualizing and observing the initial diastolic movement of the posterior mitral leaflet (72). In the normal mitral valve, the posterior leaflet moves away from the anterior leaflet during early diastole. In mitral stenosis, the posterior leaflet moves anteriorly during early diastole (Fig. 3-11).

Calcification of the mitral valve is recognized by M-mode echocardiography as thick, conglomerate, fuzzy, or shaggy echoes duplicating mitral valve motion (55). Nicolosi et al. (55) found that the best echocardiographic evidence of a calcified mitral valve is obtained by comparing the maximal thickness of the mitral valve echo (MT) with the maximal thickness of the ventricular septum (ST) (55). A MT/ST ratio of 1.5 or more had a predictive accuracy of mitral valve calcification of 87% when compared with operative findings. This predictive accuracy was somewhat less than that of roentgenography and fluoroscopy, which was 91%. Two-dimensional echocardiography is the most sensitive technique for detecting mitral valve calcification; however, its specificity is compromised by a consistent number of false positives (73).

The echocardiographic features of mitral stenosis by M-mode echocardiography are summarized in Table 3-7. Although nearly all observers agree that M-mode echocardiography is extremely valuable in confirming the presence of mitral stenosis, it is an unreliable indicator of its severity (35,71,74,75). Nichol et al. (75) reported that of 25 patients with mitral stenosis, all had a decreased E-F slope (0 to 35 mm/s). The correlation of the E-F slope with MVA at catheterization, however, was only 0.38.

The characteristic two-dimensional echocardiographic features of rheumatic mitral stenosis are increased echo density of the leaflets due to thickening (Fig. 3-12, A and B) and reduced diastolic excursion of the leaflets (Fig. 3-12B) with restricted motion of the leaflet tips due to commissural fusion, producing a domed diastolic shape of the anterior leaflet (Fig. 3-13) and a reduction in the mitral valve orifice area (Table 3-8).

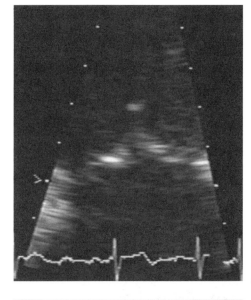

A

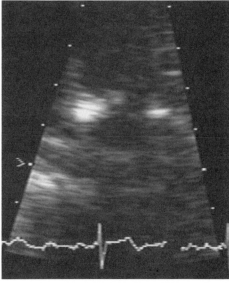

B

FIG. 3-12. A: Close-up transthoracic apical four-chamber view of mitral valve in systole. The leaflets are thickened, and the increased echocardiography density indicates the presence of calcification. B: Same mitral valve as seen in A, here in diastole. There is decreased excursion of both leaflets.

TABLE 3-7. *M-mode echocardiographic findings in mitral stenosis*

Decreased rate of diastolic closing of anterior mitral leaflet (decreased E–F slope)
Anterior motion of posterior leaflet in early diastole
Maintenance of a fixed relationship of the two leaflets to each other throughout diastole
Loss of A wave (in patients with normal sinus rhythm)
Calcification of mitral valve
Enlarged left atrium

The increased echogenicity of the leaflets initially involves the margins of the valve orifice along the leaflet commissures (Fig. 3-14). As the rheumatic pathology progresses, the increased echogenicity involves

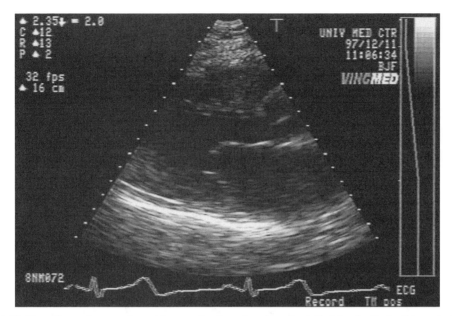

FIG. 3-13. Transthoracic parasternal long-axis view showing diastolic "doming" of a thin anterior mitral leaflet.

more of the leaflets and expands toward the annulus.

The abnormal motion of the leaflets is apparent in early diastole. Fusion of the commissures causes restriction in the motion of the tip of the anterior leaflet. However, in the early phases of the rheumatic process, the body of the anterior leaflet is pliable and continues to move anteriorly during diastole. This produces a dome-shaped leaflet, convex toward the interventricular septum (75,76) (Fig. 3-12). With progressive fibrosis and calcification the anterior leaflet becomes rigid and moves abruptly, without appearing domed.

The commissural fusion usually causes the posterior leaflet to move anteriorly during di-

TABLE 3-8. *Two-dimensional echocardiographic findings in mitral stenosis*

Increased echogenicity of the mitral leaflets
Reduced diastolic excursion of the mitral leaflets
Commissural fusion
Diastolic doming of the anterior mitral leaflet into the
  left ventricle
Reduction in mitral valve orifice area

astole with the larger anterior leaflet rather than moving posteriorly.

In mild to moderate mitral stenosis, the anterior leaflet gradually moves toward the closed position after the initial diastolic opening. The rate of this motion is slower than normal, due to the slower than normal fall in left atrial pressure. This produces the decreased E-F slope on the M-mode echocardiogram. With severe stenosis, the anterior leaflet may remain in the open position throughout diastole, due to the elevated left atrial pressure throughout diastole, and only return to the closed position with the onset of ventricular systole (75).

The two-dimensional image may be used to measure the area of the orifice of the stenotic valve (75–78). The tips of the leaflets are imaged, and the valve orifice is traced with an electronic marker. A computer calculates the area from the tracing on the video screen. Technical factors may impair the accuracy of this method. Heavily calcified leaflets may have indistinct borders that are difficult to trace. In some cases, there may be dropout of echoes, leaving gaps in the area to be traced.

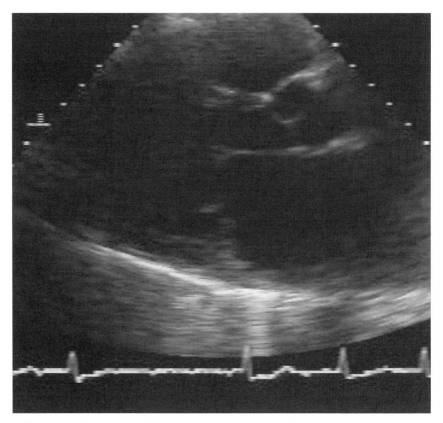

FIG. 3-14. Transthoracic parasternal long-axis view showing thickening of distal tip of anterior mitral leaflet and restricted diastolic excursion.

Despite these limitations, the two-dimensional echocardiographic measurement of valve area, when done by an experienced echocardiographer, is accurate. Wann et al. (77) reported a strong correlation with the MVA as calculated by the Gorlin and Gorlin formula in pure mitral stenosis ($R = 0.90$). Nichol et al. (75) reported an excellent correlation ($R = 0.95$) in 25 patients with pure mitral stenosis. An advantage of this technique over hemodynamic calculations using the Gorlin and Gorlin formula is that it is not influenced by mitral regurgitation, that is, mitral valve orifice size can be measured directly and accurately by two-dimensional echo in patients with mitral stenosis complicated by mitral insufficiency.

Doppler echocardiography measures the velocity of blood flow at a selected intracardiac location. Measurement of the pattern of flow across the mitral valve can diagnose the presence of stenosis, measure the pressure gradient across the valve, and estimate the area at the valve orifice.

The velocity of blood flow across the valve is directly proportional to the pressure gradient. The relationship is $P = 4V^2$, where P is the instantaneous pressure gradient between left atrium and left ventricle and V is the instantaneous peak velocity of flow across the valve. The transvalvular velocity, and hence the transvalvular pressure gradient, can be measured continuously throughout diastole. The mean of all the instantaneous diastolic gradients is the mean diastolic pressure gradient across the valve. The mean pressure gradient measured by Doppler correlates very well with the mean gradient measured by cardiac catheterization.

Flow across a normal mitral valve begins when left ventricular pressure falls below left atrial pressure in early diastole. Blood flow accelerates quickly to the peak velocity and then decelerates as left atrial emptying lowers atrial pressure and left ventricular filling raises ventricular pressure, causing a rapid drop in the pressure gradient across the valve. Late in diastole, atrial contraction raises left atrial pressure and accelerates flow across the mitral valve.

Mitral stenosis produces characteristic changes in the mitral flow velocity pattern. Mitral stenosis increases left atrial pressure throughout the cardiac cycle. This causes an increase in the early diastolic peak velocity of flow (Fig. 3-15). However, this is followed by a slower than normal rate of fall in velocity because the stenosis slows the rate at which blood flows across the valve and, consequently, slows the rate of fall of left atrial pressure. The higher left atrial pressure causes a higher than normal velocity of flow across the mitral valve throughout diastole (Fig. 3-15).

The persistent pressure gradient from the left atrium to the left ventricle eliminates the period of diastasis in mid-diastole. Left atrial and left ventricular pressures do not equalize with mitral stenosis until the onset of ventricular systole.

The velocity of flow across the mitral valve can be used to calculate the pressure gradient by the equation $P = 4V^2$. The mean gradient

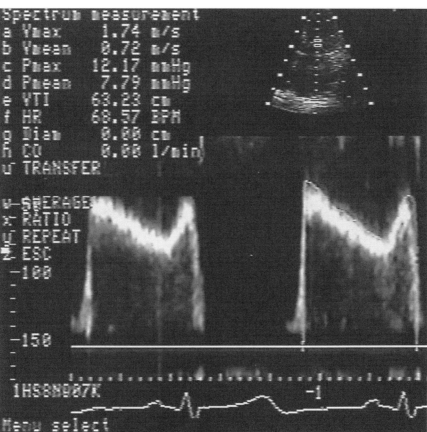

FIG. 3-15. Doppler measured flow velocity signal in diastole, measured at the tips of the mitral leaflets. The peak velocity of flow is 1.74 m/s. An increased velocity of flow is present throughout diastole. The mean diastolic gradient is 7.79 mm Hg. The time-velocity integral is also calculated.

throughout diastole can be accurately calculated (Fig. 3-15). However, the pressure gradient is affected by heart rate, cardiac output, and valvular regurgitation in addition to orifice area. Therefore, the mean diastolic gradient by itself provides only a crude estimate of valve area.

A more accurate measurement of valve area may be calculated from the pressure half-time (79–83). This is the time required for the instantaneous gradient across the valve to fall from peak value to one half of peak. As mitral stenosis becomes progressively more severe, the rate of fall of left atrial pressure during diastole slows so that more time is required for the peak pressure gradient to be reduced by one half. The pressure half-time is a simple measurement that is made by a computer installed in contemporary echocardiographic equipment (Fig. 3-16). The MVA is calculated

from the pressure half-time by the empirically derived formula

$$\text{mitral valve area (in cm}^2) = \frac{220}{\text{pressure half-time (in ms)}}$$

The pressure half-time estimate of MVA is usually sufficiently accurate for clinical use. It is not influenced by cardiac output or by the duration of diastole and is not altered by mitral regurgitation. However, the pressure half-time measurement is affected by other factors that alter the gradient between the left atrium and the left ventricle. The rate of rise of ventricular diastolic pressure will increase in a poorly compliant left ventricle. This will shorten the deceleration time, resulting in an overestimate of the MVA. Aortic insufficiency increases the rate of diastolic filling of the left ventricle, shortening the pressure half-

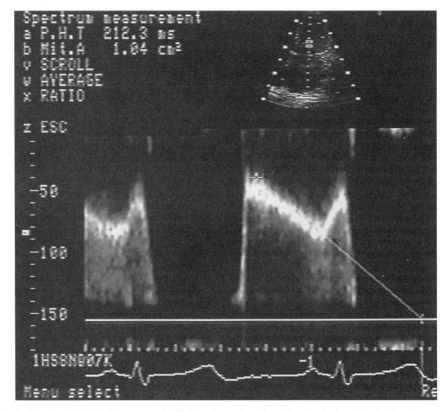

FIG. 3-16. Measurement of pressure half-time (213.3 ms) and calculation of mitral valve area (1.04 cm²), using same beat as in Fig. 3-15.

time. The pressure half-time method is not valid for several days after mitral balloon valvuloplasty (84), probably due to a decrease in left atrial pressure without a commensurate improvement in left atrial compliance.

Another method of calculating the MVA is that in the absence of valve regurgitation or an intracardiac shunt, the amount of blood flow across the mitral valve equals the amount of blood flow across the aortic valve. This relationship is called the continuity principle. The amount of blood flow across a valve is equal to the product of the valve area and the time-velocity integral (TVI) of flow across the valve. This latter measurement is easily made, using contemporary Doppler equipment, by integrating the instantaneous flow velocities over time during one cardiac cycle. The TVI across the mitral valve is measured during diastole (Fig. 3-15) and the TVI across the aortic valve is measured during systole. The area of a normal aortic valve may be easily measured from the two-dimensional echocardiographic image. Then the area of the stenotic mitral valve may be calculated using the continuity equation, as follows:

$$\text{flow across mitral valve} = \\ \text{flow across aortic valve}$$

$$\text{mitral valve area} \times \text{mitral TVI} = \\ \text{aortic valve area} \times \text{aortic TVI}$$

$$\text{mitral valve area} = \\ \frac{\textit{aortic valve area} \times \textit{aortic TVI}}{\text{mitral TVI}}$$

The continuity equation is more complicated than the pressure half-time method but is more accurate (85). The major limitation of this equation is that it is inaccurate in the presence of mitral regurgitation.

Transesophageal echocardiography provides excellent images of the mitral valve leaflets, the left atrium, and the left atrial appendage. Transthoracic imaging is usually diagnostic of mitral stenosis and can accurately assess the severity of the stenosis. However, in some cases, the transthoracic acoustic window may be inadequate. In this instance, transesophageal echocardiography provides all the anatomic and functional information needed to assess mitral stenosis. In addition, the transesophageal echocardiography visualizes the left atrium in greater detail and visualizes the left atrial appendage, which is only partially seen from the transthoracic approach. Thrombus in the left atrium is diagnosed by transthoracic echocardiography with a sensitivity of only 33% (86) to 59% (87). Transesophageal imaging detects virtually 100% of left atrial thrombi (88,89) and accurately demonstrates the location, size, shape (laminated or pedunculated), and mobility of left atrial thrombus. These anatomic features predict the potential for embolism.

The left atrial appendage is a common location of atrial thrombus. Transthoracic imaging rarely visualizes appendage thrombus (88,89). Multiplane transesophageal echocardiography visualizes most of this anatomically complex structure. Thrombus in the appendage can be accurately diagnosed by transesophageal echocardiography (88,89), but experience is needed to avoid mistaking the pectinate muscles for thrombus.

Transesophageal echocardiography may detect spontaneous echocardiography contrast in the left atrium or left atrial appendage (Fig. 3-17). This appears as a multitude of tiny echoes with a swirling motion, often described as "smoke." This phenomenon is probably due to low blood flow velocity with red blood cell rouleaux formation. In patients with mitral stenosis, spontaneous echocardiographic contrast is infrequently visualized by transthoracic imaging (90) but is commonly seen by transesophageal echocardiography. Spontaneous echocardiographic contrast is seen in most patients with AF that, in the setting of mitral stenosis, is strongly associated with left atrial or left atrial appendage thrombus and with clinical embolic events. Spontaneous echocardiographic contrast is also associated with a larger left atrium (90–92), depressed atrial and appendage contractility (93), smaller MVA (90,92,93), and absence of moderate or severe mitral regurgitation (90,93).

Spontaneous echocardiographic contrast has been observed in patients with rheumatic

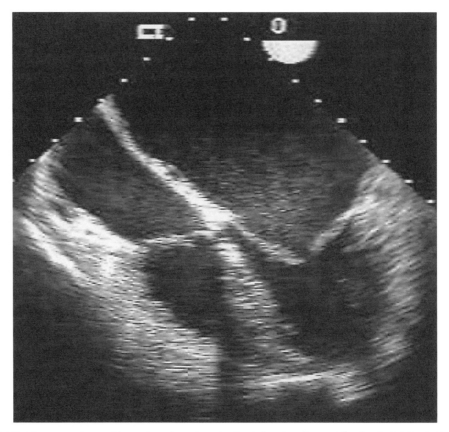

FIG. 3-17. Transesophageal four-chamber view, in diastole, showing markedly diminished excursion of only slightly thickened mitral leaflets. The multiple echoes on the atrial side of the mitral leaflets are spontaneous echocardiographic contrast. In real-time imaging, these echoes exhibit a swirling motion.

mitral stenosis who are in normal sinus rhythm. Kasliwal et al. (92) performed transesophageal echocardiography in 89 consecutive patients with mitral stenosis who were in normal sinus rhythm. Spontaneous echocardiographic contrast was seen in 51 of these patients. Of these 51 patients, 7 (14%) had left atrial or appendage thrombi, another 7 (14%) had a history of systemic embolism, and 2 (4%) had both thrombi and a history of embolism. In contrast, none of the 38 patients in sinus rhythm without spontaneous echocardiographic contrast had either thrombi or a history of embolism. These data indicate that the absence of spontaneous echocardio-

graphic contrast is associated with a very low risk of atrial thrombi or systemic embolism in patients with sinus rhythm. The presence of spontaneous echocardiographic contrast in mitral stenosis with sinus rhythm is significantly associated with systemic embolism, independent from atrial or appendage thrombus (91).

Transesophageal echocardiography is indicated before balloon valvuloplasty to evaluate the presence of left atrial thrombus. The presence of thrombus indicates a need for anticoagulation and subsequent documentation of resolution of thrombus before balloon valvuloplasty.

Transesophageal echocardiography is also indicated if there is doubt regarding the presence or severity of mitral regurgitation in a balloon valvuloplasty candidate. The distorted valve anatomy in mitral stenosis may produce an eccentric jet of regurgitation, and this may be difficult to quantify by transthoracic color Doppler. Transesophageal echocardiography can usually better characterize the mitral regurgitation. The presence of 3+ or 4+ mitral regurgitation is a contraindication to balloon valvuloplasty, because the procedure may cause additional regurgitation.

Transesophageal echocardiography may be used to guide the placement of catheters for the atrial transseptal puncture that is part of the balloon valvuloplasty procedure. The transesophageal echocardiography may also help with sizing and placement of the balloon used for the procedure.

Cardiac Catheterization

If all clinical, auscultatory, ECG, and roentgenographic findings are consistent and the two-dimensional echocardiogram and/or Doppler examinations are diagnostic of tight mitral stenosis, catheterization is needed only if there are specific questions that need to be answered (Table 3-9).

The techniques of cardiac catheterization have been well described. Left heart pressure is measured by retrograde catheterization of the left ventricle. Left atrial pressure is esti-

TABLE 3-9. *Data acquired by catheterization in patients with suspected mitral stenosis*

Confirmation, quantification of mitral valve obstruction
Detection, quantification of mitral regurgitation
Detection of complications of mitral stenosis
  Pulmonary vascular disease
  Right ventricular failure
  Tricuspid regurgitation
Status of aortic valve
Assessment of left and right ventricular function
Assessment of coronary circulation
  (in appropriate patients)

mated by accurately measuring (and confirming) the wedge pressure (9). The diastolic mitral valve gradient (Fig. 3-18) is measured simultaneously with measurement of cardiac output. The MVA is calculated as shown under Measurement of Mitral Valve Obstruction, see earlier. If the observed mitral valve gradient is small (particularly when the cardiac output is low), these measurements should be repeated during exercise. Although MVA does not change with exercise, exercise-induced increases in the mitral valve gradient and mitral valve flow decrease the errors of measurement of MVA by the Gorlin and Gorlin formula (7).

Left ventricular cineangiography is performed to determine if significant mitral regurgitation is present and to assess left ventricular function. If mitral regurgitation is present, angiographic techniques should be used to calculate the effective MVA (94). Coronary arteriography should be performed if coronary artery disease is suspected, depending on the patient's symptoms and age and the presence of risk factors for coronary artery disease. Right ventricular angiography may be appropriate if tricuspid regurgitation is suspected, particularly if pulmonary hypertension is not present. In the latter circumstance, tricuspid regurgitation may be organic rather than functional and may require surgical correction.

In addition to confirming the diagnosis of mitral stenosis, catheterization allows its quantification. As noted, calculated MVA correlates well with the symptoms of mitral stenosis. This correlation is very helpful in patients in whom the history is equivocal or uncertain. The detection and quantification of mitral regurgitation helps to determine the choice of operative procedure.

Assessment of the complications of mitral stenosis (pulmonary vascular disease, right ventricular failure) helps to assess the risks of surgical correction of mitral stenosis. Assessment of the status of the aortic valve is critical. Correction of mitral stenosis without correcting aortic stenosis has disastrous results (95).

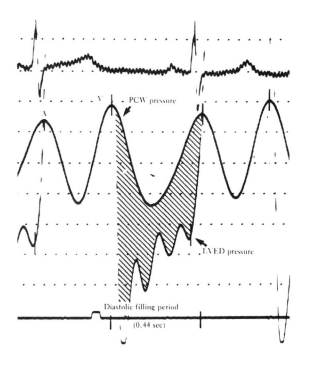

FIG. 3-18. Pressure tracing of a patient with mitral stenosis (MVA = 1.0 cm²). Note that the pulmonary capillary wedge pressure exceeds left ventricular pressure throughout the diastolic filling period. The average gradient (*shaded area*) across the mitral valve during diastole is 15 mm Hg. *LVED*, left ventricular end-diastolic pressure.

Left ventricular function is near normal in most patients with isolated mitral stenosis. If it is abnormal, coronary arteriography should be performed to determine if concomitant coronary artery disease is the cause. Some patients with pure mitral stenosis have unexplained left ventricular dysfunction, as seen by a decreased left ventricular ejection fraction (96,97). The cause of such dysfunction is uncertain. It may be due to decreased left ventricular compliance, reduced preload, or to rheumatic involvement of the myocardium. It should be noted that left ventricular dysfunction in isolated mitral stenosis rarely achieves clinical importance.

Thyroid Function Assessment

All patients with symptoms of mitral stenosis should have thyroid function assessment. Patients with thyrotoxicosis with noncritical mitral stenosis (i.e., MVA > 1.4) may become highly symptomatic when thyrotoxicosis increases mitral valve flow by causing tachycardia and increased cardiac output. In this cir-

cumstance, treatment of the hyperthyroidism may obviate the need for a cardiac operation.

DIFFERENTIAL DIAGNOSIS

Left Atrial Myxoma

Left atrial myxoma is much rarer than mitral stenosis. The incidence at autopsy is 0.03% (98). Left atrial myxomas are nearly always pedunculated and usually arise from the atrial septum in the region of the fossa ovalis (99). The most common symptom is congestive heart failure that is resistant to medical therapy. Systemic embolism may occur, and removal and microscopic examination of the embolus often leads to the correct diagnosis. The myxoma usually moves about the left atrium and may cause obstructive symptoms related to the patient's position. Systolic murmurs are more common than diastolic murmurs. An OS occasionally may be heard. AF and significant left atrial enlargement are uncommon (100).

In the past, the diagnosis of myxoma was most often made at autopsy. With the advent of cardiac surgery, the diagnosis was often made by the surgeon who was operating on a patient with apparent mitral valve disease. At the present time, the premortem diagnosis is most frequently made by echocardiography (101,102). The myxoma is seen as a series of echoes below the anterior mitral leaflet. Two-dimensional echoes are useful in recognizing the rare sessile myxoma that does not prolapse behind the mitral valve and therefore may not be visualized by M-mode echocardiography (102).

With appropriate preoperative diagnosis, left atrial myxomas may be removed surgically. The first such successful removal was by Crafoord in 1954 (103). Because myxomas may recur, follow-up echocardiography is appropriate (104).

Cor Triatriatum

The congenital anomaly cor triatriatum consists of a third atrium that receives the pulmonary veins and is separated from the true left atrium by a membrane that has one or more perforations (105). This anomaly is more frequently considered than it is actually seen. It is, in fact, a very rare lesion. Nadas and Fyler (106) described 13 cases at Children's Hospital Medical Center, Boston, from 1950 to 1970.

Patients with cor triatriatum become symptomatic very early, often in the first weeks of life (106). They present with dyspnea and signs of pulmonary vascular obstruction (107). A diastolic rumble and OS do not occur. The diagnosis is made with certainty by angiography, which visualizes the third atrium. If left atrial and wedge pressure are both measured, the latter is not found to be higher than true left atrial pressure. Surgical therapy is feasible; Brickman et al. (105) reported three successful cases of surgical excision of the membrane.

Cor triatriatum is obviously extraordinarily rare in adults and should not be confused with mitral stenosis, because it does not cause a diastolic rumble or an OS. The characteristic murmur is systolic, resulting from the passage of blood across the orifice of the intraatrial membrane (105).

Congenital Mitral Stenosis

Congenital mitral stenosis is also rare. In a literature review, Humblet et al. (108) found only 60 cases up to 1971. The stenosis may be due to a variety of anatomic abnormalities, including supravalvular rings, annular hypoplasia, and abnormality of the mitral leaflets, chordae, or papillary muscles (109). Most patients with congenital mitral stenosis present with symptoms early in life. An OS is rare, but a diastolic rumble is present in most. The cardiac catheterization findings are identical with those in rheumatic mitral stenosis. Most patients with congenital mitral stenosis have associated cardiac anomalies, particularly coarctation of the aorta and patent ductus arteriosus (108).

M-mode echocardiographic studies detect congenital mitral stenosis but do not differentiate it from rheumatic mitral stenosis (110). Two-dimensional echocardiography is very useful in delineating the anatomic cause of obstruction and its severity (110,111). The principal clinical clue to congenital mitral stenosis is the patient's age and the presence of additional congenital cardiac anomalies.

NATURAL HISTORY OF MITRAL STENOSIS WITHOUT SURGERY

At least three prospective studies of the natural history of mitral stenosis without surgery are available (37,38,112). These natural history studies have great pertinence to the evaluation of the results of and indications for the surgical or balloon valvuloplasty correction of mitral stenosis. In interpreting them, several variables must be considered. Particularly important is the degree of symptoms present when the patient is first seen.

In the series of 250 unoperated patients reported by Rowe et al. (37) (Table 3-10), 52%

TABLE 3-10. *Ten-year follow-up of 250 patients with mitral stenosis*

		Status 10 yr later		
Status at diagnosis	%	% Same	% Worse	% Dead
Asymptomatic, normal sinus rhythm (class I)	52	59	25	16
Mild symptoms, normal sinus rhythm or AF (class II)	37	21	21	58
Mild or moderate symptoms (class III)	10	4	11	85
Chronic CHF (class IV)	1	0	0	100
All patients	100	39	22	39

AF, atrial fibrillation; CHF; congestive heart failure.
From ref. 37, with permission.

were asymptomatic at the onset of the study. The average age was 28 years. The total mortality at 10 years was 39% (Table 3-10). The 10-year mortality for class III patients was 85%, however, and none of the class IV patients survived 10 years. The total mortality in the 20-year follow-up of these patients, of whom more than one half were asymptomatic when first seen, was 79% by the end of 20 years. Most deaths were due to congestive heart failure (61%) or systemic embolism (19%).

The 271 patients in the follow-up study of Olesen (38) were much older (average age, 42), and most (86%) were symptomatic at the onset of follow-up. As shown in Table 3-11, 70% were dead by 10 years. At 20 years, 83% were dead, and only 3% were unchanged from their original status. The average age at death was 48 years; 62% died of congestive heart failure and 22% died of thromboembolism.

The 20-year mortality in the Olesen series (83%) is comparable with that of the Rowe series (79%). The lower mortality at 10 years in the Rowe series is easily explained by the younger age of the patients and by the fact that more than one half were asymptomatic when first seen. In a more recent series by Rapaport (112), the 10-year mortality was 60%.

MEDICAL THERAPY OF MITRAL STENOSIS

The medical therapy of mitral stenosis consists of attempts to prevent two of its complications, systemic embolism and bacterial endocarditis, and to treat a third complication, AF, if it occurs.

Systemic embolism has already been discussed. Patients with mitral stenosis who have AF or who have already had systemic embolism require long-term anticoagulation with warfarin. Anticoagulation should be considered in patients in sinus rhythm who are aged 35 or older.

Even though bacterial endocarditis is less of a threat to the patient with pure mitral stenosis than to patients with aortic insufficiency or mitral insufficiency, these patients require antibiotic prophylaxis, as discussed in Chapter 14, in which the current guidelines for antibiotic prophylaxis to prevent recurrent rheumatic fever are also discussed.

As noted earlier, AF may occur at any point in the course of mitral stenosis. The goal of medical therapy in mitral stenosis patients with AF is to control the ventricular rate. Such control can usually be achieved with digoxin, 0.125 to 0.50 mg/day. It is prudent to measure heart rate during exercise to be certain that digitalization is adequate. Some patients require digoxin twice a day to maintain adequate control of the ventricular rate through-

TABLE 3-11. *Survival rates in unoperated on mitral stenosis*

Status	10-yr follow-up (%)	20-yr follow-up (%)
Unchanged	11	3
Deteriorated	18	12
Dead	70	83
Incomplete data	1	2

From ref. 38, with permission.

out the day. In some patients, beta-blockers in small doses may have to be added to the regimen to achieve adequate control of the ventricular rate.

A major clinical decision revolves about the indication for cardioversion in patients with mitral stenosis complicated by AF (113). In young patients with mild mitral stenosis in whom AF develops for the first time, it is usually appropriate to attempt cardioversion. If the duration of AF is more than 3 days or is unknown, anticoagulation with warfarin for 3 to 4 weeks before cardioversion is appropriate (114). If cardioversion is successful, the patient should be maintained on an antiarrhythmic agent, in addition to digoxin, to maintain sinus rhythm. Cardioversion is less likely to be successful and maintained when the left atrium is considerably enlarged (more than 45 mm) (35). Repeat cardioversion therefore is usually not indicated if the patient has reverted to AF while on adequate doses of antiarrhythmic therapy when very significant left atrial enlargement is present.

When the symptoms of pulmonary venous congestion (dyspnea, orthopnea, paroxysmal nocturnal dyspnea) occur, therapy with diuretics should be initiated and preparations for balloon valvuloplasty or mitral valve replacement (MVR) begun. These symptoms indicate that the patient is entering or is in stage 3 (Table 3-1). Such patients require relief of mitral valve obstruction. Persistent attempts at medical therapy may result in the patient progressing to stage 4 or 5. The mortality of mitral valve surgery is significantly increased if one waits until patients reach stage 4 or 5.

DEFINITIVE THERAPY FOR MITRAL STENOSIS: RELIEF OF MITRAL VALVE OBSTRUCTION

The principal symptoms of mitral stenosis are due to pulmonary venous hypertension, which is closely related to the degree of mitral valve obstruction.

The history of surgical attempts to relieve mitral valve obstruction has been summarized by Cohn and Collins (115). In 1902, Sir Lauder Brunton pointed out that severe mitral stenosis resists medical therapy and might be amenable to surgical correction. His suggestion provoked criticism but led to countless experiments in surgical laboratories throughout the world.

The first surgical attempts at relieving mitral valve obstruction, by Cutler and Levine in the 1920s (116), were made by inserting a knife into the apex of the left ventricle and blindly directing it upward toward the mitral valve. Their attempts were essentially unsuccessful.

In 1925, Souttar (117) was the first to approach the stenotic mitral valve through an incision in the left atrial appendage. His approach was successful; his patient was discharged but died of cerebral embolism 7 years later. When asked why he only did the one case, he replied, "I did not repeat the operation because I could not get another case" (118). The then current conventional wisdom was that the symptoms of mitral stenosis were due to rheumatic fever-induced damage to the heart muscle rather than mitral valve obstruction.

More than 20 years later, Harken et al. in Boston (119) and Bailey in Philadelphia (120) were successful in relieving mitral stenosis by approaching the stenotic valve with a finger inserted through an incision in the left atrial appendage.

Over the next decade, closed mitral valvuloplasty (or commissurotomy) became the established treatment of mitral stenosis. The essence of mitral valvuloplasty is to increase the size of the mitral valve orifice by mechanically splitting the fused commissures. As experience with closed mitral valvuloplasty increased, there was a progressive decrease in operative mortality (Table 3-12) (121). Most patients reported an improvement in their functional status that in some cases persisted for more than 15 years (122). However, many patients required reoperation (Table 3-13). It soon became clear that the presence of mitral valve calcification and/or significant mitral regurgitation led to suboptimal results of closed MVP.

TABLE 3-12. *Closed mitral valvuloplasty, 1948–1961: operative mortality*

	Class III		Class IV	
Case numbers	Number	Percent mortality	Number	Percent mortality
1–100	59	14	41	32
101–500	296	4	104	24
501–1000	375	1	125	19
1000–1571	485	2	86	17

From ref. 121, with permission.

The introduction of the pump oxygenator in the 1950s permitted intracardiac surgery to be performed under direct vision. This permitted open mitral valvuloplasty (123). The subsequent introduction of hemodynamically effective mechanical prosthetic valves permitted total replacement of calcified mitral valves and regurgitant mitral valves (124). Bessell et al. (125) reported a 30-year experience of MVR with a mechanical valve in 938 patients. The operative mortality over the 30-year period was 4.7%. The incidence of repeat MVR was 2.5%. Survival rates for 5, 10, 20, and 30 years were 78%, 58%, 25%, and 13%, respectively. Most surviving patients were symptomatically improved; 80% were NYHA class I or II.

Despite the low operative mortality for MVR and the excellent hemodynamics of mechanical prosthetic valves, patients must be maintained on oral anticoagulation with its risk of hemorrhage (126). Despite chronic anticoagulation, the annual risk of systemic embolism in patients with mechanical mitral valves is significant (2% to 3% per year). Of particular concern is the fact that approximately 70% of the embolic events lead to embolic stroke.

Bioprosthetic valves, most notably homograft valves from cadavers, began to be used in the mid-1960s. Their history is well described by Horowitz et al. (127). During the first 2 years after replacement, there was a low incidence of homograft failure; however, homograft valves began to deteriorate at an increasing rate 3, 4, and 5 years after operation.

The most widely used bioprosthetic valve at the present time is the Hancock Laboratories glutaraldehyde-stabilized porcine aortic valve, which is premounted on flexible polypropylene stents. Bioprosthetic or tissue valves have the distinct advantage that they do not per se require chronic anticoagulation. Anticoagulation is required only if the patient remains in AF or had recent systemic embolism or if left atrial clot was present at surgery or noted by echocardiography (126).

The operative mortality of MVR with tissue valves is comparable with replacement with mechanical valves. Postoperative cardiac catheterization has demonstrated that me-

TABLE 3-13. *Status of 729 patients 15 years following closed mitral valvuloplasty*

	Preoperative class III patients		Preoperative class IV patients	
Status	Number	Percent	Number	Percent
Improved	137	24	18	11
Unimproved	17	3	13	8
Reoperated	188	33	38	24
Dead	227	40	91	57
All patients	569	100	160	100

From ref. 122, with permission.

chanical and bioprosthetic mitral valves effectively relieve mitral valve obstruction with a postoperative MVA greater than 2.0 cm^2 in most cases (127–129).

The most important disadvantage of porcine valves is that with time they may degenerate, with resultant thickening and calcification leading to stenosis and/or insufficiency of the valve. The incidence of primary valve failure of porcine valves, that is, degeneration leading to stenosis or insufficiency without evidence of infection, is greatest in children and in adults under age 35 (130,131). As a result of these accelerated rates of primary valve failure, porcine valves are rarely indicated in children or in young adults except in women of childbearing age in whom the use of anticoagulants poses a major threat during pregnancy (132).

In adults over age 35, the annual rate of primary valve failure of porcine valves in the mitral position is very low until 4 to 5 years after MVR. After 5 years, there is a significant increase in the rate of primary valve failure. By 10 years, the incidence of valve failure requiring reoperation exceeds 20% (133,134).

For these reasons, the primary indication for bioprosthetic mitral valves is in patients with contraindications to chronic anticoagulation and, as noted, in women of childbearing age who plan future pregnancies.

Percutaneous Balloon Mitral Commissurotomy

Percutaneous balloon mitral commissurotomy (PTMC), a procedure that involves passing a balloon catheter from the right atrium through the interatrial septum into the left atrium and then across the stenotic mitral valve into the left ventricle, was reported by Inoue et al. in 1984 (135). Inflation of the balloon mechanically splits the fused commissures. This procedure, performed under local anesthesia, has had remarkable success and widespread use. PTMC can be performed with the Inoue single-balloon catheter or a double-balloon catheter. The results with the two techniques are similar (136,137). By 1996, this procedure had been performed in more than 30,000 patients worldwide (138). Most patients are from nonindustrialized nations where rheumatic fever remains prevalent. A recent report noted that more than 7,000 patients had undergone PTMC in China by 1996 (138).

Immediate Hemodynamic Results of Percutaneous Balloon Mitral Commissurotomy

As shown in Table 3-14, the immediate hemodynamic results are excellent. The MVA is

TABLE 3-14. *Hemodynamics immediately after PTMC*

Report	Years	Setting	No. of Patients (age, yr)	LA pressure (pre/post)	Gradient (pre/post, mm Hg)	MVA (pre/post, cm^2)	MVA ≥ 1.5 and MR ≤2+
Farhat et al., 1995 (139)	1987–1994	1 center, Tunisia	463 (33.0)	27/15	20/6	1.0/2.2	N.A.
Iung et al., 1996 (142)	1986–1995	1 center, Paris	1,514 (44.8)	22/13	11/5	1.0/1.9	89%
Chen and Cheng, 1995 (154)	1985–1993	120 hospitals, China	4,832 (36.8)	26/11	18/5	1.1/2.1	N.A.
Palacios, 1994 (155)	1985–1992	1 hospital, United States	564 (57.0)	25/16	15/5	0.9–2.0	79%
Feldman, 1994 (156)	1987–1993	16 centers, United States/ Canada	290 (54)	24/19	13/6	1.0/1.7	83%

PTMC, percutaneous mitral valve commissurotomy; MVA, mitral valve area; MR, mitral regurgitation; N.A., not available.

usually at least doubled and the gradient is reduced to 5 to 6 mL with a resultant postprocedure left atrial pressure that approaches
normal levels. Successful PTMC, as defined
by a postprocedure MVA of greater than 1.5
cm^2 and no more than 2+ mitral regurgitation,
occurs in approximately 80% of the patients.
The immediate hemodynamic results are
comparable with the results of closed or open
mitral valvuloplasty (139,140).

Complications

The mortality of PTMC is less than 1%
(lower than for closed MVP) and is primarily
due to cardiac perforation and cardiac tamponade. The other major complications are a
persistent atrial septal defect with a significant left to right shunt (approximately 5%)

and, as with closed MVP, the risk of perioperative embolism (2%) and procedure-induced
mitral regurgitation (2% to 5%) (Table 3-15).

Follow-Up Studies

Effective relief of mitral valve obstruction
results in a significant alleviation of symptoms. As shown in Table 3-16, at 2 to 3 years
after follow-up, more than 80% of patients are
NYHA class I or II. As with closed MVP, a
significant number of patients require repeat
PTMC or more frequently MVR because of
restenosis or an inadequate result of the initial
PTMC. Two to 3 years post-PTMC, the incidence of repeat PTMC or MVR is about 10%;
at 4 years, it was 24% in the series reported by
Dean et al. (141).

TABLE 3-15. *PTMC complications*

Report	Years	No. of Patients	Mortality (%)	ASD (%)	Perforation/ tamponade (%)	Perioperative embolism (%)	MR ≥3+ (%)
Farhat et al., 1 995 (139)	1987– 1994	463	0.4	4.8	0.7	2	4.6
Iung et al., 1996 (142)	1986– 1995	1,514	0.4	N.A.	0.3	0.3	3.4
Chen and Cheng, 1995 (154)	1985– 1993	4,832	0.12	N.A.	0.8	.5	1.4
Palacios, 1994 (155)	1985– 1992	564	0.5	N.A.	0.8	1.0	2.8
Feldman, 1994 (156)	1987– 1993	290	1.4	3.1	1.4	0	3.8

ASD, postprocedure atrial septel defect with L-R shunt >1.5/1.0; MR, mitral regurgitation; N.A., not available.

TABLE 3-16. *PTMC follow-up*

Study	No. of Patients	Mean age at PTMC (yr)	Average follow-up	Survival (%)	Class I or II (pre/ post, %)	Restenosis MVA <1.5 (%)	Repeat PTMC MVP or MVR (%)
Farhat et al., 1995 (139)	463	33	3 years	98	30 95	8	9
Chen and Cheng, 1995 (154)	4,832	37	32 months	N.A.	44 98	5.2	N.A.
Palacios, 1995 (155)	564	57	6.6 years	75	N.A.	N.A.	N.A.
Feldman, 1994 (156)	290	54	24 months	N.A.	15 80	N.A.	11
Dean et al., 1996 (141)	736	54	4 years	84	36 81	N.A.	24

PTMC, percutaneous mitral valve commissurotomy; MVA, mitral valve area; MVP, mitral valvuloplasty; MVR, mitral valve replacement; N.A., not available.

Factors Limiting the Success of Percutaneous Balloon Mitral Commissurotomy

The best results of PTMC occur in patients with pliable noncalcified valves, with mild or no subvalvular lesions and minimal mitral regurgitation. The presence of a left atrial or left ventricular clot is a contraindication to PTMC until anticoagulation results in resolution of the clot.

Calcification of the mitral valve, as detected by fluoroscopy, has a significant impact on the results of PTMC. Iung et al. (142) reported good results (postoperative MVA greater than 1.5 cm^2 with no more than 2+ MR) in 94% of 1,131 patients who had no evidence of mitral valve calcification. In contrast, only 78% of 383 patients with any detectable calcification had good results. Tuzcu et al. (143) reported a success rate of 69% in patients without calcification, compared with 59% in those with 1+ calcification, 48% with 2+, 35% with 3+, and only 33% in patients with 4+ mitral valve calcification. The long-term survival rate is lower and the incidence of repeat PTMC or MVR is significantly higher in patients with calcified valves (143,144).

Echocardiography is a significant predictor of the immediate and long-term results of PTMC. An echocardiography score developed at the Massachusetts General Hospital grades leaflet rigidity, thickening, valvular calcification, and subvalvular disease each on a scale of 0 to 4. An angiographic score approaching 16 would represent a heavily calcified, thickened, immobile valve with extensive thickening and calcification of the subvalvular apparatus (144). Such valves do not respond well to PTMC or open or closed MVP and require MVR. Palacios et al. (144) reported that the increase in MVA with PTMC is significantly greater in patients with an angiography score of 8 or less compared with those with scores more than 8 ($p < 0.01$).

Percutaneous Balloon Mitral Commissurotomy During Pregnancy

PTMC has been reported to be very successful in the treatment of severe mitral stenosis during pregnancy. Dommisse et al. (145) reported 11 women who had PTMC during pregnancy with no maternal or perinatal morbidity or mortality. In a larger series of 27 patients, Kalra et al. (146) reported one patient who required emergency MVR because of severe MR induced by PTMC and subsequently aborted at 6 months. There was no additional fetal loss, and all 27 mothers were class I at follow-up. Those results are in marked contrast to the reports of fetal loss after open mitral valvuloplasty (20% to 30%) or closed MVP (12%) (147).

Comparison of Percutaneous Balloon Mitral Commissurotomy with Surgical Valvulotomy

The reported immediate and follow-up results of patients with mitral stenosis treated with PTMC at experienced centers are clearly comparable with the published results of closed mitral valvuloplasty. Five recent randomized trials have documented that PTMC is at least as effective as closed MVP (148–152). The advantages of a procedure done under local anesthesia compared with a procedure requiring thoracotomy are apparent. The only circumstance where closed MVP may be appropriate is in some developing nations where PTMC is not available or is more expensive than closed MVP due to the cost of balloon catheters. However, Lau et al. (153) have reported that the balloon catheters may be safely reused after meticulous cleaning and sterilization, thereby decreasing the cost of the PTMC. In industrialized nations, the cost of PTMC is significantly less than surgical valvuloplasty (154).

PTMC was compared with open mitral valvuloplasty in two randomized trials (140, 152) and was found to be as effective as open mitral valvuloplasty with comparable acute complications and comparable rates of restenosis.

Choice of Therapy

The available data indicate that the definitive treatment of choice for relief of mitral

TABLE 3-17. *Indications for PTMC or open MVP/MVR*

Favors PTMC	Favors open MVP/MVR
Pliable noncalcified valve with minimal subvalvular lesions, with zero or mild MR angio score <8	Heavily calcified valve
	Nonpliable valve
	Severe subvalvular lesions
	Significant mitral regurgitation
No LA or LV clot	Angio score ≥8
	LA or LV clot
Other factors favoring PTMC	Unsuccessful PTMC
Pregnancy	
Relative contraindications to anticoagulant therapy	
Severe pulmonary hypertension	
Advanced age	
Coexistent heart or pulmonary disease	

PTMC, percutaneous mitral valve commissurotomy; MVP, mitral valvuloplasty; MVR, mitral valve replacement; LA, left atrium; LV, left ventricle; MR, mitral regurgitation.

valve obstruction in patients with pliable noncalcified valves with minimal subvalvular lesions with minimal or no mitral regurgitation is PTMC, unless there is a left atrium or left ventricle clot. At the other extreme, patients with heavily calcified nonpliable valves with severe subvalvular lesions and significant mitral regurgitation and patients with left atrium or left ventricle clot require open mitral valvuloplasty or MVR (Table 3-17).

In patients with valves that are suboptimal for PTMC, this procedure should be attempted if they are pregnant, have relative contraindications to anticoagulant therapy, or if they are at increased risk of surgery because of severe pulmonary hypertension, advanced age, or coexistent heart or lung disease.

REFERENCES

1. Bland EF, Jones TD. Rheumatic fever and rheumatic heart disease. *Circulation* 1951;4:836.
2. Roberts WC, Perloff JK. Mitral valvular disease. *Ann Intern Med* 1972;77:939.
3. Selzer A, Cohn KE. Natural history of mitral stenosis: a review. *Circulation* 1972;45:878.
4. Wood P. An appreciation of mitral stenosis. Part I. Clinical features. *Br Med J* 1954;1:1051.
5. Joswig BC, Handler JB, Vieweg WVR. Contrasting progression of mitral stenosis in Malayans versus American-born Caucasians. *Am Heart J* 1982;104:1400.
6. Silverstein DM, Hansen DP, Ojiambo HP, Griswold HE. Left ventricular function in severe pure mitral stenosis as seen at the Kenyatta National Hospital. *Am Heart J* 1980;99:727–733.
7. Gorlin R, Gorlin SG. Hydraulic formula for calculations of the area of the stenotic mitral valve, other cardiac valves, and central circulatory shunts. *Am Heart J* 1951;41:1.
8. Lewis BM, et al. Clinical and physiological correlations in patients with mitral stenosis. *Am Heart J* 1952;43:2.
9. Hellems HK, Haynes FW, Dexter L. Pulmonary capillary pressure in man. *J Appl Physiol* 1949;2:24.
10. Henry WL, Kastl DG. Echocardiographic evaluation of patients with mitral stenosis. *Am J Med* 1977;62:813.
11. Egeblad H, et al. Assessment of rheumatic mitral valve disease. *Br Heart J* 1983;49:38.
12. Dexter L, et al. Physiologic evaluation of patients with mitral stenosis before and after mitral valvuloplasty. *Trans Am Clin Climatol Assoc* 1950;62:170.
13. Bader RA, et al. Hemodynamics at rest and during exercise in normal pregnancy as studied by cardiac catheterization. *J Clin Invest* 1955;34:1524.
14. Dalen JE, et al. Pulmonary embolism, pulmonary hemorrhage and pulmonary infarction. *N Engl J Med* 1977;196:1431.
15. Spencer H. *Pathology of the Lung*. Oxford: Pergamon, 1977.
16. Dalen JE, et al. Precapillary pulmonary hypertension: its relationship to pulmonary venous hypertension. *Trans Am Clin Climatol Assoc* 1974;86:207.
17. Jordan SC. Development of pulmonary hypertension in mitral stenosis. *Lancet* 1965;2:322.
18. Wood P. An appreciation of mitral stenosis. Part II. Investigations and results. *Br Med J* 1954;1:1113.
19. Doyle AE, et al. Pulmonary vascular patterns in pulmonary hypertension. *Br Heart J* 1957;19:353.
20. Heath D, Harris P. *The Pulmonary Circulation*. Edinburgh: Churchill Livingstone, 1962.
21. Welch KJ, Johnson J, Zinsser H. The significance of pulmonary vascular lesions in the selection of patients for mitral valve surgery. *Ann Surg* 1950;132:1027.
22. Braunwald E, et al. Effects of mitral valve replacement on the pulmonary vascular dynamics of patients with pulmonary hypertension. *N Engl J Med* 1965;273:509.
23. Dalen JE, et al. Early reduction of pulmonary vascular resistance after mitral valve replacement. *N Engl J Med* 1967;277:387.
24. McIlduff JB, et al. Systemic and pulmonary hemody-

namic changes immediately following mitral valve replacement in man. *Cardiovasc Surg* 1980;21:261.

25. Zener JC, et al. Regression of extreme pulmonary hypertension after mitral valve surgery. *Am J Cardiol* 1972;30:820.

26. Dalen JE, Haynes FW, Dexter L. Life expectancy with atrial septal defect. *JAMA* 1967;200:112.

27. Gorlin R, et al. Studies of the circulatory dynamics in mitral stenosis. II. *Am Heart J* 1951;41:30.

28. Davies LG, Goodwin JF, Van Leuven BD. The nature of pulmonary hypertension in mitral stenosis. *Br Heart J* 1954;16:440.

29. Camishion RC, et al. Paralysis of the left recurrent laryngeal nerve secondary to mitral valve disease: report of two cases and literature review. *Ann Surg* 1966;163:818.

30. Arani DT, Carleton RA. The deleterious role of tachycardia in mitral stenosis. *Circulation* 1967;36:511.

31. Carleton RA, Graettinger JS. The hemodynamic role of the atria with and without mitral stenosis. *Am J Med* 1967;42:532.

32. Morganroth J, et al. Relationship of atrial fibrillatory wave amplitude to left atrial size and etiology of heart disease. *Am Heart J* 1979;97:184.

33. Garber EB, Morgan MG, Glasser SP. Left atrial size in patients with atrial fibrillation: an echocardiographic study. *Am J Med Sci* 1976;272:57.

34. Deverall PB, et al. Incidence of systemic embolism before and after mitral valvotomy. *Thorax* 1968;23:530.

35. Henry WL, et al. Relation between echocardiographically determined left atrial size and atrial fibrillation. *Circulation* 1976;53:273.

36. Ellis LB, Harken DE. Arterial embolization in relation to mitral valvuloplasty. *Am Heart J* 1961;62:611.

37. Rowe JC, et al. The course of mitral stenosis without surgery: ten- and twenty-year perspectives. *Ann Intern Med* 1960;52:741.

38. Olesen KH. The natural history of 271 patients with mitral stenosis under medical treatment. *Br Heart J* 1962;24:349.

39. Sherrid MV, Clark RD, Cohn K. Echocardiographic analysis of left atrial size before and after operation in mitral valve disease. *Am J Cardiol* 1979;43:171.

40. Coulshed N, et al. Systemic embolism in mitral valve disease. *Br Heart J* 1970;32:26.

41. Bannister RG. The risks of deferring valvotomy in patients with moderate mitral stenosis. *Lancet* 1960;2:329.

42. Levine HJ, Pauker SG, Eckman MH. Antithrombotic therapy in valvular heart disease. Fourth ACCP Consensus Conference on Antithrombotic Therapy. *Chest* 1995;108:360S.

43. Braunwald E. Valvular heart disease. In: Isselbacher KJ, et al., eds. *Principles of Internal Medicine*, 9th ed. New York: McGraw-Hill, 1979:1097.

44. Rackley CF, Edwards JF, Karp RB. Mitral valve disease. In: Hurst W, ed. *The Heart*, 6th ed. New York: McGraw-Hill, 1986:761.

45. Waller BF, McManus BM, Roberts WC. Mitral valve stenosis produced by or worsened by active bacterial endocarditis. *Chest* 1982;82:498.

46. Levine SA. *Clinical Heart Disease*, 5th ed. Philadelphia: W.B. Saunders, 1958.

47. Legler JF, Benchimol A, Dimond EG. The apex car-

diogram in the study of the 2-OS interval. *Br Heart J* 1963;25:246.

48. Craige E. Phonocardiographic studies in mitral stenosis. *N Engl J Med* 1957;257:650.

49. Ravin A, et al. Diagnosis of tight mitral stenosis. *JAMA* 1952;149:1079.

50. Criley JM, Hermer JAJ. The crescendo presystolic murmur of mitral stenosis with atrial fibrillation. *N Engl J Med* 1971;285:1284.

51. Sokolow M, McIlroy MB. *Clinical Cardiology*, 2nd ed. Los Altos, CA: Lange Medical Publications, 1979.

52. DeSanctis JRW, Dean DC, Bland EF. Extreme left atrial enlargement. *Circulation* 1964;29:14.

53. Plaschkes J, et al. Giant left atrium in rheumatic heart disease: a report of 18 cases treated by mitral valve replacement. *Ann Surg* 1971;174:194.

54. Chen JTT, et al. Correlation of roentgen findings with hemodynamic data in pure mitral stenosis. *Am J Roentgenol Radium Ther Nucl Med* 1968;102:280.

55. Nicolosi GL, Pugh DM, Dunn M. Sensitivity and specificity of echocardiography in the assessment of valve calcification in mitral stenosis. *Am Heart J* 1979;98:171.

56. Pomerance A. Pathological and clinical study of calcification of the mitral valve ring. *J Clin Pathol* 1970;23:354.

57. D'Crus IA, et al. Clinical manifestations of mitral annulus calcification with emphasis on its echocardiographic features. *Am Heart J* 1977;94:367.

58. Mellino M, et al. Echographic-quantified severity of mitral annulus calcification: prognostic correlation to related hemodynamic, valvular, rhythm, and conduction abnormalities. *Am Heart J* 1982;103:222.

59. Labovitz AJ, et al. Frequency of mitral valve dysfunction from mitral annular calcium as detected by Doppler echocardiography. *Am J Cardiol* 1985;55:133.

60. Osterberger LE, et al. Functional mitral stenosis in patients with massive mitral annular calcification. *Circulation* 1981;64:472.

61. Nair, CK, et al. High prevalence of symptomatic bradyarrhythmias due to atrioventricular node-fascicular and sinus node-atrial disease in patients with mitral annular calcification. *Am Heart J* 1982;103:226.

62. Hollenberg G, Gross S. Endocarditis. *N Y State J Med* 1979;79:1579.

63. Korn D, DeSanctis RW, Sell S. Massive calcifications of the mitral annulus. *N Engl J Med* 1962;267:900.

64. Kronzon I, et al. Two-dimensional echocardiography in mitral annulus calcification. *AJR Am J Roentgenol* 1980;134:355.

65. Forman MB, et al. Mitral annular calcification in chronic renal failure. *Chest* 1984;85:367.

66. Gedgaudas E, Kieffer SA, Erikson C. Left atrial calcification. *Am J Roentgenol Radium Ther Nucl Med* 1968;102:293.

67. Seltzer RA, Harthorne JW, Austen WG. The appearance and significance of left atrial calcification. *Am J Roentgenol Radium Ther Nucl Med* 1967;100:307.

68. Slutsky RA, et al. Extravascular lung water in patients with mitral stenosis: relationship to pulmonary capillary wedge pressure and Kerley B lines. *Radiology* 1984;153:317.

69. Moore CB, et al. The relationship between pulmonary

arterial pressure and roentgenographic appearance in mitral stenosis. *Am Heart J* 1959;58:576.

70. Edler I, Gustafson A. Ultrasonic cardiogram in mitral stenosis. *Acta Med Scand* 1957;159:85.

71. Pridie RB, Oakley CM. Echocardiographic evaluation of the mitral valve. *Prog Cardiovasc Dis* 1978;21:92.

72. Duchak JM Jr, Chang S, Feigenbaum H. The posterior mitral valve echo and the echocardiographic diagnosis of mitral stenosis. *Am J Cardiol* 1972;29:628.

73. Zanolla L, et al. Two-dimensional echocardiographic evaluation of mitral valve calcification. *Chest* 1982; 82:154.

74. Cope GD, et al. A reassessment of the echocardiogram in mitral stenosis. *Circulation* 1975;52:664.

75. Nichol PM, Gilbert BW, Kisslo JA. Two-dimensional echocardiographic assessment of mitral stenosis. *Circulation* 1977;55:120.

76. Martin RP, et al. Reliability and reproducibility of two-dimensional echocardiographic measurement of the stenotic mitral valve orifice area. *Am J Cardiol* 1979; 43:560.

77. Wann LS, et al. Determination of mitral valve area by cross-sectional echocardiography. *Ann Intern Med* 1978;88:337.

78. Henry WL, et al. Measurement of mitral orifice area in patients with mitral valve disease by real-time two-dimensional echocardiography. *Circulation* 1975;51: 827.

79. Hatle L, Angelsen B, Tromsdal A. Non-invasive assessment of atrioventricular pressure half-time by Doppler ultrasound. *Circulation* 1979;60:1096.

80. Knutsen KM, et al. Doppler ultrasound in mitral stenosis. *Acta Med Scand* 1982;211:433.

81. Thuillez C, et al. Pulsed Doppler echocardiographic study of mitral stenosis. *Circulation* 1980;61:381.

82. Stamm RB, Martin RP. Quantification of pressure gradients across stenotic valves by Doppler ultrasound. *J Am Coll Cardiol* 1983;2:707.

83. Libanott AJ, Rodbard S. Atrioventricular pressure half-time. *Circulation* 1968;38:144.

84. Thomas JD, et al. Inaccuracy of mitral pressure half-time immediately after percutaneous mitral valvotomy. *Circulation* 1988;78:980.

85. Nakatani S, et al. Value and limitations of Doppler echocardiography in the quantification of stenotic mitral valve area: comparison of the pressure half-time and the continuity equation methods. *Circulation* 1988;77:78.

86. Schweizer P, Bardos P, Erbel R, et al. Detection of left atrial thrombi by echocardiography. *Br Heart J* 1981; 45:148.

87. Shrestha NK, Moreno FL, Narciso FV, et al. Two-dimensional echocardiographic diagnosis of left atrial thrombus in rheumatic heart disease: a clinicopathologic study. *Circulation* 1983;67:341.

88. Aschenberg W, Schluter M, Kremer P, et al. Transesophageal two-dimensional echocardiography for the detection of left atrial appendage thrombus. *J Am Coll Cardiol* 1986;7:163.

89. Mugge A, Daniel WG, Haverich A, Lichtlen PR. Diagnosis of noninfective cardiac mass lesions by two-dimensional echocardiography: comparison of the transthoracic and transesophageal approaches. *Circulation* 1991;83:70.

90. Beppu S, Yasuharu N, Sakakibara H, et al. Smoke-like

echo in the left atrial cavity in mitral valve disease: its features and significance. *J Am Coll Cardiol* 1985;6: 744.

91. Daniel WG, Nellessen U, Schroder E, et al. Left atrial spontaneous echo contrast in mitral valve disease: an indicator for an increased thromboembolic risk. *J Am Coll Cardiol* 1988;11:1204.

92. Kasliwal RR, Mittal S, Kanojia A, et al. A study of spontaneous echo contrast in patients with rheumatic mitral stenosis and normal sinus rhythm: an Indian perspective. *Br Heart J* 1995;74:296.

93. Li Y-H, Hwang J-J, Ko Y-L, et al. Left atrial spontaneous echo contrast in patients with rheumatic mitral valve disease in sinus rhythm. *Chest* 1995;108:99.

94. Askenazi J, et al. Mitral valve area in combined mitral stenosis and regurgitation. *Circulation* 1976;34:480.

95. Uricchio JF, Likoff W. Effect of mitral commissurotomy on coexisting aortic-valve lesions. *N Engl J Med* 1957;256:199.

96. Feigenbaum H, et al. Evaluation of the left ventricle in patients with mitral stenosis. *Circulation* 1966;34:462.

97. Gash AK, et al. Left ventricular ejection performance and systolic muscle function in patients with mitral stenosis. *Circulation* 1983;67:148.

98. Bulkley BH, Hutchins GM. Atrial myxomas: a fifty-year review. *Am Heart J* 1979;97:639.

99. Newman HA, Cordell AR, Prichard RW. Intracardiac myxomas. Literature review and report of six cases, one successfully treated. *Am Surg* 1966;32:219.

100. Alridge HE, Greenwood WF. Myxoma of the left atrium. *Br Heart J* 1960;22:189.

101. Lappe DL, Bulkley BH, Weiss JL. Two-dimensional echocardiographic diagnosis of left atrial myxoma. *Chest* 1978;74:55.

102. Martinez EC, Giles TD, Burch GE. Echocardiographic diagnosis of left atrial myxoma. *Am J Cardiol* 1974; 33:281.

103. Crafoord C. In discussion of Andrus et al. In: Lam CR, ed. *International Symposium on Cardiovascular Surgery: Physiology, Diagnosis and Techniques. Proceedings of symposium held at Henry Ford Hospital, Detroit, MI*. Philadelphia: W.B. Saunders, 1955:202.

104. Walton JA Jr, Kahn DR, Willis PW III. Recurrence of left atrial myxoma. *Am J Cardiol* 1972;29:872.

105. Brickman RD, et al. Cor triatriatum. *J Thorac Cardiovasc Surg* 1970;60:523.

106. Nadas AS, Fyler DC. *Pediatric Cardiology*, 3rd ed. Philadelphia: W.B. Saunders, 1972.

107. Ehrich DA, et al. Cor triatriatum: report of case in a young adult with special reference to the echocardiographic features and etiology of the systolic murmur. *Am Heart J* 1977;94:217.

108. Humblet L, et al. Observations, cliniques, la stenose mitrale congenitale. *Acta Cardiol* 1971;26:500.

109. Smallhorn J, et al. Congenital mitral stenosis. *Br Heart J* 1981;45:527.

110. Driscoll DJ, Gutgesell HP, McNamara DG. Echocardiographic features of congenital mitral stenosis. *Am J Cardiol* 1978;42:259.

111. Vitarelli A, et al. Echocardiographic assessment of congenital mitral stenosis. *Am Heart J* 1984;108:523.

112. Rapaport E. Natural history of aortic and mitral valve disease. *Am J Cardiol* 1975;35:221.

113. Lown B. Electrical reversion of cardiac arrhythmias. *Br Heart J* 1967;29:469.

114. Laupacis A, Albers G, Dalen J, et al. Antithrombotic therapy in atrial fibrillation. Fourth ACCP Consensus Conference on Antithrombotic Therapy. *Chest* 1995; 108:352S.

115. Cohn LH, Collins JJ Jr. Surgical treatment of mitral stenosis: a medical milestone. *N Engl J Med* 1973; 289:1035.

116. Cutler EC, Levine SA. Cardiotomy and valvulotomy for mitral stenosis. Experimental observations and clinical notes concerning an operated case with recovery. *Boston Med Surg J* 1923;188:1024.

117. Souttar HS. The surgical treatment of mitral stenosis. *Br Med J* 1925;2:603.

118. Khan MN. The relief of mitral stenosis. *Tex Heart Inst J* 1996;23:258.

119. Harken DE, et al. The surgical treatment of mitral stenosis. I. Valvuloplasty. *N Engl J Med* 1948;239:801.

120. Bailey CP. The surgical treatment of mitral stenosis (mitral commissurotomy). *Dis Chest* 1949;15:377.

121. Ellis LB, Harken DE. Closed valvuloplasty for mitral stenosis. *N Engl J Med* 1964;270:643.

122. Ellis LB, et al. Fifteen- to twenty-year study of one thousand patients undergoing closed mitral valvuloplasty. *Circulation* 1973;48:357.

123. Housman LB, et al. Prognosis of patients after open mitral commissurotomy. *J Thorac Cardiovasc Surg* 1977;73:742.

124. Starr A, et al. Mitral valve replacement. *Circulation* 1976;54[Suppl III]:47.

125. Bessell JR, Gower G, Craddock DR, Stubberfield J, Maddern GJ. Thirty years experience with heart valve surgery: isolated mitral valve replacement. *Aust N Z J Surg* 1996;66:806.

126. Stein PD, Alpert JS, Copeland J, Dalen JE, Goldman S, Turpie AGG. Antithrombotic therapy in patients with mechanical and biological prosthetic heart valves. *Chest* 1995;108:371S.

127. Horowitz MS, et al. Mitral valve replacement with the glutaraldehyde-preserved porcine heterograft. *J Thorac Cardiovasc Surg* 1974;67:885.

128. Hannah H III, Reis RL. Current status of porcine heterograft prostheses. *Circulation* 1976;54[Suppl III]: 27.

129. Johnson AD, et al. Functional evaluation of the porcine heterograft in the mitral position. *Circulation* 1975; 50[Suppl I]:40.

130. Magilligan DJ Jr, et al. Natural history of the porcine bioprosthetic heart valve. *Henry Ford Hosp Med J* 1982;30:113.

131. Walker WE, et al. Early experience with the Ionescu-Shiley pericardial xenograft valve. *J Thorac Cardiovasc Surg* 1983;86:570.

132. Cohn LH, et al. Early and late risk of mitral valve replacement: a 12-year concomitant comparison of the porcine bioprosthetic and prosthetic disc mitral valves. *J Thorac Cardiovasc Surg* 1985;90:872–881.

133. Magilligan DJ Jr, et al. The porcine bioprosthetic valve twelve years later. *J Thorac Cardiovasc Surg* 1985; 89:499–507.

134. Gallo I, Ruiz B, Duran CG. Isolated mitral valve replacement with the Hancock porcine bioprosthesis in rheumatic heart disease: analysis of 213 operative survivors followed up 4.5 to 8.5 years. *Am J Cardiol* 1984;53:178.

135. Inoue J, Owaki T, Nakamura T, Kitamon F, Miyamoto N. Clinical application of transvenous mitral commissurotomy by a new balloon catheter. *J Thoracic Cardiovasc Surg* 1984;87:394.

136. Zhang HP, Gamra H, Allen JW, Lau FYK, Ruiz CE. Comparison of late outcome between Inoue balloon and double-balloon techniques for percutaneous mitral valvotomy in a matched study. *Am Heart J* 1995; 130:340.

137. Trevino AJ, Ibarra M, Garcia A, et al. Immediate and long-term results of balloon mitral commissurotomy for rheumatic mitral stenosis: comparison between Inoue and double-balloon techniques. *Am Heart J* 1996; 131:530–536.

138. Cheng TO. Percutaneous balloon mitral valvuloplasty: the why, the when, the what, and the which [editorial]. *Cathet Cardiovasc Diagn* 1996;37:353.

139. Farhat MB, Betbout F, Gamra H, et al. Results of percutaneous double-balloon mitral commissurotomy in one medical center in Tunisia. *Am J Cardiol* 1995; 76:1266.

140. Reyes VP, Raju BS, Wynne J, et al. Percutaneous balloon valvuloplasty compared with open surgical commissurotomy for mitral stenosis. *N Engl J Med* 1994; 331:961.

141. Dean LS, Mickel M, Bonan R, et al. Four-year follow-up of patients undergoing percutaneous balloon mitral commissurotomy. *J Am Coll Cardiol* 1996;28:1452.

142. Iung B, Cormier B, Ducimetiere P, et al. Immediate results of percutaneous mitral commissurotomy: a predictive model on a series of 1514 patients. *Circulation* 1996;94:2124.

143. Tuzcu EM, Block PC, Griffin B, Dinsmore R, Newell JB, Palacios IF. Percutaneous mitral balloon valvotomy in patients with calcific mitral stenosis: immediate and long-term outcome. *J Am Coll Cardiol* 1994;23:1604.

144. Palacios IF, Tuzcu ME, Weyman AE, Newell JB, Block PC. Clinical follow-up of patients undergoing percutaneous mitral balloon valvotomy. *Circulation* 1995; 91:671.

145. Dommisse J, Commerford PJ, Levetan B. Balloon valvuloplasty for severe mitral valve stenosis in pregnancy. *S Afr Med J* 1996;86:1194.

146. Kalra GS, Arora R, Khan JA, Nigam M, Khalillulah M. Percutaneous mitral commissurotomy for severe mitral stenosis during pregnancy. *Cathet Cardiovasc Diagn* 1994;33:28.

147. Oto MA, Kabukcu M, Ovunc K, et al. Percutaneous balloon valvuloplasty for severe mitral stenosis in pregnancy: four case reports. *J Vasc Dis* 1997;48:463.

148. Farhat MB, Ayari M, Maatouk F, et al. Percutaneous balloon versus surgical closed and open mitral commissurotomy: seven-year follow-up results of a randomized trial. *Circulation* 1998;97:245–250.

149. Turi ZG, Reyes VP, Raju BS, et al. Percutaneous balloon versus surgical closed commissurotomy for mitral stenosis: a prospective, randomized trial. *Circulation* 1991;83:1179.

150. Patel JJ, Sharma D, Mitha AS, et al. Balloon valvuloplasty versus closed commissurotomy for pliable mitral stenosis: a prospective hemodynamic study. *J Am Coll Cardiol* 1991;18:1318.

151. Arora R, Nair M, Kalra GS, Nigam M, Kkhalillulah M. Immediate and long-term results of balloon and surgical closed mitral valvotomy: a randomized comparative study. *Am Heart J* 1993;125:1091.

152. Bueno R, Anrade P, Nercolini D, et al. Percutaneous mitral valvuloplasty versus open mitral valve commissurotomy: results of a randomized clinical trial. *J Am Coll Cardiol* 1993;21:429A.

153. Lau K-W, Ding Z-P, Hung J-S. Percutaneous transvenous mitral commissurotomy versus surgical commissurotomy in the treatment of mitral stenosis. *Clin Cardiol* 1997;20:99.

154. Chen C-R, Cheng TO. Percutaneous balloon mitral valvuloplasty by the Inoue technique: a multicenter study of 4832 patients in China. *Am Heart J* 1995; 129:1197.

155. Palacios IF. Percutaneous mitral balloon valvotomy for patients with mitral stenosis. *Curr Opin Cardiol* 1994 9:164–175.

156. Feldman T. Hemodynamic results, clinical outcome, and complications of Inoue balloon mitral valvotomy. *Cathet Cardiovasc Diagn* 1994;2:2.

4

Chronic Mitral Regurgitation

Maurice Enriquez-Sarano, Hartzell V. Schaff, Abdul Jamil Tajik, and Robert L. Frye

Division of Cardiovascular Diseases, Mayo Clinic, Rochester, Minnesota 55905

Mitral regurgitation (MR) is defined as the abnormal ejection of blood from the left ventricle (LV) to the left atrium (LA), inducing an LV and LA volume overload commensurate to the degree of MR. The management of chronic MR has considerably changed recently because the etiology is now dominated by degenerative and ischemic causes in developed countries; because of recent developments of transesophageal echocardiography, color flow imaging, and quantitative methods of assessment of the degree of MR; because of improved understanding of the impact of LV function on outcome; and, most importantly, because of the advances in conservative surgery.

NORMAL MITRAL STRUCTURE AND FUNCTION

The mitral valve is a complex structure with four components (1–5):

1. The annulus is asymmetric with a fixed portion (corresponding to the anterior leaflet) shared with the aortic annulus (3), called the fibrosa, and a dynamic portion (4) (corresponding to the posterior leaflet) that represents most of the circumference of the annulus.
2. The anterior and posterior leaflets are thin and asymmetric. The anterior leaflet has the greatest length of tissue but occupies the smaller portion of the circumfer-

ence of the annulus than does the posterior leaflet (1,3). The main mechanism preventing MR is a sufficient area of coaptation of the rough zones of atrial surface of the leaflets in systole (3).
3. The chordae attach each papillary muscle to the corresponding commissure area and the adjacent halves of both leaflets (2) and maintain the two leaflets in a position allowing coaptation.
4. The two papillary muscles and the adjacent wall attach the mitral apparatus to the LV.

In most etiologies of MR dysfunction, more than one anatomic element occurs that underlines the complexity of conservative surgery for restoration of normal mitral function (5).

Mitral competence during systole is normally ensured, first by a large area of coaptation between leaflets, allowing high friction resistance to abnormal valve movement, and second by the systolic position of the anterior leaflet parallel to the direction of blood flow.

ETIOLOGY AND MECHANISM OF CHRONIC MITRAL REGURGITATION

Chronic MR may be the result of a slowly progressing valvular disease such as in rheumatic disease. It may also be observed as a consequence of lesions acutely constituted, such as valvular perforations or ruptured chor-

TABLE 4-1. *Mechanisms of MR*

Etiology	Mechanism	Echocardiographic appearance
Postinflamatory	Retraction	Thickened chordae/leaflets
Rheumatic	Thickening	Normal or restricted motion
Lupus erythematosus		
Anticardiolipin syndrome		
Postradiation		
Degenerative	Prolapsed leaflets	Prolapsing/Flail leaflets
Mitral valve prolapse	Ruptured chords	Redundant tissue
Idiopathic ruptured chordae		Ruptured chords
Marfan's syndrome		
Ehlers-Danlos syndrome		
Traumatic MR		
Myocardial disease	Dilatation of annulus	Normal leaflets
Ischemic (chronic)	Tenting of leaflets	Reduced motion of leaflets
Cardiomyopathies		
Infiltrative disease	Thickened leaflet	Thickened leaflets
Amyloid disease	Loss of coaptation	Reduced motion
Hurler's disease		
Encasing disease	Immobilization of leaflets	Thickened leaflets and chordae
Hypereosinophilic syndrome	Thickened leaflets	Restricted motion
Endomyocardial fibrosis		
Carcinoid disease		
Ergot lesions		
Diet-drug lesions		
Endocarditis	Destructive lesions	Perforations
		Flail leaflets
Congenital	Cleft leaflet	Cleft leaflet
	Transposed valve	Tricuspid valve

MR, mitral regurgitation.

dae that did not cause acute symptoms but secondarily by virtue of adaptive processes reach the chronic stage of MR. Because in most cases the exact timing of occurrence of these acute lesions is unknown, the definition of an absolute duration of MR to establish the chronic nature of MR has not been developed. A simplified classification of MR mechanisms using valvular movements has been described (6), but the mechanisms of MR are complex and often multiple and should be analyzed with each etiology (Table 4-1).

Rheumatic Mitral Regurgitation

This is often associated with some degree of stenosis and fusion of the commissures, but in approximately 10% of rheumatic mitral valve disease it is pure without associated stenosis (7). Severe rheumatic MR requiring surgical correction is still frequent in developing countries but is now rare in developed countries

(8,9). The underlying lesion is retractile fibrosis of the valvular apparatus, causing loss of leaflet coaptation (10). The secondary dilatation of the mitral annulus tends to further decrease the contact between leaflets. Elongated or ruptured cords are infrequent.

Degenerative Mitral Regurgitations

These causes are often associated with valve prolapse, an abnormal movement of the leaflets into the LA during systole due to inadequate chordal support (elongation or rupture), and excessive valvular tissue (9). In Western countries, mitral prolapse is the most frequent lesion observed during surgery for severe MR (8,9). Degenerative MR can be separated into three categories:

1. The mitral valve prolapse (11) syndrome, which may have an hereditary component (12). Macroscopically there is a marked increase in valve area and length (9) with

interchordal hooding involving a large area of the leaflets (13), and secondary ruptured chordae may occur. Microscopically the valves are myxomatous, with deposition of mucopolysaccharides in a thickened spongiosa layer encroaching on the fibrosa layer (14). Annular myxomatous changes may lead to dilatation and calcification. The myxomatous infiltration may also involve the other cardiac valves and result in regurgitation of these valves.

2. The degenerative "primary" ruptured chordae involve more often the posterior than the anterior leaflet and occur more often in men than in women (15). There is usually no excessive tissue (9), but enlargement of the annulus may occur as in any MR. The involved leaflet may present with a myxomatous infiltration (16), but the other leaflet usually remains normal (17). Calcification of the mitral annulus (18), or systemic hypertension, may precede the occurrence of the ruptured chordae. Isolated ruptured cord may occasionally be due to blunt thoracic trauma and endocarditis (secondary forms).

3. Degenerative MR without prolapse is usually mild and due to sclerosis of the valve or calcification of the mitral annulus (19), and the MR is secondary to deformation of the valves or annulus.

Infective Endocarditis

Infective endocarditis involving the mitral valve may cause acute MR. However, surgery for severe MR can often be performed at the chronic stage of the disease. Vegetations may produce mild MR by interposition between the leaflets. Severe endocarditic MR is usually related to ruptured cords and less frequently to the destruction of mitral tissue involving either the edges of the leaflets or a perforation (20).

Ischemic and Functional Mitral Regurgitation

Chronic ischemic and functional MR, due to transient or permanent papillary muscle dysfunction (21), to LV dilatation (22), isolated or with an aneurysm, to cardiomyopathies, or to myocarditis, have in common the same mechanism. The abnormal shape or systolic contraction of the LV produces an excessive traction on the chordae mainly transmitted to the anterior leaflet, resulting in an abnormal anterior position in systole of this leaflet with a consequent reduction of the area of coaptation (23,24).

Other Causes of Chronic Mitral Regurgitation

MR is observed frequently with color flow imaging, even in normal patients, but clinically significant chronic MR may be found in connective tissue disorders, Marfan's syndrome (25), Ehlers-Danlos syndrome (26), pseudoxanthoma elasticum, osteogenesis imperfecta, Hurler's disease, systemic lupus erythematosus (27), and anticardiolipin syndrome (28); penetrating or nonpenetrating cardiac trauma (29); myocardial disease such as hypertrophic cardiomyopathy (30) or sarcoidosis (31); endocardial disease such as hypereosinophilic syndrome (32), endocardial fibroelastosis, and carcinoid tumors (33); iatrogenic causes, such as that due to ergot-derivative (34) or anorexigen (35) related lesions; congenital lesions such as cleft mitral valve isolated or associated with persistent atrioventricular canal, corrected transposition with or without Ebstein abnormality of the left atrioventricular valve (36); and cardiac tumors.

PATHOPHYSIOLOGY

The abnormal coaptation of the mitral leaflets creates a *regurgitant orifice* during systole. The systolic pressure gradient between the LV and the LA is the driving force of the regurgitant flow that results in a *regurgitant volume*. This regurgitant volume represents a percentage of the total ejection of the LV and may be expressed as the *regurgitant fraction*. The regurgitant volume creates a volume overload by entering the LA in systole and the LV in diastole, modifying LV loading and function.

Timing of Regurgitation

The pressure gradient between the LV and atrium begins with the mitral closure simultaneous to the first heart sound and persists after the closure of aortic valve and the second heart sound until the mitral valve opens (37). Throughout that period, the timing of MR parallels that of the effective regurgitant orifice (ERO). In clinically significant MR, the ERO is usually present throughout systole and the MR is holosystolic beginning with S_1 and finishing after S_2 (37). However, the ERO area may vary, and the interactions of these changes with that of the regurgitant gradient during systole are complex.

Angiographic studies suggested that most MR occurs in early systole, but small changes in LV volumes are observed during that period (38). Experimental data suggest that a progressive decrease in ERO occurs parallel to the decrease of ventricular volume during systole (37), an observation consistent with the confinement of MR to early systole in patients with small degrees of MR. More recently, the proximal isovelocity surface area method, which allows instantaneous measurement of regurgitant flow, studied the dynamics of the ERO during systole (39,40). Rheumatic lesions appear mostly stable throughout systole (39), but functional MR appears to vary often in degree with larger orifices during isovolumic contraction and relaxation during which a reduced ventricular pressure may lead to decreased coaptation of leaflets (23). Conversely, a valve prolapse may appear late in systole, below a specific LV volume (41). Analysis using the flow convergence method has shown that in patients with valve prolapse, the ERO increases exponentially throughout systole whether a flail segment is present or not (40). Interestingly, the regurgitant volume does not follow a totally similar course and tends to increase from early to

mid-systole, but in late systole it declines despite the increased orifice due to the marked decrease in gradient (40). Despite these variations of the ERO, the measure of the instantaneous orifice in mid-systole correlates well to the mean ERO area (39,40).

Degree and Repercussion of Regurgitation

The area of the ERO is an essential determinant of the degree of volume overload and thus of the dilatation of LV and LA (42). However, the resultant volume overload (regurgitant volume) depends also on the magnitude of the regurgitant gradient and its duration. For example, the volume overload observed in patients with MR is usually less severe than in aortic regurgitation (43,44), although the regurgitant gradient and ERO (42) are usually larger than in aortic regurgitation. Such differences are related to a duration of regurgitation during the cardiac cycle, which is usually shorter in mitral than in aortic regurgitation (42).

The degree of MR is not fixed and may vary with interventions (45). Vasodilators tend to decrease the degree of MR (46), but the change in ERO area rather than that of the ventriculoatrial gradient is the main mechanism of this effect; in functional (47,48) and organic MR (49), the ERO may change acutely after alterations of LV volumes and contractility (49). The ERO increases with increased afterload or ventricular volume, decreases with decreased afterload or improved contractility, but is not influenced by changes in heart rate (50).

With MR, the regurgitant energy produced by the LV translates into two components, the kinetic energy (regurgitant volume) and the potential energy (elevation of atrial pressure). The typical LA pressure change in the V wave reflects a reduced late systolic atrial compliance (51) and may reach extremely high levels in patients with severe MR but is not specific for MR (52) and can be observed solely as a result of changes in the LA pressure–volume relationship (53). In chronic MR, the LA is more dilated and compliant than in acute

MR. Consequently, the V wave is less prominent and the LA pressure may be normal even with severe MR (54).

Left Ventricular Remodeling

In patients with MR, the LV is dilated but less so than in aortic regurgitation of comparable degree (43,55). The end-diastolic LV volume and wall stress are increased (55). The end-systolic volume is increased in chronic MR, but end-systolic wall stress is nevertheless usually normal (56,57). The LV is more spherical in diastole and systole than in normal patients (38), especially with large volumes or reduced function. After correction of the MR, the shape of the ventricle tends to normalize (58). The myocardial mass is increased in patients with MR, proportionate to the degree of LV dilatation (58).

LV function is difficult to characterize because of the changes in preload and afterload. It has been suggested that normalization of the ejection fraction to the preload would provide an appropriate assessment of LV function (59,60). Afterload is more difficult to assess because the regurgitation toward the LA may decrease the instantaneous impedance to ejection, but the measure of afterload provided by end-systolic wall stress is within the normal range (56,57). However, the usual inverse correlation between end-systolic wall stress and ejection fraction is also observed in MR (61). Complex indices using the afterload such as the end-systolic wall stress (62) or maximum elastance (56) normalized to the LV volume have been proposed and may be sensitive to subtle changes in function.

LV dysfunction is a frequent complication of MR that carries a poor prognosis (63,64). Although interstitial fibrosis is present in advanced LV failure (65), the exact mechanism of LV dysfunction remains mysterious. Experimentally, LV dysfunction is not due to changes in coronary blood flow (66). Changes in myofiber contractility parallel the changes in global LV function (67) and are associated with reduced myofiber content (68), but the

cause of the myofiber dysfunction is yet to be determined. In animal models, LV dysfunction is reversible after correction of MR (68) in contrast to the progressive deterioration seen in humans (63,64), raising the question of the validity of the current models of chronic MR.

Diastolic LV function is difficult to analyze in MR due to increase in filling volume. LV relaxation is frequently prolonged, but chamber stiffness is usually reduced due to the enlarged cavity size (69). Age and decreased systolic function (69) are associated with increased chamber stiffness, which is a possible determinant of the age-related hemodynamic alterations observed in MR (70).

Functional Mitral Regurgitation

In patients with functional MR due to chronic ischemic heart disease or cardiomyopathy, the primary disease involves the LV, which is often poorly contracting, and the normal mitral leaflet. However, the MR does not appear to be directly determined by the degree of LV dysfunction and appears to be more dependent on local ventricular remodeling (71–73). In ischemic or functional as opposed to organic (due to primary valvular disease) MR, the regurgitant volume is usually small (74), and the LV dilatation is not proportional to the degree of MR (42). Nevertheless, functional MR is of clinical significance, is associated with higher LA pressure (75) and volume (42), is a marker of advanced myocardial disease (76,77), and is associated with higher efficacy of vasodilators (78) in these patients.

CLINICAL PRESENTATION

The clinical presentation of chronic MR, including symptoms, physical findings, electrocardiographic changes, and radiographic changes, is determined by the degree and the cause of the MR and by the function and compliance of the LA and ventricle (Table 4-2).

TABLE 4-2. *Clinical presentations of chronic MR*

	MVP syndrome	Organic MR	Functional MR
Symptoms	Chest pain	Fatigue	CHF
Physical examination	Mid-systolic click, end-systolic murmur	Loud holosystolic murmur, S_3	Soft early systolic murmur S_4, S_3
ECG	ST-T changes	Atrial fibrillation	Q waves, LBBB
CXR	Pectus excavatum	Cardiomegaly, LA enlargement	Cardiomegaly, pulmonary edema

MR, mitral regurgitation; MVP, mitral valve prolapse; CHF, congestive heart failure; ECG, electrocardiogram; LBBB, left bundle branch block; CXR, chest x-ray; LA, left atrium.

Symptoms

Patients with mild MR usually have no symptoms. Severe MR may be associated with no or minimal symptoms for years (7). Fatigue due to the low cardiac output and mild dyspnea on exertion are the usual symptoms and are rapidly improved by rest (79). Severe dyspnea on exertion or, more rarely, paroxysmal nocturnal dyspnea, frank pulmonary edema, or even hemoptysis (7,79) may also be observed. Such severe symptoms may be triggered by new onset of atrial fibrillation, an increase in the degree of MR, the occurrence of new endocarditis or ruptured chordae (80), or a change in ventricular compliance or function. Progression of symptoms may not be observed despite progression of hemodynamic alterations because of the efficacy of diuretic treatment or because of the progressive self-limitation of physical activity. The severity of symptoms is more related to the hemodynamic tolerance than the degree of MR (81).

In the transition from acute to chronic MR, dramatic symptoms often present at onset such as pulmonary edema or congestive heart failure (80,82,83) and progressively subside either spontaneously due to increased compliance of the LA or with administration of diuretics.

Sudden death is rarely the revealing manifestation of chronic MR (84) but is a dreaded and not infrequent complication of severe MR, even when asymptomatic (85).

Sex distribution has changed parallel to the changes in the etiology of MR (7). With the decrease in rheumatic heart disease, severe MR is now predominantly seen in males (65% to 75%). As degenerative diseases of the mitral valve are more common later in life, the mean age of patients has been steadily increasing (most frequently in the sixth decade of life).

Physical Examination

Blood pressure is usually normal. Carotid upstroke is brisk, and this impression is further increased by the reduced ejection time of severe MR.

Cardiac palpation may show a laterally displaced, diffuse, brief cardiac apex impulse in patients with enlarged LV. An apical thrill is characteristic of severe MR. A right ventricular heave at the left sternal border is observed with right ventricular dilatation and may be difficult to distinguish from the LA lift due to the dilated expansive LA, which is more substernal and lower.

The first heart sound is merged within the murmur but is usually normal and may be increased in rheumatic heart disease. The second heart sound is usually normal. The presence of a third heart sound is directly related to the volume of MR and LV dilatation in patients with organic MR (86,87). It is often associated with an early diastolic rumble due to the increased mitral flow in diastole that may be present and prolonged even in the absence of mitral stenosis. The third heart sound and diastolic rumble are low-pitched sounds and may be difficult to detect without careful auscultation performed in the left lateral decubitus position. The S_3 is more noticeable with expiration. In patients with ischemic and/or functional MR, the third heart sound corresponds more often to restrictive LV filling (87). An atrial gallop is heard mainly in MR of recent onset (88) and in patients with ischemic/functional MR if the sinus rhythm is maintained. Mid-systolic clicks are markers of mitral valve prolapse, occurring simultaneously with the prolapse (41), and are due to the sudden tension of the chordae.

The hallmark of MR is the systolic murmur. In MR of at least moderate degree, the murmur is holosystolic, including the first and the second heart sound. If an opening snap or a third heart sound is mistakenly interpreted as being the second heart sound, the murmur may appear mid-systolic. Only a careful examination beginning at the base of the heart to identify the second heart sound and progressing toward the apex will allow clear recognition of the nature of the murmur. The murmur is of the blowing type but may be harsh, especially in mitral valve prolapse. The maximum intensity of the murmur is usually at the apex, and it may radiate to the axilla in patients with rheumatic or anterior leaflet prolapse regurgitation. In patients with prolapse of the posterior leaflet, the jet of MR is usually superiorly and medially directed and the murmur radiates toward the base of the heart (89). The murmur may be heard in the back, in the neck, and sometimes on the skull. If the murmur radiates to the base, it may be difficult to distinguish from the murmur of aortic stenosis or obstructive cardiomyopathy and pharmacologic maneuvers, showing that the murmur decreases with amyl nitrite and increases with methoxamine, which strongly suggests MR. The murmur does not increase with postextrasystolic beats, probably because the regurgitant flow is unchanged due to the combination of a decreased ERO (49) and increased regurgitant gradient. The murmur usually parallels the degree of MR; this correlation is weaker in ischemic or functional MR (90).

Murmurs of shorter duration usually correspond to mild MR; they may be mid-to-late systolic in patients with mitral valve prolapse or early systolic in patients with functional MR.

Electrocardiogram

The most frequent feature of MR is atrial fibrillation, which was found in approximately 60% to 75% (7) of earlier series and is now present in 40% to 50% of surgically corrected MR (91). Patients in sinus rhythm may present with signs of LA enlargement. LV hypertrophy is more rarely seen and may be associated with secondary ST-T abnormalities (92). Right ventricular hypertrophy is uncommon. The electrocardiogram, especially in acute MR, may be entirely normal. In patients with mitral valve prolapse syndrome, nonspecific ST-T wave changes may be observed. In patients with ischemic MR Q waves in the inferior leads or a left bundle branch block are often noted (Fig. 4-1).

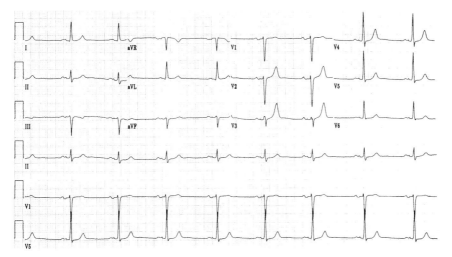

FIG. 4-1. Electrocardiogram of a patient with severe chronic mitral regurgitation. Note the left atrial enlargement.

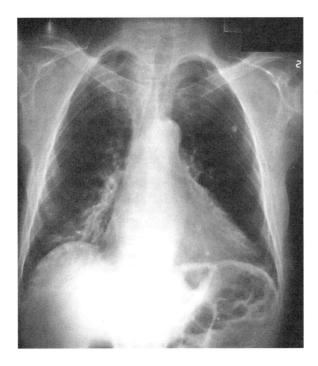

FIG. 4-2. Chest radiography of a patient with severe chronic mitral regurgitation. Note the nonspecific cardiomegaly.

Chest Roentgenogram

Patients with mitral valve prolapse or Marfan's syndrome may present with pectus excavatum or scoliosis. Cardiomegaly with LA and atrial appendage dilatation may be present in chronic MR or in patients with ischemic/functional MR. Although valvular calcifications are rare (18), annular calcifications seen as a C-shaped density below the posterior leaflet are frequent. Giant left atria are usually seen in severe mixed mitral valve disease (93). Signs of pulmonary hypertension or pulmonary edema are infrequently observed in patients with chronic MR (Fig. 4-2).

LABORATORY TESTS

Doppler Echocardiography

Doppler echocardiography is now the major tool in the assessment of patients with MR. Doppler echocardiography assesses the morphologic lesions of the mitral valve, the degree of MR, and the ventricular and atrial function.

Morphology

Rheumatic MR is characterized by thickening of the leaflets, mainly at their tips, and chordae (94). The posterior leaflet has reduced mobility, whereas the anterior leaflet has normal mobility and may be doming if commissural fusion is associated with MR. A valvular prolapse is usually not present unless a ruptured chordae or active rheumatic carditis are present (95). Similar lesions are observed in lupus or anticardiolipin syndrome (27,28) in which transesophageal echocardiography may also show small vegetations on the atrial side of the leaflets.

In *degenerative MR*, there are three critical lesions to be defined. First, a valvular prolapse is defined by the passage of valvular tissue beyond the plane of the annulus. Because of the saddle shape of the mitral annulus (96), the apical four-chamber view may overestimate the presence of valvular prolapse. Therefore, long-axis views are critical to this diagnosis (Fig. 4-3). Transesophageal echocardiography can be useful for the diagnosis of prolapse if standard imaging is of mediocre quality (97).

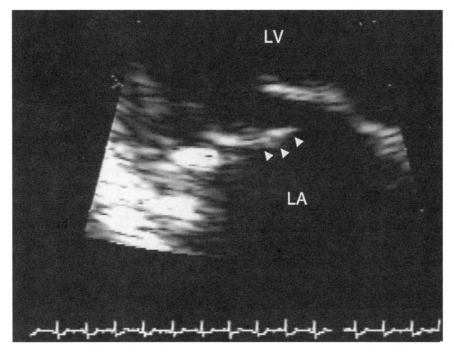

FIG. 4-3. Two-dimensional echocardiogram of a patient with flail posterior leaflet of the mitral valve (**arrows**) shown in an enlarged view. *LV*, left ventricle; *LA*, left atrium.

The prolapse may involve one (most frequently the posterior) or both leaflets. The initial direction of the jet confirms the predominant lesion (98), with jets centrally directed in equal bileaflet prolapse or directed inferior and externally in predominant anterior leaflet prolapse or directed superiorly and medially in predominant posterior leaflet prolapse (Fig. 4-4). A flail leaflet is diagnosed on the basis of complete loss of leaflet coaptation in the regurgitant area (98). Flail leaflets can usually be diagnosed by transthoracic echocardiography but are more clearly delineated by transesophageal echocardiography (99). Also, ruptured chordae may be better diagnosed by the transesophageal approach (Fig. 4-5) (100).

Second, diffuse myxomatous changes are diagnosed on the basis of diffusely thickened leaflets (101) with excessive valvular tissue. And third, mitral annular calcification may limit the possibility of conservative surgery if extensive and severe.

Endocarditic MR, the usual mechanism for MR (i.e., flail leaflets), is usually clearly demonstrated by transthoracic echocardiography. Perforations of a leaflet are more difficult to diagnose. Mitral annular abscesses are rare and are best detected by transesophageal echocardiography (102). Vegetations can be seen on leaflets or on ruptured cords by the transthoracic approach, but transesophageal echocardiography is of superior sensitivity (103).

Mitral annular (24,104) dilation is not specific (74) for *ischemic/functional MR*, but the amplitude of its systolic descent is reduced (105). Essential diagnostic observations are the regional or global LV dysfunction (104) and normal or mildly sclerotic leaflet tissue. The characteristic apical displacement of the anterior leaflet with tenting (73) is due to the abnormal tension on the principal chordae (106) and results, in combination with the annular enlargement, in in-

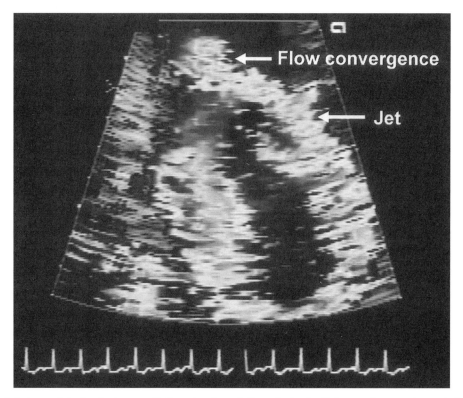

FIG. 4-4. Large jet of mitral regurgitation due to a flail posterior leaflet seen in an enlarged view of the left atrium. The flow convergence is seen proximal to the regurgitant orifice in the left ventricle and the jet in the left atrium. Note the wraparound of the jet in the left atrium.

complete leaflet coaptation (24,104) with a central jet of MR (74).

In other causes of MR, some characteristic features may be observed related to etiology. In obstructive cardiomyopathy, the systolic anterior motion of the mitral valve is associated with a loss of coaptation and the jet of MR is directed inferior and externally. If the jet is directed medially and superiorly, one should strongly suspect the association of ruptured cord of the posterior leaflet (107). In eosinophilic heart disease, characteristic infiltration of the region below the posterior leaflet by thrombus can be demonstrated with immobilization of the posterior leaflet and resultant MR. Other aspects such as calcification of the mitral annulus (108) and sclerosis with nodular calcification of the leaflet, can also be clearly demonstrated by transthoracic echocardiography.

Assessment of Severity of Regurgitation

There are several semiquantitative methods used to assess the severity of MR (Table 4-3). First, color flow imaging of the jet demonstrates the origin and direction of the jet (98). The jet length, the ratio of the jet area to the LA area (109), or more simply the jet area (110) has been suggested as a good index of severity of MR. Small jets such as those seen in normal subjects consistently correspond to mild MR (74). However, color flow imaging has significant limitations, technical but also, more importantly, intrinsically related to the nature of regurgitant jets. The extent of a jet is determined by its momentum and thus as much by regurgitant velocity as by regurgitant flow. Also, jets are constrained by the LA and expand more in large atria (74,109). The eccentric jets of valve prolapse (111) impinge

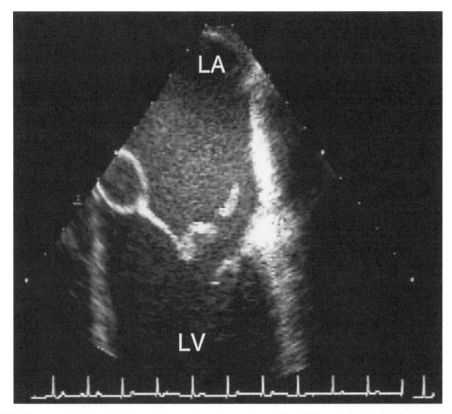

FIG. 4-5. Transesophageal echocardiography of a patient with a flail anterior leaflet to which the ruptured chord is still attached.

TABLE 4-3. *Assessment of severity of MR*

Clinical
  Systolic thrill
  Murmur intensity
  S₃
  Diastolic rumble
Laboratory
  Qualitative
    Large jet ≥8 cm² (echo-Doppler)
    Pulmonary vein reversal (Doppler, angio)
    Dense contrast in LA (angio)
  Quantitative
    Criteria
      Regurgitant volume ≥60 mL
      Regurgitant fraction ≥50%
      ERO ≥40 mm²
    Method
      Doppler echocardiography
        Quantitative Doppler
        Quantitative 2D-echo
        PISA
      Radionuclide angiography
      Quantitative LV angiography

MR, mitral regurgitation; LA, left atrium; ERO, effective regurgitant orifice; 2D, two-dimensional; PISA, proximal isovelocity surface area; LV, left ventricle.

on the LA wall (112) and tend to underestimate the MR (74,113). The central jets of ischemic and/or functional MR expand markedly in the enlarged LA and tend to overestimate the MR (74). Transesophageal echocardiography usually shows larger jets but does not suppress these limitations of color flow imaging.

With another method, the density of the continuous wave Doppler signal (114) grossly reflects the degree of MR in that it is determined by the number of moving red blood cells within the beam of ultrasound. However, eccentric jets are often captured on a short length and are often of low density. Finally, pulmonary venous velocity profile assesses the degree of MR (115,116). Systolic reversal of flow in the pulmonary veins is a strong argument for severe MR. Unfortunately, there is an important interaction between MR severity, direction of the jet, LA pressure, and the

occurrence of pulmonary venous flow reversal (117). This sign may be absent or asymmetric in severe MR (117). It is not specific
for severe MR and may be observed in patients with elevated LA pressure or markedly
enlarged LA (Fig. 4-6).

There are also quantitative methods and the
goal here is to measure parameters that will
reflect the degree of MR. The volume overload can be expressed as the regurgitant volume (difference between the total and forward
stroke volume) per beat or the regurgitant
fraction that is the proportion to the LV ejection volume regurgitated into the LA. The regurgitant lesion can be expressed as the ERO
area and calculated as ERO = regurgitant
flow/regurgitant velocity or ERO = regurgitant volume/regurgitant TVI, where TVI is the

time velocity integral of the regurgitant jet
(42,118).

The practical quantitation of MR can be
performed using various methods. Quantitative Doppler is based on the calculation of the
mitral and aortic stroke volumes using
pulsed-wave Doppler (119,120). The principle is simple and applicable in most cases, but
the measurement of the mitral stroke volume
is technically demanding, with a significant
learning phase (119). Quantitative two-dimensional echocardiography is of similar
principle but is based on measurement of LV
volumes for total stroke volume calculation
(121). Conversely, the proximal isovelocity
surface area method directly measures the regurgitant flow by analyzing the flow convergence region proximal to the regurgitant ori-

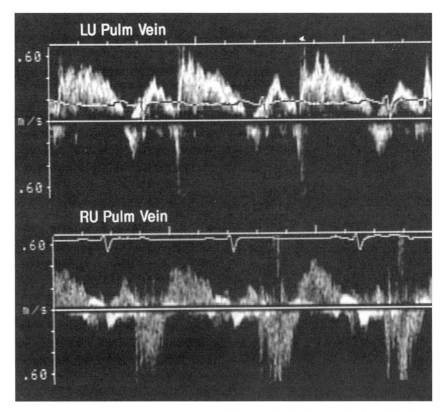

FIG. 4-6. Pulmonary venous flow velocities recorded from the left upper (*LU*) and right upper (*RU*) pulmonary veins using transesophageal echocardiography in a patient with severe mitral regurgitation, showing systolic flow reversal in the right but not the left vein.

fice and is based on the principle of conservation of mass (122). Because color flow mapping allows precise determination of the velocity in the flow convergence region, the regurgitant flow can be calculated (123). Using the regurgitant flow and the regurgitant velocities, the ERO and the regurgitant volume can be calculated (118,124). This method is simple and accurate if the assumptions are respected (125). The vena contracta method measures the smallest jet width immediately below the regurgitant orifice (126) and provides an estimate of the radius of the ERO (127). This method is simple, and although not providing physiologic quantitative data, it appears to correlate well with the ERO area (128).

The gradation of MR using these quantitative indices suggests that regurgitant volume (60 mL), regurgitant fraction (50%), and ERO (40 mm²) represent severe MR (129). Vena contracta width (0.5 cm) appears to represent severe MR (130).

Assessment of Left Ventricular and Atrial Function

Guided M-mode diameter is used for the assessment of the LV size, mass, and wall stress (91,131–133). The ejection fraction can be calculated (134) or estimated (135). The estimation of both ejection fraction and wall stress can be accurately obtained by these methods, but diameters tend to have a larger range of error with increasing LV size (136), and for the assessment of LV remodeling it is preferable to use the LV volumes measured by two-dimensional echocardiography (137,138). The M-mode measurement of the LA diameter is limited by the asymmetric shape of that cavity. LA area or volume can be simply measured by two-dimensional echocardiography (139).

Radionuclide Studies

Radionuclide angiography can be used to estimate the LV end-diastolic and end-systolic volume and the right ventricular and LV ejection fraction. The detection of exercise-induced LV dysfunction is frequent (140). However, the significance of such measurement on the long-term prognosis has not been analyzed in large series of patients. The comparison of the counts measured over the right ventricle and LV allow the calculation of the regurgitant fraction.

Cardiac Catheterization

Cardiac catheterization is used to assess the hemodynamic status, the severity of MR, the LV function, and coronary anatomy. In our practice, cardiac catheterization is rarely needed for confirmation of echocardiographic diagnosis but is often indicated to detect coronary disease before surgery.

The major hemodynamic consequences of MR are a reduced cardiac output and an elevated left atrial pressure. However, the left atrial pressure may be normal because of the compensatory effect of left atrial enlargement (54), and marked pulmonary hypertension is rare (141). Similarly, a large V wave is less frequent in chronic than in acute MR and is not specific for MR (52).

The degree of MR can be assessed by LV selective angiography and can be qualitatively graded in three or four grades on the basis of the degree and persistence of opacification of the LA (142). This classic method has limitations similar to all qualitative methods (143). The quantitation of MR can be obtained by comparing the angiographic stroke volume to the forward stroke volume as calculated by the Fick or by the thermodilution methods (144) to calculate the regurgitant volume and fraction. The angiographic stroke volume usually overestimates the true stroke volume, and correction factors have been used to minimize the overestimation of the regurgitant volume. Angiographic quantitation of MR is difficult and has a potentially high range of error (145) that cannot be verified by use of combined methods or by repeating the measurements. In our practice, left ventricular angiography for documentation of severity of MR is rarely used.

The assessment of LV function can be performed using quantitative angiography. LV volumes correlate strongly with the regurgitant volume (146), duration of MR (147), etiology of MR, and LV function. The most frequently used indices of LV function are the end-systolic volume (in part determined by the degree of MR) and the ejection fraction. Both have been shown to be useful for prognostic purposes (64,148). The association of high-fidelity pressure recording with LV angiography allows the calculation of more complex indices of LV compliance in diastole (69) and of systolic wall stress (62,149) and elastance (56). The additional value of these complex measurements has been investigated in small groups of patients and remains to be defined in larger populations.

Regional wall motion abnormalities have been observed in MR even without coronary lesions. Selective coronary angiography is, at present, the only technique allowing definition of the coronary anatomy. Coronary stenoses may be present even in the absence of angina (150,151), and coronary angiography is performed ordinarily in patients older than 40 years (152).

Strategy for Use of Laboratory Testing

It is not necessary to perform all these tests in all patients with MR. Transthoracic Doppler echocardiography confirms the diagnosis of MR, demonstrates associated valvular disease, provides a unique assessment of the morphologic lesions of the mitral valve, and is performed in most cases for the initial diagnostic assessment, for follow-up, and for presurgical assessment. Transesophageal echocardiography provides high-resolution imaging, but its incremental value has not been fully documented (100). In our practice it is reserved preoperatively for patients in whom lesions (especially if endocarditis is suspected) or severity of MR are uncertain but is used on a large scale intraoperatively to monitor the results of valve repair (96–98,101).

Coronary angiography is indicated as a presurgical procedure depending on age. LV angiography is not mandatory unless there is concern regarding the validity of echocardiographic studies (153). Although discrepancies between color flow Doppler and angiography may be observed (154), the understanding of the pitfalls of color Doppler (74) and more recently the introduction of quantitative methods have reduced the need for redundant tests. Also, the analysis of LV function provided by routine LV angiography does not appear to add significant information to the noninvasive data (91). However, tests should be used on an individual basis according to patient characteristics and the results of noninvasive studies.

MANAGEMENT

Principles

Surgical treatment is reserved for patients with severe MR. In these patients, the most relevant question is the timing of the surgical indication, which is influenced by the natural history of the disease and by the outcome of the surgical correction of MR (Table 4-4).

TABLE 4-4. *Determinants of outcome*

Unoperated patients	Operated patients
Age	Age
Symptoms	Preoperative symptoms
Pulmonary hypertension	Atrial fibrillation
AV-O_2 difference	Coronary artery disease
LV ejection fraction	LV ejection fraction
LV end-diastolic volume	LV end-systolic dimension
	LA size?
	Valve repair

AV-O_2, anteriovenous oxygen difference; LV, left ventricle; LA, left atrium.

Natural History

The natural history of MR remains ill defined due to the imprecise assessment of the degree of MR. Nevertheless, it appears that in populations including mostly patients with mild MR, whether due to rheumatic disease (155) or mitral valve prolapse (156), the prognosis is usually excellent. Conversely, in patients with more severe MR conservatively managed, the 10-year survival rate has been reported to be 60% (157) or 46% (158). A 5-year survival rate as low as 27% (159) has been noted, underlining the potential problems related to selection bias and to comparison with expected survival in assessing the natural history of MR. In our experience with patients with flail mitral leaflets who uniformly have severe MR (99,111), at 10 years, survival was 57%, which represents an excess mortality as compared with the expected survival (160) (Fig. 4-7).

The predictors of poor survival in patients medically treated are severe symptoms (New York Heart Association [NYHA] classes III and IV) (158), even if these symptoms are transient and improved by medical treatment (160); pulmonary hypertension; markedly increased LV end-diastolic volume or arteriovenous difference in O_2 (161); and reduced ejection fraction (160,162). Several important points should be noted. First, the threshold of ejection fraction associated with a marked excess mortality is 60% and therefore patients with ejection fraction between 50% and 60%, who are usually considered to have a normal LV function, should be considered at high risk in the context of MR (160). Second, there is no single subgroup at very low risk among patients with severe MR, even if they present with no or minimal symptoms or with an ejection fraction of at least 60% (160).

The probability of sudden death is important to consider before delaying surgery.

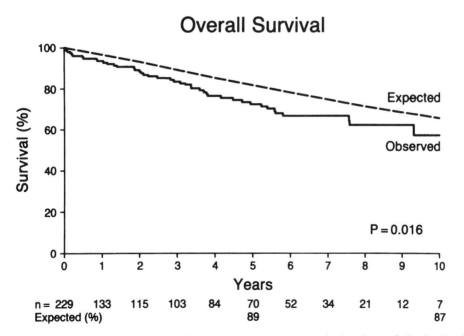

FIG. 4-7. Long-term survival of patients diagnosed with mitral regurgitation due to flail mitral leaflets. The observed survival is noted as a solid line and the expected survival as a dashed line. Note the significant excess mortality in the patients with mitral regurgitation. Reproduced with authorization of the Massachusetts Medical Society. (From ref. 160.)

Such a devastating complication can occur (163), and is more common if ventricular function is decreased (84), but may also occur in asymptomatic patients with a normal ejection fraction (164). The rate of 1.5% per year was observed in our experience in patients with severe MR (85). However, because of relatively small populations, these rates have a wide confidence interval. Nevertheless, the poor predictability of the occurrence of sudden death (85,164) is another incentive for early surgery.

The comparison of the prognosis in medically and surgically treated patients shows a trend in favor of surgical treatment (164), especially early surgery (160), with definite improvement of outcome of patients with decreased systolic LV function (161,165).

In patients initially asymptomatic with severe MR, approximately 10% per year develop symptoms (166) that may be hastened by atrial fibrillation (7). Morbidity was high in our experience with severe MR; at 10-year follow-up, heart failure occurred in 63% and atrial fibrillation in 30% of patients initially in sinus rhythm (160). Conversely, the rates of endocarditis and thromboembolism are low. At 10 years, 90% of the patients had either died or undergone surgery (160), confirming that in these patients surgery for relief of severe MR is ultimately needed and that delays may be catastrophic or seriously compromise long-term results (Fig. 4-8).

In patients with mitral prolapse, the development of severe MR occurs usually with a long delay after the initial diagnosis of the murmur (167), is rare before the age of 50, but its incidence increases thereafter and more so in men (15). The progression, determinants, and most accurate method of monitoring LV dysfunction in patients medically treated are not well characterized.

The natural history of functional MR (i.e., due to global or localized left ventricular dysfunction) is also not well known. However, the current evidence suggests that the presence of MR is a predictor of excess mortality both in patients with cardiomyopathy (168) or with ischemic heart disease (76). The patterns of progression of functional MR have not been well described.

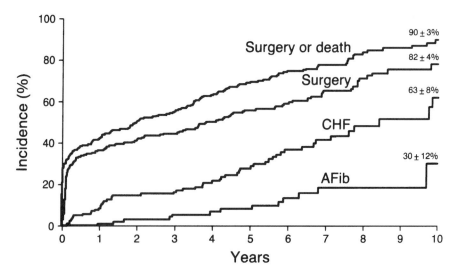

FIG. 4-8. Cardiovascular events occurring after the diagnosis of mitral regurgitation due to flail leaflets. Note the high rates of complications, in particular at 10 years 90% of patients either died or were operated. *AFib*, atrial fibrillation; *CHF*, congestive heart failure. Reproduced with authorization of the Massachusetts Medical Society. (From ref. 160.)

Treatment

Medical Treatment

Prevention of infective endocarditis using the appropriate prophylaxis is necessary in patients with MR (169). Young patients with rheumatic MR should receive rheumatic fever prophylaxis. In patients with atrial fibrillation, rate control is achieved using digoxin and/or beta-blockers. Long-term maintenance of sinus rhythm after cardioversion in patients with severe MR or enlarged LA is usually not possible under conservative management. However, return to sinus rhythm after surgery is possible in patients with atrial fibrillation of short duration (170). Oral anticoagulation should be used in patients with atrial fibrillation. Beta-blockers are the drug of choice in patients with the mitral valve prolapse syndrome and palpitations or chest pain. Diuretic treatment is extremely useful for the control of heart failure and for the chronic control of symptoms, especially dyspnea.

Marked afterload reduction decreases the degree of MR (46), not only by reducing the LV systolic pressure but also by decreasing the ERO area (47,48). Angiotensin-converting enzyme inhibitors have been demonstrated to improve survival in patients with symptomatic LV dysfunction (171). The presence of functional MR may well be a marker for accrued efficacy of these medications in these patients (78,172–174).

Chronic afterload reduction is more controversial for therapy in organic chronic MR (175). The hemodynamic effect of either hydralazine or angiotensin-converting enzyme inhibitors have been analyzed in small series of mostly mild or moderate MR (176–178), and their efficacy in obtaining reductions of regurgitant volume is controversial (179–181) and the effect at most modest. In addition, although no change in ejection fraction was observed, a negative inotropic effect is possible (182). The use of blockers of angiotensin II receptors is also limited. In our preliminary experience, a trend for decrease in the degree of MR was observed that appeared nevertheless moderate in magnitude (183). More prospective and long-term studies are needed to assess the role of vasodilators and in particular of the blockers of the renin-angiotensin system in the treatment of chronic organic MR.

Surgical Treatment

There are two main surgical options: mitral valve reconstruction and mitral valve replacement.

Mitral Valve Reconstruction

The reconstruction of an incompetent mitral valve is almost always possible (approximately 85% to 90% of patients referred for primary correction of acquired MR at the Mayo Clinic). The frequency with which valve repair can be used in patients with MR varies with experience of the operating team and the spectrum of underlying valve disease; repair is more often feasible in patients with degenerative valve disease than in patients with MR caused by rheumatic valvulitis or endocarditis.

Valvular Procedure. In patients with leaflet prolapse, immobilization of this prolapsing section can be obtained by plicating it (184) or by excising (6) the section and then repairing the leaflet. This will overcome the problem of localized prolapse. However, the resulting reduction in area of the leaflet could reduce coaptation and induce residual MR; therefore, annuloplasty is a routine part of the repair. Resection or plication of prolapsing sections is most successful with posterior leaflet prolapse. In patients with anterior leaflet prolapse, the risk of residual MR is higher if the plication or resection is not combined with subvalvular procedures (97). Other repairable leaflet abnormalities include congenital clefts and acquired perforation. A perforation in a leaflet as a result of infective endocarditis, especially if located at the base of the anterior leaflet, may be closed by using a patch of pericardium or synthetic material.

Subvalvular Procedure. In patients with elongated chordae, chordal shortening may be necessary to ensure the appropriate coaptation of the leaflets. Major recent progress has been the introduction of transposition of chordae and of artificial chordae that have made the anterior leaflet prolapse as repairable as the posterior leaflet prolapse (185,186).

Annular Procedure. Annular dilatation, almost constantly associated with MR, is treated by reduction in the circumference of the mitral orifice (i.e., annuloplasty). The annuloplasty should be placed in the region of the annulus supporting the posterior leaflet to preserve the area of anterior leaflet. Commissural annuloplasty has been used (187,188), but this approach tended to distort the valve. The concept of concentrically shortening the posterior mitral annulus by suturing it to a cloth-covered rigid ring was developed by Carpentier et al. (6). Recently, flexible annuloplasty rings have been developed to preserve the changes in shape of the mitral annulus during systole (189). In general, results with the Carpentier ring annuloplasty have been favorable, but LV outflow obstruction associated with abnormal systolic anterior motion of the anterior mitral leaflet has been reported in 6% to 10% of patients (190–192). This complication is mainly due to hypovolemia and hypercontractility due to excessive use of inotropes (97), but the incidence of this complication may be lower with flexible rings, which may better preserve LV function (193).

Intraoperative Assessment of Valve Repair. It is important to assess the adequacy of mitral valve reconstruction before completion of the operation. When satisfactory repair cannot be achieved, it is preferable to replace the valve immediately. To assess the presence of residual MR, the most recent and currently preferred technique is transesophageal echocardiography (96,97), which can be performed without interrupting or interfering with the surgical procedure and is used routinely (97). If, with an appropriate blood pressure and ventricular filling, only trace or mild MR is noted by color flow imaging, the intervention is considered satisfactory. In some cases, a systolic anterior motion of the mitral

valve complicated by intraventricular flow obstruction may be observed, which can usually be corrected by discontinuation of inotropes and fluid replacement (97).

Mitral Valve Replacement

When reconstruction of the mitral valve is considered impossible or, if attempted, is unsuccessful, then replacement must be performed. The dilemma is the choice between a mechanical valve of excellent durability but with the hazard of thromboembolism and a biologic valve with undefined long-term durability (194) but less tendency to cause thromboembolism (195). In patients with atrial fibrillation (195), chronic anticoagulant therapy is necessary even after replacement with a bioprosthesis, so that avoiding anticoagulation is not relevant in choosing a prosthesis (196).

Postoperative Outcome

Valve repair, by preserving the normal valvular tissue, is preferable to valve replacement (6). Compared with prosthetic replacement, mitral valve reconstruction has a lower operative mortality (197,198). Direct comparison of the results of valve repair and replacement is difficult (198), because the patients undergoing a valve repair are usually at a less advanced stage of the disease than patients undergoing valve replacement (197). It appears, however, that survival and LV function (199) after mitral valve reconstruction for MR are superior to that observed after insertion of a prosthetic valve (197), even after adjustment for all baseline differences. Better ventricular function with valvuloplasty may be due to preservation of chordae tendineae and papillary muscles (199,200). Also, valve repair has the same low rate of reoperation as valve replacement (197), mostly due to the development of new lesions (201). Therefore, valve repair should be the preferred procedure for surgical correction of MR (Fig. 4-9).

Operative mortality has been reported to be in the range of 5% to 12% (194,202) for pa-

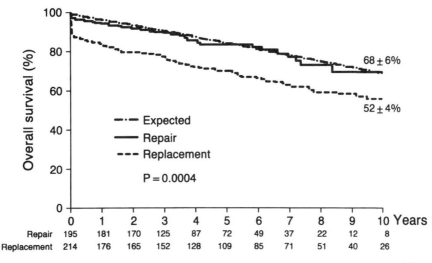

FIG. 4-9. Long-term survival after surgical correction of organic mitral regurgitation. The patients who underwent valve replacement displayed significant excess mortality in compared with patients who underwent valve repair and compared with expected survival. Reproduced with authorization of the American Heart Association.

tients undergoing operation in earlier series, but most patients had prosthetic valve replacement rather than reconstruction. Age, symptoms, and the association of coronary disease remain the most important predictors of operative mortality (91,203). The operative risk is lower in the current era, less than 1% in patients younger than 75 years with organic MR operated at the Mayo Clinic, whether they had valve repair or replacement (91,204). In patients older than 75 years, the operative mortality is around 5% but may vary considerably depending on the degree of heart failure at surgery and the presence of coronary disease (203). It should be noted that LV function is not a predictor of operative mortality and that patients with organic MR and with even markedly depressed LV function have a reasonable chance of surviving surgery (91).

The effect of surgical correction of MR on long-term survival has not been documented by randomized trials. In general, patients operated on for MR have lower survival rates than do those treated for mitral stenosis. However, observational studies suggest that surgical treatment performed at any time results in improved long-term survival (160). Reported long-term survivorship ranges from 75% (194,202,205) to around 50% at 5 years, and these numbers are difficult to reconcile because of age differences between the reported series. In our experience, the survival after valve repair is markedly superior to that obtained after valve replacement (197). Remarkably, patients operated in classes I and II display a survival that is not only superior to those with severe preoperative symptoms, but also not different from the expected survival in the general population (204).

Most long-term survivors after mitral valve replacement for MR show a symptomatic improvement by at least one functional class and some become asymptomatic (206). However, with time the incidence of postoperative congestive heart failure increases (38% at 10 years in operative survivors) and is most often (two thirds of cases) due to residual LV dysfunction after surgery (207). Valvular or prosthetic dysfunction explain the heart failure in approximately one third of cases (207). Postoperative congestive heart failure has a dismal prognosis and should be prevented as much as possible (207), including by early correction of the MR.

The most frequent cause of mortality after surgical correction of MR is LV dysfunction (91) due to chronic irreversible myocardial damage (58,63,64,208) (Fig. 4-10). LV dysfunction occurs in our experience in 40% of patients overall and 32% of those with organic MR (63). Most patients demonstrate a decrease in ejection fraction after successful valve replacement (58,59,63,131,202), probably due to the cumulative effect of several factors: preoperative myocardial damage due to the volume overload; occasional myocardial insult sustained during operation; postoperative changes in loading conditions, especially preload; and alteration of the papillary muscle annular connection after transection of the subvalvular apparatus.

The relationship between pre- and postoperative LV function (Fig. 4-11) (56,58,63,64, 131,148,209) and between preoperative LV function and postoperative survival (62,91, 132,208,210) underlines the fact that LV dysfunction is present preoperatively in most patients presenting with this complication postoperatively. However, the altered loading conditions of MR make the precise assessment of LV function difficult, and multiple and complex indices have been proposed (56,59–62). Nevertheless, despite these altered loading conditions, the simple preoperative ejection fraction is a useful independent predictor of postoperative ejection fraction (58,63,64) and survival (91). In general, one can estimate that the postoperative ejection fraction likely will decrease by approximately 10% early after valve replacement (58,63,64). However, there is a significant individual variation, and more decline can be observed in patients with markedly increased end-systolic diameter (63), volume (64,148), or wall stress (63,209) or in patients with severe symptoms, prolonged duration of MR, or coronary disease (63). A markedly reduced preoperative ejection fraction (less than 50%) is associated with a high late mortality (91), but nevertheless surgery provides a better outcome than medical treatment (161,165). Even a "borderline" ejection fraction (50% to 60%) is associated with an excess late mortality. The best outcome with surgery is obtained in

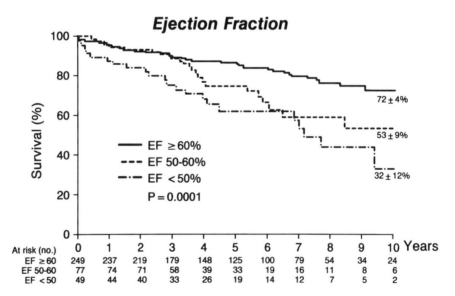

FIG. 4-10. Postoperative survival according to preoperative ejection fraction in patients with chronic organic mitral regurgitation. Note the significant and major differences between the three subsets. Reproduced with authorization from the American Heart Association. (From ref. 160.)

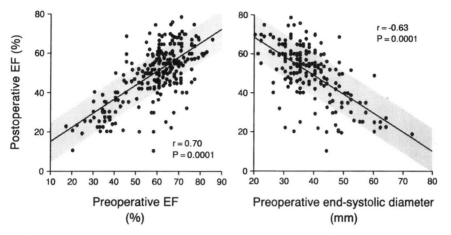

FIG. 4-11. Correlations between postoperative ejection fraction (*y* axis) and preoperative ejection fraction (**left graph**) and preoperative end-systolic diameter (**right graph**) obtained by echocardiography. Note the significant correlations but with wide scatter characterized by the occurrence of unexpected left ventricular dysfunction. Reproduced with authorization of the *Journal of the American College of Cardiology.*

patients with no or minimal symptoms and an ejection fraction of at least 60% (63,91). In these patients, even accounting for operative mortality, the long-term survival is identical to age- and sex-expected survival in the general population (91). The excellent results observed at that stage are an essential incentive for early surgery (Fig. 4-10).

The fortuitous association of coronary artery disease with organic MR is frequent, mostly due to the age of patients operated for chronic MR (151). Despite the almost universal combination of coronary bypass grafting and mitral operation in patients with this association (211,212), a continued postoperative excess mortality is noted in these patients (203). The utilization of the internal mammary artery as a conduit for the bypass grafting appears, similarly to the results observed in isolated coronary disease (213), to minimize the excess mortality due to associated coronary atherosclerosis (203).

The reoperation rates are not different after valve repair and replacement (197). The most frequent causes of reoperation for prosthetic valves are thrombotic occlusion or repeated thromboembolism, primary degeneration, and periprosthetic regurgitation. With regard to valve repair, freedom from reoperation is ap-

proximately 90% at 10 years in our experience (197). The major cause of reoperation is the appearance of new lesions such as ruptured chordae (201). Progression of rheumatic lesions is also a major cause of failure of repairs with rheumatic valves (214). The stability of repair of rheumatic lesions is the most questionable aspect and limits the possibility of early surgery in these patients (215).

Atrial fibrillation when present preoperatively usually persists postoperatively, unless of brief duration (170), but the excess risk due to this arrhythmia appears to be modest (91,170), although it requires anticoagulation. The role of the Maze procedure is not perfectly defined yet, because it may restore atrial activity but conversely is a source of additional operative time and possibly morbidity (216).

Late risk of thromboembolism after valve replacement is not different whether MR or other types of mitral valve disease were corrected (196). Differences in thromboembolic risk after valve repair and valve replacement have been variably estimated (197,198,205) but appear to favor valve repair. After valve repair, anticoagulation is recommended permanently only if atrial fibrillation persists; the occurrence of bleeding is more uncommon in these patients than in those receiving a prosthesis (197).

The outcome after surgical correction of functional MR has been reported in a short series (217). It appears that symptoms may improve after surgery, but survival is limited by the primary myocardial disease. The postoperative outcome in patients with chronic ischemic MR is characterized by a relatively high operative (211,218) and excess long-term mortality (207), due to the presence of LV dysfunction and coronary atherosclerosis in addition to the MR.

Indications for Surgery

Based on the most recent data regarding the natural history of MR treated with and without surgery, the indications for surgery can be outlined according to the etiology, symptoms, and LV function.

Ischemic or Functional Mitral Regurgitation. In patients with cardiomyopathy, the surgical indications have remained relatively restrictive to patients with severe MR and marked symptoms of heart failure. Recent reports have suggested that surgical reduction of the degree of MR by valve repair (219) or by left ventricular reduction and valve repair (220) may provide symptomatic relief. The long-term outcome of these procedures compared with cardiac transplantation needs to be assessed further.

In patients with chronic ischemic MR, two schematic situations can be encountered based on the need for revascularization due to angina or extensive reversible ischemia. First, for patients in whom there is no clearly defined indication for bypass surgery, the usual requirements to recommend surgery for ischemic MR are the severe nature of the MR and the presence of frank symptoms due, at least in part, to the MR. Second, for patients in whom there is a definite indication for coronary bypass surgery, the requirements are less stringent, and it is conceivable to correct moderate MR, even if it is not directly responsible for the symptoms at presentation (221).

Organic Mitral Regurgitation. In patients with organic MR, surgical indications have been evolving toward earlier interventions that appear to provide an improved outcome (222). It is now widely accepted that some subsets of asymptomatic patients should be referred to surgery (223). The indications for surgery should be individualized but can be schematically summarized three ways. First, traditional indications are for patients with severe symptoms (functional NYHA class III or IV), even if these symptoms are transient or markedly improved by medical treatment. These patients benefit from a remarkable postoperative functional improvement but display an excess postoperative mortality independent of other baseline characteristics (204). Second. advanced indications are used for patients with no or minimal symptoms (functional NYHA class I or II) but with signs of overt LV dysfunction (LV ejection fraction less than 60%, end-systolic diameter more than 45 mm in our practice). In these patients, the suppression of the volume overload is expected to prevent further myocardial deterioration, but the overt LV dysfunction is associated with an excess postoperative mortality independent of other baseline characteristics (64,91,132).

Finally, early indications are for patients with severe MR and no or minimal symptoms (functional NYHA class I or II) and with no sign of LV dysfunction (ejection fraction more than 60%). The rationale for this type of indication are as follows: the risk of LV dysfunction secondary to the volume overload, which implies a worse outcome but for which there are no simple, precise, and sensitive methods of detection; the notable mortality occurring under conservative management and in particular the relatively high risk of sudden death; the almost unavoidable need for surgery in patients with severe MR; and the recent progress of surgery that provides with increasing frequency *a restitutio ad integrum*. These patients can expect the best results of surgery and in particular, after the immediate postoperative phase, a survival identical to that of the general population (91). Surgery is, in our opinion, a reasonable option in this subgroup but remains widely discussed (224). However, because surgery in these patients is justified neither by symptoms nor by LV dysfunction, certain conditions should be fulfilled. Both the operative mortality in the institution where such an indication is contemplated and the operative risk for the individual patient involved should be minimal (1% to 2%). The valvular lesions as determined by echocardiography should be highly repairable and the surgeon performing the intervention should have extensive experience with all forms of valve repair. Intraoperative transesophageal echocardiography should be performed by experienced physicians to monitor the repair procedure and to help with decisions warranted by an imperfect result. Quantitation of MR should be performed systematically in these patients preoperatively using multiple noninvasive techniques to determine objectively the degree of MR and affirm that surgery is warranted.

CONCLUSION

Remarkable progress has been achieved in the past decade regarding our management of patients with severe MR. Recommendations for early surgery must be based on careful documentation of the severity of the MR and recognition that the low operative mortality rates and high successful repair rates are not shared equally by all surgeons.

REFERENCES

1. Rusted I, Scheifley C, Edwards J. Studies of the mitral valve. I. Anatomic features of the normal mitral valve and associated structures. *Circulation* 1952;6:825–831.
2. Lam J, Ranganathan N, Wigle E, Silver M. Morphology of the human mitral valve. I. Chordae tendineae: a new classification. *Circulation* 1970;41:449–458.
3. Ranganathan N, Lam J, Wigle E, Silver M. Morphology of the human mitral valve. II. The valve leaflets. *Circulation* 1970;41:459–467.
4. Ormiston J, Shah P, Tei C, Wong M. Size and motion of the mitral valve annulus in man. II. Abnormalities in mitral valve prolapse. *Circulation* 1982;65:713–719.
5. Carpentier A. Cardiac valve surgery—the French correction. *J Thorac Cardiovasc Surg* 1983;86:323–337.
6. Carpentier A, Chauvaud S, Fabiani J, et al. Reconstructive surgery of mitral valve incompetence: ten year appraisal. *J Thorac Cardiovasc Surg* 1980;79: 338–348.
7. Selzer A, Katayama F. Mitral regurgitation: clinical patterns, pathophysiology and natural history. *Medicine (Baltimore)* 1972;51:337–366.
8. Olson L, Subramanian R, Ackermann D, Orszulak T, Edwards W. Surgical pathology of the mitral valve: a study of 712 cases spanning 21 years. *Mayo Clin Proc* 1987;62:22–34.
9. Waller B, Morrow A, Maron B, et al. Etiology of clinically isolated, severe, chronic, pure mitral regurgitation: analysis of 97 patients over 30 years of age having mitral valve replacement. *Am Heart J* 1982;104: 276–288.
10. Edwards J, Burchell H. Pathologic anatomy of mitral insufficiency. *Mayo Clin Proc* 1958;33:497–509.
11. Wooley C, Baker P, Kolibash A, Kilman J, Sparks E, Boudoulas H. The floppy, myxomatous mitral valve, mitral valve prolapse, and mitral regurgitation. *Prog Cardiovasc Dis* 1991;33:397–433.
12. Pini R, Greppi B, Kramer-Fox R, Roman M, Devereaux R. Mitral valve dimensions and motion and familial transmission of mitral valve prolapse with and without mitral leaflet billowing. *J Am Coll Cardiol* 1988;12:1423–1431.
13. Lucas R, Edwards J. The floppy mitral valve. *Curr Probl Cardiol* 1982;7:1–48.
14. Guthrie R, Edwards J. Pathology of the myxomatous mitral valve: nature, secondary changes and complications. *Minn Med* 1976;59:637–647.
15. Wilcken D, Hickey A. Lifetime risk for patients with mitral valve prolapse of developing severe valve regurgitation requiring surgery. *Circulation* 1988;78: 10–14.
16. Hickey A, Wilcken D, Wright J, Warren B. Primary (spontaneous) chordal rupture: relation to myxomatous valve disease and mitral valve prolapse. *Am Coll of Cardiol* 1985;5:1341–1346.
17. Van Der Bel-Kahn J, Duren D, Becker A. Isolated mitral valve prolapse: chordal architecture as an anatomic basis in older patients. *J Am Coll Cardiol* 1985; 5:1335–1340.
18. Byram M, Roberts W. Frequency and extent of calcific deposits in purely regurgitant mitral valves: analysis of 108 operatively excised valves. *Am J Cardiol* 1983;52: 1059–1061.
19. Bloor C. Valvular heart disease in the elderly. *J Am Geriatr Soc* 1982;30:466–472.
20. Buchbinder N, Roberts W. Left-sided valvular active infective endocarditis. A study of forty-five necropsy patients. *Am J Med* 1972;53:20–35.
21. Godley R, Wann L, Rogers E, Feigenbaum H, Weyman A. Incomplete mitral leaflet closure in patients with papillary muscle dysfunction. *Circulation* 1981;63: 565–571.
22. Ballester M, Jajoo J, Rees S, Rickards A, McDonald L. The mechanism of mitral regurgitation in dilated left ventricle. *Clin Cardiol* 1983;6:333–338.
23. He S, Fontaine A, Schwammenthal E, Yoganathan A, Levine R. Integrated mechanism for functional mitral regurgitation. *Circulation* 1997;96:1826–1834.
24. Boltwood C, Tei C, Wong M, Shah P. Quantitative echocardiography of the mitral complex in dilated cardiomyopathy: the mechanism of functional mitral regurgitation. *Circulation* 1983;68:498–508.
25. Pyeritz R, Wappel M. Mitral valve dysfunction in the Marfan syndrome: clinical and echocardiographic

study of prevalence and natural history. *Am J Med* 1983;74:797–807.

26. Leier C, Call T, Fulkerson P, Wooley C. The spectrum of cardiac defects in the Ehlers-Danlos syndrome, types I and III. *Ann Intern Med* 1980;92:171–178.

27. Galve E, Candell-Reira J, Pigrau C, Permanyer-Miralda G, Gardia-Del-Castillo H, Soler-Soler J. Prevalence, morphologic types, and evolution of cardiac valvular disease in systemic lupus erythematosus. *N Engl J Med* 1988;319:817–823.

28. Galve E, Ordi J, Barquinero J, Evangelista A, Vilardell M, Soler-Soler J. Valvular heart disease in the primary antiphospholipid syndrome. *Ann Intern Med* 1992; 116:293–298.

29. Mazzuco A, Rizzoli G, Faggian G, et al. Acute mitral regurgitation after blunt chest trauma. *Arch Intern Med* 1983;143:2326–2329.

30. Kinoshita N, Nimura Y, Okamoto M, Miyatake K, Nagata S, Sakakibara H. Mitral regurgitation in hypertrophic cardiomyopathy. Non-invasive study by two dimensional Doppler echocardiography. *Br Heart J* 1983;49:574–583.

31. Burstow D, Tajik A, Bailey K, DeRemee R, Taliercio C. Two-dimensional echocardiographic findings in systemic sarcoidosis. *Am J Cardiol* 1989;63:478–482.

32. Gottdiener J, Maron B, Schooley R, Harley J, Roberts W, Fauci A. Two-dimensional echocardiographic assessment of the idiopathic hypereosinophilic syndrome. Anatomic basis of mitral regurgitation and peripheral embolization. *Circulation* 1983;67:572–578.

33. Pellikka P, Tajik A, Khandheria B, et al. Carcinoid heart disease. Clinical and echocardiographic spectrum in 74 patients. *Circulation* 1993;87:1188–1196.

34. Redfield M, Nicholson W, Edwards W, Tajik A. Valve disease associated with ergot alkaloid use: echocardiographic and pathologic correlations. *Ann Intern Med* 1992;117:50–52.

35. Connolly H, Crary J, McGoon M, et al. Valvular heart disease associated with fenfluramine-phentermine. *N Engl J Med* 1997;337:581–588.

36. Bauer E, Lasker A, Von Segesser L, Turina M. Conservative surgery of congenital isolated mitral valve anomalies in children. *Helv Chir Acta* 1990;57: 557–561.

37. Yellin E, Yoran C, Sonnenblick E, Gabbay S, Frater R. Dynamic changes in the canine mitral regurgitant orifice area during ventricular ejection. *Circ Res* 1979; 45:677–683.

38. Vokonas P, Gorlin R, Cohn P, Herman M, Sonnenblick E. Dynamic geometry of the left ventricle in mitral regurgitation. *Circulation* 1973;48:786–796.

39. Schwammenthal E, Chen C, Benning F, Block M, Breithardt G, Levine R. Dynamics of mitral regurgitant flow and orifice area. Physiologic application of the proximal flow convergence method: clinical data and experimental testing. *Circulation* 1994;90:307–322.

40. Enriquez-Sarano M, Sinak L, Tajik A, Bailey K, Seward J. Changes in effective regurgitant orifice throughout systole in patients with mitral valve prolapse. A clinical study using the proximal isovelocity surface area method. *Circulation* 1995;92:2951–2958.

41. Mathey D, Decoodt P, Allen H, Swan H. The determinants of onset of mitral valve prolapse in the systolic click-late systolic murmur syndrome. *Circulation* 1976;53:872–878.

42. Enriquez-Sarano M, Seward J, Bailey K, Tajik A. Effective regurgitant orifice area: a noninvasive doppler development of an old hemodynamic concept. *J Am Coll Cardiol* 1994;23:443–451.

43. Tyrrell M, Ellison R, Hugenholtz P, Nadas A. Correlation of degree of left ventricular volume overload with clinical course in aortic and mitral regurgitation. *Br Heart J* 1970;32:683–690.

44. Dodge H, Baxley W. Left ventricular volume and mass and their significance in heart disease. *Am J Cardiol* 1969;23:528–537.

45. Borgenhagen D, Serur J, Gorlin R, Adams D, Sonnenblick E. The effects of left ventricular load and contractility on mitral regurgitant orifice size and flow in the dog. *Circulation* 1977;56:106–113.

46. Chatterjee K, Parmley W, Swan H, Berman G, Forrester J, Marcus H. Beneficial effects of vasodilator agents in severe mitral regurgitation due to dysfunction of subvalvular apparatus. *Circulation* 1973;48: 684–690.

47. Keren G, Bier A, Strom J, Laniado S, Sonnenblick E, LeJemtel T. Dynamics of mitral regurgitation during nitroglycerin therapy: a Doppler echocardiographic study. *Am Heart J* 1986;112:517–525.

48. Keren G, Laniado S, Sonnenblick E, LeJemtel T. Dynamics of functional mitral regurgitation during dobutamine therapy in patients with severe congestive heart failure: a Doppler echocardiographic study. *Am Heart J* 1989;118:748–754.

49. Yoran C, Yellin E, Becker R, Gabbay S, Frater R, Sonnenblick E. Dynamic aspects of acute mitral regurgitation: effects of ventricular volume, pressure and contractility on the effective regurgitant orifice area. *Circulation* 1979;60:170–176.

50. Yoran C, Yellin E, Hori M, et al. Effects of heart rate on experimentally produced mitral regurgitation in dogs. *Am J Cardiol* 1983;52:1345–1349.

51. Grose R, Strain J, Cohen M. Pulmonary arterial V waves in mitral regurgitation: clinical and experimental observations. *Circulation* 1984;69:214–222.

52. Fuchs R, Heuser R, Yin F, Brinker J. Limitations of pulmonary wedge V waves in diagnosing mitral regurgitation. *Am J Cardiol* 1982;49:849–854.

53. Snyder R, Glamann B, Lange R, et al. Predictive value of prominent pulmonary arterial wedge V waves in assessing the presence and severity of mitral regurgitation. *Am J Cardiol* 1994;73:568–570.

54. Braunwald E, Awe W. The syndrome of severe mitral regurgitation with normal left atrial pressure. *Circulation* 1963;27:29–35.

55. Wisenbaugh T, Spann J, Carabello B. Differences in myocardial performance and load between patients with similar amounts of chronic aortic versus chronic mitral regurgitation. *J Am Coll Cardiol* 1984;3: 916–923.

56. Starling M, Kirsch M, Montgomery D, Gross M. Impaired left ventricular contractile function in patients with long-term mitral regurgitation and normal ejection fraction. *J Am Coll Cardiol* 1993;22:239–250.

57. Kontos GJ, Schaff H, Gersh B, Bove A. Left ventricular function in subacute and chronic mitral regurgitation. Effect on function early postoperatively. *J Thorac Cardiovasc Surg* 1989;98:163–169.

58. Enriquez-Sarano M, Hannachi M, Jais J, Acar J. Résultats hémodynamiques et angiographiques après cor-

rection chirurgicale de l'insuffisance mitrale: a propos de 51 cathétérismes itératifs. *Arch Mal Coeur* 1983;76: 1194–1203.

59. Wisenbaugh T. Does normal pump function belie muscle dysfunction in patients with chronic severe mitral regurgitation?. *Circulation* 1988;77:515–525.

60. Mirsky I, Corin W, Murakami T, Grimm J, Hess O, Krayenbuehl H. Correction for preload in assessment. *Circulation* 1988;78:68–80.

61. Corin W, Monrad E, Murakami T, Nonogi H, Hess O, Krayenbuehl H. The relationship of afterload to ejection performance in chronic mitral regurgitation. *Circulation* 1987;76:59–67.

62. Carabello B, Nolan S, McGuire L. Assessment of preoperative left ventricular function in patients with mitral regurgitation: value of the end-systolic wall stress-end-systolic volume ratio. *Circulation* 1981;64: 1212–1217.

63. Enriquez-Sarano M, Tajik A, Schaff H, et al. Echocardiographic prediction of left ventricular function after correction of mitral regurgitation: results and clinical implications. *J Am Coll Cardiol* 1994;24:1536–1543.

64. Crawford M, Souchek J, Oprian C, et al. Determinants of survival and left ventricular performance after mitral valve replacement. *Circulation* 1990;81: 1173–1181.

65. Fuster V, Danielson M, Robb R, Broadbent J, Brown AJ, Elveback L. Quantitation of left ventricular myocardial fiber hypertrophy and interstitial tissue in human hearts with chronically increased volume and pressure overload. *Circulation* 1977;55:504–508.

66. Carabello B, Nakano K, Ishihara K, Kanazawa S, Biederman R, Spann JJ. Coronary blood flow in dogs with contractile dysfunction due to experimental volume overload. *Circulation* 1991;83:1063–1075.

67. Urabe Y, Mann D, Kent R, et al. Cellular and ventricular contractile dysfunction in experimental canine mitral regurgitation. *Circ Res* 1992;70:131–147.

68. Spinale F, Ishihra K, Zile M, De Fryte G, Crawford F, Carabello B. Structural basis for changes in left ventricular function and geometry because of chronic mitral regurgitation and after correction of volume overload. *J Thorac Cardiovasc Surg* 1993;106:1147–1157.

69. Corin W, Murakami T, Monrad E, Hess O, Krayenbuehl H. Left ventricular passive diastolic properties in chronic mitral regurgitation. *Circulation* 1991;83: 797–807.

70. Clancy K, Iskandrian A, Hakki A, Nestico P, DePace N. Age-related changes in cardiovascular performance in mitral regurgitation: analysis of 61 patients. *Am Heart J* 1985;109:442–447.

71. Kono T, Sabbah H, Rosman H. Left ventricular shape is the primary determinant of functional mitral regurgitation in heart failure. *J Am Coll Cardiol* 1992;20: 1594–1598.

72. Nass O, Rosman H, Al-Khaled N, et al. Relation of left ventricular chamber shape in patients with low ejection fraction to severity of functional mitral regurgitation. *Am J Cardiol* 1995;76:402–404.

73. Yiu S, Enriquez-Sarano M, Seward J. Localized left ventricular remodeling determines the degree of functional mitral regurgitation in left ventricular dysfunction. *Circulation* 1997;96:I-83(abst).

74. Enriquez-Sarano M, Tajik A, Bailey K, Seward J. Color flow imaging compared with quantitative doppler assessment of severity of mitral regurgitation: influence of eccentricity of jet and mechanism of regurgitation. *J Am Coll Cardiol* 1993;21:1211–1219.

75. Enriquez-Sarano M, Rossi A, Seward J, Bailey K, Tajik A. Determinants of pulmonary hypertension in left ventricular dysfunction. *J Am Coll Cardiol* 1997; 29:153–159.

76. Hickey M, Smith L, Muhlbaier L, et al. Current prognosis of ischemic mitral regurgitation. Implications for future management. *Circulation* 1988;78-I:51–59.

77. Lehman K, Francis C, Dodge H. Mitral regurgitation in early myocardial infarction. Incidence, clinical detection, and prognostic implications. *Ann Intern Med* 1992;117:10–17.

78. Stevenson L, Bellil D, Grover-McKay M, et al. Effects of afterload reduction (diuretics and vasodilators) on left ventricular volume and mitral regurgitation in severe congestive heart failure secondary to ischemic or idiopathic dilated cardiomyopathy. *Am J Cardiol* 1987; 60:654–658.

79. Bentivoglio L, Uricchio J, Goldberg H. Clinical and hemodynamic features of advanced rheumatic mitral regurgitation. *Am J Med* 1961;30:372–381.

80. Roberts W, Braunwald E, Morrow A. Acute severe mitral regurgitation secondary to ruptured chordae tendineae: clinical, hemodynamic, and pathologic considerations. *Circulation* 1966;33:58–70.

81. Leung D, Griffin B, Snader C, Luthern L, Thomas J, Marwick T. Determinants of functional capacity in chronic mitral regurgitation unassociated with coronary artery disease or left ventricular dysfunction. *Am J Cardiol* 1997;79:914–920.

82. Ronan JJ, Steelman R, DeLeon AJ, Waters T, Perloff J, Harvey W. The clinical diagnosis of acute severe mitral insufficiency. *Am J Cardiol* 1971;27:284–290.

83. Selzer A, Kelly JJ, Vannitamby M, Walker P, Gerbode F, Kerth W. The syndrome of mitral insufficiency due to isolated rupture of the chordae tendineae. *Am J Med* 1967;43:822–836.

84. Kligfield P, Hochreiter C, Niles N, Devereux R, Borer J. Relation of sudden death in pure mitral regurgitation, with and without mitral valve prolapse, to repetitive ventricular arrythmias and right and left ventricular ejection fractions. *Am J Cardiol* 1987;60:397–399.

85. Grigioni F, Enriquez-Sarano M, Ling LH, Bailey KR, Seward JB, Tajik AJ, Frye RL. Sudden death in mitral regurgitation due to flail leaflet. *J Am Coll Cardiol* (in press).

86. Folland E, Kriegel B, Henderson W, Hammermeister K, Sethi G. Implications of third heart sounds in patients with valvular heart disease. The Veterans Affairs Cooperative Study on Valvular Heart Disease. *N Engl J Med* 1992;327:458–462.

87. Horn R, Sarano M, Seward J. The significance of an audible S3 is different in aortic or mitral regurgitation, and LV dysfunction: a quantitative Doppler echocardiographic study. *J Am Coll Cardiol* 1996;116a (abstract).

88. Cohen L, Mason D, Braunwald E. Significance of an atrial gallop sound in mitral regurgitation. A clue to the diagnosis of ruptured chordae tendineae. *Circulation* 1967;35:112–118.

89. Antman E, Angoff G, Sloss L. Demonstration of the mechanism by which mitral regurgitation mimics aortic stenosis. *Am J Cardiol* 1978;42:1044–1048.

90. Desjardins V, Enriquez-Sarano M, Tajik A, Bailey D,

Seward J. Intensity of murmurs correlates with severity of valvular regurgitation. *Am J Med* 1996;100: 149–156.

91. Enriquez-Sarano M, Tajik A, Schaff H, Orszulak T, Bailey K, Frye R. Echocardiographic prediction of survival after surgical correction of organic mitral regurgitation. *Circulation* 1994;90:830–837.

92. Glick B, Roberts W. Usefulness of total 12-lead QRS voltage in diagnosing left ventricular hypertrophy in clinically isolated, pure, chronic, severe mitral regurgitation. *Am J Cardiol* 1992;70:1088–1092.

93. Plaschkes J, Borman J, Merin G, Milwidsky H. Giant left atrium in rheumatic heart disease: a report of 18 cases treated by mitral valve replacement. *Ann Surg* 1971;174:194–201.

94. Mintz G, Kotler M, Parry W, Segal B. Statistical comparison of M mode and two dimensional echocardiographic diagnosis of flail mitral leaflets. *Am J Cardiol* 1980;45:253–259.

95. Marcus R, Sareli P, Pocock W, et al. Functional anatomy of severe mitral regurgitation in active rheumatic carditis. *Am J Cardiol* 1989;63:577–584.

96. Dahm M, Iversen S, Schmid F, Drexler M, Erbel R, Oelert H. Intraoperative evaluation of reconstruction of the atrioventricular valves by transesophageal echocardiography. *J Thorac Cardiovasc Surg* 1987; 35:140–142.

97. Freeman W, Schaff H, Khanderia B, et al. Intraoperative evaluation of mitral valve regurgitation and repair by transesophageal echocardiography: incidence and significance of systolic anterior motion. *J Am Coll Cardiol* 1992;20:599–609.

98. Sheikh K, Bengtson J, Rankin J, de Bruijn N, Kisslo J. Intraoperative transesophageal Doppler color flow imaging used to guide patient selection and operative treatment of ischemic mitral regurgitation. *Circulation* 1991;84:594–604.

99. Himelman R, Kusumoto F, Oken K, et al. The flail mitral valve: echocardiographic findings by precordial and transesophageal imaging and Doppler color flow mapping. *J Am Coll Cardiol* 1991;17:272–279.

100. Hozumi T, Yoshikawa J, Yoshida K, Yamaura Y, Akasaka T, Shakudo M. Direct visualization of ruptured chordae tendineae by transesophageal two-dimensional echocardiography. *J Am Coll Cardiol* 1990;16:1315–1319.

101. Reichert S, Visser C, Moulijn A, et al. Intraoperative transesophageal color-coded Doppler echocardiography for evaluation of residual regurgitation after mitral valve repair. *J Thorac Cardiovasc Surg* 1990;100: 756–761.

102. Daniel W, Mugge A, Martin R, et al. Improvement in the diagnosis of abscesses associated with endocarditis by transesophageal echocardiography. *N Engl J Med* 1991;324:795–800.

103. Shively B, Gurule F, Roldan C, Leggett J, Schiller N. Diagnostic value of transesophageal compared with transthoracic endocardiography in infective endocarditis. *J Am Coll Cardiol* 1991;18:391–397.

104. Izumi S, Miyatake K, Beppu S, et al. Mechanism of mitral regurgitation in patients with myocardial infarction: a study using real-time two-dimensional Doppler flow imaging and echocardiography. *Circulation* 1987;76:777–785.

105. Keren G, Sonnenblick E, LeJemtel T. Mitral annulus

motion. Relation to pulmonary venous and transmitral flows in normal subjects and in patients with dilated cardiomyopathy. *Circulation* 1988;78:621–629.

106. Otsuji Y, Handschumacher M, Schwammenthal E, et al. Insights from three dimensional echocardiography into the mechanism of functional mitral regurgitation. *Circulation* 1997;96:1999–2008.

107. Roberts W, Kishel J, McIntosh C, Cannon RI, Maron B. Severe mitral or aortic valve regurgitation, or both, requiring valve replacement for infective endocarditis complicating hypertrophic cardiomyopathy. *J Am Coll Cardiol* 1992;19:365–371.

108. Schott C, Kotler M, Parry W, Segal B. Mitral annular calcification. Clinical and echocardiographic correlations. *Arch Intern Med* 1977;137:1143–1150.

109. Helmcke F, Nanda N, Hsiung M, et al. Color Doppler assessment of mitral regurgitation with orthogonal planes. *Circulation* 1987;75:175–183.

110. Spain M, Smith M, Grayburn P, Harlamert E, DeMaria A. Quantitative assessment of mitral regurgitation by Doppler color flow imaging: angiographic and hemodynamic correlations. *J Am Coll Cardiol* 1989;13:585–590.

111. Pearson A, St. Vrain J, Mrosek D, Labovitz A. Color Doppler echocardiographic evaluation of patients with a flail mitral leaflet. *J Am Coll Cradiol* 1990;16: 232–239.

112. Cape E, Yoganathan A, Weyman A, Levine R. Adjacent solid boundaries alter the size of regurgitant jets on Doppler color flow maps. *J Am Coll Cardiol* 1991;17: 1094–1102.

113. Chen C, Thomas J, Anconina J, et al. Impact of impinging wall jet on color Doppler quantification of mitral regurgitation. *Circulation* 1991;84:712–720.

114. Utsunomiya T, Patel D, Doshi R, Quan M, Gardin J. Can signal intensity of the continuous wave Doppler regurgitant jet estimate severity of mitral regurgitation? *Am Heart J* 1992;123:166–171.

115. Castello R, Pearson A, Lenzen P, Labovitz A. Effect of mitral regurgitation on pulmonary venous velocities derived from transesophageal echocardiography color-guided pulsed Doppler imaging. *J Am Coll Cardiol* 1991;17:1499–1506.

116. Klein A, Obarski T, Stewart W, et al. Transesophageal Doppler echocardiography of pulmonary venous flow: a new marker of mitral regurgitation severity. *J Am Coll Cardiol* 1991;18:518–526.

117. Enriquez-Sarano M, Dujardin K, Tribouilloy C, et al. Determinants of pulmonary venous flow reversal in mitral regurgitation and its usefulness in determining the severity of the mitral regurgitation. *Am J Cardiol* (in press).

118. Vandervoort P, Rivera J, Mele D, et al. Application of color Doppler flow mapping to calculate effective regurgitant orifice area. An in vitro study and initial clinical observations. *Circulation* 1993;88:1150–1156.

119. Enriquez-Sarano M, Bailey K, Seward J, Tajik A, Krohn M, Mays J. Quantitative Doppler assessment of valvular regurgitation. *Circulation* 1993;87:841–848.

120. Rokey R, Sterling L, Zoghbi W, et al. Determination of regurgitant fraction in isolated mitral or aortic regurgitation by pulsed Doppler two-dimensional echocardiography. *J Am Coll Cardiol* 1986;7:1273–1278.

121. Blumlein S, Bouchard A, Schiller N, et al. Quantitation of mitral regurgitation by Doppler echocardiography. *Circulation* 1986;74:306–314.

122. Bargiggia G, Tronconi L, Sahn D, et al. A new method for quantitation of mitral regurgitation based on color flow Doppler imaging of flow convergence proximal to regurgitant orifice. *Circulation* 1991;84:1481–1489.

123. Chen C, Koschyk D, Brockhoff C, et al. Noninvasive estimation of regurgitant flow rate and volume in patients with mitral regurgitation by Doppler color mapping of accelerating flow field. *J Am Coll Cardiol* 1993;21:374–383.

124. Enriquez-Sarano M, Miller FJ, Hayes S, Bailey K, Tajik A, Seward J. Effective mitral regurgitant orifice area: clinical use and pitfalls of the proximal isovelocity surface area method. *J Am Coll Cardiol* 1995;25:703–709.

125. Nozaki S, Shandas R, DeMaria N. Requirement for accurate measurement of regurgitant stroke volume by the combined continuous-wave Doppler and color Doppler flow convergence method. *Am Heart J* 1997;133:19–28.

126. Tribouilloy C, Shen W, Quere J, et al. Assessment of severity of mitral regurgitation by measuring regurgitant jet width at its origin with transesophageal Doppler color flow imaging. *Circulation* 1992;85:1248–1253.

127. Mele D, Vandervoort P, Palacios I, et al. Proximal jet size by Doppler color flow mapping predicts severity of mitral regurgitation. *Circulation* 1995;91:746–754.

128. Hall S, Brickner M, Willett D, Irani W, Afridi I, Grayburn P. Assessment of mitral regurgitation by Doppler color flow mapping of the vena contracta. *Circulation* 1997;95:636–642.

129. Dujardin K, Enriquez-Sarano M, Bailey K, Nishimura R, Seward J, Tajik A. Grading of mitral regurgitation by quantitative Doppler echocardiography—calibration by left ventricular angiography in routine clinical practice. *Circulation* 1997;96:3409–3415.

130. Heinle S, Hall S, Brickner E, Willett D, Grayburn P. Comparison of vena contracta width by multiplane transesophageal echocardiography with quantitative Doppler assessment of mitral regurgitation. *Am J Cardiol*. 1998;81:175–179.

131. Schuler G, Peterson K, Johnson A, et al. Temporal response of left ventricular performance to mitral valve surgery. *Circulation* 1979;59:1218–1231.

132. Wisenbaugh T, Skudicky D, Sareli P. Prediction of outcome after valve replacement for rheumatic mitral regurgitation in the era of chordal preservation. *Circulation* 1994;89:191–197.

133. Zile M, Gaasch W, Carroll J, Levine J. Chronic mitral regurgitation: predictive value of preoperative echocardiographic indexes of left ventricular function and wall stress. *J Am Coll Cardiol* 1984;3:235–242.

134. Quinones M, Waggoner A, Reduto L. A new, simplified and accurate method for determining ejection fraction with two-dimensional echocardiography. *Circulation* 1981;64:744–753.

135. Rich S, Sheikh A, Gallastegui J, Kondos G, Mason T, Lam W. Determination of left ventricular ejection fraction by visual estimation during real-time two-dimensional echocardiography. *Am Heart J* 1982;104:603–606.

136. Dujardin K, Enriquez-Sarano M, Rossi A, Bailey K, Seward J. Echocardiographic assessment of left ventricular remodeling: are left ventricular diameters suitable tools? *J Am Coll Cardiol* 1997;30:1534–1541.

137. Schiller N, Shah P, Crawford M, et al. Recommendations for quantitation of the left ventricle by two-dimensional echocardiography. American Society of Echocardiography Committee on Standards, Subcommittee on Quantitation of Two-Dimensional Echocardiograms. *J Am Soc Echocardiogr* 1989;2:358–367.

138. Gorge G, Erbel R, Brennecke R, Rupprecht H, Todt M, Meyer J. High resolution two-dimensional echocardiography improves the quantification of left ventricular function. *J Am Soc Echocardiogr* 1992;5:125–134.

139. Ren J, Kotler M, DePace N, et al. Two-dimensional echocardiographic determination of left atrial emptying volume: a noninvasive index in quantifying the degree of nonrheumatic mitral regurgitation. *J Am Coll Cardiol* 1983;2:729–736.

140. Lavie C, Lam J, Gibbons R. Effects of exercise on left ventricular volume and output changes in severe mitral regurgitation. A radionuclide angiographic study. *Chest* 1989;96:1086–1091.

141. Alexopoulos D, Lazam C, Borrico S, Fiedler L, Ambrose J. Isolated chronic mitral regurgitation with preserved systolic left ventricular function and severe pulmonary hypertension. *J Am Coll Cardiol* 1989;14:319–322.

142. Sellers R. Left retrograde cardioangiography in acquired heart disease: technique, indications and interpretations in 700 cases. *Am J Cardiol* 1964;14:437–447.

143. Croft C, Lipscomb K, Mathis K, et al. Limitations of qualitative angiographic grading in aortic or mitral regurgitation. *Am J Cardiol* 1984;53:1593–1598.

144. Sandler H, Dodge H, Hay R, Rackley C. Quantitation of valvular insufficiency in man by angiocardiography. *Am Heart J* 1963;65:501–513.

145. Lopez J, Hanson S, Orchard R, Tan L. Quantification of mitral valvular incompetence. *Cathet Cardiovasc Diagn* 1985;11:139–152.

146. Kennedy J, Yarnall S, Murray J, Figley M. Quantitative angiography. IV. Relationships of left atrial and ventricular pressure and volume in mitral valve disease. *Circulation* 1970;41:817–824.

147. Baxley W, Kennedy J, Feild B, Dodge H. Hemodynamics in ruptured chordae tendinae and chronic rheumatic mitral regurgitation. *Circulation* 1973;48:1288–1294.

148. Borow K, Green L, Mann T, et al. End systolic volume as a predictor of postoperative left ventricular performance in volume overload from valvular regurgitation. *Am J Med* 1980;68:655–663.

149. Wisenbaugh T, Yu G, Evans J. The superiority of maximum fiber elastance over maximum stress-volume ratio as an index of contractile state. *Circulation* 1985;72:648–653.

150. Ramsdale D, Bennett D, Bray C, Ward C, Beton D, Faragher E. Angina, coronary risk factors and coronary artery disease in patients with valvular disease: a prospective study. *Eur Heart J* 1984;5:716–726.

151. Enriquez-Sarano M, Klodas E, Garratt KN, et al. Secular trends in coronary atherosclerosis—analysis in patients with valvular regurgitation. *N Engl J Med* 1996;335:316–322.

152. Ramsdale D, Bray C, Bennett D, Ward C, Beton D, Faragher E. Routine coronary angiography is unnecessary in all patients with valvular heart disease. *Z Kardiol* 1986;75:61–67.

153. Leitch J, Mitchell A, Harris P, Fletcher P, Bailey B. The effect of cardiac catheterization upon management of advanced aortic and mitral regurgitation. *Eur Heart J* 1991;12:602–607.

154. Slater J, Gindea A, Freedberg R, et al. Comparison of cardiac catheterization and Doppler echocardiography in the decision to operate in aortic and mitral valve disease. *J Am Coll Cardiol* 1991;17:1026–1036.

155. Wilson M, Lim W. The natural history of rheumatic heart disease in the third, fourth, and fifth decades of life. I. Prognosis with special reference to survivorship. *Circulation* 1957;16:700–712.

156. Nishimura R, McGoon M, Shub C, Miller F, Ilstrup D, Tajik A. Echocardiographically documented mitral-valve prolapse. Long-term follow-up of 237 patients. *N Engl J Med* 1985;313:1305–1309.

157. Rappaport E. Natural history of aortic and mitral valve disease. *Am J Cardiol* 1975;35:221–227.

158. Munoz S, Gallardo J, Diaz-Gorrin J, Medina O. Influence of surgery on the natural history of rheumatic mitral and aortic valve disease. *Am J Cardiol* 1975;35: 234–242.

159. Horstkotte D, Loogen F, Kleikamp G, Schulte H, Trampisch H, Bircks W. Effect of prosthetic heart valve replacement on the natural course of isolated mitral and aortic as well as multivalvular diseases. Clinical results in 783 patients up to 8 years following implantation of the Björk-Shiley tilting disc prosthesis. *Z Kardiol* 1983;72:494–503.

160. Ling H, Enriquez-Sarano M, Seward J, et al. Clinical outcome of mitral regurgitation due to flail leaflets. *N Engl J Med* 1996;335:1417–1423.

161. Hammermeister K, Fisher L, Kennedy W, Samuels S, Dodge H. Prediction of late survival in patients with mitral valve disease from clinical, hemodynamic, and quantitative angiographic variables. *Circulation* 1978; 57:341–349.

162. Ramanathan K, Knowles J, Connor M, et al. Natural history of chronic mitral insufficiency: relation of peak systolic pressure/end-systolic volume ration to morbidity and mortality. *J Am Coll Cardiol* 1984;3: 1412–1416.

163. Chesler E, King R, Edwards J. The myxomatous mitral valve and sudden death. *Circulation* 1983;67: 632–639.

164. Delahaye J, Gare J, Viguier E, Delahaye F, De Gevigney G, Milon H. Natural history of severe mitral regurgitation. *Eur Heart J* 1991;12[Suppl B]:5–9.

165. Hochreiter C, Niles N, Devereux R, Kligfield P, Borer J. Mitral regurgitation: relationship of noninvasive descriptors of right and left ventricular performance to clinical and hemodynamic findings and to prognosis in medically and surgically treated patients. *Circulation* 1986;73:900–912.

166. Rosen S, Borer J, Hochreiter C, et al. Natural history of the asymptomatic/minimally symptomatic patient with with severe mitral regurgitation secondary to mitral valve prolapse and normal right and left ventricular performance. *Am J Cardiol* 1994;74:374–380.

167. Kolibash AJ, Kilman J, Bush C, Ryan J, Fontana M, Wooley C. Evidence for progression from mild to severe mitral regurgitation in mitral valve prolapse. *Am J Cardiol* 1986;58:762–767.

168. Blondheim D, Jacobs L, Kotler M. Dilated cardiomyopathy with mitral regurgitation: decreased survival despite a low frequency of left ventricular thrombus. *Am Heart J* 1991;122:763–771.

169. Shulman S, Amren D, Bisno A, et al. Prevention of bacterial endocarditis. A statement for health professionals by the Committee on Rheumatic Fever and Bacterial Endocarditis of the Council on Cardiovascular Diseases in the Young of the American Heart Association. *Am J Dis Child* 1985;139:232–235.

170. Chua Y, Schaff H, Orszulak T, Morriss J. Outcome of mitral valve repair in patients with preoperative atrial fibrillation. Should the maze procedure be combined with mitral valvuloplasty? *J Thorac Cardiovasc Surg* 1994;107:408–415.

171. SOLVD Investigators. Effect of enalapril on survival in patients with reduced left ventricular ejection fractions and congestive heart failure. *N Engl J Med* 1991;325:293–302.

172. Evangelista-Masip A, Bruguera-Cortada J, Serrat-Serradell R. Influence of mitral regurgitation on the response to captopril therapy for congestive heart failure caused by idiopathic dilated cardiomyopathy. *Am J Cardiol* 1992;69:373–376.

173. Hamilton M, Stevenson L, Child J, Moriguchi J, Walden J, Woo M. Sustained reduction in valvular regurgitation and atrial volumes with tailored vasodilator therapy in advanced congestive heart failure secondary to dilated (ischemic or idiopathic) cardiomyopathy. *Am J Cardiol* 1991;67:259–263.

174. Stevenson L, Brunken R, Belil D, et al. Afterload reduction with vasodilators and diuretics decreases mitral regurgitation during upright exercise in advanced heart failure. *J Am Coll Cardiol* 1990;15:174–180.

175. Levine H, Gaasch W. Vasoactive drugs in chronic regurgitant lesions of the mitral and aortic valves. *J Am Coll Cardiol* 1996;28:1083–1091.

176. Greenberg B, Massie B, Brundage B, Botvinick E, Parmley W, Chatterjee K. Beneficial effects of hydralazine in severe mitral regurgitation. *Circulation* 1978;58:273–279.

177. Schon H, Schroter G, Blomer H, Schomig A. Beneficial effects of a single dose of quinapril on left ventricular performance in chronic mitral regurgitation. *Am J Cardiol* 1994;73:785–791.

178. Schanzenbacher P, Liebau G. Effect of captopril on left ventricular dynamics in patients with chronic left ventricular volume overload. *Klin Wochenschr* 1983;61: 343–347.

179. Marcotte F, Honos G, Walling A, et al. Effect of angiotensin converting enzyme inhibitor therapy in mitral regurgitation with normal left ventricular function. *Can J Cardiol* 1997;13:479–485.

180. Tishler M, Rowan M, LeWinter M. Effect of enalapril on left ventricular mass and volumes in asymptomatic chronic, severe mitral regurgitation secondary to mitral valve prolapse. *Am J Cardiol* 1998;82:242–245.

181. Rothlisberger C, Sareli P, Wisenbaugh T. Comparison of single dose nifedipine and captopril for chronic severe mitral regurgitation. *Am J Cardiol* 1994;73:978–981.

182. Wisenbaugh T, Essop R, Rothlisberger C, Sareli P. Effects of a single oral dose of captopril on left ventricular performance in severe mitral regurgitation. *Am J Cardiol* 1992;69:348–353.

183. Dujardin K, Enriquez-Sarano M, Seward J. A prospective trial on the effects of losartan on the degree of mitral regurgitation. *Circulation* 1997;96:I-468(abst).

184. McGoon D. Repair of mitral insufficiency due to ruptured chordae tendineae. *J Thorac Cardiovasc Surg* 1960;39:357–362.

185. Frater R, Gabbay S, Shore D, Factor S, Strom J. Reproducible replacement of elongated or ruptured mitral valve chordae. *Ann Thorac Surg* 1983;35:14–28.

186. Lessana A, Escorsin M, Romano M, et al. Transposition of posterior leaflet for treatment of ruptured main chordae of the anterior mitral leaflet. *J Thorac Cardiovasc Surg* 1985;89:804–806.

187. Reed G, Fooley R, Moggio R. Durability of measured mitral annuloplasty: seventeen-year study. *J Thorac Cardiovasc Surg* 1980;79:321–325.

188. Kay C, Kay J, Zubiate P, Yokoyama T, Mendez M. Mitral valve repair for mitral regurgitation secondary to coronary artery disease. *Circulation* 1986;74:188–198.

189. Duran C, Revuelta J, Gaite L, Alonso C, Fleitas M. Stability of mitral reconstructive surgery at 10–12 years for predominantly rheumatic valvular disease. *Circulation* 1988;78:I91–I96.

190. Schiabone W, Cosgrove D, Lever H, Stewart W, Salcedo E. Long-term follow-up of patients with left ventricular outflow tract obstruction after Carpentier ring mitral valvuloplasty. *Circulation* 1988;78:60–66.

191. Galler M, Kronzon I, Slater J, et al. Long-term follow-up after mitral valve reconstruction: incidence of postoperative left ventricular outflow obstruction. *Circulation* 1986;74:I99–I103.

192. Mihaileanu S, Marino J, Chauvaud S, et al. Left ventricular outflow obstruction after mitral valve repair (Carpentier's technique). Proposed mechanisms of disease. *Circulation* 1988;78:I78–I84.

193. David T, Komeda M, Pollick C, Burns R. Mitral valve annuloplasty: the effects of the type on left ventricular function. *Ann Thorac Surg* 1989;47:524–528.

194. Cohn L, Allred E, Cohn L, et al. Early and late risk of mitral valve replacement: a 12-year concomitant comparison of the porcine bioprosthetic and prosthetic disc mitral valves. *J Thorac Cardiovasc Surg* 1985;90:872–880.

195. Pumphrey C, Fuster V, Chesebro J. Systemic thromboembolism in valvular heart disease and prosthetic heart valves. *Mod Concepts Cardiovasc Dis* 1982;51:131–136.

196. Edmunds LJ. Thromboembolic complications of current cardiac valvular prostheses. *Ann Thorac Surg* 1982;34:96–106.

197. Enriquez-Sarano M, Schaff H, Orszulak T, Tajik A, Bailey K, Frye R. Valve repair improves the outcome of surgery for mitral regurgitation. *Circulation* 1995;91:1264–1265.

198. Perier P, Deloche A, Chauvaud S, et al. Comparative evaluation of mitral valve repair and replacement with Starr, Bjork, and porcine valve prostheses. *Circulation* 1984;70:I187–I192.

199. Goldman M, Mora F, Guarino T, Fuster V, Mindich B. Mitral valvuloplasty is superior to mitral valve replacement for preservation of left ventricular function: an intraoperative two-dimensional echocardiographic study. *J Am Coll Cardiol* 1987;10:568–575.

200. David T, Burns R, Bacchus C, Druck M. Mitral regurgitation with and without preservation of chordae tendinae. *J Thorac Cardiovasc Surg* 1984;88:718–725.

201. Cerfolio R, Orszulak T, Pluth J, Harmsen W, Schaff H. Reoperation after valve repair for mitral regurgitation: early and intermediate results. *J Thorac Cardiovasc Surg* 1996;111:1177–1183.

202. Kay J, Zubiate P, Mendez M, Vanstrom N, Yokoyama T. Mitral valve repair for significant mitral insufficiency. *Am Heart J* 1978;95:253–262.

203. Tribouilloy C, Enriquez-Sarano M, Schaff H, et al. Excess mortality due to coronary artery disease after valvular surgery. Secular trends in valvular regurgitation and effect of internal mammary bypass. *Circulation* 1998;98:II108–II115.

204. Tribouilloy C, Enriquez-Sarano M, Schaff H, et al. Impact of preoperative symptoms on survival after surgical correction of organic mitral regurgitation: rationale for optimizing surgical indications. *Circulation* 1999;99:400-S.

205. Orszulak T, Schaff H, Danielson G, et al. Mitral regurgitation due to ruptured chordae tendineae. Early and late results of valve repair. *J Thorac Cardiovasc Surg* 1985;89:491–498.

206. McGoon M, Fuster V, McGoon D, Pumphrey C, Pluth J, Elveback L. Aortic and mitral valve incompetence: long-term follow-up (10–19 years) of patients treated with the Starr-Edward prosthesis. *J Am Coll Cardiol* 1984;3:930–938.

207. Enriquez-Sarano M, Schaff H, Orszulak T, Bailey K, Tajik A, Frye R. Congestive heart failure after surgical correction of mitral regurgitation. A long-term study. *Circulation* 1995;92:2496–2503.

208. Phillips H, Levine F, Carter J, et al. Mitral valve replacement for isolated mitral regurgitation: analysis of clinical course and late postoperative left ventricular ejection fraction. *Am J Cardiol* 1981;48:647–654.

209. Zile M, Gaasch W, Levin H. Left ventricular stress-dimension-shortening relations before and after correction of chronic aortic and mitral regurgitation. *Am J Cardiol* 1985;56:99–105.

210. Reed D, Abbott R, Smucker M, Kaul S. Prediction of outcome after mitral valve replacement in patients with symptomatic chronic mitral regurgitation. The importance of left atrial size. *Circulation* 1991;84:23–34.

211. Ashraf S, Shaukat N, Odom N, Keenan D, Grotte G. Early and late results following combined coronary bypass surgery and mitral valve replacement. *Eur J Cardiothorac Surg* 1994;8:57–62.

212. Kay P, Nunley D, Grunkemeier G, Pinson C, Starr A. Late results of combined mitral valve replacement and coronary bypass surgery. *J Am Coll Cardiol* 1985;5:29–33.

213. Cameron A, Davis K, Green G, Schaff H. Coronary bypass surgery with internal thoracic artery grafts: effects on survival over a 15 year period. *N Engl J Med* 1996;334:216–219.

214. Turner E, Wisenbaugh T, Sinovich V, Cronje S, Sareli P. Morphologic patterns in patients undergoing reoperation after repair of rheumatic mitral regurgitation. *Am J Cardiol* 1993;5:455–457.

215. Antunes M, Magalhaes M, Colsen P, Kinsley R. Valvuloplasty for rheumatic mitral valve disease: a surgical challenge. *J Thorac Cardiovasc Surg* 1987;94:44–56.

216. Cox J, Boineau J, Schuessler R, Kater K, Lappas D. Five-year experience with the Maze procedure for atrial fibrillation. *Ann Thorac Surg* 1993;56:814–824.

217. Bach D, Bolling S. Early improvement in congestive

heart failure after correction of secondary mitral re-gurgitation in end-stage cardiomyopathy. *Am Heart J* 1995;129:1165–1170.

218. Flameng W, Herijgers P, Szécsi J, Sergeant P, Daenen W, Scheys I. Determinants of early and late results of combined valve operations and coronary artery bypass graftings. *Ann Thorac Surg* 1996;61:621–628.

219. Bolling S, Deeb G, Brunsting L, Bach D. Early outcome of mitral valve reconstruction in patients with end-stage cardiomyopathy. *J Thorac Cardiovasc Surg* 1995;109:676–682.

220. Batista R, Verde J, Nery P, et al. Partial left ventriculectomy to treat end-stage heart disease. *Ann Thorac Surg* 1997;64:634–638.

221. Cohn L, Rizzo R, Adams D, et al. The effect of pathophysiology on the surgical treatment of ischemic mitral regurgitation: operative and late risks of repair versus replacement. *Eur J Cardiothorac Surg* 1995;9: 568–574.

222. Ling L, Enriquez-Sarano M, Seward J, et al. Early surgery in patients with mitral regurgitation due to partial flail leaflet: a long-term outcome study. *Circulation* 1997;96:1819–1825.

223. Bonow R, Carabello B, DeLeon A, et al. ACC/AHA guidelines for the management of patients with valvular heart disease. *Circulation* 1998;98:1949–1984.

224. Ross J. The timing of surgery for severe mitral regurgitation. *N Engl J Med* 1996;335:1456–1458.

5

Acute Mitral Regurgitation

Blase A. Carabello

Department of Medicine, Baylor College of Medicine;
Veterans Affairs Medical Center, Houston, Texas 77030

The mitral valve is comprised of the valve leaflets, the chordae tendineae, the papillary muscles, and the mitral annulus. Although acute mitral regurgitation can be caused by abnormalities in any of these four structures, practically speaking it is more useful to classify acute mitral regurgitation based on pathophysiology rather than anatomy. Thus, primary nonischemic mitral regurgitation, primary ischemic mitral regurgitation, and secondary mitral regurgitation differ from one another in cause and outcome. Each occurs in a different cardiac setting and requires a different approach to therapy, mandating that they each be treated separately. By way of definition, the designation "primary" indicates one or more of the four primary valve components noted above that is responsible for valvular incompetence. The term "secondary" implies ventricular dilatation or segmental wall motion abnormalities rather than the valve components that are responsible for the regurgitation.

ACUTE PRIMARY NONISCHEMIC MITRAL REGURGITATION

The common causes of acute primary nonischemic mitral regurgitation are spontaneous chordal rupture and mitral valve perforation (Table 5-1) (1). Chordal rupture occurs in patients with myxomatous degeneration of the mitral valve where tensile strength of the chordae tendineae is reduced, during infective endocarditis, and occasionally in previously apparently normal subjects. Leaflet perforation usually is due to infective endocarditis. Occasionally, either blunt or penetrating trauma can also damage the mitral valve.

Pathophysiology

In acute primary mitral regurgitation, a previously normal left ventricle and left atrium are suddenly burdened with a severe volume overload constituted by normal forward flow returning from the pulmonary veins combined with the volume regurgitated into the left atrium from the left ventricle (Fig. 5-1) (2). The volume overload stretches existing sarcomeres toward their maximum, in turn increasing end-diastolic volume and at the same time maximizing utilization of the Frank-Starling mechanism. This increase in preload allows the left ventricle to increase its volume output. End-systolic volume decreases because the new alternative pathway for ejection

TABLE 5-1. *Causes of acute nonischemic mitral regurgitation*

Chordal rupture
Infective endocarditis
Myxomatous valvular degeneration
Trauma
Hypovolemia in mitral valve prolapse

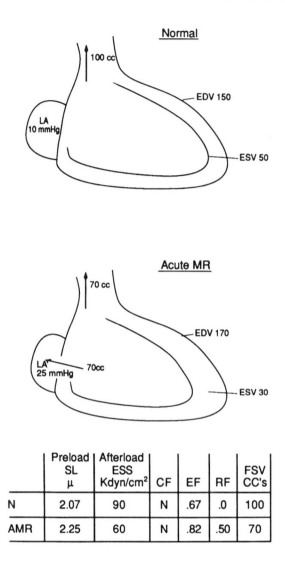

FIG. 5-1. Normal physiology (*N*) is compared with that of acute mitral regurgitation (*AMR*). The acute volume overload on the left ventricle increases preload (sarcomere length, *SL*) and thus end-diastolic volume (*EDV*) increases. The new pathway for ejection into the left atrium (*LA*) facilitates left ventricular ejection and end-systolic volume (*ESV*) decreases as afterload (end-systolic stress, *ESS*) decreases. The favorable loading conditions present increase ejection fraction (*EF*), whereas contractile function (*CF*) remains normal. Because 50% of the total stroke volume is regurgitated into the left atrium (regurgitant fraction, *RF*, 0.5), forward stroke volume (*FSV*) is reduced. (From ref. 2, with permission.)

	Preload SL μ	Afterload ESS Kdyn/cm²	CF	EF	RF	FSV CC's
N	2.07	90	N	.67	.0	100
AMR	2.25	60	N	.82	.50	70

into the left atrium reduces left ventricular afterload and enhances ejection. Increased preload and decreased afterload produce a substantial increase in total stroke volume. However, in severe mitral regurgitation more than half of this stroke volume is ejected into the left atrium, and thus forward stroke volume is actually reduced despite the increase in total stroke volume.

At the same time, the volume overload on the unprepared left atrium increases left atrial and pulmonary venous pressures, in turn leading to pulmonary congestion. At this time the patient suffers all the manifestations of heart failure (pulmonary congestion and reduced cardiac output), yet ventricular contractility is normal or even increased by increased sympathetic tone. It will not be until eccentric hypertrophy and ventricular dilatation develop, allowing a much greater increase in total stroke volume at a lower filling pressure, that compensation will occur.

Diagnosis

The patient with acute severe mitral regurgitation is nearly always symptomatic. In some cases the patient can pinpoint the moment of chordal rupture by the onset of severe dyspnea and weakness. Occasionally, chordal rupture is associated with chest pain. Orthopnea, paroxysmal nocturnal dyspnea, and fatigue also accompany acute mitral regurgitation. During the history interview, clues to etiology should be sought, including a history of mitral valve prolapse or a recent febrile illness consistent with endocarditis.

Detection of acute mitral regurgitation during physical examination is more subtle than is detection of chronic mitral regurgitation (Table 5-2). Because eccentric hypertrophy has not had time to develop, the apical impulse is not displaced nor impressively hyperdynamic. S_1 is reduced in intensity. Because of reduced forward stroke volume, early closing of the aortic valve may increase the normal splitting of the second heart sound. Rapid left ventricular filling of the high volume stored in the left atrium during systole results in a third heart sound. A palpable atrial filling wave may be present. The holosystolic murmur prominent in chronic mitral regurgitation may be unimpressive in acute mitral regurgitation. The high-pressure V wave generated by regurgitation of a large volume into a small left atrium causes rapid equilibration between left ventricular and left atrial pressures early in systole, in turn reducing the driving gradient for regurgitation and shortening the murmur. An apical thrill may be noted. Murmur intensity does not vary with the RR interval (3). In disease involving the posterior leaflet, the regurgitant jet is directed anteriorly, creating a murmur that may mimic aortic stenosis. In anterior leaflet involvement, the posteriorly projected jet may cause the murmur to be referred to the back. In some cases, the murmur may be entirely absent or very difficult to appreciate.

Apart from the diagnosis of mitral regurgitation itself, the physical examination should also focus on clues regarding the etiology of acute mitral regurgitation (i.e., a search should be made for the mucocutaneous manifestations of endocarditis, etc.).

Laboratory Examination

The electrocardiogram usually demonstrates normal sinus rhythm; atrial fibrillation is rare in acute disease, whereas it is common in chronic disease (Table 5-2). Nonspecific ST and T wave abnormalities may be present. These may be more marked in the inferior leads if mitral valve prolapse syndrome is the cause of the patient's acute mitral regurgitation (4).

The chest x-ray gives important clues to the diagnosis. Because left ventricular and left atrial dilatation have not yet occurred, the cardiac silhouette is usually normal in configuration and size. The finding of pulmonary congestion with a normal-sized heart has a limited differential diagnosis, including acute mitral regurgitation, severe coronary disease and extensive ischemia, acute aortic regurgitation, and conditions causing left ventricular concentric hypertrophy or infiltration with attendant diastolic dysfunction.

Echocardiography

Echocardiography is indispensable in making the diagnosis. The three major objectives

TABLE 5-2. *Acute severe vs. chronic severe mitral regurgitation*

	Acute	Chronic
Symptoms	Almost always present, usually severe	May be absent
Cardiac palpation	Unremarkable	Displaced dynamic apical impulse
S_1	Soft	Soft or normal
Murmur	Early systolic to holosystolic	Holosystolic
Electrocardiogram	Normal	LVH and atrial fibrillation common
CXR	Normal cardiac silhouette; pulmonary edema	Enlarged heart; normal lung fields
Echocardiogram therapy	Normal LA and LV vasodilators	Enlarged LA and LV surgery

LA, left atrium; LV, left ventricle.

of echocardiography in acute mitral regurgitation are to derive the specific pathology responsible for the mitral regurgitation, to assess the hemodynamic severity of the lesion, and to search for coexisting cardiac pathology. By establishing the etiology of the mitral regurgitation, both medical and surgical therapies are facilitated. In endocarditis, for example, although in some cases the diagnosis may have already been established by other clinical tests, in other cases identification of valvular vegetations during echocardiography makes the diagnosis for the first time (5). Further, different types of valvular pathoanatomy make repair rather than replacement of the valve more or less feasible. In posterior chordal rupture, repair is almost always accomplished, but if mitral regurgitation is due to severe bacterial damage to the anterior leaflet, repair may be impossible. In addition to assessment of the mitral valve, pathology of the other cardiac valves should be sought because disease there may complicate management by adding an additional hemodynamic burden and the need for additional cardiac surgery.

The severity of acute mitral regurgitation is estimated during color flow Doppler interrogation of the valve. Other clues to lesion severity present in *chronic* mitral regurgitation such as left atrial and ventricular enlargement are not likely to be present in *acute* mitral regurgitation. Color flow Doppler examination detects changes in the velocity of blood flow created at the regurgitant orifice. Even in the most severe mitral regurgitation, the orifice area is relatively small; thus, a large pressure gradient exists between the left ventricle and left atrium, and this pressure difference accelerates blood flow as it enters the regurgitant orifice on the ventricular side. The high-velocity jet entrains red blood cells on the atrial side of the valve, causing an area of high velocity disturbance in the left atrium.

Several methods based on characteristics of the regurgitant jet exist for quantifying the severity of mitral regurgitation, a testimony to the fact that none of these methods has gained universal acceptance. Subjective grading of the amount of atrial flow disturbance is most widely used because it is easily practiced. It is also the least accurate method of establishing regurgitant severity. Usually, trivial versus severe mitral regurgitation can be assessed in this fashion, but intermediate grades of mitral regurgitation are more difficult to establish. Jet mapping is an attempt to better quantify the severity of mitral regurgitation by measuring the area of disturbed flow either as an absolute area or as an area relative to left atrial size (6). Initially, this method was greeted with enthusiasm and seemed to increase the accuracy of the assessment. However, several pitfalls in the method have been defined, raising the question as to whether it increases accuracy of assessment enough to justify time devoted to flow mapping. Machine settings, jet angulation, and jet velocity may all confound flow mapping (7–9).

More recently, the proximal isovelocity surface area method has been used to evaluate regurgitation severity (10–20). As blood flows from the left ventricle to the left atrium, it converges to form a hemispherical jet (Fig. 5-2). At the outer edge of the convergence zone, the area of the jet is large and the velocity is slow. From there, velocity increases and area decreases. By measuring the radius of the jet, the jet area is calculated as area $= 2\pi r^2$. The velocity of the jet is determined at the point of aliasing by the machine display. By multiplying area and velocity, actual regurgitant flow can be calculated and used as an index of severity. Although this method is an advance over subjective assessment, it is limited because in some cases the hemisphere is hard to define and the radius is hard to measure. Further, the method only measures peak instantaneous flow, and thus total regurgitant flow cannot be calculated. However, by dividing peak flow by peak flow velocity, the regurgitant orifice area can be calculated. It is presumed that larger orifice areas are conductive of greater mitral regurgitation and thus orifice area can be used as an index of regurgitation severity.

Another method for assessing regurgitant severity is quantitative Doppler echocardiog-

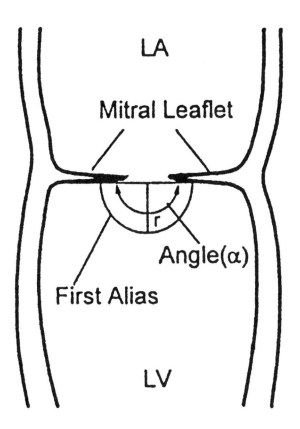

FIG. 5-2. The concept of the proximal isovelocity surface area method is shown. As flow enters the regurgitant orifice, the jet develops a hemispheric shape. By knowing the radius (*r*) of the hemisphere, its area (*a*) can be calculated ($a = 2\pi r^2$). By knowing the velocity of blood at that point, instantaneous flow calculated as velocity times area can also be estimated as an index of the severity of mitral regurgitation. *LA*, left atrium; *LV*, left ventricle. (From ref. 13, with permission.)

raphy (21,22). In this method, total left ventricular output is calculated as diastolic mitral valve area times the diastolic mitral time-velocity integral. This product represents the total flow entering the left ventricle during diastole. Forward flow is then calculated as the product of aortic outflow tract area times the systolic aortic time-velocity integral. The difference between the two products equals regurgitant flow. Regurgitant flow divided by total flow is equal to the regurgitant fraction. Although accurate, this time intensive method has not gained widespread use.

A simpler technique that shows promise is to measure the size of the vena contracta, the area of the jet at its smallest aperture (23). This area reflects the regurgitant orifice area and thus is a measure of the anatomic size of the regurgitant orifice.

In many cases, transthoracic echocardiography is sufficient to diagnose the etiology of the condition and assess lesion severity. However, in some cases transthoracic echocardio-graphy may underestimate the severity of regurgitation or fail to image the mitral valve well. In these cases, transesophageal echocardiography offers an excellent view of the mitral valve and a potentially more accurate assessment of the amount of regurgitation present. In cases where there is a disparity between the clinical and echocardiographic assessment of lesion severity, transesophageal echocardiography may clarify the situation.

Cardiac Catheterization

In patients with severe hemodynamic instability, bedside right heart catheterization is usually performed to further assess the lesion hemodynamically. Acute mitral regurgitation increases both the left atrial and pulmonary artery pressures. The large regurgitant volume entering a small left atrium creates a large increase in left atrial pressure during systole (a large V wave). Although of some help diagnostically, a large V wave neither confirms nor refutes the diagnosis of severe acute mitral regurgitation. Cases in which large V waves exist in the absence of mitral regurgitation include acute congestive heart failure, which causes left atrial hypertension that magnifies the height of the V wave, and acute ventricular septal rupture, which also increases flow into the left atrium. This latter condition may be especially confusing diagnostically because it also causes a loud systolic murmur in the presence of a left atrial V wave. Thus, large V waves do not always indicate severe mitral regurgitation. On the other hand, the Swan-Ganz catheter, which is long and small in bore, is not ideal for high-fidelity hemodynamic recordings, and its utility is blunted even more when the catheter is connected to its transducer by long tubing connections. Overdamping of the system is particularly marked at high heart rates and thus the operator may fail to record a large V wave even if one were present in the left atrium.

If still uncertain after noninvasive examination, the amount of mitral regurgitation can be further assessed during cardiac catheterization (24). Severity is gauged semiquantitatively during left ventriculography according to how much radiopaque contrast is delivered into the left atrium during systole. Unlike color flow Doppler examination, actual flow is visualized during ventriculography instead of flow velocity. However, this technique has many of the same drawbacks as color flow Doppler interrogation. It is usually excellent at distinguishing between severe and mild mitral regurgitation, whereas middle grades of severity are often left in doubt.

Quantitative angiography offers another approach to the problem of quantification. Total left ventricular stroke volume is calculated as the difference between angiographic end-diastolic volume and end-systolic volume. Volumes are calculated using the area-length method or Simpson's rule. Forward flow is calculated using the thermodilution or the Fick techniques. Forward stroke volume is cardiac output determined by these techniques divided by heart rate. The difference between total and forward stroke volume is equal to the regurgitant volume. Forward stroke volume divided by total stroke volume is equal to the regurgitant fraction. In theory this should be an excellent technique for establishing regurgitant severity. Typically, regurgitant fractions of greater than 40% are severe enough to cause symptoms and require therapy (25,26). Unfortunately, the attention to detail needed to calculate left ventricular volumes angiographically is frequently omitted in today's busy interventional cardiac catheterization laboratory. The result is that volumes calculated in this manner are often inaccurate and thus provide little advantage in the quantification of mitral regurgitation.

Medical Therapy

The therapy of acute mitral regurgitation is aimed at reducing regurgitant volume, thereby reducing left atrial and pulmonary venous hypertension while concomitantly increasing forward stroke volume. Arterial vasodilators such as sodium nitroprusside form the cornerstone of such therapy (27). Arterial vasodilatation reduces vascular resistance, thereby preferentially increasing forward flow while simultaneously decreasing regurgitant flow. At the same time, reduced left ventricular volume may help to partially restore mitral valve competence (28). Intravenous infusion of nitroprusside is particularly useful in these potentially unstable patients because its very short half-life allows easy dose titration. With placement of a Swan-Ganz catheter, the dose of nitroprusside can be regulated to optimally increase forward flow while decreasing left atrial pressure and yet maintaining systemic blood pressure.

However, it should be noted that ferrocyanate, a metabolite of sodium nitroprusside, can lead to intoxication and even death (29). Intoxication is usually heralded by tinnitus and nausea. It may progress to uncontrolled muscular movements, delirium, and coma. Ferrocyanate intoxication is usually encountered when doses of a microgram per kilogram per minute are infused for more than 48 hours. Because ferrocyanate is excreted renally, vigilance for intoxication is particularly important in patients with renal failure. In addition to watching for the clinical signs of ferrocyanate intoxication, daily monitoring of plasma levels is warranted in situations where high doses are infused for a prolonged period of time.

In patients whose severe mitral regurgitation causes hypotension, vasodilators cannot be infused because hypotension may be exacerbated. In such patients, intraaortic balloon counterpulsation restores mean arterial blood pressure while reducing afterload and increasing forward output (27). In patients with this degree of instability, preparation for urgent valve surgery should be made once stabilization has been acquired.

Surgical Therapy

Obviously, surgical therapy is directed at reestablishing mitral valve competence. Until a decade ago, a mitral valve prosthesis would have been inserted after the native valve was excised. Although this operation does achieve valvular competence, it also incurs the risks of prosthetic valves (thromboembolism, relative stenosis, and valve failure) and also causes left ventricular damage. This latter aspect derives from the fact that the valve apparatus is an integral part of the ventricle that helps coordinate contraction and maintains the efficient elliptical shape of the left ventricle (30–33). Therefore, chordal transection injures the ventricle and virtually always reduces left ventricular ejection fraction postoperatively (33–36). Thus, whenever possible, the mitral valvular apparatus and continuity between the leaflets and papillary muscles should be preserved. Either mitral valve repair or replacement with chordal preservation accomplishes this goal. The latter operation is used when the native valve is too badly damaged to be repaired. In that case, as much

of the native leaflet and the chordal attachments are preserved and a valve prosthesis is inserted inside the native leaflets.

ACUTE ISCHEMIC MITRAL REGURGITATION

Acute ischemic mitral regurgitation must be differentiated from acute nonischemic mitral regurgitation in patients with coronary artery disease. Acute ischemic mitral regurgitation implies that the mitral regurgitation is due to effects of myocardial ischemia on left ventricular and annular geometry or on papillary muscle function. On the other hand, many patients with other causes of mitral regurgitation such as myxomatous degeneration may also have coronary artery disease. The presence of coronary disease might worsen the overall prognosis of such patients (37), but because the coronary disease is not the cause of the mitral regurgitation, it means the mitral regurgitation will be treated in the same way that primary nonischemic mitral valve disease is treated.

Acute ischemic mitral regurgitation may occur at the time of acute myocardial infarction. Alternatively, mitral regurgitation that is due to the effects of myocardial ischemia may develop remotely after the infarct as ventricular remodeling occurs, causing papillary muscle displacement and annular dilatation.

Mechanisms of Ischemic Mitral Regurgitation

From a mechanistic standpoint, the simplest form of acute mitral regurgitation due to ischemic heart disease is that of papillary muscle rupture. Either an entire papillary muscle may rupture, leading to pulmonary edema, shock, and usually death, or one head of a papillary muscle may rupture, causing severe but more manageable mitral regurgitation. Papillary muscle infarction and rupture is much more common during inferoposterior myocardial infarction than during anterior myocardial infarction (38,39). Increased pos-

terior papillary muscle damage probably relates to a more tenuous blood supply to the
posterior medial papillary muscle compared
with the multiple blood supplies to the anterior papillary muscle. Further, the posterior
papillary muscle is almost always involved in
posterior infarction (40), whereas the anterior
papillary muscle may be spared in anterior infarction. Papillary muscle rupture from infarction usually occurs between the second
and fifth day after the event. The overwhelming loss of integrity of the mitral valve apparatus in papillary muscle rupture leads to a
flail leaflet and severe mitral regurgitation
that almost always necessitates urgent surgical correction.

More difficult to understand is the mitral
regurgitation that occurs in ischemic heart
disease in the absence of overt papillary muscle necrosis. Although such mitral regurgitation is often said to be due to papillary muscle dysfunction, dysfunction by itself is rarely
an actual cause of mitral regurgitation. Although it is true that the papillary muscle fails
to shorten during ischemia or infarction, the
increase in leaflet travel of 1 to 2 mm pro-

duced in this fashion is usually not enough to
allow regurgitation because the area of leaflet
coaptation is generous and tolerant of this
amount of chordal lengthening (41,42).
Rather, asymmetric changes in annular shape
(Fig. 5-3), asymmetric annular dilatation, and
dysnergic ventricular contraction altering the
position of the papillary muscles (Fig. 5-4)
contribute in concert to mitral regurgitation in
the acute ischemic phase (43–45).

In experimental models, myocardial damage inadequate to cause acute mitral regurgitation may lead to mitral regurgitation in 4 to
6 weeks as left ventricular dilatation and
change in papillary muscle position leads to
failure of leaflet coaptation (41). Thus, the
amount of left ventricular damage required to
cause ischemic mitral regurgitation varies
widely. In one instance, a tiny myocardial infarction leading to papillary muscle necrosis
and rupture could be enough damage to cause
severe mitral regurgitation. In other cases,
substantial damage is required to produce
asymmetric ventricular contraction and left
ventricular dilatation, in turn leading to mitral
regurgitation.

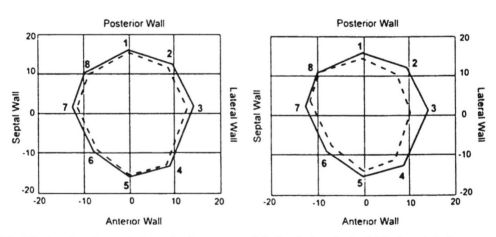

FIG. 5-3. Annular size and shape is demonstrated during ischemia (*solid line*) and during normal
conditions (*dotted line*). During ischemia there is asymmetric enlargement of the annulus most
marked during systole. (From ref. 44, with permission.)

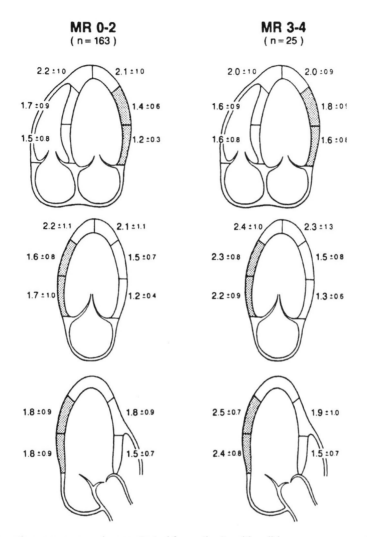

FIG. 5-4. Wall motion scores are demonstrated for patients with mild versus severe mitral regurgitation. As can be seen, wall motion is substantially worse in severe MR. Worsened wall motion contributes both to the severity of the mitral regurgitation and to increased mortality. (From ref. 45, with permission.)

Diagnosis

Acute severe ischemic mitral regurgitation should be considered in any case of shock or congestive heart failure accompanying myocardial infarction, especially in the presence of a new murmur. However, occasionally severe ischemic mitral regurgitation occurs without the presence of a heart murmur. As noted earlier, in any case of severe acute mitral regurgitation, the presence of a high V wave results in the rapid equilibration of left ventricular and left atrial pressures, decreasing the length of the murmur and diminishing its impact on the physical examination. The electrocardiogram is almost always abnormal, although it may often fail to be diagnostic of acute myocardial infarction because posterior infarction, the usual cause of acute ischemic mitral regurgitation, is often less obvious electrocardiographically. As in other cases of acute mitral regurgitation, pulmonary edema together with a normal-sized heart is common. Echocardiography is extremely important in demonstrating the wall motion abnormalities that are usually responsible for the mitral regurgitation and in demonstrating the mitral regurgitation itself. As noted earlier, sometimes transthoracic echocardiography underestimates the severity of the regurgitation that is visualized better during transesophageal echocardiography. In the case of papillary muscle rupture, a flail leaflet will be noted, but the diagnosis of papillary muscle rupture itself is often hard to make echocardiographically.

Except in dire emergencies, cardiac catheterization to implement coronary arteriography should be performed because every effort to revascularize existing coronary disease will be made at the time of the mitral valve operation. Except in the case of total papillary muscle rupture, intraaortic balloon counterpulsation is extremely effective in stabilizing the patient so that cardiac catheterization can be accomplished.

Therapy

Most patients with severe acute mitral regurgitation have it persistently. Occasionally, in some patients, acute mitral regurgitation is episodic, occurring during ischemia and resolving as ischemia resolves. In this latter group, it might be possible to treat the mitral regurgitation by revascularization alone either percutaneously or during surgery. However, in patients with acute persistent mitral regurgitation, a definitive mitral valve operation must be performed in tandem with coronary revascularization after patients have been stabilized.

Unlike nonischemic mitral regurgitation where mitral valve repair is almost always favored, there is no unanimous opinion regarding the surgical approach to acute ischemic mitral regurgitation. Irrespective of approach, operative mortality is high, ranging from 10% to 70%, although one recent report noted only

a 4% operative risk (46). High operative mortality stems from the severe hemodynamic compromise of patients suffering both acute myocardial infarction and acute mitral regurgitation simultaneously. In a study of both acute and chronic ischemic mitral regurgitation, Cohn et al. (47) found an operative mortality of approximately 9% for both repair and replacement. However, long-term survivorship was much better for mitral valve replacement in which the mitral apparatus was preserved than for pure mitral valve repair. Mitral valve repair may fail to be superior to replacement in this condition because usually the valve itself is not pathologically involved but rather the mitral regurgitation is created by ventricular segmental wall motion abnormalities and local annular dilatation, situations not necessarily correctable at the time of repair. On the other hand, Bolling et al. (46) reported on 100 consecutive patients with severe ischemic mitral regurgitation. The early mortality was 4% with an additional 6% mortality at 25 months.

Prognosis

The presence of even mild mitral regurgitation occurring acutely after myocardial infarction substantially worsens prognosis. Lamas et al. (48), reporting for the SAVE Investigators (Fig. 5-5), found that the presence of mitral regurgitation during ventriculography in patients with an ejection fraction of less than 0.4 substantially worsened prognosis. Patients with mitral regurgitation had a 29% mortality during the 3.5-year follow-up versus 12% for patients not demonstrating mitral regurgitation. The combined end point of heart failure mortality or recurrent myocardial infarction was 47% in patients with mitral regurgitation versus 29% in patients without mitral regurgitation. Because the mitral regurgitation in this study was mostly mild in nature, it was presumably not the extra hemodynamic burden that the regurgitation placed on the ventricle but rather that mitral regurgitation was a marker of severe regional dyssynergy and cardiac dilatation that was associated with the

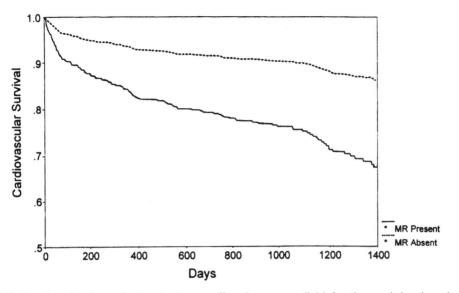

FIG. 5-5. Survivorship for patients who have suffered a myocardial infarction and developed mitral regurgitation is shown. (From ref. 48, with permission.)

poor result. Not unexpectedly, when the mitral regurgitation is more severe, the risk is even higher. Thus, Tcheng et al. (49) found that in patients with severe ischemic mitral regurgitation immediately after a myocardial infarction, 30-day mortality was 24%, whereas over half of these patients were dead 1 year after the infarction. In this case, the additional hemodynamic burden of the mitral regurgitation and more severe left ventricular dysfunction probably contributed to the very poor prognosis of these patients.

In summary, severe acute ischemic mitral regurgitation is usually a life-threatening event requiring immediate stabilization and early surgery. Operative mortality is high, but the best operation for this complication of myocardial infarction has not yet been established. However, it appears that mitral valve replacement with chordal preservation together with myocardial revascularization may be just as effective or even superior to mitral valve repair in this circumstance. Even when less severe nonsurgical mitral regurgitation develops acutely, the prognosis worsens, presumably because its presence indicates more extensive myocardial damage with more regional wall motion abnormality, ventricular dilatation, and annular dilatation.

ACUTE SECONDARY MITRAL REGURGITATION IN CARDIOMYOPATHY

As cardiomyopathy progresses, it leads to left ventricular enlargement and remodeling. At some point in this process, there is usually enough increase in left ventricular size that malalignment of the papillary muscles leads to mitral regurgitation. Although the course of this progression is often unknown, it seems clear that in some cases, mitral regurgitation may develop acutely in this process and is one of the causes for decompensation or of recurrent heart failure in the patient with cardiomyopathy. In fact, when mitral regurgitation accompanies dilated cardiomyopathy, both hemodynamics and prognosis worsen (50). If the patient has been followed for a long period of time, it may be possible to recognize that the mitral regurgitation is a consequence of cardiomyopathy by history. However, in other cases where a patient presents for the first time with a dilated left ventricle, reduced left ventricular function, and severe mitral regurgitation, it may be hard to tell whether cardiomyopathy caused the mitral regurgitation or if mitral regurgitation caused the cardiomyopathy.

Transesophageal echocardiography may be helpful in resolving this issue because a structural valvular abnormality usually indicates that it was the mitral regurgitation that was primary. Finding no specific valvular abnormality, it might be assumed that the myopathy was primary and that the mitral regurgitation was secondary. The effect of medical therapy in this type of mitral regurgitation is unclear. In one study, medical therapy with vasodilators and diuretics reduced left ventricular volume and restored mitral valve competence, in turn improving cardiac index while decreasing left ventricular volume (51). Implicit in these results is that regurgitant volume decreased as forward flow increased. A recent study confirmed these results (52).

Although it might seem intuitive that valvular surgery would be ineffective in treating mitral regurgitation due to myopathy because the myopathy itself would not be treated by surgery, Bach et al. (53) demonstrated encouraging surgical results. In their series of patients with secondary mitral regurgitation and very low ejection fraction (0.15), a simple mitral valve annuloplasty resulted in no operative deaths, a 70% 1-year survival rate, and a significant reduction in cardiac volume and an increase in ejection fraction in those people who did survive.

At the current time there are no data to help distinguish whether medical versus surgical therapy is superior in the treatment of secondary mitral regurgitation. It should be noted that acute mitral regurgitation occurring in cardiomyopathy may be a cause of decompensation. Such patients should initially be treated with vasodilators and diuretics. If this therapy fails, some thought should be given to mitral valve annuloplasty in selected centers where this procedure can be achieved at low mortality.

REFERENCES

1. Waller BF, Howard J, Fess S. Pathology of mitral valve stenosis and pure mitral regurgitation. Part II. *Clin Cardiol* 1994;17:395.
2. Carabello BA. Mitral regurgitation, Part 1. Basic pathophysiologic principles. *Mod Concepts Cardiovasc Dis* 1988;57:53.
3. Karliner JS, et al. Haemodynamic explanation of why the murmur of mitral regurgitation is independent of cycle length. *Br Heart J* 1973;35:397.
4. Lobstein HP, et al. Electrocardiographic abnormalities and coronary arteriograms in the mitral click-murmur syndrome. *N Engl J Med* 1973;289:127.
5. Durack DT, et al. New criteria for diagnosis of infective endocarditis: utilization of specific echocardiographic findings. Duke Endocarditis Service. *Am J Med* 1994; 96:200.
6. Spain MG, et al. Quantitative assessment of mitral regurgitation by Doppler color flow imaging: angiographic and hemodynamic correlations. *J Am Coll Cardiol* 1989;13:585.
7. Shah PM. Quantitative assessment of mitral regurgitation. *J Am Coll Cardiol* 1989;13:591.
8. Chen CG, et al. Impact of impinging wall jet on color Doppler quantification of mitral regurgitation. *Circulation* 1991;84:712.
9. Sahn DJ. Instrumentation and physical factors related to visualization of stenotic and regurgitant jets by Doppler color flow mapping. *J Am Coll Cardiol* 1988;12:1354.
10. Simpson IA, et al. Spatial velocity distribution and acceleration in serial subvalve tunnel and valvular obstructions: an in vitro study using Doppler color flow mapping. *J Am Coll Cardiol* 1989;13:241.
11. Recusani F, et al. A new method for quantification of regurgitant flow rate using color Doppler flow imaging of the flow convergence region proximal to a discrete orifice. An in vitro study. *Circulation* 1991;83:594.
12. Bargiggia GS, et al. A new method for quantification of mitral regurgitation based on color flow Doppler imaging of flow convergence proximal to regurgitant orifice. *Circulation* 1991;84:1481.
13. Pu M, et al. Quantification of mitral regurgitation by the proximal convergence method using transesophageal echocardiography. Clinical validation of a geometric correction for proximal flow constraint. *Circulation* 1995;92:2169.
14. Vandervoort PM, Rivera JM, Mele D, et al. Application of color Doppler flow mapping to calculate effective regurgitant orifice area. An in vitro study and initial clinical observations. *Circulation* 1993;88:1150.
15. Enriquez-Sarano M, et al. Effective mitral regurgitant orifice area: clinical use and pitfalls of the proximal isovelocity surface area method. *J Am Coll Cardiol* 1995;25:703.
16. Simpson IA, et al. Current status of flow convergence for clinical applications: is it a leaning tower of "PISA"? *J Am Coll Cardiol* 1996;27:504.
17. Shandas R, et al. Experimental studies to define the geometry of the flow convergence region: laser Doppler particle tracking and color Doppler imaging. *Echocardiography* 1992;9:43.

18. Weintraub R, et al. Comparison of flow convergence (FC) calculations using color Doppler flow mapping (CD) and phase velocity encoded MRI: an in vitro study. *Circulation* 1991;84[Suppl II]:II-636(abst).

19. Enriquez-Sarano EM, et al. Effective regurgitant orifice area: a noninvasive Doppler development of an old hemodynamic concept. *J Am Coll Cardiol* 1994;23:443.

20. Pu M, et al. Quantification of mitral regurgitation by the proximal convergence method using transesophageal echocardiography. Clinical validation of a geometric correction for proximal flow constraint. *Circulation* 1995;92:2169.

21. Enriquez-Sarano EM, et al. Quantitative Doppler assessment of valvular regurgitation. *Circulation* 1993; 87:841.

22. Lewis JF, et al. Pulsed Doppler echocardiographic determination of stroke volume and cardiac output: clinical validation of two new methods using the apical window. *Circulation* 1984;70:425.

23. Hall SA, et al. Assessment of mitral regurgitation severity by Doppler color flow mapping of the vena contracta. *Circulation* 1997;95:636.

24. Slater J, et al. Comparison of cardiac catheterization and Doppler echocardiography in the decision to operate in aortic and mitral valve disease. *J Am Coll Cardiol* 1991; 17:1026.

25. Eckberg DL, et al. Mechanics of left ventricular contraction in chronic severe mitral regurgitation. *Circulation* 1973;47:1252.

26. Nagatsu M, et al. The effects of complete versus incomplete mitral valve repair in experimental mitral regurgitation. *J Thorac Cardiovasc Surg* 1994;107:416.

27. Horstkotte D, et al. Diagnostic and therapeutic considerations in acute, severe mitral regurgitation: experience in 42 consecutive patients entering the intensive care unit with pulmonary edema. *J Heart Valve Dis* 1993; 2:512.

28. Yoran C, et al. Mechanism of reduction of mitral regurgitation with vasodilator therapy. *Am J Cardiol* 1979; 43:773.

29. Carabello BA, et al. *Cardiology Pearls.* Philadelphia: Hanley & Belfus, 1994:209.

30. Hansen DE, et al. Physiologic role of the mitral apparatus in left ventricular regional mechanics, contraction synergy, and global systolic performance. *J Thorac Cardiovasc Surg* 1989;97:521.

31. Rushmer RF. Initial phase of ventricular systole: asynchronous contraction. *Am J Physiol* 1956;184:188.

32. Sarris GE, et al. Restoration of left ventricular systolic performance after reattachment of the mitral chordae tendineae. The importance of valvular-ventricular interaction. *J Thorac Cardiovasc Surg* 1988;95:969.

33. Goldman ME, et al. Mitral valvuloplasty is superior to valve replacement for preservation of left ventricular function: an intraoperative two-dimensional echocardiographic study. *J Am Coll Cardiol* 1987;10:568.

34. David TE, et al. Mitral valve replacement for mitral regurgitation with and without preservation of chordae tendineae. *J Thorac Cardiovasc Surg* 1984;88:718.

35. Hennein HA, et al. Comparative assessment of chordal

36. Rozich JD, et al. Mitral valve replacement with and without chordal preservation in patients with chronic mitral regurgitation: mechanism for differences in postoperative ejection performance. *Circulation* 1992;86: 1718.

37. Lytle BW. Impact of coronary artery disease on valvular heart surgery. *Cardiol Clin* 1991;9:301.

38. Wei JY, et al. Papillary muscle rupture and fatal acute myocardial infarction. *Ann Intern Med* 1979;90:149.

39. Nishimura RA, et al. Papillary muscle rupture complicating acute myocardial infarction: analysis of 17 patients. *Am J Cardiol* 1983;51:373.

40. Heikkila J. Mitral incompetence as a complication of acute myocardial infarction. *Acta Med Scand Suppl* 1967;475:1.

41. Llaneras MR, et al. A large animal model of ischemic mitral regurgitation. *Ann Thorac Surg* 1994;57:432.

42. Kaul S, et al. Mechanism of ischemic mitral regurgitation. An experimental evaluation. *Circulation* 1991;84: 2167.

43. Gorman JH III, et al. Distortions of the mitral valve in acute ischemic mitral regurgitation. *Ann Thorac Surg* 1997;64:1026.

44. Glasson JR, et al. Three-dimensional dynamics of the canine mitral annulus during ischemic mitral regurgitation. *Ann Thorac Surg* 1996;62:1059.

45. Van Dantzig JM, et al. Pathogenesis of mitral regurgitation in acute myocardial infarction: importance of changes in left ventricular shape and regional function. *Am Heart J* 1996;131:865.

46. Bolling SF, et al. Mitral valve reconstruction in elderly, ischemic patients. *Chest* 1996;109:35.

47. Cohn LH, et al. The effect of pathophysiology on the surgical treatment of ischemic mitral regurgitation: operative and late risks of repair versus replacement. *Eur J Cardiothorac Surg* 1995;9:568.

48. Lamas GA, et al. for the Survival and Ventricular Enlargement Investigators. Clinical significance of mitral regurgitation after acute myocardial infarction. *Circulation* 1997;96:827.

49. Tcheng JE, et al. Outcome of patients sustaining acute ischemic mitral regurgitation during myocardial infarction. *Ann Intern Med* 1992;117:18.

50. Junker A, et al. The hemodynamic and prognostic significance of echo-Doppler-proven mitral regurgitation in patients with dilated cardiomyopathy. *Cardiology* 1993;83:14.

51. Greenberg BH, et al. Beneficial effects of hydralazine in severe mitral regurgitation. *Circulation* 1978;58:273.

52. Stevenson LW, et al. Afterload reduction with vasodilators and diuretics decreases mitral regurgitation during upright exercise in advanced heart failure. *J Am Coll Cardiol* 1990;15:174.

53. Bach DS, et al. Improvement following correction of secondary mitral regurgitation in end-stage cardiomyopathy with mitral annuloplasty. *Am J Cardiol* 1996;78: 966.

6

Syndrome of Mitral Valve Prolapse

Robert A. O'Rourke

Department of Medicine/Cardiology, The University of Texas Health Science Center,
San Antonio, Texas 78284-7872

The mitral valve prolapse (MVP) syndrome is a very common cardiac disorder. It has been estimated to occur in as many as 15 million Americans (1). This entity is now diagnosed more frequently, even in asymptomatic patients, because its auscultatory features have become well recognized and its characteristic echocardiographic findings are frequently detected during echocardiographic studies for other reasons.

Mid-systolic clicks were first reported in the late 19th century and originally were thought to be pericardial or extracardiac in origin (2–5). Subsequently, late systolic murmurs were described in otherwise healthy subjects and were associated with a normal long-term prognosis. Therefore, this murmur also was attributed to an extracardiac source (2–5). In 1961, Reid (6) postulated that the mid-systolic click and late systolic murmur were due to mitral regurgitation (MR), and in 1963 Barlow et al. (7) confirmed this hypothesis by left ventricular (LV) cineangiography. In 1965, intracardiac (left atrial [LA]) phonocardiogram studies confirmed the mitral valve origin of the systolic click and late systolic murmur (8). During the past three decades, considerable information obtained from pathologic studies, cineangiography, and echocardiography have demonstrated coincidently that this common syndrome is associated with systolic prolapse of one or both mitral valve leaflets into the left atrium (9–12).

Recognition of the MVP syndrome may be difficult because of the extreme variability of its clinical manifestations. However, it is an important cause of incapacitating chest pain and refractory arrhythmias in certain patients (13). The abnormal components of the mitral valve apparatus are a potential site for endocarditis, and some patients may develop severe MR as a result of endocarditis and/or ruptured chordae (5,13).

DEFINITION, ETIOLOGY, AND PATHOLOGY

MVP is defined as the systolic billowing of one or both mitral leaflets into the left atrium with or without MR. It is the most common form of valvular heart disease and occurs in 2% to 6% of the population (1–5,13). MVP often occurs as a clinical syndrome associated with little or no MR but is also the most common cause of significant MR and the most frequent substrate for mitral valve endocarditis in the United States. MR stemming from MVP often is associated with unique clinical characteristics when compared with the other causes of MR (14,15).

The mitral valve apparatus is a complex structure composed of the mitral annulus, valve leaflets, chordae tendineae, papillary muscles, and the supporting LV, LA, and aortic walls (16) (Fig. 6-1). Disease processes involving any one or more of these structures

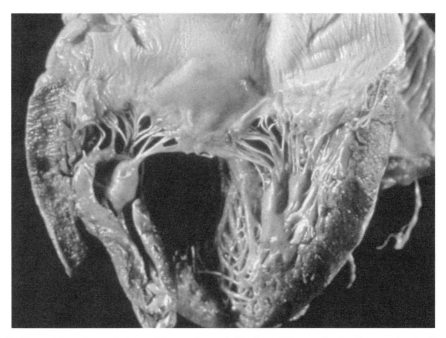

FIG. 6-1. Normal heart specimen cut open through the left atrium, mitral valve, and anterior wall of left ventricle. The functional components of the mitral valve apparatus are the left atrium, mitral valve annulus, posterior mitral valve leaflet, anterior mitral valve leaflet, anterolateral papillary muscle, chordae tendineae, posteromedial papillary muscle, and left ventricular wall. (From ref. 2, with permission.)

may cause valve apparatus dysfunction and prolapse of the mitral leaflets toward the left atrium during systole when LV pressure exceeds LA pressure. When MR is produced from any cause, there is a tendency for progressive dysfunction of the entire mitral apparatus over time, because of increasing LA and LV dilatation that further disrupts the mitral apparatus. Thus, "MR begets MR" (17). In any particular situation, it may be difficult to identify which one of six functional components was initially responsible for the development of MR.

The complexity of the mitral valve apparatus provides an explanation for secondary prolapse in certain conditions that affect one or more of the components of the mitral apparatus (such as ruptured mitral chordae). There is, however, considerable evidence that a disorder of mitral valve leaflets exists in which there are specific pathologic changes causing redundancy of mitral leaflets and

their prolapse into the left atrium during systole. This is the *primary* form of MVP (Table 6-1) (3,13,18).

In primary MVP there is interchordal hooding due to redundancy of the leaflets that involve both the rough and clear zones (Fig. 6-2). The height of the interchordal hooding usually exceeds 4 mm and involves at least one half of the anterior leaflet and/or at least two thirds of the posterior mitral leaflet. The characteristic microscopic feature of primary MVP is marked proliferation (not "degeneration") of the spongiosa, the delicate myxomatous connective tissue between the atrialis (a thick layer of collagen and elastic tissue forming the atrial aspect of the leaflet) and the fibrosa or ventricularis (composed of dense layers of collagen) that forms the basic support of the leaflet (Fig. 6-3) (12). In primary MVP, myxomatous proliferation of the acid mucopolysaccharide-containing spongiosa tissue causes focal interruption of the fibrosa (Fig.

TABLE 6-1. *Classification of mitral valve prolapse*

Primary MVP
  Familial
  Nonfamilial
  Marfan's syndrome
  Other connective tissue diseases
Secondary MVP
  Coronary artery disease
  Rheumatic heart disease
  Reduced LV dimensions[a]
    Hypertrophic cardiomyopathy
    Atrial septal defect
    Pulmonary hypertension
    Anorexia nervosa
    Dehydration
    Straight back syndrome/pectus excavatum
  "Flail" mitral valve leaflet(s)
Normal variant
  Inaccurate auscultation
  "Echocardiographic heart disease"

[a]From ref. 18, with permission.
MVP; mitral valve prolapse; LV; left ventricle.
From ref. 3, with permission.

6-3). Secondary effects of the primary MVP syndrome include fibrosis of the surfaces of the mitral valve leaflets, thinning and/or elongation of chordae tendineae, and ventricular friction lesions. Fibrin deposits often form in the mitral valve-LA angle (12).

The primary form of MVP may occur in families where it appears to be inherited as an autosomal dominant trait with varying penetrance (19,20). However, no consistent chromosomal abnormalities have yet been identified in patients with MVP, and the syndrome of MVP commonly occurs in isolated cases (21). Primary MVP is usually present in patients with Marfan's syndrome (12) and often occurs in other heritable connective tissue diseases such as Ehlers-Danlos syndrome (22), pseudoxanthoma elasticum (23), and osteogenesis imperfecta (24). Marfan's syn-

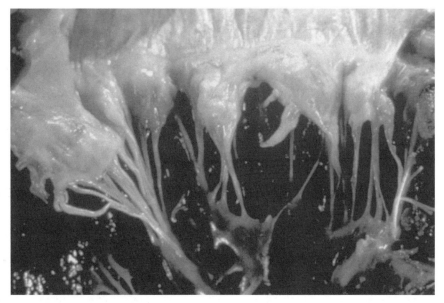

FIG. 6-2. Pathologic specimen of a prolapsing mitral valve. The gross pathologic changes in primary mitral valve prolapse are leaflet redundancy and interchordal hooding, increased valve surface area, thinning and elongation (and rupture) of the chordae tendineae, and ventricular friction lesions secondary to excess leaflet and chordal mobility. In this specimen, the left atrium and left ventricle have been cut and opened such that the posterior leaflet is viewed directly. Interchordal hooding involves the anterior and posterior leaflets. The chordae tendineae are thin and elongated. Chordal rupture involves the anterolateral scallop of the posterior leaflet. (From Prabhu SD, O'Rourke RA. Mitral valve prolapse. In: Rahimtoola SH, ed. *Atlas of Heart Diseases. Valvular Heart Disease.* St. Louis: Mosby, 1997:10.1–10.18 and Dr. Steven Bailey, The University of Texas Health Science Center at San Antonio, with permission.)

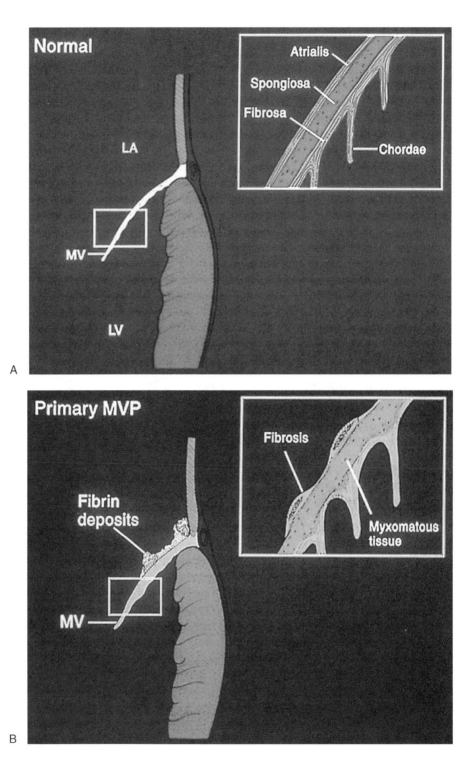

drome also has an autosomal dominant mode of inheritance.

Many clinical investigators have speculated that primary MVP syndrome represents a generalized disorder of connective tissue. Thoracic skeletal abnormalities, including straight thoracic spine and pectus excavatum, frequently are associated with this syndrome (25,26). The mitral valve primordium undergoes differentiation between the 35th and 42nd days of fetal life when chondrification and ossification of the vertebrae and thoracic cage are beginning (26). Detrimental factors in this period might affect both the mitral valve and the bones of the thoracic cage. Interestingly, rats fed a diet containing large amounts of peas of the genus *Lathyrus* develop both bony abnormalities and myxomatous changes in their valve leaflets (15). Accordingly, it has been suggested that the primary MVP syndrome may be a connective tissue disorder resulting from fetal exposure to toxic agents during the early part of pregnancy (15).

It has also been postulated that MVP may be due to defective embryogenesis of cell lines of mesenchymal origin. The coexistence of primary MVP with increased frequency in patients with von Willebrand disease and other coagulopathies, primary hypomastia, and various connective tissue diseases has been used to support this concept (27,28).

Secondary forms of MVP occur in which myxomatous proliferation of the spongiosa portion of the mitral valve leaflet is absent (Table 6-1). Experimental studies in animals and serial evaluations in patients with known ischemic heart disease occasionally have documented unequivocal MVP after an acute coronary syndrome (or occlusion of a coronary artery) that was previously absent (29–31). In most patients with coronary artery disease and MVP, however, the two entities are coincident but unrelated.

Several recent studies indicate that valvular regurgitation secondary to MVP may result from postinflammatory changes (without myxomatous proliferation), including those after rheumatic fever (32–34). In surgically excised valves, histologic studies have shown fibrosis with vascularization and scattered infiltration of lymphocytes and plasmacytes *without myxomatous proliferation* of the spongiosa. The anterior mitral leaflet is more likely to prolapse with rheumatic carditis.

MVP has been observed in patients with hypertrophic cardiomyopathy in whom posterior secondary MVP may result from a disproportionally small LV cavity, altered papillary muscle alignment, or a combination of factors (14,35). Secondary MVP (without myxomatous proliferation) may also occur in association with reduced LV volumes due to atrial septal defect, pulmonary hypertension,

FIG. 6-3. Histopathology of primary MVP. **A:** The normal mitral valve (*MV*) is composed of three layers: the atrialis, a thin layer of collagen and elastic tissue along the atrial aspect of the leaflet; the fibrosa (ventricularis), a denser layer of collagen along the ventricular aspect; and the spongiosa, the fine myxomatous connective tissue layer between the two. **B:** In primary mitral valve prolapse, dissolution of collagen bundles occurs primarily with secondary myxomatous proliferation of the spongiosa and interruption of the fibrosa and fibrosis of the atrial and ventricular surfaces of the valve. These secondary effects appear to occur as a response to repeated stress on the valve apparatus. Focal endothelial disruption occurs commonly and may provide a site for thrombus formation. Fibrin deposits often form at the mitral valve-left atrial angle. Similar histologic changes can occur in the chordae tendineae and result in chordal thinning and rupture. Myxomatous degeneration of the annulus can occur as well, especially in patients with connective tissue disorders, resulting in annular dilation and calcification and worsening of mitral regurgitation. *LV,* left ventricle. (From Prabhu SD, O'Rourke RA. Mitral valve prolapse. In: Rahimtoola SH, ed. *Atlas of Heart Diseases. Valvular Heart Disease.* St. Louis: Mosby, 1997:10.1–10.18, with permission.)

anorexia neurosa, dehydration, or straight back syndrome (18,36,37). The mitral valve leaflet is usually normal. However, there may also be an association between atrial septal defect and primary MVP (12). MVP may occur secondary to ruptured chordae tendineae as a flail or partially flail mitral leaflet whether spontaneous or due to infective endocarditis.

Patients with primary and secondary MVP must be distinguished from those with no heart disease but who have misinterpreted findings on cardiac auscultation or echocardiography (1–5). Inaccurate interpretation can result in an incorrect diagnosis of MVP, particularly in patients who are hyperkinetic during physical examination, two-dimensional echocardiography, or both. Other auscultatory findings, such as a split first heart sound, an S_4–S_1 complex, an S_2–S_3 complex, or a systolic ejection sound, may be misinterpreted as mid-systolic clicks. Patients with mild-to-moderate billowing of one or both nonthickened mitral leaflets toward the left atrium with leaflet coaptation on the ventricular side of the mitral annulus and no or minimal MR by Doppler echocardiography are probably normal. Unfortunately, many such patients with neither a mid-systolic click nor a murmur of MR are frequently diagnosed as having the MVP syndrome.

PATHOPHYSIOLOGY

In patients with MVP, there is often LA and LV enlargement depending on the presence and extent of MR (38). The mitral valve supporting apparatus is often affected in patients with Marfan's syndrome; the mitral annulus often is calcified, usually dilated, and fails to reduce its circumference by the usual 30% during LV systole. The hemodynamic effects of mild to moderate MR on cardiac function are no different than those from other etiologies of MR.

Autonomic nervous system dysfunction is apparent in many patients with primary MVP (14,39–43). In 1979, Gaffney et al. (39)

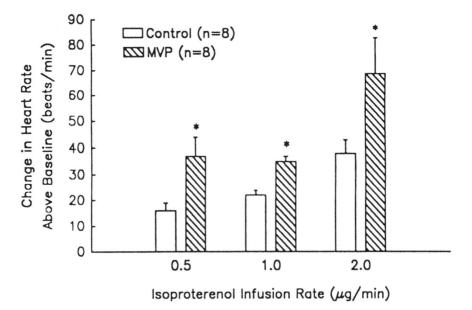

FIG. 6-4. Effect of isoproterenol infusion on heart rate in control and mitral valve prolapse (MVP) subjects. MVP value is significantly greater than control value, $p < 0.01$. Baseline heart rate (before isoproterenol infusion) was equivalent in MVP subjects and control subjects (58 ± 4 vs. 60 ± 3 beats/min, respectively; $p > 0.05$). (From ref. 44, with permission.)

demonstrated a reduced heart rate slowing with intravenous phenylephrine and an abnormal diving reflex heart rate response in patients with MVP compared with age-matched control subjects. Patients with MVP also had a less than normal lower extremity pooling of blood in response to lower body negative pressure (39). An increased incidence of heightened vagal tone and of prolonged QT interval on the electrocardiogram (ECG) occurs in patients with MVP. Measurements of serum and 24-hour urine epinephrine and norepinephrine levels often are increased in patients with symptomatic MVP compared with age-matched control subjects (40,41). Patients with MVP often have an increased heart rate and contractility response to intravenous isoproterenol (4,44) (Fig. 6-4). The incidence of high-affinity β-receptors in the lymphocytes of patients is greater with MVP, and the increment in cyclic adenosine monophosphate with isoproterenol stimulation is augmented as compared with normal individuals (44). Patients with MVP often have postural phenomena such as orthostatic tachycardia and hypotension. Low intravascular volume and/or an abnormality in the renin–aldosterone axis have been postulated to explain the orthostatic changes (46,47).

ASSOCIATED ABNORMALITIES

In postmortem studies, tricuspid valve prolapse that is associated with a similar interchordal hooding and histologic evidence of mucopolysaccharide proliferation and collagen dissolution occurs in up to 40% of patients with primary MVP (3,12). This high incidence of primary tricuspid valve prolapse at necropsy has been also demonstrated by two-dimensional echocardiography and right atrial phonocardiograms (5). Pulmonic valve prolapse and aortic valve prolapse due to myxomatous proliferation occur in approximately 10% and 2% of patients with MVP, respectively (12).

The frequent finding of thoracic skeletal abnormalities and autonomic nervous system dysfunction in patients with MVP has been noted above. There appears to be both an increased incidence of secundum atrial septal defect in patients with MVP and an increased likelihood of primary MVP in patients with atrial septal defects that cannot be explained by a chance occurrence and does not represent only stretching of a patent fossa ovalis (12,47). An association between left-sided atrioventricular bypass tracts and supraventricular tachycardias has also been described in patients with MVP (48).

CLINICAL PRESENTATION

History

The diagnosis of MVP is most often made by cardiac auscultation in asymptomatic patients or by echocardiography being performed for some other reason. Occasionally, the patient may be referred because of a family history of cardiac disease, including MVP. Less often, the patient is assessed because of an abnormal resting ECG.

One or more of the common symptoms that occur in patients with the MVP syndrome often results in medical evaluation. The most common presenting complaint is *palpitation*, the usual source being ventricular premature beats. However, various supraventricular arrhythmias are also frequent, and the most common sustained tachycardia is paroxysmal reentry junctional tachycardia (5). Ventricular tachycardia has been documented in some patients and symptomatic bradyarrhythmias in others. Palpitation is often reported by patients at a time when continuous ambulatory electrocardiographic recordings show no arrhythmias.

Chest discomfort is a frequent complaint of patients with MVP. It is an atypical chest pain and most patients have no coexistent ischemic heart disease; the discomfort rarely resembles classic angina pectoris. Occasionally, it is recurrent and can be incapacitating. The etiology of the chest discomfort is unknown; it could represent true myocardial ischemia produced by abnormal tension on the papillary muscles and supporting ventricular wall by the prolapsing mitral leaflets in some cases. In one study, the pain could be reproduced by elevating the systemic arterial pressure with intravenous phenylephrine (49). Coronary artery spasm has been reported in patients with MVP but is probably not the cause of most episodes of atypical chest pain (50).

Fatigue and dyspnea are common symptoms in patients with MVP but occur in many patients without severe MR. Objective exercise testing usually fails to show an impaired exercise tolerance, and many patients exhibit distinct episodes of hyperventilation (3,5). Neuropsychiatric complaints often are voiced by patients with MVP. Some patients have panic attacks and others frank manic-depressive syndromes (51). Both MVP and panic attacks occur relatively frequently. Accordingly, the occurrence of the two syndromes in the same individual would be expected to occur frequently by chance rather than panic attacks necessarily being part of the primary MVP syndrome.

There is an increased incidence of cerebral ischemic syndromes in patients with MVP, and some develop stroke syndromes (52–58). Amaurosis fugax, homonymous field loss, and retinal artery occlusion have been described, and occasionally the visual loss persists (59). These signs likely are due to embolization of platelets and fibrin deposits that occur on the LA side of the mitral valve leaflets (12,10).

Physical Examination

The diagnosis of MVP may be considered because of the presence of thoracic skeletal abnormalities; the most common are scoliosis, pectus excavatum, straightened thoracic spine, and narrowed anterior-posterior diameter of the chest (61). Some patients with MVP may show signs that are more typical of Marfan's syndrome, such as arachnodactyly.

The principal feature on cardiac auscultation is the mid-systolic click, a high-pitched sound of short duration (Fig. 6-5). The mid-systolic click may be soft or loud and varies in its timing according to LV loading conditions and contractility. It is due to the sudden tensing of the mitral valve apparatus as the leaflets billow into the LA during systole. Multiple systolic clicks may be generated by different portions of the mitral leaflets that prolapse at differing times during systole (62). The major differentiating features of the mid-systolic click of mitral prolapse from that due to other causes (e.g., aneurysm of the ventricular septum, atrial myxomas, pericarditis) is that its timing during systole may be altered by maneuvers that change hemodynamic conditions (see below).

The mid-systolic click is frequently followed by a late systolic murmur, usually medium- to high-pitched and most audible at the apex (Fig. 6-6). Occasionally, the murmur has a musical or honking quality. The character and intensity of the murmur also vary under certain conditions, from brief and almost inaudible to holosystolic and loud.

Dynamic auscultation is often useful for establishing the clinical diagnosis of the MVP syndrome (2,3,5). Changes in the LV end-diastolic volume lead to changes in the timing of the mid-systolic click and murmur. When end-diastolic volume is decreased, the critical volume is achieved earlier in systole and the click–murmur complex occurs shortly after the first heart sound (Fig. 6-7).

In general, any maneuver that decreases the end-diastolic LV volume increases the rate of ventricular contraction or that decreases the resistance to LV ejection of blood causes the MVP to occur early in systole and the systolic click and murmur to move toward the first heart sound (Fig. 6-8). By contrast, any maneuver that augments the volume of blood in the ventricle reduces myocardial contractility or that increases LV afterload lengthens the time from the onset of systole to the initiation of MVP and the systolic click and/or murmur move toward the second heart sound. Maneuvers causing the click and/or murmur to occur earlier in systole include standing from the supine position, submaximal isometric handgrip exercise, the Valsalva maneuver, and amyl nitrite inhalation (Fig. 6-8). Those that cause the click and murmur to move toward the second heart sound include squatting from the upright position (Fig. 6-9) and maneuvers that slow the heart rate.

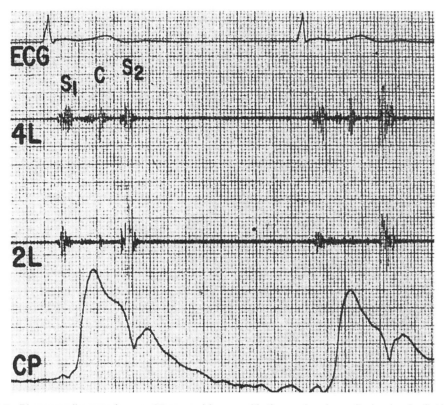

FIG. 6-5. Phonocardiogram from a 23-year-old man with the prolapsing mitral valve leaflet(s) syndrome. The mid-systolic click occurs in the characteristic location after the upstroke of the carotid pulse. *ECG*, electrocardiogram; *4L*, fourth left interspace at 100 cycles per second; *2L*, second left intercostal space at 100 cycles per second; *CP*, carotid pulse tracing; S_1, first heart sound; S_2, second heart sound; *C*, click. (From ref. 2, with permission.)

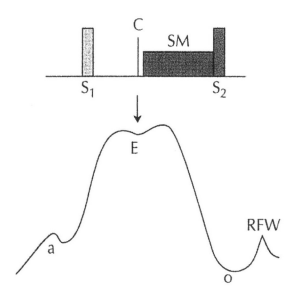

FIG. 6-6. Schematic representation of a simultaneous phonocardiogram and apex cardiogram with a systolic phonocardiogram and a notch (*E*) on the apexcardiogram (ACG) at the time of the click as left ventricular "A" wave at the time of left atrium contraction. *RFW*, rapid ventricular filling wave. (From Prabhu SD, O'Rourke RA. Mitral valve prolapse. In: Rahimtoola SH, ed. *Atlas of Heart Diseases. Valvular Heart Disease.* St. Louis: Mosby, 1997: 10.1–10.18, with permission.)

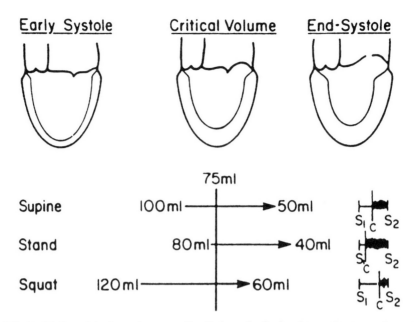

FIG. 6-7. Effect of left ventricular volume on the timing of mitral valve prolapse and accompanying murmur. In the upper panels, three phases of left ventricular systole are illustrated. In early systole, there is coaptation of the leaflets and no prolapse; when a critical ventricle volume of 75 mL is reached, valve prolapse commences and progresses until the end of systole. In the lower panel, three body positions are indicated; the corresponding change in volume and timing of the click–murmur are shown. The critical volume for prolapse remains constant. When the critical volume occurs earlier, the onset of click–murmur is earlier. When the critical volume occurs later, the onset of the click–murmur is later. Abbreviations same as in Fig. 6-5. (From ref. 4, with permission.)

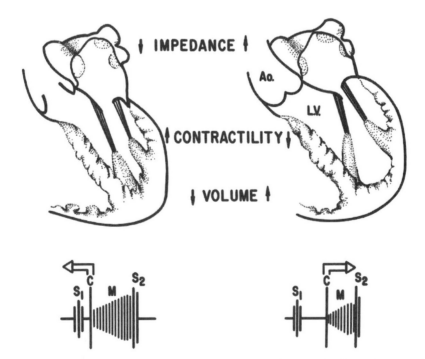

FIG. 6-8. Diagrammatic representation of the influence of the three major hemodynamic factors on the mitral valve apparatus and the mid-systolic click late systolic murmur. *Ao,* aorta; *LV,* left ventricle.

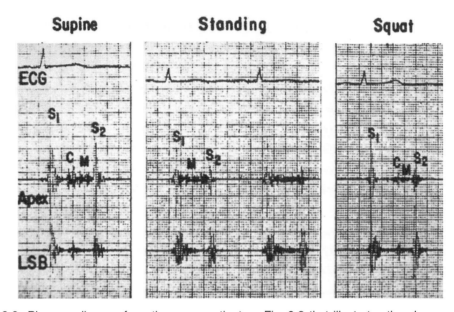

FIG. 6-9. Phonocardiogram from the same patient as Fig. 6-3 that illustrates the changes in the click–murmur complex with changes in position. **Left:** Supine phonocardiogram at 100 cycles per second from the apex and the lower left sternal border (*LSB*). The late systolic murmur begins after the mid-systolic clicks. **Middle:** Movement of the click–murmur complex toward the first heart sound in the standing position. The murmur is pansystolic and the click no longer is present. **Right:** Effect of a rapid squat. The click–murmur complex moves toward the second heart sound and the murmur diminishes in intensity. (From ref. 2, with permission.)

Electrocardiogram

The ECG is often normal in patients with MVP. The most common abnormality in the MVP syndrome is the presence of ST-T wave depression or T wave inversion in the inferior leads (II, III, aVF) (63) (Fig. 6-10). These changes may have been attributed to ischemia of the inferior wall due to traction on the posteromedial papillary muscle by the prolapsing mitral leaflets. Sometimes ST-T wave changes are present only during interventions that induce prolapse earlier in systole, such as sitting or standing. More unusual ECG changes include prominent U waves, peaked T waves in the mid-precordial leads, and prolongation of the QT interval.

The MVP syndrome is associated with an increased incidence of false-positive *exercise electrocardiographic* ST-T wave depressions in patients with normal coronary arteries, especially females. Myocardial perfusion imaging with thallium or technetium sestamibi has been useful for differentiating false from true abnormal exercise ECG findings in patients with MVP (13).

Although arrhythmias may be observed on the resting ECG or during treadmill or bicycle exercise, they are detected more reliably by *continuous ambulatory electrocardiographic* recordings. Although the reported incidence of documented arrhythmias is higher in patients with MVP (40% to 75%), most arrhythmias detected are not life threatening (2,51,64). Patients with ST-T wave changes in the inferior ECG leads appear to have a higher incidence of serious ventricular arrhythmias on ambulatory recordings (65).

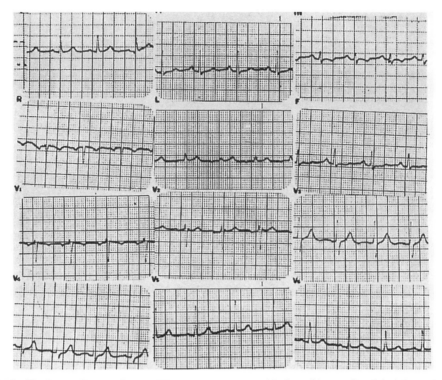

FIG. 6-10. Electrocardiogram from a 32-year-old woman with the mid-systolic click–late systole murmur syndrome showing T wave changes in leads III and aVF. This patient was hospitalized because of severe chest pain, and coronary arteriography was normal. Her left ventricular cineangiogram demonstrated marked prolapse of the posterior mitral valve leaflet. (From ref. 2, with permission.)

Echocardiography

Two-dimensional and Doppler echocardiography are the most useful noninvasive tests for defining MVP. The M-mode echocardiographic definition of MVP includes no more than a 2-mm posterior displacement of one or both leaflets or holosystolic posterior "hammocking" of more than 3 mm (Fig. 6-11). On two-dimensional echocardiography, systolic displacement of one or both mitral leaflets, in the parasternal long-axis view, particularly when they coapt on the atrial side of the annular plane, indicates a high likelihood of MVP. There is disagreement concerning the reliability of echocardiographic diagnosis of MVP when observed in only the apical four-chamber view (66,67). The diagnosis of MVP is even more certain when the leaflet thickness is more than 5 mm. Leaflet redundancy

is often associated with an enlarged mitral annulus and elongated chordae tendineae (64). On Doppler velocity recordings, the presence or absence of MR is an important consideration, and MVP is more likely when the MR is detected as a high-velocity eccentric jet in late systole (18).

At present, there is no consensus on the two-dimensional echocardiographic criteria for MVP. Because echocardiography is a tomographic cross-sectional technique, no single view should be considered diagnostic. The parasternal long-axis view permits visualization of the medial aspect of the anterior mitral leaflet and middle scallop of the posterior leaflet (Fig. 6-12). If the findings of prolapse are localized to the lateral scallop in the posterior leaflet, they would be best visualized by the apical four-chamber view. All available echocardiographic views should be used with

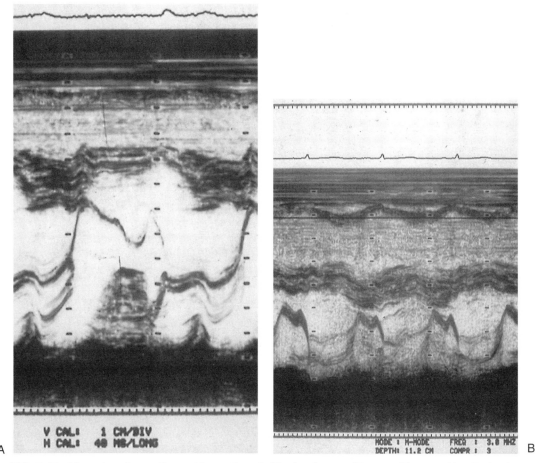

FIG. 6-11. M-mode echocardiographic studies. **A:** Tracing from a 41-year-old man with mitral valve prolapse. There is late systolic posterior displacement of both mitral valve leaflets. **B:** Tracing from a 54-year-old woman with predominantly anterior leaflet prolapse. Significant holosystolic hammocking is seen. Both patients had evidence of leaflet thickening. Each division is 1 cm. (From Prabhu SD, O'Rourke RA. Mitral valve prolapse. In: Rahimtoola SH, ed. *Atlas of Heart Diseases. Valvular Heart Disease.* St. Louis: Mosby, 1997:10.1–10.18, with permission.)

the provision that billowing of the anterior leaflet alone in the four-chamber apical view is not evidence of prolapse; however, a displacement of the posterior leaflet or the coaptation point in any view, including the apical view, suggests the diagnosis of prolapse. The echocardiographic criteria for MVP should include structural changes such as leaflet thickening, redundancy, annular dilatation, and chordal elongation. Often, the two-dimensional echo shows evidence of coincident tricuspid valve prolapse (Fig. 6-13).

Patients with echocardiographic evidence for MVP but without evidence of thickened/redundant leaflets or definite MR are more difficult to classify. If such patients have clinical auscultatory findings of MVP, then the echocardiogram usually confirms the diagnosis. The American College of Cardiologists/American Heart Association (ACC/AHA) recommendations for echocardiography in MVP prolapse are listed in Table 6-2.

Although the echocardiogram is a confirmatory test for diagnosing MVP, it is not al-

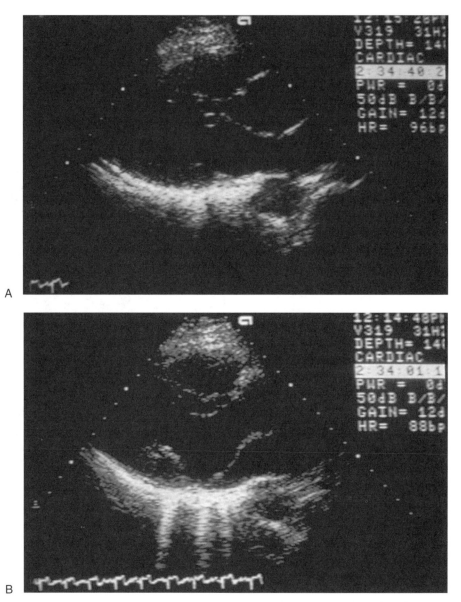

FIG. 6-12. Two-dimensional echocardiographic and Doppler ultrasound studies. Two-dimensional study from a 51-year-old man with predominately anterior mitral leaflet prolapse. **A:** The diastolic frame reveals a large thickened anterior leaflet in the parasternal long-axis (*PLAX*) view. **B:** The systolic frame shows billowing of the anterior leaflet beyond the annular plane and excessive posterior displacement of the coaptation point. (From Prabhu SD, O'Rourke RA. Mitral valve prolapse. In: Rahimtoola SH, ed. *Atlas of Heart Diseases. Valvular Heart Disease.* St. Louis: Mosby, 1997: 10.1–10.18, with permission.)

ways abnormal. Nevertheless, echocardiography is useful for defining LA size, LV size and function, and the extent of mitral leaflet redundancy, thereby defining patients at high risk for complications and for detecting asso-

ciated lesions such as secundum atrial septal defect. Doppler echocardiography is helpful for the detection and semiquantitation of MR. Although there is controversy concerning the need for echocardiography in patients with

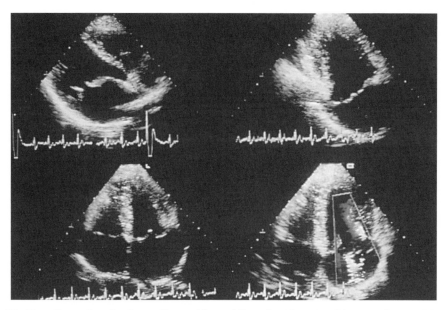

FIG. 6-13. Two-dimensional echocardiographic and Doppler ultrasound images from a 55-year-old man with classic mitral valve prolapse and associated tricuspid valve prolapse. The parasternal long-axis view shows significant leaflet thickening of both mitral leaflets. The upper left presents the apical long-axis view showing prolapse of both leaflets and the coaptation point beyond the annular plane in the lower left panel. The apical four-chamber view displays a systolic prolapse of both the mitral and tricuspid valves in the upper right panel. Doppler mapping in the left atrium demonstrates central mitral regurgitation in the lower right panel. Tricuspid regurgitation was noted as well (not shown). (From Prabhu SD, et al. Mitral valve prolase. In: Rahimtoola, SH, ed. *Atlas of Heart Disease. Valvular Heart Disease.* St. Louis: Mosby, 1997; 10.1–10.18, with permission.)

TABLE 6-2. *Recommendations for echocardiography in mitral valve prolapse*

Indication	Class
1. Diagnosis, assessment of hemodynamic severity of MR, leaflet morphology, and ventricular compensation in patients with physical signs of MVP.	I
2. To exclude MVP in patients who have been given the diagnosis where there is no clinical evidence to support the diagnosis.	I
3. To exclude MVP in patients with first-degree relatives with known myxomatous valve disease.	IIa
4. Risk stratification in patients with physical signs of MVP or known MVP.	IIa
5. To exclude MVP in patients in the absence of physical findings suggestive of MVP or a positive family history.	III
6. Routine repetition of echocardiography in patients with MVP with no or mild regurgitation and no changes in clinical signs or symptoms.	III

Class I:[a] Conditions for which there is evidence and/or general agreement that a given procedure or treatment is useful and effective.

Class II: Conditions for which there is conflicting evidence and/or a divergence of opinion about the usefulness/efficacy of a procedure or treatment.

Class IIa: Weight of evidence/opinion is in favor of usefulness/efficacy.

Class IIb: Usefulness efficacy is less well established by evidence/opinion.

Class III: Conditions for which there is evidence and/or general agreement that the procedure/treatment is not useful/effective and in some cases may be harmful.

[a]From ACC-AHA Clinical Practice Guidelines for Valvular Heart Disease (in press).
MR, mitral regurgitation; MVP, mitral valve prolapse.

TABLE 6-3. *Use of echocardiography for risk stratification in mitral valve prolapse*

Study	No. of Patients	Features examined	Outcome	p
Nishimura et al., 1985 (68)	237	MV leaflet ≥5 mm	1 sum of sudden death, endocarditis and cerebral embolus	<0.02
		LVID ≥60 mm	1 MVR (26% vs. 3.1%)	<0.001
Zuppiroli et al., 1994 (69)	119	MV leaflet >5 mm	1 complex ventricular arrhythmia	<0.001
Babuty et al., 1994 (70)	58	Undefined MV thickening	No relation to complex ventricular arrhythmias	NS
Takamoto et al., 1991 (71)	142	MV leaflet ≥3 mm, redundant, low echo density	1 ruptured chordae (48 vs. 5%)	
Marks et al., 1989 (66)	456	MV leaflet ≥5 mm	1 endocarditis (3.5 vs. 0%)	<0.02
			1 moderate-severe MR (11.9 vs. 0%)	<0.001
			1 MVR (6.6 vs. 0.7%)	<0.02
			1 stroke (7.5 vs. 5.8)	NS
Chandraratna et al., 1984 (72)	86	MV leaflets >5.1 mm	1 cardiovascular abnormalities (60 vs. 6%)	
			(Marfan vs syndrome, TVP, MR, dilated descending aorta)	<0.001

MV, mitral valve; LVID, left ventricular internal diameter; MVR, mitral valve replacement; MR, mitral regurgitation; TVP, tricuspid valve prolapse.
From ref. 74, with permission.

classic auscultatory findings of MVP, the usefulness of echocardiography for risk stratification in patients with MVP has been demonstrated in at least six published studies (66,68–72) (Table 6-3). All patients with MVP should have an initial echocardiogram. Serial echocardiograms usually are not necessary in the asymptomatic patient with MVP unless there are clinical indications of severe or worsening MR.

The use of echocardiography as a screening test for MVP in patients with or without symptoms who have no systolic click or murmur on serial carefully performed auscultatory examinations is not *recommended* (73). The likelihood of finding a prolapsing mitral valve in such patients is extremely low (73). Most patients with or without symptoms who have negative dynamic cardiac auscultation and "mild MVP" by echocardiography should not be diagnosed as having MVP.

As indicated earlier, two-dimensional echocardiography is useful for determining LA size, LV size and function, and the extent of mitral leaflet redundancy and for detecting associated lesions such as secundum atrial septal defect. Doppler echocardiography is valuable for the detection and semiquantitation of MR

as well. Serial echocardiograms may be useful in certain patients with murmurs, especially holosystolic murmurs, because quantitation of MR by examination alone is more difficult. However, repeat echocardiogram status is not necessary in those with mild MR and no change in symptoms (Table 6-2). In a carefully performed study comparing auscultatory findings with echocardiographic results in patients with clinical evidence of MVP, the amount of billowing of one or both mitral leaflets into the left atrium, the level of the leaflets coaptation point, and the presence or absence of moderate or severe MR were each important considerations in deciding on the likelihood of MVP and its severity (74).

Chest Roentgenogram

Posterior-anterior and lateral chest roentgenograms usually show normal cardiopulmonary findings. The skeletal abnormalities described earlier can be seen (26) (Figs. 6-14 and 6-15). When severe MR is present, both LA and LV enlargement often result. Various degrees of pulmonary venous congestion are present when left heart failure results. Acute chordal rupture with a sudden

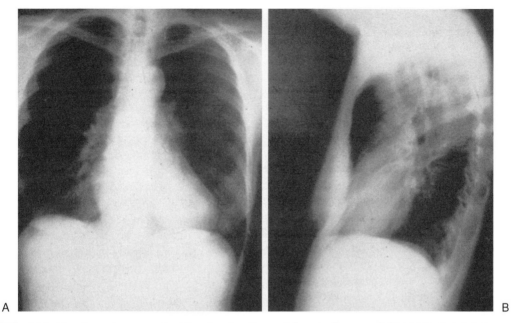

A

B

FIG. 6-14. Chest roentgenography. The chest radiograph is usually normal. Thoracic skeletal abnormalities may be visualized. This radiograph is from a 26-year-old woman with mitral valve prolapse and reveals mild scoliosis on the posteroanterior view **(A)** and pectus excavatum on the lateral view **(B)**. The mitral annulus may be calcified, especially in adult patients with Marfan's syndrome. In patients with progressive mitral regurgitation, left atrial and left ventricular enlargement can be seen. Pulmonary venous congestion and pulmonary edema are present in patients with heart failure. (From ref. 2, with permission.)

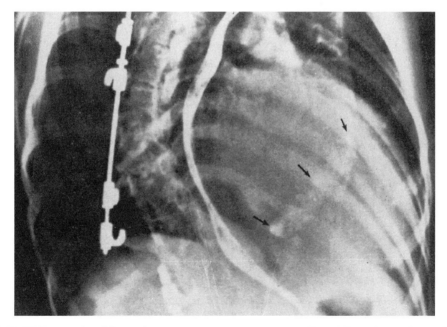

FIG. 6-15. Right anterior oblique chest x-ray from a young male with the Marfan's syndrome. The arrows point to the large calcified mitral annulus in this patient. Left ventricular cineangiogram demonstrated marked prolapse of the posterior mitral valve leaflet. (From ref. 2, with permission.)

increase in the amount of MR may present as pulmonary edema without obvious LV or LA dilatation. Calcification of the mitral annulus may be seen (Fig. 6-15), particularly in adults with Marfan's syndrome.

Myocardial Perfusion Scintigraphy

Exercise myocardial perfusion imaging with thallium or technetium-based radioisotopes has been recommended as an adjunct to exercise ECG for determining the presence or absence of coexistent myocardial ischemia in patients with MVP (3,75). Most MVP patients with clinical evidence of coronary artery disease have an abnormal exercise scintigram. On the other hand, a negative scintigram in such patients does not exclude ischemia as the basis for the chest pain nor does it completely exclude coronary artery disease as the etiology (13).

Cardiac Catheterization

Cardiac catheterization is rarely used as a diagnostic technique for MVP. Also, contrast ventriculography is unnecessary for determining LV function because it usually can be quantitated by two-dimensional echocardiography or radionuclide ventriculography. Although contrast cineventriculography is often useful for assessing the severity of MR, cardiac catheterization and angiography are most commonly used in patients with MVP to exclude the possibility of coronary artery disease.

Intracardiac pressures and cardiac output are usually normal in uncomplicated MVP; however, these measurements become progressively more abnormal as MR becomes more severe. LV angiography usually confirms the presence of prolapse of the mitral valve (2,5). The right anterior oblique projection is best for observing prolapse of the three scallops of the posterior leaflet; the left anterior oblique view is necessary for the adequate evaluation of prolapse of the anterior leaflet.

LV wall motion is usually normal in patients with primary MVP, but some patients show abnormal contraction patterns in the absence of coronary artery diseases (2) (Fig. 6-16). These

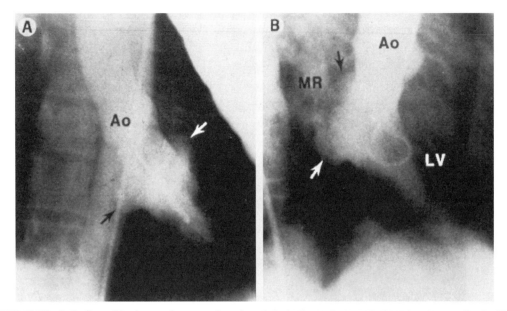

FIG. 6-16. A: Left ventricular angiogram at end-systole in the anteroposterior view in a patient with prolapse of all three scallops of the posterior mitral valve leaflet, which results in a "doughnut-like" configuration (*arrows*). Also note the "hourglass" deformity of the left ventricular silhouette. **B:** Same angiogram in the lateral view, which shows the prolapsing scallops of the posterior leaflet (*arrows*) and the resultant mitral regurgitation. (From ref. 2, with permission.)

contraction abnormalities usually represent indentation of the LV at the point of attachment of the papillary muscles; it is thought to be due to abnormal traction on the papillary muscles and buckling of the ventricular wall. Patients with the most severe prolapse more commonly exhibit abnormal ventricular cavities during systole, and wall motion abnormalities frequently disappear after successful mitral valve replacement or repair (35). Coronary arteriography is usually normal in patients with primary MVP and no congenital anomalies of the coronary vessels have been associated with this syndrome.

Electrophysiologic Testing

The indications for electrophysiologic testing in a patient with MVP are similar to those in general practice (i.e., recurrent unexplained syncope, sudden death survivors, symptomatic complex ventricular ectopy, and the presence of preexcitation syndromes) (14). Upright tilt studies with monitoring of blood pressure and rhythm may be valuable in patients with light-headedness or syncope and in diagnosing autonomic dysfunction (14).

NATURAL HISTORY, PROGNOSIS, AND COMPLICATIONS

In most patient studies, the MVP syndrome is associated with a benign prognosis (76–82) (Fig. 6-17, Table 6-4). The age-adjusted survival rate for both males and females with MVP is similar to that in patients without this common clinical entity. The gradual progression of MR in patients with mitral prolapse, however, may result in progressive dilatation of the LA and LV. LA dilatation often results

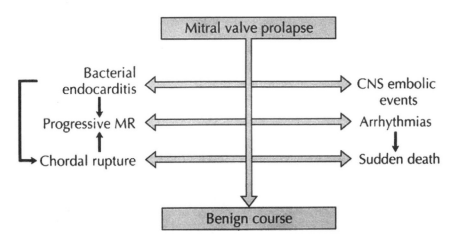

FIG. 6-17. Overview of the clinical course in mitral valve prolapse (MVP). Most patients with MVP follow a benign course and their age-adjusted survival is similar to persons without MVP. However, serious complications can occur in 10% to 10% of patients. These include infective endocarditis, chordal rupture, progressive mitral regurgitation (MR), life-threatening arrhythmias, neurologic and embolic events, and sudden death. The risk of infective endocarditis is five to eight times greater in patients with MVP than in the general population, and MVP is the leading underlying diagnosis in patients with endocarditis. Progressive MR is often accelerated by infective endocarditis or chordal rupture. The overall incidence of ophthalmologic and central nervous system (CNS) embolic events is generally low. An increase in risk for CNS events associated with MVP is detectable in patients who do not have other cerebrovascular risk factors, especially young women. Sudden death is the least common complication of MVP and occurs mainly in patients with significant MR, reduced ventricular function, and malignant ventricular arrhythmias. (From Prabhu SD, O'Rourke RA. Mitral valve prolapse. In: Rahimtoola SH, ed. *Atlas of Heart Diseases. Valvular Heart Disease.* St. Louis: Mosby, 1997:10.1–10.18, with permission.)

TABLE 6-4. *Complications of MVP*

	N	No. of complications	Follow-up (yr)	Incidence of complications (%/yr)	Patient-years
Allen et al., 1974 (76)	62	8	13.8	0.9	856
Mills et al., 1985 (77)	53	8	23.7	1.1	1,256
Bisset et al., 1990 (78)	109	2	6.9	0.3	752
Nishimura et al., 1985 (68)	236	27	6.2	1.9	1,469
Vered et al., 1985 (79)	42	8	5.1	3.7	214
Duren et al., 1988 (80)	300	62	6.1	3.4	1,830
Zuppiroli et al., 1995 (81)	316	26	8.5	1.0	2,686

in atrial fibrillation and moderate to severe MR eventually results in LV dysfunction and the development of congestive heart failure (5). Pulmonary hypertension may occur with associated right ventricular dysfunction. In some patients with an initially prolonged asymptomatic interval, the entire process may enter an accelerated phase as a result of LV dysfunction, atrial fibrillation, and in certain instances ruptured mitral valve chordae (3,5). The latter occurs more commonly in males and with increasing age (3,5,13).

Several long-term prognostic studies suggest that complications occur most commonly in patients with a mitral systolic murmur, thickened redundant mitral valve leaflets, or increased LV or LA (Fig. 6-18) (14,81,82). In a prospective follow-up study of 237 asymptomatic patients with MVP documented by echocardiography, sudden death occurred in 6 patients (68). In a multivariant analysis of echocardiographic findings, the presence or absence of redundant mitral valve leaflets by M-mode echocardiography was the only vari-

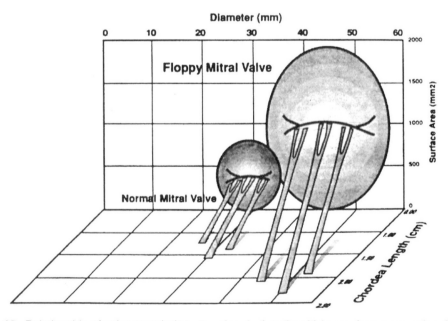

FIG. 6-18. Relationship of valve morphology to valve dysfunction. Valve surface area, valve diameter, and chordal length are all increased in mitral valve prolapse. The mitral valve is thus inordinately large relative to the left ventricular chamber and does not maintain normal coaptation/apposition during systole. This results in prolapse and valvular regurgitation. (From ref. 45, with permission.)

able associated with sudden death. Ten patients sustained a cerebral embolic event, six of whom were in atrial fibrillation with LA enlargement.

Marks et al. (66) confirmed these data in a retrospective two-dimensional echocardiographic study from 456 patients with MVP. Two groups of patients were compared: those with thickening and redundancy of the mitral valve leaflet and those without leaflet thickening. Complications, or a history of complications, were more prevalent in those with leaflet thickening and redundancy than in those without leaflet thickening. The incidence of stroke, however, was similar in the two groups.

Long-term follow-up studies in patients with MVP associated with a floppy myxomatous mitral valve permit several conclusions (14). Serious complications occur in some patients with MVP, predominantly in those with diagnostic auscultatory findings. Also, redundant mitral valve leaflets and increased LV size are associated with more serious complications. Finally, men and those over 50 years of age are at increased risk of complications, including severe MR requiring surgery (14).

Sudden death is the least common but obviously the most severe complication of MVP. Although infrequent, the highest incidence of sudden death has been reported in the familial form of MVP. Some of these patients have had QT prolongation. Also, patients with MVP with severe autonomic dysfunction and excessive vagotonia resulting in bradyarrhythmias and asystole have been reported (14,83,84). Because arrhythmias are likely to be the usual cause of sudden death in patients with MVP, it seems prudent to limit ambulatory ECG recordings to those patients at highest risk. Many believe that patients with ECG ST-T wave changes are more likely to have complex ventricular arrhythmias (12,14). Certainly, any patients with symptoms suggestive of arrhythmia or who have arrhythmias noted during physical examination or on the resting ECG should be evaluated further.

Infective endocarditis is a serious complication of MVP (10,14,85), and MVP is the leading predisposing cardiovascular diagnosis in most series of patients reported with endocarditis. Because the absolute incidence of endocarditis is extremely low for the entire MVP population, there has been considerable debate concerning the risk of endocarditis in MVP (85,86). Although there is general agreement that MVP patients with murmurs and/or thickened redundant valves confirmed by echocardiography or cineangiography should receive antibiotic prophylaxis, some authorities state that patients with isolated systolic clicks and no murmurs do not need antibiotic prophylaxis for endocarditis (76). The dynamic nature of MVP, with variable physical findings on different examinations, makes it difficult to make judgments on the basis of the presence or absence of a systolic murmur. With the increasing use of color-flow echo-Doppler studies, MR has often been observed in patients in whom no murmur is heard (77,78). Because endocarditis can cause destruction of even a mildly affected valve, antibiotic prophylaxis could be warranted in most cases when the diagnosis of MVP seems certain (5).

As indicated above, progressive MR occurs frequently in patients with long-standing MVP. In some patients, fibrin emboli cause visual problems consistent with involvement of the ophthalmic or posterior cerebral circulation (59). There is an increased likelihood of cerebral vascular accidents of various types in patients under age 45 who have MVP than would be expected in a similar population without MVP (52–58). Therefore, it has been recommended that antiplatelet drugs such as aspirin or anticoagulants are administered to patients who have MVP and suspected cerebral nervous system emboli (see below). However, neither antiplatelet drugs nor anticoagulants should be prescribed routinely for patients with MVP because the incidence of embolic phenomena is very low.

MANAGEMENT

Asymptomatic Patients

Reassurance is a major part of the management of patients with MVP, most of whom are

TABLE 6-5. *Recommendations for antibiotic endocarditis prophylaxis for patients with mitral valve prolapse undergoing procedures associated with bacteremia*

Indication	Class
1. Patients with characteristic systolic click-murmur complex.	I
2. Patients with isolated systolic click and echo evidence of MVP and MR.	I
3. Patients with isolated systolic click, echo evidence of high-risk MVP.	IIa
4. Patients with isolated systolic click and no or equivocal evidence of MVP	III

MVP, mitral valve prolapse; MR, mitral regurgitation.
From ref. 13, with permission.

asymptomatic or have no cardiac symptoms and lack a high-risk profile. These patients with mild or no symptoms, and findings of milder forms of prolapse should be reassured of the benign prognosis. A normal lifestyle and regular exercise is encouraged (1–5,14).

Antibiotic prophylaxis for the prevention of infective endocarditis during procedures associated with bacteremia is recommended for most patients in whom the diagnosis of MVP is definite (see above). There has been some disagreement concerning whether patients with an isolated systolic click and no systolic murmur should undergo endocarditis prophylaxis. The ACC/AHA recommendations for antibiotic endocarditis for patients with MVP are listed in Table 6-5.

Symptomatic Patients

Some patients consult their physicians because of one or more of the common symptoms that occur in patients with this syndrome; palpitations, often reported at a time when continuous ambulatory electrocardiographic recordings show no arrhythmias; atypical chest pain that rarely resembles classic angina pectoris; dyspnea and fatigue, when objective exercise testing often fails to show any impairment in exercise tolerance; and neuropsychiatric complaints with many patients having panic attacks and similar syndromes (13). Transient cerebral ischemic episodes occur with increased incidence in

patients with MVP, and some patients develop stoke syndromes. Reports of amarous fugax, homonymous field loss, and retinal artery occlusion have been described; occasionally, the visual loss persists (2,5,14).

The roles of cardiac auscultation and echocardiography in the assessment of symptomatic patients with MVP are the same as in patients without symptoms. The indications for antibiotic prophylaxis to prevent endocarditis are also unchanged.

Patients with MVP and palpitations associated with mild tachyarrhythmias or increased adrenergic symptoms and those with chest pain, anxiety, or fatigue often respond to therapy with beta-blockers (5,64). In many cases, however, the cessation of stimulants such as caffeine, alcohol, and cigarettes may be sufficient to control symptoms. In patients with recurrent palpitations, continuous or event-activated ambulatory ECG recordings may reveal the presence or absence of arrhythmias at the time of symptoms and indicate appropriate treatment of existing arrhythmias. The indications for electrophysiologic testing are similar to those in the general population (e.g., aborted sudden death, recurrent syncope of unknown cause, and symptomatic or sustained ventricular tachycardia) (14).

Cardiac catheterization is not required for the diagnosis of MVP. It is helpful in evaluating associated conditions (e.g., coronary artery disease, atrial septal defect) and may be needed to assess the hemodynamic effects of severe MR (as well as coronary artery anatomy) before consideration for valve repair or replacement.

Orthostatic symptoms due to postural hypotension and tachycardia are best treated with volume expansion, preferably by liberalizing fluid and salt intake. Mineralocorticoid therapy or clonidine may be needed in severe cases and wearing support stockings may be beneficial (14).

Daily aspirin therapy (80 to 325 mg/day) is recommended for MVP patients with documented focal neurologic events who are in sinus rhythm with no atrial thrombi (Table 6-6). Such patients also should avoid cigarettes and

TABLE 6-6. *Recommendations for aspirin and oral anticoagulants in mitral valve prolapse*

Indication	Class
1. Aspirin therapy for cerebral transient ischemic attacks (TIAs).	I
2. Warfarin therapy for patients in atrial fibrillation with age ≥65 yr, hypertension, MR murmur, or history of heart failure.	I
3. Aspirin therapy for patients in atrial fibrillation <65 years old with no history of MR, hypertension, or heart failure.	I
4. Warfarin therapy for poststroke patients.	I
5. Warfarin therapy for TIAs despite aspirin therapy.	IIa
6. Aspirin therapy in poststroke patients with contraindications to anticoagulants.	IIa
7. Aspirin therapy for patients in sinus rhythm with echocardiographic evidence of high-risk MVP.	IIb

MR, mitral regurgitation; MVP, mitral valve prolapse. From ref. 13, with permission.

oral contraceptives. Long-term anticoagulation therapy with warfarin is recommended for poststroke patients with MVP and for MVP patients with recurrent transient ischemic attacks on aspirin therapy (international normalized ratio [INR] 2 to 3). In MVP patients with atrial fibrillation, warfarin therapy is indicated in patients at least 65 years old and those with MR, hypertension, or a history of heart failure (INR 2 to 3). Aspirin therapy is satisfactory in patients with atrial fibrillation who are less than 65 years old, have no MR, and have no history of hypertension or heart failure. Daily aspirin therapy also is often recommended for patients with high-risk echocardiographic characteristics (13).

A normal lifestyle and regular exercise is encouraged for most patients with MVP, especially those who are asymptomatic. Restriction from competitive sports is recommended when moderate LV enlargement, LV dysfunction, uncontrolled tachyarrhythmias, long QT interval, unexplained syncope, prior sudden death, or aortic root enlargement is present individually or in combination (13). A familial occurrence of MVP should be explained to the patient and is particularly important in those with associated disease who are at greater risk for complications. There is no contraindication to pregnancy based on the diagnosis of MVP alone.

Asymptomatic patients with MVP and no significant MR can be evaluated clinically every 3 to 5 years (13). Serial echocardiography is not necessary in most of these patients and is obtained only if there is the development of symptoms consistent with cardiovascular disease, a change in physical findings suggesting the development of significant MR, and in patients who have high-risk characteristics on the initial echocardiogram. Patients who have high-risk characteristics, including those with moderate to severe MR, should be followed once a year.

Patients with severe MR with symptoms and/or impaired LV systolic function require cardiac catheterization and evaluation for mitral valve surgery. The thickened redundant mitral valve often can be repaired rather than replaced, with a lower operative mortality and excellent short- and long-term results (13,90–94). Follow-up studies also suggest lower thrombotic and endocarditis risk with valve repair than with prosthetic valves.

Surgical Considerations

Management of the patient with MVP may require valve surgery, particularly in those patients who develop a flail mitral leaflet due to rupture of chordae tendineae or their marked elongation (95). Most such valves can be repaired successfully by surgeons experienced with mitral valve repair, especially when the posterior leaflet of the mitral valve is predominantly affected. Symptoms of heart failure, the severity of MR, the presence or absence of atrial fibrillation, LV systolic function, LV end-diastolic and end-systolic volumes, and pulmonary artery pressure (rest and exercise) all influence the decision to recommend mitral valve surgery. Recommendations for surgery in patients with MVP and MR are the same as for those with other forms of nonischemic severe MR and include class III and IV symptoms, LV ejection fraction less than 60%, and/or marked increases in LV end-diastolic and end-systolic volumes. If mitral repair is likely to be successful, severe MR with class II symptoms or atrial fibrillation may be an appropriate reason for surgical referral (13).

REFERENCES

1. Harvey WP. *Clinical Pearls.* New Jersey: Laennec Publishing, 1993.
2. O'Rourke RA, Crawford MH. The systolic click-murmur syndrome: clinical recognition and management. *Curr Probl Cardiol* 1976;1:1–60.
3. O'Rourke RA. The mitral valve prolapse syndrome. In: Chizner MA, ed. *Classic Teachings in Clinical Cardiology.* New Jersey: Laennec Publishing, 1996:1049–1070.
4. Crawford MH, O'Rourke RA. Mitral valve prolapse syndrome. In: Isselbacher KJ, Adams RD, Braunwald E, et al., eds. *Update I. Harrison's Principles of Internal Medicine.* New York: McGraw-Hill, 1981:91–152.
5. O'Rourke RA. Mitral valve prolapse syndrome. In: Alexander RA, Schlant RA, Fuster VF, et al., eds. *Hurst's The Heart.* New York: McGraw-Hill 1998: 1821–1831.
6. Reid JV. Mid-systolic clicks. *S Afr Med J* 1961;35: 353–357.
7. Barlow JB, Pocok WA, Marchand P, Denny M. The significance of late systolic murmurs. *Am Heart J* 1963; 66:443–452.
8. Read RC, Thal AP, Wendt VE. Symptomatic valvular myxomatous transformation (the floppy valve syndrome). *Circulation* 1965;32:897–910.
9. Criley JM, Lewis KB, Humphries JO, Ross RS. Prolapse of the mitral valve: clinical and cine-angiocardiographic findings. *Br Heart J* 1966;28:488–496.
10. Barlow JB, Bosman CK, Pocock WA, Marchland P. Late systolic murmurs and non-ejection ("mid-late") systolic clicks: an analysis of 90 patients. *Br Heart J* 1968; 30:203–218.
11. Pomerance A. Ballooning deformity (mucoid degeneration) of atrioventricular valves. *Br Heart J* 1969; 31:343–351.
12. Lucas RV Jr, Edwards JE. The floppy mitral valve. *Curr Probl Cardiol* 1982;7:1–48.
13. Bonow R, Carabello B, DeLeon AC, Jr., et al. ACC-AHA Guidelines for the management of patients with valvular heart disease. *JACC* 1998;32:1486–1588.
14. Fontana ME, Sparks EA, Boudoulas H, Wooley CF. Mitral valve prolapse and the mitral valve prolapse syndrome. *Curr Probl Cardiol* 1991;16:309–375.
15. Crawford MH, O'Rourke RA. Mitral valve prolapse syndrome. In: Isselbacher KJ, Adams RD, Braunwald E, eds. *Update I. Harrison's Principles of Internal Medicine.* New York: McGraw-Hill, 1981:91–152.
16. Perloff JK, Roberts WC. The mitral apparatus: functional anatomy of mitral regurgitation. *Circulation* 1972;46:227–239.
17. Burchell HB, Edwards JE. Rheumatic mitral insufficiency. *Circulation* 1953;7:747–756.
18. Levine HJ, Isner JM, Salem DN. Primary versus secondary mitral valve prolapse: clinical features and implications. *Clin Cardiol* 1982;5:371–375.
19. Devereux RB, Brown WT, Kramer-Fox R, Sachs I. Inheritance of mitral valve prolapse: effect of age and sex on gene expression. *Ann Intern Med* 1982;97:826–832.
20. Shell WE, Walton JA, Clifford ME, Willis PW III. The familial occurrence of the syndrome of mid-late systolic click and late systolic murmur. *Circulation* 1969;39: 327–337.
21. Savage DD, Garrison RJ, Devereux RB, et al. Mitral valve prolapse in the general population. I. Epidemiologic features: The Framingham Study. *Am Heart J* 1983;106:571–576.
22. Leier CV, Call TD, Fulkerson PK, Wooley CF. The spectrum of cardiac defects in the Ehlers-Danlos syndrome, types I and III. *Ann Intern Med* 1980;92:171–178.
23. Lebwohl MG, Distefano D, Prioleau PG, Uram M, Yannuzzi LA, Fleischmajer R. Pseudoxanthoma elasticum and mitral-valve prolapse. *N Engl J Med* 1982;307: 228–231.
24. Schwarz T, Gotsman MS. Mitral valve prolapse in osteogenesis imperfecta. *Isr J Med Sci* 1981;17: 1087–1088.
25. Salomon J, Shah PM, Heinle RA. Thoracic skeletal abnormalities in idiopathic mitral valve prolapse. *Am J Cardiol* 197;36:32–36.
26. Bon Tempo CP, Ronan JA Jr. Radiographic appearance of the thorax in systolic click late systolic murmur syndrome. *Am J Cardiol* 1975;36:27–31.
27. Pickering NJ, Brody JI, Barrett MJ. von Willebrand syndromes and mitral valve prolapse. *N Engl J Med* 1981; 305:131–134.
28. Rosenberg CA, Derman GH, Grabb WC, et al. Hypomastia and mitral valve prolapse. Evidence of a linked embryologic and mesenchymal dysplasia. *N Engl J Med* 1983;309:1230–1232.
29. Tei C, Sakamaki T, Shah PM, et al. Mitral valve prolapse in short-term experimental coronary occlusion: a possible mechanism of ischemic mitral regurgitation. *Circulation* 1983;68:183–189.
30. Crawford MH. Mitral valve prolapse due to coronary artery disease. *Am J Med* 1977;62:447–451.
31. Hendren WG, Nemec JJ, Lytle BW, et al. Mitral valve repair for ischemic mitral insufficiency. *Ann Thorac Surg* 1991;52:1246–1251.
32. Tomaru T, Uchida Y, Mohri N, Mori W, Furuse A, Asano K. Postinflammatory mitral and aortic valve prolapse: a clinical and pathological study. *Circulation* 1987;76: 68–76.
33. Lembo NJ, Dell Italia LJ, Crawford MH, Miller JF, Richards KL, O'Rourke RA. Mitral valve prolapse in patients with prior rheumatic fever. *Circulation* 1988; 77:830–836.
34. Marcus RH, Sareli P, Pocock WA, et al. Functional anatomy of severe mitral regurgitation in active rheumatic carditis. *Am J Cardiol* 1989;63:577–584.
35. Crawford MH, O'Rourke RA. Mitral valve prolapse: a cardiomyopathic state? *Prog Cardiovasc Dis* 1984;27: 133–139.
36. Lax D, Eicher M, Goldberg SJ. Mild dehydration induces echocardiographic signs of mitral valve prolapse in healthy females with prior normal cardiac findings. *Am Heart J* 1992;124:1533–1540.
37. Aufderheide S, Lax D, Goldberg SJ. Gender differences in dehydration-induced mitral valve prolapse. *Am Heart J* 195:129:83–86.
38. Fakuda N, Oki T, Iuchi A, et al. Predisposing factors for severe mitral regurgitation in idiopathic mitral valve prolapse. *Am J Cardiol* 1995;76:503–507.
39. Gaffney FA, Karlsson ES, Campbell W, et al. Autonomic dysfunction in women with mitral valve prolapse syndrome. *Circulation* 1979;59:894–901.

40. Boudoulas H, Reynolds JC, Mazzaferri E, Wooley CF. Mitral valve prolapse syndrome: the effect of adrenergic stimulation. *J Am Coll Cardiol* 1983;2:638–644.

41. Boudoulas H, Reynolds JC, Mazzaferri E, Wooley CF. Metabolic studies in mitral valve prolapse syndrome. *Circulation* 1980;61:1200–1205.

42. Gaffney FA, Bastian BC, Lane LB, et al. Abnormal cardiovascular regulation in the mitral valve prolapse syndrome. *Am J Cardiol* 1983;52:316–320.

43. Davies AO, Mares A, Pool JL, Taylor AA. Mitral valve prolapse with symptoms of beta-adrenergic hypersensitivity. Beta2-adrenergic receptor supercoupling with desensitization of isoproterenol exposure. *Am J Med* 1987;82:193–201.

44. Anwar A, Kohn SR, Dunn JF, et al. Altered beta-adrenergic receptor function in subjects with symptomatic mitral valve prolapse. *Am J Med Sci* 1991;302:89–97.

45. Fontana ME, Pence HL, Leighton RF, Wooley CF. The varying clinical spectrum of the systolic click-late systolic murmur syndrome. *Circulation* 1970;41:807–816.

46. Santos AD, Puthenpurakal MK, Ahmad H, Wallace WA, Matthew PK, Hilal A. Orthostatic hypotension: a commonly unrecognized cause of symptoms in mitral valve prolapse. *Am J Med* 1981;71:746–750.

47. Betriu A, Wigle ED, Felderhof CH, McLoughlin MJ. Prolapse of the posterior leaflet of the mitral valve associated with secundum atrial septal defect. *Am J Cardiol* 1975;35:363–369.

48. Josephson ME, Horowitz LM, Kastor JA. Paroxysmal supraventricular tachycardia in patients with mitral valve prolapse. *Circulation* 1978;57:111–119.

49. LeWinter MM, Hoffman Jr, Shell WE, et al. Phenylephrine-induced atypical chest pain in patients with prolapsing mitral valve leaflets. *Am J Cardiol* 1974;34:12–18.

50. Sabom MB, Curry RC Jr, Pepine CJ, Christie LG, Conti CR. Ergonovine testing for coronary artery spasm in patients with angiographic mitral valve prolapse. *Cathet Cardiovasc Diagn* 1978;4:265–274.

51. Mazza DL, Martin D, Spacavento L, Jacobsen J, Gibbs HL. Prevalence of anxiety disorders in patients with mitral valve prolapse. *Psychiatry* 1986;143:349–352.

52. Barnett HJ, Jones MW, Boughner DR, Kostuk WJ. Cerebral ischemic events associated with prolapsing mitral valve. *Arch Neurol* 1976;33:777–782.

53. Boughner DR, Barnett HJM. The enigma of the risk of stroke in mitral valve prolapse. *Stroke* 1985;16:175–177.

54. Barletta GA, Gagliardi R, Benvenuti L, Fantini F. Cerebral ischemic attacks as a complication of aortic and mitral valve prolapse. *Stroke* 1985;16:219–223.

55. Jones HR Jr, Nagger CZ, Seljan MP, Downing LL. Mitral valve prolapse and cerebral ischemic events. A comparison between a neurology population with stroke and a cardiology population with mitral valve prolapse observed for five years. *Stroke* 1982;13:451–453.

56. Barnett HJM, Boughner DR, Taylor DW, Cooper PE, Kostuk VJ, Nichol PM. Further evidence relating mitral valve prolapse to cerebral ischemic event. *N Engl J Med* 1980;302:139–144.

57. Petty GW, Orencia AJ, Khandheria BK, Whisnant JP. A population-based study of stroke in the setting of mitral valve prolapse: risk factors and infarct subtype classification. *Mayo Clin Proc* 1994;69:632–634.

58. Orencia AJ, Petty GW, Khandheria BK, O'Fallon WM, Whisnant JP. Mitral valve prolapse and the risk of stroke after initial cerebral ischemia. *Neurology* 1995;45:1083–1086.

59. Wilson LA, Keeling PW, Malcolm AD, Russel RW, Webb-Peploe MM. Visual complications of mitral leaflet prolapse. *Br Med J* 1977;2:86–88.

60. Chesler E, King RA, Edwards JE. The myxomatous mitral valve and sudden death. *Circulation* 1983;67:632–639.

61. Tamura K, Fukada Y, Ishizaki M, Masuda Y, Yamanaka N, Ferrans, VJ. Abnormalities in elastic fibers and other connective tissue components of floppy mitral valve. *Am Heart J* 1995;29:1149–1158.

62. Weis AJ, Salcedo EE, Stewart WJ, Level HM, Klein AL, Thomas JD. Anatomic explanation of mobile systolic clicks: Implications for the clinical and echocardiographic diagnosis of mitral valve prolapse. *Am Heart J* 1995;129:314–320.

63. Bhutto ZR, Barron JT, Liebson PR, et al. Electrocardiographic abnormalities in mitral valve prolapse. *Am J Cardiol* 1992;70:265–266.

64. Winkle RA, Lopes MG, Goodman DJ, Fitzgerald JW, Schroeder JS, Harrison DC. Propranolol for patients with mitral valve prolapse. *Am Heart J* 1977;93:422–427.

65. Schaal SF. Ventricular arrhythmias in patients with mitral valve prolapse. *Cardiovasc Clin* 1992;22:307–316.

66. Marks AR, Choong CY, Sanfilippo AJ, Ferre M, Weyman AE. Identification of high-risk and low-risk subgroups of patients with mitral-valve prolapse. *N Engl J Med* 1989;320:1031–1036.

67. Shah PM. Echocardiographic diagnosis of mitral valve prolapse. *J Am Soc Echocardiogr* 1994;7:286–293.

68. Nishimura RA, McGoon MD, Shub C, Miller FA, Ilstrup DM, Tajik AJ. Echocardiographically documented mitral-valve prolapse. Long-term follow-up of 237 patients. *N Engl J Med* 1985;313:1305–1309.

69. Zuppiroli A, Mori F, Favilli S, et al. Arrhythmias in mitral valve prolapse: relation to anterior mitral leaflet thickening, clinical variables, and color Doppler echocardiographic parameters. *Am Heart J* 1994;128:919–927.

70. Babuty D, Cosnay P, Breuillac JC, et al. Ventricular arrhythmia factors in mitral valve prolapse. *PACE Pacing Clin Electrophysiol* 1994;17:1090–1099.

71. Takamoto T, Nitta M, Tsujibayashi T, Taniguchi K, Marumo F. The prevalence and clinical features of pathologically abnormal mitral valve leaflets (myxomatous mitral valve) in the mitral valve prolapse syndrome: an echocardiographic and pathological comparative study. *J Cardiol Suppl* 1991;25:75–86.

72. Chandraratna PAN, Nimalasuriya A, Kawanishi D, Duncan P Rosin B, Rahimtoola SH. Identification of the increased frequency of cardiovascular abnormalities associated with mitral valve prolapse by two-dimensional echocardiography. *Am J Cardiol* 1984;54:1283–1285.

73. Cheitlin MD, Alpert JS, Armstrong WF, et al. ACC/AHA guidelines for the clinical application of echocardiography. *Circulation* 1977;95:1686–1744.

74. Krivokapich J, Child JS, Dadourian BJ, Perloff JK. Reassessment of echocardiographic criteria for diagnosis of mitral valve prolapse. *Am J Cardiol* 1988;61:131–135.

75. Klein GJ, Kostuk WJ, Bougher DR, et al. Stress myocardial imaging in mitral leaflet prolapse syndrome. *Am J Cardiol* 1978;42:746–750.

76. Allen H, Harris A, Leatham A. Significance and prognosis of an isolated late systolic murmur: a 9- to 22-year followup. *Br Heart J* 1974;36:525–532.

77. Mills P, Rose J, Hollingsworth J, Amara I, Craige E. Long-term prognosis of mitral-valve prolapse. *N Engl J Med* 1985;313:1305–1309.

78. Bisset GS III, Schwartz DC, Meyer RA, James FW, Kaplan S. Clinical spectrum and long-term follow-up of isolated mitral valve prolapse in 199 children. *Circulation* 1990;62:423–429.

79. Vered Z, Oren S, Rabinowitz B, Meltzer RS, Neufeld NH. Mitral valve prolapse: quantitative analysis and long-term follow-up. *Isr J Med Sci* 1985;21:644–648.

80. Duren DR, Becker AE, Dunning AJ. Long-term follow-up of idiopathic mitral valve prolapse in 300 patients: a prospective study. *J Am Coll Cardiol* 1988;11:42–47.

81. Zuppiroli A, Rinaldi M, Kramer-Fox R, Favilli S, Roman MJ, Devereux RB. Natural history of mitral valve prolapse. *Am J Cardiol* 1995;75:1028–1032.

82. Fukada N, Oki T, Iuchi A, et al. Predisposing factors for severe mitral regurgitation in idiopathic mitral regurgitation. *Am J Cardiol* 1995;76:503–507.

83. Stoddard MF, Prince CR, Dillon S, Longaker RA, Monnes GT, Liddell NE. Exercise-induced mitral regurgitation is a predictor of morbid events in subjects with mitral valve prolapse. *J Am Coll Cardiol* 1995;25:693–699.

84. Gooch AS, Vicencio F, Maranbao V, Goldberg H. Arrhythmias and left ventricular asynergy in the prolapsing mitral leaflet. *Am J Cardiol* 1972;29:601–620.

85. Clemens JD, Horwitz RI, Jaffe CC, Feinstein AR, Stanton BF. A controlled evaluation of the risk of bacterial endocarditis in persons with mitral valve prolapse. *N Engl J Med* 1982;307:776–781.

86. Devereux RB, Frary CJ, Kramer-Fox R, Roberts RB, Ruchlin HS. Cost-effectiveness of infective endocarditis prophylaxis for mitral valve prolapse with or without a mitral regurgitant murmur. *Am J Cardiol* 1994;74:1024–1029.

87. Dajani AS, Bisno AL, Chung KJ, et al. Prevention of bacterial endocarditis. Recommendations by the American Heart Association. *JAMA* 1990;264:2919–2922.

88. Stroke Prevention in Atrial Fibrillation Study Investigators. Preliminary report of the Stroke Prevention in Atrial Fibrillation Study. *N Engl J Med* 1990;322:863–868.

89. Hart RG, Halperin JL. Atrial fibrillation and stroke: revisiting the dilemmas. *Stroke* 1994;25:1337–1341.

90. Cosgrove DM, Stewart WJ. Mitral valvuloplasty. *Curr Probl Cardiol* 1989;14:359–415.

91. Kirklin JW. Mitral valve repair for mitral incompetence. *Mod Concepts Cardiovasc Dis* 1987;56:7–11.

92. Cohn LH, Couper GS, Aranki SF, Rizzo RJ, Kinchla NM, Collins JJ Jr. Long-term results of mitral valve reconstruction for regurgitation of the myxomatous mitral valve. *J Thorac Cardiovasc Surg* 1994;107:143–150.

93. Eishi K, Kawazoe K, Sasako Y, Kosakai Y, Kitoh Y, Kawashima Y. Comparison of repair techniques for mitral valve prolapse. *J Heart Valve Dis* 1994;3:432–438.

94. Perier P, Clausnizer B, Mistarz K. Carpentier sliding leaflet technique for repair of the mitral valve: early results. *Ann Thorac Surg* 1994;57:383–386.

95. Ling LH, Enriquez-Sarano M, Seward JB, et al. Clinical outcome of mitral regurgitation due to flail leaflet. *N Engl J Med* 1996;335:1417–1423.

7

Aortic Stenosis

Gilbert E. Levinson† and Joseph S. Alpert

†Deceased. Department of Medicine, University of Arizona
College of Medicine, Tucson, Arizona 85724-5035

Various aortic valvular, subvalvular, and supravalvular lesions encroach significantly on the effective orifice for left ventricular ejection and thereby increase ventricular afterload (i.e., add to the normal impedance to ventricular emptying). These lesions include congenital and acquired valvular deformities; supravalvular aortic bands, membranes, and constrictions; discrete fibrous ridges and diffuse fibromuscular thickening in the outflow tract of the left ventricle; and the complex of anatomic and physiologic abnormalities that constitute hypertrophic cardiomyopathy.

PATHOPHYSIOLOGIC FEATURES

By narrowing the outflow orifice, the various aortic lesions all cause a systolic ejection murmur (1). In addition, the systolic overload they impose on the left ventricle evokes certain compensations (i.e., mechanisms to permit normal ventricular emptying and thereby to maintain cardiac output). The physiologic compensations are an increase in the pressure generated by the left ventricle, with a resultant gradient between that chamber and the aorta and a prolongation of the systolic ejection period. No measurable gradient develops until the area of the aortic valve is reduced by 50%. The anatomic compensation is an increase in contractile mass (i.e., left ventricular hypertrophy). As long as these compensations suffice to

maintain normal ventricular emptying, the patient with aortic outflow obstruction exhibits no signs of cardiac failure and may be entirely asymptomatic. If left ventricular contractility is impaired or if there is a progressive increase in obstruction, or if the contractile reserve (i.e., capacity for compensatory hypertrophy) is exhausted, the end-systolic volume rises and an additional compensation, namely, dilatation with augmented fiber stretch (the Frank-Starling mechanism), attempts to maintain output. When this preload reserve is exhausted, no further compensations are available, and pump failure ensues (1).

The compensatory mechanisms have consequences other than maintenance of output. Left ventricular hypertrophy is associated with reduced diastolic ventricular compliance (Δvolume/Δpressure) because of increased wall stiffness and impaired myocardial relaxation. Although mean left ventricular diastolic pressure is only slightly increased as a result of this, late diastolic filling necessitates an increased force of atrial contraction, with resultant prominence of the left atrial A wave ("atrial kick") and elevation of left ventricular end-diastolic pressure. The associated clinical consequences are a prominent fourth heart sound (S_4) and deterioration in pump performance if atrial contraction is lost secondary to atrial fibrillation or heart block. Clinical heart failure can develop if an appropriate timed atrial contraction is lost.

Individuals with marked left ventricular hypertrophy may exhibit the syndrome of diastolic heart failure in which left ventricular systolic function is maintained in the face of severely abnormal diastolic function. Clinical heart failure is often present in these individuals who are frequently elderly women with exuberant left ventricular hypertrophy and aortic stenosis.

The increased left ventricular muscle mass also raises myocardial oxygen consumption and, in experimental models, increases the intercapillary distance for oxygen diffusion. Left ventricular systolic hypertension further raises myocardial oxygen need while at the same time impedes systolic coronary perfusion. Prolongation of systole raises myocardial oxygen consumption while at the same time limits the duration of diastole, the phase of the cardiac cycle in which most coronary blood flow normally occurs. These "side effects" of the compensatory mechanisms set the stage for episodic or sustained imbalance between myocardial oxygen supply and demand. Acute imbalance may be manifested by anginal attacks, paroxysmal arrhythmias (with possible acute reduction in cardiac output and resultant syncope), episodes of acute nonarrhythmic power failure (with possible resultant syncope), or sudden death. Prolonged imbalance may cause patchy myocardial fibrosis, with exacerbation or impairment of diastolic or systolic performance. Left ventricular systolic function depends on myocardial contractility, preload, and afterload. Thus, abnormal left ventricular ejection fraction in patients with aortic stenosis can be the result of reduced intrinsic myocardial function, reduced preload (e.g., loss of atrial systole) and/or a preload–afterload mismatch (e.g., arterial hypertension). However, most patients with aortic stenosis have normal left ventricular systolic function.

Myocardial supply–demand imbalance of blood flow can produce ischemia in the absence of obstructive coronary artery disease. Julius et al. (1a) attributed myocardial ischemia in this setting to inadequate left ventricular hypertrophy, high systolic and diastolic wall stresses, and reduced coronary flow reserve. Episodic or chronic hypoxia and left ventricular systolic hypertension both may damage the conduction system; therefore, patients with outflow obstructions exhibit a very high incidence of conduction disturbances. The lesions that obstruct left ventricular outflow have in common the features shown in Table 7-1.

In addition to these general and shared characteristics, each outflow obstructing lesion exhibits unique distinguishing features reflecting the locus of the lesion, its cause and pathologic anatomic features, and the probability of associated disorders, sequelae, and

TABLE 7-1. *Cardinal manifestations of left ventricular outflow obstructions*

Systolic ejection murmur
S_4
Prolonged ejection period
Left ventricular hypertrophy
Gradient between left ventricle and aorta
Possibility of
  Paroxysmal symptoms: chest pain, syncope
  Sudden death
  Prolonged preservation of pump function
  Ultimate left heart failure

TABLE 7-2. *Lesions obstructing left ventricular outflow*

Valvular aortic stenosis
  Acquired
    Postinflammatory (usually rheumatic)
    Fibrocalcific deformity of a congenital bicuspid aortic valve
    Fibrocalcific deformity of a three-cusped aortic valve
  Unusual causes
    Obstructive infectious endocarditis vegetation
    Familial hypercholesterolemia
    Paget's disease
    Rheumatoid arthritis
    Ochronosis
    Radiation
  Congenital
    Unicuspid unicommisural valve
    Three-cusped valve with fusion of commissures
    Hypoplastic annulus
Nonvalvular aortic stenosis
  Subvalvular
    Discrete fibromembranous
    Diffuse fibromuscular (tunnel)
    Muscular (hypertrophic subaortic stenosis)
  Supravalvular
    Hourglass
    Hypoplastic
    Membrane

TABLE 7-3. *Differential diagnosis of aortic stenosis: history*

Type of stenosis	Age when murmur noted	Age when symptomatic	Family history of murmur	Family history of sudden childhood death	Personal past history
Acquired nonrheumatic	Early to late adulthood	Middle age to old age	Rare	None	None
Acquired rheumatic	Late childhood to early adulthood	Early adulthood to middle age	Occasional	None	Acute rheumatic fever (common)
Hypertrophic subaortic	Early childhood to late adulthood	Any age	Common	Occasional	None
Congenital valvular	Infancy to childhood (frequently at birth, 50% by 1 yr, almost all by age 8 yr)	Rare	None	None	None
Congenital subvalvular		Childhood to middle age	Rare	None	Infantile hypercalcemia or renal failure (uncommon but diagnostic)
Congenital supravalvular			Common	Occasional	

TABLE 7-4. *Differential diagnosis of aortic stenosis: physical findings*

Type of stenosis	Maximum murmur and thrill	Aortic ejection sound	Aortic component of second sound	Regurgitant diastolic murmur	Arterial pulse
Acquired nonrheumatic	Second right ICS; sternal border to neck; may be at apex in the aged	Uncommon	Decreased or absent	Common	Delayed upstroke; anacrotic notch; ±small amplitude
Acquired rheumatic		Uncommon	Decreased or absent	Common	
Hypertrophic subaortic	Fourth left ICS; sternal border to apex (±regurgitant systolic murmur at apex)	Rare	Normal or decreased	Very rare	Brisk upstroke, sometimes bisferiens
Congenital valvular	Second right ICS; sternal border to neck (along left sternal border in some infants)	Very common in children, disappearing with decrease in valve mobility with age	Normal or increased in childhood; decreased with decrease in valve mobility with age	Uncommon in child; not uncommon in adult	Delayed upstroke; anacrotic notch; ±small amplitude
Congenital subvalvular	Discrete: like valvular; tunnel; left sternal border	Rare	Not helpful (normal, increased, decreased or absent)	Almost all	
Congenital supravalvular	First right ICS; sternal border to neck and sometimes to medial aspect of right arm; occasionally greater in neck than in chest	Rare	Normal or decreased	Uncommon	Rapid upstroke in right carotid, delayed in left carotid; right arm pulse pressure greater than left

ICS, intercostal space.

TABLE 7-5. *Differential diagnosis of aortic stenosis: laboratory and other findings*

Type of stenosis	Aortic valve calcium	Ascending aortic dilatation	Echocardiographic features	Gradient	Angiographic features	Other diagnostic features
Acquired nonrheumatic	Usual	Usual	Eccentric aortic valve closure plus features of rheumatic lesion (see below)	Left ventricle/aorta	Calcified aortic valve with decreased mobility; cylindrical cavity; ±coronary or mitral annular calcification	Aortic regurgitation, often severe
Acquired rheumatic	Common	Usual	Concentric left ventricular hypertrophy; calcified leaflets; fluttering of anterior mitral leaflet if aortic regurgitation present; wide ascending aorta	Left ventricle/aorta	Calcified aortic valve with decreased mobility; cylindrical cavity ± mitral leaflet calcification	Aortic regurgitation, often severe; mitral disease common
Hypertrophic subaortic	None	Absent or mild	ASH; SAM; midsystolic closure; adynamic septum; decreased E-F slope; anterior mitral valve	Left ventricle/left ventricle	Dynamic stenosis, subvalvular; banana-shaped cavity; anterior mitral leaflet; ± cavity obliteration	Apical double impulse; ECG: WPW or Qs simulating myocardial infarction; bifid apex impulse; abnormal post-PVC pulse pressure; murmur decrease with squatting, increased with Valsalva maneuver
Congenital valvular	Related to age	Common	Diastolic closure is perpendicular rather than parallel to aortic walls	Left ventricle/aorta	Central or eccentric jet; ±dome-shaped valve	Coarctation; other congenital heart disease
Congenital subvalvular	None	Usually absent or mild	Concentric left ventricular hypertrophy; membrane or ridge or diffuse outflow narrowing; very early partial systolic closure of aortic valve; fluttering of aortic valve cusps	Left ventricle/left ventricle	Membrane or ridge below aortic valve or long, narrow outflow tract	Shone's or Noonan's syndrome; coarctation; mitral regurgitation; other congenital heart disease
Congenital supravalvular	None	Absent	Concentric left ventricular hypertrophy; abnormality in ascending aorta	Aorta/aorta	Membrane, ridge, hourglass deformity, or hypoplasia of aorta; prominant coronaries	Elfin face; retardation; peripheral pulmonary artery stenosis; coarctation; other congenital heart disease

ASH, asymetric septal hypertrophy; SAM, systolic anterior motion; ECG, electrocardiogram; WPW, Wolff Parkinson White; Q, q-waves; PVC, premature ventricular contraction.

complications. The lesions may be classified as in Table 7-2. The clinical and laboratory findings in the various lesions are summarized in Tables 7-3, 7-4, and 7-5.

VALVULAR AORTIC STENOSIS

Valvular aortic stenosis is by far the most common cause of left ventricular outflow obstruction. All acquired aortic stenosis and 70% of congenital aortic stenosis are valvular (1). Moreover, except for mitral regurgitation secondary to myocardial disease, valvular aortic stenosis is the most common fatal cardiac valve lesion (2).

Etiology and Pathogenesis

About one third of cases are associated with mitral stenosis or incompetence, and there is considerable evidence that these cases are rheumatic in origin (3). The pathologic features are inflammation, commissural fusion, and secondary calcification. The other two thirds of cases are isolated lesions (aortic stenosis with or without aortic regurgitation), and most of these are nonrheumatic in origin (4,5). In patients presenting with clinically pure stenosis or stenosis accompanied by mild regurgitation, fibrocalcific deformity of a congenital bicuspid valve accounts for about one half, postinflammatory fibrocalcific disease (including rheumatic disease) for about one third, degenerative calcification of an aging valve or of a congenitally unicommissural valve for about one sixth, and the remainder are indeterminate in cause (6). In patients presenting with significant degrees of both stenosis and regurgitation, calcification of congenitally bicuspid valves accounts for some cases, but most are caused by postinflammatory disease that includes but is not necessarily confined to rheumatic valvulitis (7,8). As the U.S. population ages, degenerative calcific aortic stenosis is increasingly common.

In the pediatric age group, infancy through mid-adolescence, most cases of isolated valvular aortic stenosis are the result of a congenital deformity that has been described clinically as a bicuspid valve with fusion of one commissure (9,10). In autopsy reports it has been described as a unicuspid unicommissural valve with a false second commissure due to a congenital raphe (11,12). Such valves are inherently stenotic, they are stenotic at birth, usually calcified by age 30 (ordinarily with worsening of the stenosis and often with consequent development of aortic regurgitation), three times more prevalent in men than women, and occur mostly in infancy and early childhood. A few cases in this age group are due to hypoplasia of the aortic annulus (13) or to commissural fusion(s) in a three-cusped or four-cusped valve.

In later childhood through mid-adolescence, there is an increasing incidence of aortic stenosis due to fibrotic deformation of a congenital bicuspid valve or, less commonly, of a congenitally malformed tricuspid valve (2). The bicuspid anomaly is of particular importance, especially in adult life, because it is, next to the floppy mitral valve, the most common major congenital cardiac malformation. It has a possible frequency as high as 2% of all live births and a 4:1 male preponderance (14). Such valves are not inherently stenotic but suffer connective tissue alterations secondary to their abnormal stresses with movement and perhaps also to superficial deposition of microthrombi generated by turbulence (12,15). The result is a stenotic valve due to fibrosis and calcification of the cusps and not to commissural fusion. How often this occurs is not known, but Fenoglio et al. (16) suggested that in patients beyond age 20 who were born with bicuspid valves, about one third of the valves cause no hemodynamic derangement, one third become stenotic, and in one third regurgitation develops, usually secondary to infective endocarditis but occasionally without such infection (17). Sabet et al. (17a) studied 542 patients with bicuspid aortic valves who required aortic valve replacement: 75% had aortic stenosis, 13% had aortic regurgitation, and 10% had mixed stenosis and regurgitation. Almost all bicuspid valves that become stenotic are calcified by age 30

(14). Coexisting congenital anomalies are rare except for coarctation of the aorta, which Roberts (14) observed in 5 of 85 patients with bicuspid valves over the age of 14. Congenital bicuspid aortic valve is an important risk factor for type I and II aortic dissections that have been reported to occur nine times more often in persons with bicuspid valves than in those with three-cusped valves (18).

Congenital malformations underlie most cases of isolated valvular stenosis between ages 15 and 65, 10% being unicuspid and 60% bicuspid. Among the remaining 30%, it is probable that inequalities in cusps, commissures, or both, in at least some of these three-cusped valves, are the basis for a wear-and-tear fibrocalcific degenerative process (19). This process appears to be the cause of most cases of isolated calcific aortic stenosis over the age of 65 in which Roberts et al. (20) found 90% of the valves to be tricuspid and only 10% bicuspid. This degenerative process is very common and results in some degree of calcification in 30% and an aortic outflow murmur in 69% of people in their nineties (21,22). In most such cases, however, although the leaflets are thickened and somewhat rigid (aortic sclerosis), significant obstruction to outflow is not present. Stewart et al. (22a) studied the relation between aortic valve fibrosis and calcification in more than 5,000 patients aged 65 and above. They noted that 26% of patients had nonobstructive sclerosis of the aortic valve, whereas 2% had aortic stenosis. In patients aged 75 or above, 37% had sclerosis and 2.6% had stenosis. Most important was their observation that the presence of aortic sclerosis/stenosis in these individuals correlated with the presence of traditional risk factors for atherosclerosis (e.g., hypertension, smoking, and hypercholesterolemia). Thus, the atherosclerotic process undoubtedly plays a role in the development of three-cusped, degenerative, calcific aortic stenosis. Consistent with this relationship is the observation that *Chlamydia pneumoniae* is frequently present in aortic stenotic valves affected with degenerative calcific disease (22b, 22c).

A number of investigators have reported on the rate of progression of aortic stenosis. Considerable variation exists from patient to patient with mean reduction in aortic valve area usually in the vicinity of 0.1 cm^2/yr (22d). Predictors of progression include jet velocity, rate of change of jet velocity, and clinical status (22e).

Rare causes of valvular aortic stenosis include systemic lupus erythematosus, especially after steroid therapy; Fabry's disease and ochronosis (in both of which metabolic products accumulate in the valve cusps); type II (familial) hyperlipoproteinemia; encroachment on the valve orifice by bulky vegetations of infective endocarditis; and damage secondary to radiotherapy (23–32). Figures 7-1 and 7-2 show the normal valve and several stenotic valves.

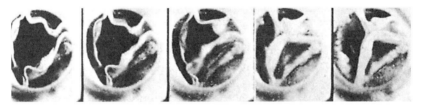

FIG. 7-1. Normal aortic valve photographed from above. The valve is seen in the fully open systolic position in the photograph on the extreme left and in the closed position in diastole in the photograph on the extreme right. Note the presence of three cusps, the systolic orifice in the shape of an equilateral triangle, the complete coaptation of the leaflets in diastole, and the leaflet flexibility indicated by the sequence of pictures from left to right. (From McMillan IKR. Aortic stenosis: a postmortem cinephotographic study of valve action. *Br Heart J* 1955;17:56, with permission.)

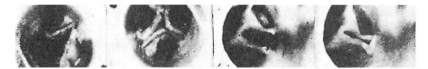

FIG. 7-2. Stenotic aortic valves photographed from above. The two photographs on the left show a calcified three-cusped aortic valve in the fully open and fully closed positions. Note the irregularity of the systolic orifice and the incomplete coaptation of the leaflets in diastole. The two photographs on the right show a calcified bicuspid valve in the fully open and fully closed positions. Note the small "fish-mouth" orifice in systole and the incomplete diastolic closure. Both valves exemplify calcific aortic stenosis and regurgitation. (From McMillan IKR. Aortic stenosis: a postmortem cinephotographic study of valve action. *Br Heart J* 1955;17:56, with permission.)

Clinical Presentation

History

In the compensated phase, the patient may be entirely asymptomatic or may suffer from syncope, dizziness, or angina pectoris, all generally associated with effort (1). Dizziness and syncope may occur at any age; angina increases in incidence with increasing age. Dizziness or syncope occurs in 15% to 30% of symptomatic patients and may result from an abrupt fall in cardiac output during effort without compensatory increase in systemic vascular resistance, an abrupt fall in systemic vascular resistance in the presence of a fixed output, or an arrhythmia (33–37a). Schwartz et al. (38) identified two phases of effort syncope. The first lasts 20 to 40 seconds and is associated with sudden hypotension, dizziness, pallor, and the disappearance of heart sounds and murmur but persistence of regular rhythm. The second, occurring after 40 seconds, is characterized by arrhythmias, apnea or Cheyne-Stokes breathing, cyanosis, and sometimes convulsions. It is important to note that the briefer episodes may consist only of light-headedness or "graying out," generally referred to as near syncope.

Angina is more frequent with aortic stenosis than with any other valve lesion and is usually a typical angina of effort (33). It occurs in about two thirds of patients with severe aortic stenosis (39,40). Only about one half of these angina patients have high-grade coronary artery stenoses (lumen narrowing of at least 70% to 75%) (39–41). Although it is possible that lesser degrees of lumen narrowing (e.g., 50%) may cause significant coronary hemodynamic abnormalities in patients with severe aortic stenosis, some aortic stenosis patients have very little angiographically demonstrable coronary artery disease (1a,42).

The mechanism of angina pectoris in patients without significant coronary artery disease has been the subject of extensive investigation. Among patients with severe aortic stenosis and normal coronary arteries, those with and without angina pectoris do not differ in resting coronary blood flow per unit of left ventricular muscle; luminal diameter of the coronary vessels on angiography; coronary sinus blood flow and lactate; echocardiographically or ventriculographically measured left ventricular wall thickness, chamber size, systolic and diastolic wall stress, and mass; or electrocardiogram (ECG) voltage (43–49). Some reports suggest that patients with angina differ from those without angina in having a smaller aortic valve area, higher resting left ventricular systolic pressure and transvalvular gradient, and lower ratio of the diastolic pressure-time index to the systolic pressure-time index (an estimate of the subendocardial supply-and-demand ratio) (45,49–51). Others describe no differences at rest in patients with and without angina in the ratio of diastolic to systolic pressure-time indices or in the aortic gradient and valve area (46,49). As noted earlier, Julius et al. (1a) ascribed myocardial ischemia to reduced coronary flow reserve, lessened degrees of left ventricular hypertrophy, and higher wall stresses.

With the metabolic stress of isoproterenol or pacing, most patients with aortic stenosis and normal coronary arteries exhibit evidence of ischemia (i.e., lactate production or decreased lactate extraction (44,47,48). Moreover, despite comparable increases in coronary blood flow, patients with angina have, during isometric exercise, a significantly lower subendocardial supply-and-demand ratio than do those who are pain free (46). This ischemia may be due in part to a deficit in flow. Direct intraoperative measurements of postocclusive flow rates in arteries perfusing the left ventricle support the concept of decreased coronary reserve (i.e., vasodilatory capacity) in patients with aortic stenosis (52). This could be due to a failure of the coronary microvasculature to grow apace with the increased left ventricular mass, resulting in an increase in minimal coronary vascular resistance with a corresponding decrease in capacity to dilate in response to stress (52). The concept of a decreased coronary vascular reserve in aortic stenosis has also been suggested by others and could apply to left ventricular hypertrophy due to any pressure overload (53–57). The ischemia could also be due in part to an increase in demand representing greater severity of the valve lesion and higher left ventricular systolic pressure and aortic gradient during stress (50,58). Finally, the hypertrophic heart appears to have a greater susceptibility than normal to ischemic damage. In an experimental animal model of valvular aortic stenosis, preischemic and ischemic endocardial blood flow and subendocardial high-energy phosphate stores and baseline mitochondrial function were lower than normal, and the hypertrophied hearts of animals with experimental aortic stenosis suffered ischemic contracture sooner than controls (59). Thus, increased myocardial demand, decreased subendocardial supply, and enhanced susceptibility to supply-and-demand imbalance all appear to contribute to the angina in patients with aortic stenosis and no significant coronary artery disease.

With long-standing and severe valvular narrowing, if the patient does not succumb to a myocardial infarction or a lethal arrhythmia and has not already presented with dizziness, syncope, or angina, failure of the left ventricle is virtually inevitable (1,33,34). In this case, the patient presents with the classic symptoms of left ventricular failure: fatigue, cough, progressive dyspnea on exertion, orthopnea, and paroxysmal nocturnal dyspnea.

Some patients may have infective endocarditis. This is a particular risk for younger patients because the stenotic aortic valve is increasingly calcified with age, and the incidence of infective endocarditis diminishes as the extent of calcification increases (14). If endocarditis occurs, regardless of the underlying pathologic condition, destruction of valve tissue is likely to lead to an important component of aortic regurgitation. The patient with endocarditis may present with fever of unknown origin, sudden left ventricular failure due to valve destruction, or cerebral or other systemic embolism.

Embolization may occur, in the absence of infective endocarditis, because of calcific microemboli and perhaps because of thrombotic microemboli (15,60,61). Emboli involving heart, kidney, or brain are the most common and are usually clinically silent (60,61). Cerebral manifestations may occur as either transient ischemic attacks or infarction with brief or prolonged deficits, including aphasia, lateralized numbness or weakness, slurred speech, hemiparesis, and hemianopsias (62). In addition, calcium emboli to the central retinal artery or one of its branches may occur, presenting with amaurosis fugax or a prolonged visual deficit associated with an irregular pure white body in the occluded retinal vessel (63–66). Retinal emboli may be recurrent and bilateral (67).

Some patients may have severe, even massive, gastrointestinal bleeding, which may be recurrent or chronic, with no source discernible by barium studies or by upper and lower gastrointestinal endoscopy. The association between aortic stenosis and gastrointestinal bleeding of undetermined source, first noted in two letters to the editor in the *New England Journal of Medicine* (68,69), is very clearly real. In several large series, 25% to 30% of patients with gastrointestinal bleeding in whom the source could not be determined by barium studies and endoscopy had aortic stenosis (70,71). The hemorrhagic lesion is an arteriovenous malformation, usually termed angiodysplasia, occurring predominantly in the right colon and also in the small bowel and stomach (72–74). Selective mesenteric angiography may identify an early draining vein (i.e., one that fills during the arterial phase) and/or a series of tortuous and dilated arterial branches (72). In a sizable fraction of patients, however, one or more angiograms and laparotomies may fail to reveal a bleeding site (71,74,75). If the aortic stenosis is not of high grade, endoscopic electrocoagulation can be attempted in cases where the bleeding site is found, and blind resection of the ascending colon has been used in cases where the site cannot be found (73,74). If the aortic stenosis is severe, aortic valve replacement should be performed and gastrointestinal bleeding, however recurrent or massive, will usually cease (75–78).

Whether the initial symptom is dizziness, syncope, angina pectoris, frank myocardial infarction, arrhythmia, progressive dyspnea, fatigue, fever, acute pulmonary edema, neurologic or visual deficit, or gastrointestinal bleeding, a history of known heart murmur for many years or even decades is common. In patients who have congenital unicuspid valves, a murmur usually has been heard at birth or in infancy, and most (but not all) of these patients present by age 30. With bicuspid valves, a murmur usually has been heard in childhood, youth, or early adulthood, and the patient may present in any of these periods or at age 65 or over. Most patients in the latter group have a degenerative (wear-and-tear) lesion that was manifest as an ejection systolic murmur in middle age. Except for coincidence or instances of erroneous diagnosis, none of the patients with these causes of isolated aortic valvular stenosis gives a history consistent with acute rheumatic fever. When such a history is obtained, the patient almost always is over 30 years of age, and attention

should be given to the probable concurrence of a mitral lesion, especially mitral stenosis (which is not necessarily hemodynamically significant but is important in confirming the etiologic diagnosis). If the mitral component is significant, a history of long-standing murmur is much less likely to be obtained because the mitral lesion probably demanded earlier clinical attention because of dyspnea, marked fatigue, paroxysmal atrial fibrillation, and/or systemic emboli (79). There is a history of antecedent acute rheumatic fever in most of these patients (5).

Finally, a few asymptomatic patients may be referred for evaluation because of an abnormal finding on a screening examination, such as a chest roentgenogram or an ECG. Here also there may be a history of a long-standing murmur that was interpreted as functional, innocent, or unimportant or for which no further evaluation had previously been recommended.

Physical Findings

Except in patients over 65 and in those with rheumatic lesions (multivalvular with probable history of rheumatic fever), examination (1,33,80–82) usually reveals a male patient with a systolic murmur. (This reflects the fact that most congenital aortic valve malformations occur in males; in rheumatic- and geriatric-group patients, this disparity is not seen.) The murmur (Fig. 7-3) is of the ejection type, beginning after the first heart sound (S_1) (at the end of isometric contraction), crescendo-decrescendo, harsh, maximal at the second right sternal edge, radiating to the carotids and to the lower left sternal edge, and often accompanied by a thrill. Because of its intensity and site of origin (at the threshold of the systemic arterial circulation), the murmur is widespread in radiation; it is sometimes heard over the entire thorax, the frontal sinuses, or the abdominal aorta. The intensity, duration, and configuration of the murmur bear a rough relation to the severity of the stenosis. Soft short murmurs suggest a lesser severity than do loud long ones, as do murmurs that reach

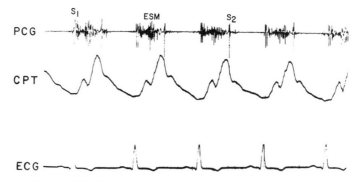

FIG. 7-3. Phonocardiogram (PCG), indirect carotid pulse tracing (CPT), and electrocardiogram in a patient with valvular aortic stenosis. The PCG shows the typical diamond-shaped ejection systolic murmur of left ventricular outflow obstruction occurring after the first heart sound (S_1). The CPT shows the delayed peak and an unusually prominent anacrotic notch on the prolonged upstroke, indicating a hemodynamically significant fixed obstruction.

maximum intensity in early rather than late systole. In some patients (especially infants and the elderly), the murmur is best heard at the apex. In senile, degenerative, calcific stenosis, the apical murmur may be of a musical "cooing dove" character. Except in a patient with a very low cardiac output (who, if aortic stenosis is the cause, is probably moribund), the absence of a murmur rules out a diagnosis of hemodynamically significant valvular aortic stenosis.

The systolic murmur may be accompanied by a high-pitched, blowing, decrescendo diastolic murmur, indicating the presence of aortic regurgitation. This finding does not establish the valve as the site of the outflow obstruction, because regurgitant diastolic murmurs are common in discrete membranous or diffuse fibromuscular subvalvular stenosis and are present in some patients with supravalvular obstruction. It also suggests that hypertrophic cardiomyopathy is not the cause of the obstruction, because regurgitant diastolic murmurs in that disorder are very rare (82).

In some patients there may also be a regurgitant systolic murmur representing ruptured mitral chordae tendineae. In one report, severe aortic stenosis was present in 8% of a large consecutive series of surgical cases with ruptured chordae (83). Most had extensive mitral annular calcification and no evidence of rheumatic or myxomatous mitral pathology. These data suggest that coincidental mitral annular calcification or extension of aortic valve calcium into the mitral annulus, in conjunction with high left ventricular systolic pressures, predisposes the patient with aortic stenosis to rupture of the mitral chordae tendineae.

In younger patients, in whom calcific immobilization of the valve has not occurred, there may be an ejection sound (84) (Fig. 7-4). This early systolic click is, when present, a valuable clue to the valvular locus of the obstruction. In the pediatric age group its absence should lead to a suspicion of nonvalvular stenosis, because the ejection sound is rare in this type of stenosis but common in the inherently stenotic unicuspid valve, which constitutes 60% of valvular stenosis through age 15. Above that age, the absence of the sound is of little diagnostic help, but its presence points to a valvular locus of a lesion of only mild or moderate severity with cusps that are still mobile (84).

The aortic component (A_2) of the second heart sound (S_2) is delayed because of the prolongation of systolic ejection and is absent or diminished in intensity with immobility or limited mobility of the cusps (Fig. 7-4). When, despite a severe degree of stenosis, the

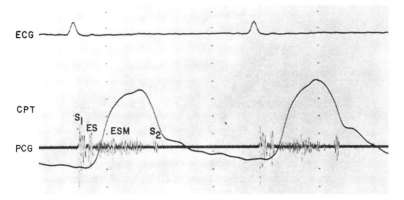

FIG. 7-4. The electrocardiogram, phonocardiogram, and carotid pulse tracing in a patient with valvular aortic stenosis. Note the high anacrotic shoulder and late peak of the carotid pulse, which indicate a hemodynamically significant fixed obstruction; the ejection sound (ES), which follows the S_1, precedes the ejection systolic murmur, and indicates the valvular locus of the obstruction; and the second heart sound (S_2), which is single in the beats shown and was not observed to split in long recordings. An ES is observed in almost all patients with noncalcified aortic stenosis and in about one half with calcific aortic stenosis. (Figure taken from ref. 84.)

A_2 is still audible, its lateness may give rise to paradoxical splitting of the S_2. Because higher degrees of narrowing are associated with progressively less cusp mobility in adults, S_2 in severe valvular aortic stenosis is typically single. An A_2 of normal intensity is found in only about 10% of patients with hemodynamically significant calcific aortic stenosis.

In general, auscultation in valvular stenosis serves to demonstrate the presence of the lesion and provides some clues as to severity (chiefly singularity of the S_2 or a diminished A_2 but also the loudness, duration, and shape of the murmur and paradoxical splitting). Other indexes of severity are found elsewhere in the physical examination, especially in sphygmomanometry and palpation of the systemic arteries and precordium.

The arterial blood pressure in the asymptomatic patient or the patient suffering only nonrespiratory symptoms (angina, syncope, or dizziness but not dyspnea, cough, or orthopnea) is usually normal. After all, the cardiac output and stroke volume are maintained by the compensatory mechanisms that have been described. Only when these no longer suffice to compensate for the overload and the patient (or, more properly, the lesion) is "de-

compensated" do stroke volume and, concomitantly, systolic and pulse pressures fall. Thus, the classic "pulsus parvus," or small pulse, is a sign not of aortic stenosis but of decompensated aortic stenosis and is usually accompanied by other evidence of left ventricular failure. Indeed, because loss of elasticity of the aortic wall with a corresponding widening of pulse pressure caused by elevation of systolic pressure is an accompaniment of aging, a wide pulse pressure with normal diastolic pressure is typical of the middle-aged or elderly patient with compensated aortic stenosis (85). Moreover, aortic stenosis does not protect against hypertensive vascular disease. That most common cardiovascular affliction may coexist with the valvular lesion, and the patient may have elevated systolic and diastolic blood pressures, although it is most unusual for systolic pressures in such cases to exceed 200 mm Hg (33,86). Finally, if pulse pressure in a patient with high-grade aortic stenosis is widened and diastolic pressure reduced, the valve lesion usually has a significant component of regurgitation. There is a tendency in such cases to underestimate the magnitude of the leak on the basis of bedside signs. Moderately severe and severe aortic re-

gurgitation may not, in the presence of comparable grades of aortic stenosis, be associated with impressive lowering of aortic diastolic pressure and widening of pulse pressure
(87). Before cardiac catheterization and angiocardiography, major clues to the presence
of an important leak include the popliteal-
brachial systolic pressure difference and the
presence of cardiomegaly without symptoms
or signs of left ventricular failure (87).

Prolongation of the ejection phase ordinarily is evident from palpation of the arterial
pulse (1,33,82,86). A slow rise of the arterial
pressure, the "pulsus tardus," sometimes with
systolic vibrations or "shudder," can be felt
best at the carotid artery and, although subject
to appreciable observer error (88), can be a
valuable sign of hemodynamically significant
stenosis. Conversely, the presence of a normally brisk carotid upstroke in valvular aortic
stenosis is evidence against a significant degree of obstruction. Occasionally, however,
with rigid vessels or associated aortic regurgitation, the carotid upstroke may be brisk despite high-grade aortic stenosis. Systolic vibrations or shudder of the carotid pulse
represent the presence of a transmitted murmur and do not correlate with the severity of
the stenosis (89). One report indicates that the
prolonged ejection phase in significant aortic
stenosis can be detected with a high sensitivity, specificity, and predictive accuracy by a
distinct lag between the initial systolic thrust
at the apex and the peak of the carotid pulse
(90). This sign appears to be easier to elicit
than the classic pulsus tardus.

Left ventricular hypertrophy is evident as a
sustained thrusting or heaving apex impulse.
Because, until failure occurs, the hypertrophy
is not accompanied by dilatation, there is no
cardiomegaly, and the apex impulse is not displaced. The apical thrust or heave may be present before unequivocal findings of left ventricular hypertrophy are evident in the ECG.
Indeed, physical examination, except in cases
of very heavy chest muscularity, adiposity, or
pulmonary emphysema, is so sensitive to the
presence of left ventricular hypertrophy that
the absence of an apical thrust or heave in aor-

tic stenosis strongly suggests that, on a scale
of 1+ to 4+, the lesion is mild (1+) or at most
moderate (2+) in severity. Conversely, in the
absence of other left ventricular overloads
(such as hypertension or mitral regurgitation),
which might be responsible for the finding, a
definite apical thrust or heave, even with a
negative ECG, suggests that aortic stenosis is
moderately severe (3+) or severe (4+).

With failure, the increase in left ventricular
chamber size results in displacement of the
apex impulse downward and to the left. This
finding in a patient with the murmur, thrill,
delayed carotid upstroke, and abnormal S_2,
typical of valvular aortic stenosis, indicates
decompensation even in the absence of symptoms. In addition to palpable or percussible
cardiomegaly, there is, with decompensation,
a narrowing of pulse pressure and a ventricular diastolic gallop, and there may be dependent lung rales.

Other physical signs of high-grade stenosis
include occasional prominence of a jugular
venous A wave, thought to reflect diminished
right ventricular compliance secondary to
ventricular septal hypertrophy, and evidence
(on inspection, palpation, or auscultation) of
the prominent left atrial kick (81,82).

Laboratory Findings

Electrocardiogram

The ECG is useful in assessing severity and
in documenting important sequelae (33,38,91,
92). Most patients with high-grade (moderately severe or severe) stenosis show either
QRS or ST-T abnormalities consistent with left
ventricular hypertrophy, although the full left
ventricular hypertrophy with "strain" pattern is
seen in no more than half (93). The higher the
gradient across the aortic valve, the more likely
is the strain or "systolic overload" pattern (38,
92). In one study, the total 12-lead QRS amplitude in millimeters was similar to the left ventricular systolic pressure in millimeters of mer-
cury in most patients with pure aortic valve
disease and no evidence of mitral, coronary, or
myocardial disease (94). Thus, subtraction of

brachial systolic cuff pressure from total 12-lead QRS amplitude is a noninvasive predictor of the peak systolic pressure gradient across the aortic valve. As is the case with evidence of left ventricular hypertrophy on physical examination, the ECG finding does not indicate severity of the stenosis in the presence of hypertension or mitral regurgitation but is significant evidence of a high-grade lesion in their absence. An ECG with normal QRS complexes, S-T segments, and T waves suggests a mild or, at most, moderate stenosis but does not entirely rule out a severe lesion, because 9% of patients with aortic stenosis who die suddenly have a normal ECG (17,22).

Electrocardiographic evidence of left atrial hypertrophy may be seen without accompanying mitral valve disease in severe aortic stenosis (95). It reflects a significant and sustained elevation of left ventricular diastolic pressure, which may occur with marked ventricular hypertrophy accompanied by myocardial fibrosis and invariably occurs in the decompensated lesion. Although left atrial hypertrophy in a patient with aortic stenosis should raise suspicion of an associated mitral lesion, mitral lesions are typically associated with left atrial enlargement (seen on chest roentgenograms) and hypertrophy (seen on the ECG), whereas the left atrium in isolated aortic stenosis is seldom dilated.

Abnormalities in conduction are more common in aortic stenosis than in any other valve lesion, with the exception of mitral regurgitation secondary to left ventricular myocardial damage. First-degree atrioventricular block, bundle branch block, and intraventricular conduction disturbances are fairly common, and complete heart block may be seen (33,85,96). These sequelae may result from septal trauma incident to high intramyocardial tensions, from hypoxic damage to the conducting fibers, or from extension of valvular calcification into the fibrous septum. In addition, ventricular dysrhythmias can be demonstrated by ambulatory ECG monitoring in most patients with valvular aortic stenosis (37a.) Their frequency and grade are not related to the severity of the stenosis but correlate significantly with deficits in myocardial function (97).

The rhythm is usually normal sinus. Except in elderly patients and those with left ventricular failure, atrial fibrillation suggests a concomitant mitral lesion.

Roentgenogram

The roentgenographic features of compensated valvular aortic stenosis are concentric hypertrophy of the left ventricle, poststenotic dilatation of the aorta, and calcification of the valve cusps (Figs. 7-5 and 7-6).

Concentric hypertrophy is manifested roentgenographically by a rounding of the lower left border of the heart shadow in the posteroanterior view without an increase in the cardiothoracic ratio. Normally, the lower left-heart border is an arc of a circle that extends beyond the right-heart border. With concentric hypertrophy, the rounded lower left-heart border is an arc of a much smaller circle, all of which lies within the cardiac shadow. With decompensation and associated left ventricular dilatation, the left ventricular dimensions increase. The cardiac apex is displaced leftward, inferiorly, and posteriorly. Cardiomegaly is evident in the posteroanterior projection and the cardiac apex overlies the spine in the left anterior oblique projection. The lung fields may show pulmonary venous congestion.

Dilatation of the aorta may be seen in the posteroanterior chest film but is more readily identified in the left anterior oblique projection. It is confined to the ascending aorta and seen in about 80% of cases of valvular aortic stenosis (33,98). Its absence should raise suspicion of nonvalvular stenosis or coexisting mitral stenosis (79). The magnitude of the dilatation is not correlated with severity. The significance of the finding is in localization of the outflow obstruction, because it is not found with supravalvular stenoses and is uncommon and usually mild when present in subvalvular stenoses.

Calcification of the valve cusps is a most important finding. Its presence points to a valvular locus of the obstruction. It may be seen as early as adolescence and with increas-

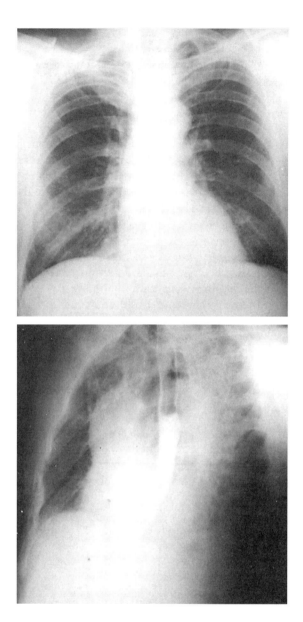

FIG. 7-5. Chest roentgenograms in the posteroanterior projection **(top)** and left anterior oblique projection **(bottom)** of a patient with valvular aortic stenosis. The posteroanterior view shows rounding of the left ventricular salient consistent with concentric hypertrophy but no cardiomegaly. The left anterior oblique view reveals enlargement of the left ventricle, shown as considerable overlapping of the spine by that chamber, and a dilated ascending aorta typical of valvular obstruction.

ing frequency with age. Its absence has no diagnostic importance in the child, adolescent, or young adult but in the patient over 40 years of age virtually rules out a diagnosis of hemodynamically significant valvular stenosis (98,99). The uncommon exceptions are patients, usually women, with combined mitral and aortic stenosis (79,82). On chest films, aortic valve calcification is difficult to detect in posteroanterior views because it is superimposed on the shadow of the spine. It should be anticipated in the lateral or oblique projec-

tions. It is more readily detected fluoroscopically, where valve motion and aperture narrowing enhance visibility. The conclusion that calcification is absent in a given patient cannot be based on films alone even with a full cardiac series, including oblique projections.

It is of the utmost importance to recognize that the routine posteroanterior and lateral chest roentgenograms may be within normal limits in hemodynamically significant, compensated, isolated valvular aortic stenosis. The heart shadow is not changed in size but only in

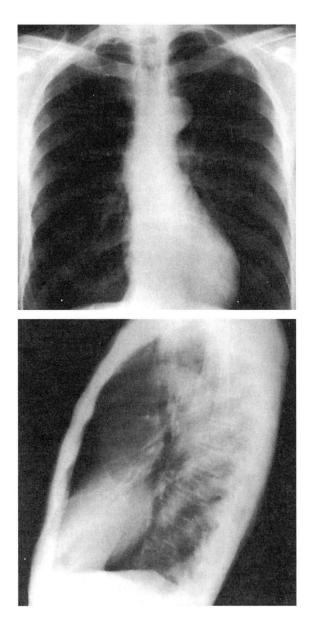

FIG. 7-6. Chest roentgenograms in the posteroanterior **(top)** and lateral **(bottom)** projections in a patient with valvular aortic stenosis. The posteroanterior film shows rounding of the left ventricular salient consistent with concentric hypertrophy and a dilated ascending aorta. There is no cardiomegaly. The lateral view confirms the poststenotic dilatation of the ascending aorta and shows aortic valvular calcification.

configuration, and the rounding of the lower left-heart border may be subtle or may be masked by an apical fat pad. The poststenotic dilatation may be equivocal in all views but the left anterior oblique. The valvular calcification may be invisible on the posteroanterior view and uninterpretable (because of superimposition of hilar shadows) on the lateral view. The pulmonary vascular markings are normal. Thus, significant aortic stenosis cannot be ruled out on the basis of normality in the routine posteroanterior and lateral chest films,

and, of equal importance, cardiomegaly in the normotensive patient with isolated aortic stenosis indicates a decompensated lesion. This sign of left ventricular myocardial failure may antedate symptoms and may occur with a normal cardiac output (maintained by the Frank-Starling mechanism).

M-mode Echocardiogram

The M-mode echocardiogram may show poststenotic dilatation of the aorta, left ventric-

ular mural thickening, dilatation of the left ventricular cavity in the patient with myocardial
failure, and abnormalities in the valve leaflets.
The presence of poststenotic dilatation points to
the valvular site of the obstruction. The magnitude of dilatation offers no help in assessment
of severity. Left ventricular wall thickening is,
of course, the hallmark of the higher grade of
lesion, and the echocardiogram is equal in
specificity and superior in sensitivity to the
ECG for diagnosis of left ventricular hypertrophy (100). Moreover, an estimate of left ventricular systolic pressure can be derived from
measurements relating left ventricular wall
thickness to left ventricular cavity dimensions.
The difference between this pressure and the
systolic arterial blood pressure measured con-
ventionally with a cuff provides an estimate of
the aortic systolic gradient (101–104). Although such estimates may not have enough accuracy to be used as a substitute for cardiac
catheterization data, the method may be useful
in distinguishing patients with milder lesions,
in whom invasive studies can be deferred, from
those in whom a definitive catheterization procedure should be performed (101–106). In addition, this technique may be helpful in following the clinical course of patients preoperatively
or postoperatively, although one study has
shown such measurements to be unreliable in
the postoperative period (106).

The underlying assumption in the above
studies is that a chronic pressure overload elic-
its an increase in ventricular wall thickness such
that peak systolic wall stress remains constant
and normal. This assumption is valid only for
the compensated state, and end-systolic thickness-to-radius ratios correlated poorly with left
ventricular systolic pressure when applied to
patients in whom aortic stenosis was accompanied by heart failure, reduced ejection fraction,
or coronary disease (107). End-diastolic measurements have, however, been shown to be
useful in predicting the severity of aortic stenosis, even in the presence of left ventricular dysfunction (107,108). An elevated end-diastolic
thickness-to-radius ratio in conjunction with
aortic valve calcification has been reported to
be highly sensitive and specific for the diagnosis of aortic stenosis in adult patients (107).

Echocardiographic measurements of intracavitary dimensions can, like roentgenographic
findings, be useful in diagnostic, prognostic,
and management decisions by indicating the
absence of dilatation in the compensated lesion
and the presence of dilatation, perhaps even before symptoms or fall in cardiac output occur,
in the patient with myocardial dysfunction in
whom overt pump failure has not yet occurred.
More sophisticated assessments of myocardial
function are possible by estimating echocardiographically the rate of change in cavity dimensions during filling and ejection.

With regard to the valve structure itself, the
echocardiogram can identify the nature of the
lesion and, within limits, estimate its severity. In
the nonstenotic three-cusped valve (Figs. 7-7
and 7-8), leaflet coaptation in diastole is represented by a thin linear echo midway between
and parallel to the walls of the aorta. Systole is
represented by the abrupt separation of this single central echo into two thin, parallel, linear
echoes, one approaching the anterior wall of
the aorta and the other the posterior wall. These
are believed to represent the anterior and posterior leaflets of the aortic valve, with the lateral leaflet being invisible. When, in addition
to these echoes of leaflet position, echoes corresponding to the movement of the leaflets at
the beginning and at the end of systole are also
recorded, the resultant figure is a parallelo-
gram. Sometimes the opening and closing
movements are so rapid that they are not
recorded, and one sees only the single midline
echo representing diastolic coaptation and the
dual systolic echoes representing the separated
leaflets. Fine oscillations ("flutter") of one or
both leaflets are commonly seen in the normal
valve and in valves that, although somewhat
stenotic, retain a considerable pliancy. Although the absence of valve flutter on the M-
mode echocardiogram is of no diagnostic significance, its presence is reported to be strong
evidence against severe aortic stenosis (109).

With congenital aortic stenosis, in most patients due to the presence of the inherently obstructive unicuspid valve, the systolic M-
mode echocardiogram is often extremely
confusing because of the dome shape of the
valve and the variable traversal path of the

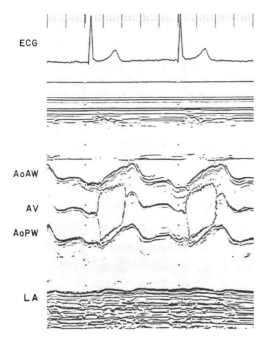

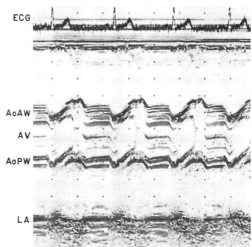

FIG. 7-7. Echocardiogram of normal aortic valve. Two aortic leaflets are seen to separate and move toward the aortic walls in systole and to come together in diastole. The systolic echoes are two thin parallel lines, and the diastolic echo is a single line roughly midway between the aortic walls. Note the fine oscillations ("flutter"), especially evident in the anterior leaflet. *AoAW* and *AoPW*, anterior and posterior walls of the aorta; *AV*, aortic valve; *LA*, left atrium.

FIG. 7-8. Echocardiogram in a patient with "aortic sclerosis" (thickening, sometimes with calcification, of the aortic cusps but without systolic obstruction). The echoes of two aortic leaflets are seen in apposition with the aortic walls in systole, producing a fully open "box" demonstrating the absence of stenosis. In diastole, the single thin line of normal closure is replaced by multiple heavy echoes corresponding to the thickened leaflets. *AoAW* and *AoPW*, anterior and posterior walls of the aorta; *AV*, aortic valve; *LA*, left atrium.

beam through the dome (110). In diastole, however, the M-mode echocardiogram reveals a striking and diagnostic departure from the normal: Instead of the single thin line midway between and parallel to the aortic walls, valve closure is represented by multiple lines perpendicular to the aortic walls (111).

With the bicuspid valve, before extensive calcification, immobilization, and obstruction have occurred, the systolic echoes are similar to those seen in the normal person, but diastole is characterized by an eccentric closure line appreciably closer to one aortic wall than the other (Fig. 7-9). This reflects the significant difference in the size of the two leaflets that usually characterizes the bicuspid deformity. An aortic eccentricity index has been developed to facilitate identification of the bicuspid

valve (112). The index (the ratio of the radius of the aortic root to the shortest distance to the aortic wall in diastole) normally lies between 1.0 and 1.2, but in three fourths of bicuspid valves it exceeds 1.3 and usually ranges from 1.5 to 4.5 (113). Because the bicuspid valve is not inherently stenotic but becomes so as a result of wear-and-tear degeneration with thickening and calcification, the echocardiogram of the severely stenotic bicuspid valve may show only loss of the fine vibratory motion of systolic leaflet echoes (indicating thickening), replacement of the normal slender leaflet echoes by multiple dense echoes in diastole and sometimes also in systole (indicating calcification), and diminished leaflet excursion, but not the eccentricity of closure.

The stenotic three-cusped valve (Fig. 7-10)—because it too is the result of long-standing pathologic changes with thickening and calcification—exhibits dense and multiple echoes

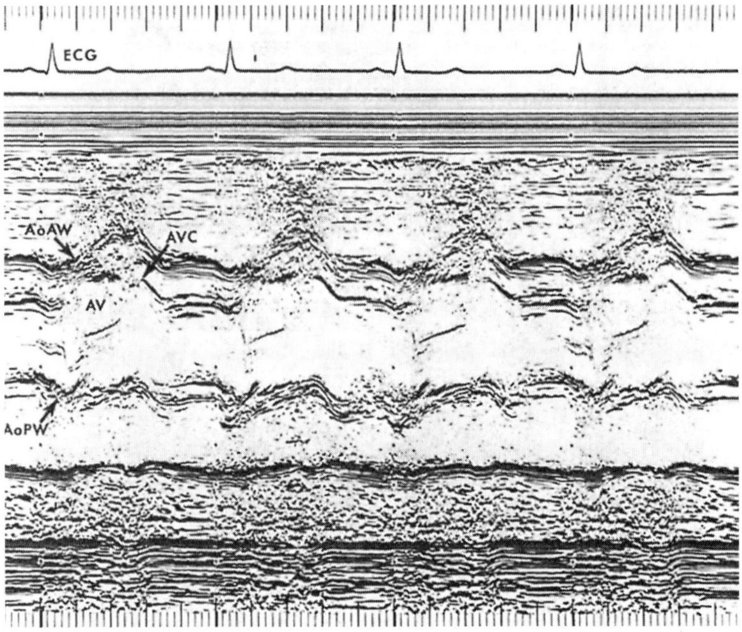

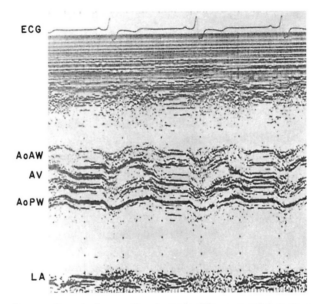

FIG. 7-9. Echocardiogram of a bicuspid aortic valve (*AV*). Note the eccentric echo of aortic valve closure (*AVC*) that lies much closer to the anterior wall of the aorta (*AoAW*) than to the posterior (*AoPW*). The eccentricity index (the ratio of aortic radius to the distance between AVC and the closest aortic wall) is 3.5, or about three times the upper limit of normal. In systole, because the posterior leaflet does not come close to the AoPW, the valve opening is also eccentric and smaller than normal. Finally, the multiple diastolic echoes demonstrate leaflet thickening.

FIG. 7-10. Echocardiogram in valvular aortic stenosis. The essential features are the thickened echoes of the aortic valve (*AV*) throughout systole and diastole, the small "box" produced by movement of the leaflets toward the anterior and posterior aortic walls (*AoAW* and *AoPW*) during systole, and the multiple echoes during diastole. *LA*, left atrium.

and diminished leaflet excursion with no other special features. The demonstration of leaflet thickening and calcification is of importance in identifying the valve as the seat of disease. The absence of multiple and dense echoes in middle age and in later life virtually excludes a diagnosis of hemodynamically significant valvular aortic stenosis. Although measurements of cusp separation (interecho distance in systole) have been suggested as useful in estimating the severity of stenosis, their usefulness is limited by uncertainty concerning the path of the beam across the valve and by the presence of multiple echoes (114,115).

Two-dimensional Echocardiography

Two-dimensional (2D) echocardiography is the best noninvasive test for defining the various pathologic and pathophysiologic aspects of aortic stenosis. This technique permits the aortic valve to be inspected in a long-axis view (Fig. 7-11), which observes the outflow tract, valve, and ascending aorta, and a short-axis view (Fig. 7-12), which is directed at the valve orifice. The maximum separation of the aortic

cusps in systole, in the long-axis view, can be measured in most patients. In the short-axis view, direct measurement of the area of the valve orifice is possible in only a small minority; however, in most patients, the short-axis view provides very useful information concerning leaflet mobility. In general, the two views provide complementary data that have a high predictive value for the severity of stenosis in both children and adults (116–118). In congenital aortic stenosis, the 2D echocardiogram can provide a good picture of the entire dome of the unicuspid valve and even permit an estimate of the extent of narrowing of the orifice located at the apex of the dome (111) (Fig. 7-11). With regard to the bicuspid valve (Fig. 7-12), the technique is indeterminate as to the number of cusps in 25%, but, excluding these, it is sensitive and highly specific for the diagnosis of bicuspid aortic valve (119). Because the 25% of patients in whom the number of cusps is indeterminate by 2D echocardiogram is not the same 25% of patients who have a falsely negative eccentricity index by M-mode echocardiography, the two echocardiographic techniques succeed in identifying most patients with bicuspid valves.

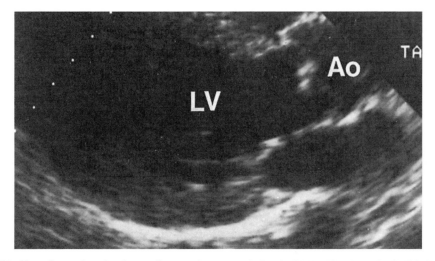

FIG. 7-11. Two-dimensional echocardiogram in congenital valvular aortic stenosis. In this long-axis view, recorded during systole, the doming of the stenotic aortic valve can be seen between the left ventricle (*LV*) and the aorta (*Ao*). The valve leaflets are thickened and a minute orifice can be seen at the top of the dome.

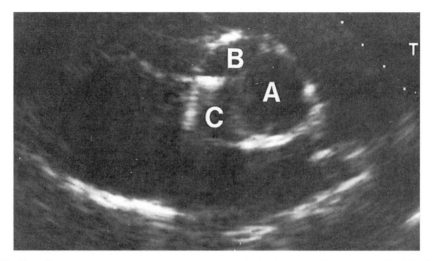

FIG. 7-12. Two-dimensional echocardiogram in congenital valvular aortic stenosis. In this short-axis view, obtained from the suprasternal notch, an eccentric opening (*A*) can be seen to the right of two aortic cusps (*B, C*) between which lies a fused raphe. To the right of the eccentric opening (*A*) is a rudimentary third cusp.

Doppler Ultrasound

Doppler ultrasound, performed in conjunction with 2D echocardiography, has revolutionized noninvasive diagnosis in valvular heart disease (120,121). Two techniques, pulsed wave and continuous wave, are used and may be used independently or in conjunction with simultaneous or interrupted 2D imaging (122–124). Both techniques are accurate for detecting the presence of valvular stenosis or regurgitation by recording abnormal turbulence (123,124). In aortic stenosis, multiple velocity vectors in the area of turbulence cause the Doppler signal to have a wide spectral broadening that has been shown to be almost 100% sensitive and specific in detecting left ventricular outflow obstruction (125). The continuous-wave mode (Fig. 7-13) permits the recording of a peak flow velocity (*V*) from which the maximal instantaneous pressure gradient (*PG*) can be calculated from a modified Bernoulli equation as $PG = 4V^2$ (126,127).

The gradients derived from the peak Doppler velocity have an excellent correlation with pressure gradients measured at cardiac catheterization (126–128). Moreover, studies

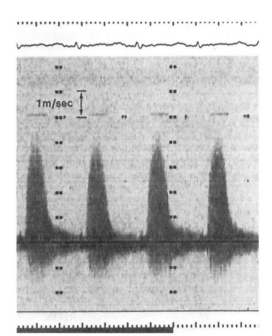

FIG. 7-13. Doppler tracing in the continuous-wave mode recorded from the suprasternal notch in a child with severe valvular aortic stenosis. The peak velocity is 4 m/s, giving an estimated peak systolic gradient of 64 mm Hg.

in an *in vitro* model have shown that the pressure gradients and orifice areas calculated from Doppler measurements accurately reflect the actual gradients and areas except for the smallest orifices (129). The latter produce sprays rather than jets with a resultant underestimation of gradient; however, this occurs at stenoses of such high grade that the error is not clinically meaningful (129).

In addition to providing accurate estimation of peak instantaneous gradient, Doppler echocardiography can permit calculation of cardiac output. Measurement of the average velocity of flow across a normal valve or through a normal large vessel, when the cross-sectional area is known, allows calculation of output as the product of area and mean velocity of blood flow. Reasonably accurate estimates of cardiac output have been obtained in animals and in humans (130–134). Reports of studies using Doppler methods to measure peak systolic gradient and transvalvular flow suggest that these noninvasive measurements may, for the purpose of assessing the outflow obstruction, make cardiac catheterization unnecessary (135,136).

In using and interpreting Doppler data, the following should be noted:

1. In left ventricular outflow obstruction, localization of the site of obstruction as valvular, subvalvular, or supravalvular is best accomplished with pulsed Doppler (127,137).
2. In estimation of peak gradient by continuous-wave Doppler, the transducer position and direction should be adjusted so that the Doppler beam is as nearly as possible parallel to the maximal velocity vector. This is probably easier to accomplish in infants and children than in adults (138). In practice, the underestimation of velocity is very small (less than 10%) if the Doppler angle, which equals zero when the beam is parallel to the maximal velocity vector, is less than 25 degrees. Larger angles, however, yield significant underestimates of both velocity and gradient (121).

3. Not all patients can be examined from any one of the usual windows: apical, right parasternal, or suprasternal. The supravalvular windows (right parasternal and suprasternal) are the most reliable in younger patients (127). In adults, multiple windows should be used to ascertain the maximal Doppler-derived gradient (139).
4. Continuous-wave ultrasound can underestimate, but not overestimate, the peak systolic gradient (127).
5. Aortic regurgitation can be detected by either the pulsed-wave or continuous-wave Doppler technique; however, Doppler methodology has not yet allowed quantification of regurgitant flow (120). In mixed aortic stenosis and regurgitation, the aortic valve area in systole cannot be estimated by Doppler echocardiography.

Doppler color-flow mapping permits the observer to visualize flow toward and away from the transducer as different colors with relative velocities represented by varying shades of these colors (140,140a,141). The extended-range pulsed-Doppler technique attempts to incorporate the precise volume-sampling capability of pulsed-wave Doppler with the higher velocity-detection capability of continuous-wave Doppler (142,143). Color mapping is particularly useful in evaluating patients with combined regurgitation and stenosis. The extended-range pulsed-Doppler system permits better estimation of high velocities and precise localization of stenotic lesions. Almost all patients can have an accurate determination of aortic valve area within 0.3 cm^2 by means of transthoracic or transesophageal echo-Doppler (143).

Cardiac Catheterization

In aortic stenosis as in other valvular lesions, the definitive diagnostic procedure is cardiac catheterization. The aims of the study are confirmation of the diagnosis of left ventricular outflow obstruction, localization of the obstructing lesion, estimation of the severity of the obstruction, determination of the presence or absence of other valve lesions, assessment of the functional status of the left ventricle, and evaluation of the coronary circulation. In many patients, aortic valve area and even left ventricular function will be determined; echocardiographic catheterization in these individuals may, therefore, be limited to coronary angiography (143a). The fundamental datum establishing the presence of outflow obstruction is the systolic gradient between the left ventricle and the aorta (Figs. 7-14 and 7-15). Documentation of the location of the obstruction is obtained by a continuous pressure recording during slow withdrawal of a catheter from the left ventricle into the aorta. In the case of obstruction located at the valve, the diagnostic datum is an abrupt transition from left ventricular to aortic pressure (Fig. 7-16). Severity of the obstruction is determined by calculating the effective area of the systolic orifice from the

formula of Gorlin and Gorlin. This estimate requires measurements as nearly simultaneous as possible of the systolic gradient and the aortic transvalvular flow. When there is no aortic regurgitation, the transvalvular flow equals cardiac output. The latter may be measured by either the indicator dilution method or the Fick method. When aortic regurgitation is present, an estimate of the volume of the leak is required for valid and accurate estimation of the systolic orifice area, because transvalvular flow is the sum of the forward and regurgitant flows. In most cases of mixed aortic valve lesions, other available data make accurate measurement of transvalvular flow unnecessary. Where necessary, however, it can be obtained either by indicator dilution or by nearly simultaneous measurement of total stroke volume from a left ventriculogram and forward stroke volume by the Fick method or by indicator dilution (144–147).

Data that bear on the functional status of the left ventricle include the rate of rise

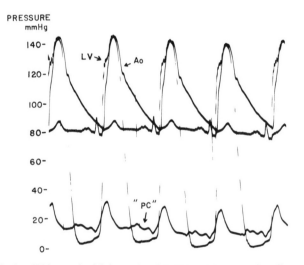

FIG. 7-14. Left ventricular (*LV*), aortic (*Ao*), and pulmonary artery wedge (i.e., pulmonary capillary [*PC*]) pressures recorded at cardiac catheterization in a patient with mitral stenosis but no stenosis at the aortic valve. A gradient between PC and LV pressures throughout diastole and a prominent A wave in the PC indicate the mitral stenosis. The LV and Ao tracings show no difference in peak systolic pressure; a small difference (LV higher than Ao) during systolic ejection, which begins when LV pressure crosses the Ao pressure and ends at peak systolic pressure; and a corresponding small difference (Ao higher than LV) during protodiastole, which begins at the end of ejection and ends with aortic valve closure at the aortic incisura. The positive and negative gradients corresponding to ejection and protodiastole are usually immeasurably small.

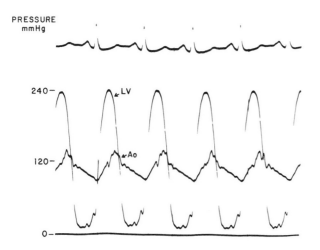

FIG. 7-15. Left ventricular (*LV*) and aortic (*Ao*) pressures in a patient with severe valvular aortic stenosis. There is a large gradient throughout systole, and the aortic pulse shows the anacrotic notch and delayed peak typical of a fixed obstruction in the left ventricular outflow tract.

(*dP/dt*) of the left ventricular pressure obtained by electronic differentiation of the ventricular pressure pulse, left ventricular volume measured by indicator dilution or quantitative angiocardiography, and various derived measurements or indexes of ventricular chamber and muscle performance (147–155). The state of the coronary circulation is evaluated by selective coronary cinefluorography and by assessment of segmental left ventricular wall function.

The simplest approach technically and an entirely satisfactory one is to insert an arterial catheter by the retrograde approach into the left ventricle and a venous catheter into the pulmonary capillary wedge position. After simultaneous recording of the pulmonary capillary wedge pressure, left ventricular pressure,

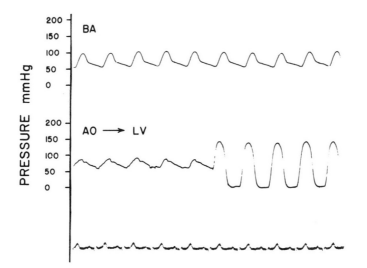

FIG. 7-16. Left ventricular (*LV*), aortic (*Ao*), and brachial arterial (*BA*) pressures in a patient with valvular aortic stenosis. The BA pressure is recorded from a Cournand needle, and the Ao and LV pressures are recorded through a catheter. The Ao pressure shows the slow upstroke typical of a fixed obstruction. During passage of the catheter from Ao to LV, the obstruction is shown to be at the aortic valve, with no evidence of a subvalvular or supravalvular gradient.

and left ventricular dP/dt, the venous catheter is withdrawn into the pulmonary artery and the arterial catheter is slowly pulled back, with constant recording, across the aortic valve. Cardiac output may then be measured by the Fick method or by indicator dilution with injection into the pulmonary artery and sampling from the aorta.

Aortography is the next step. If opaque dye is seen to cross the aortic valve, the severity of the regurgitation can be graded 1+ (mild) to 4+ (severe) from the aortogram on the basis of published criteria (156). From reported data on the regurgitant and total flows (measured by indicator dilution) corresponding to each of the angiographic grades of severity, the measured cardiac output can be amended to provide a range within which total aortic valve flow probably falls in that patient (145).

The arterial catheter can then be advanced again across the aortic valve for left ventriculography. The latter confirms the site of obstruction at the valve, across which a thin jet of opacified blood is ejected into the aorta, and demonstrates the presence or absence of mitral regurgitation, provides a semiquantitative measure of the leak if mitral regurgitation is present, permits an assessment of left ventricular wall thickness and movement, and provides an estimate of left ventricular end-diastolic and end-systolic volumes (151).

If aortic regurgitation is shown to be present by aortography and there is a need for quantitative estimation of the volume of the leak, the left ventriculogram should be immediately followed by a repeat measurement of cardiac output. The aortic leak can then be quantitatively estimated as the difference between total stroke volume (end-diastolic volume minus end-systolic volume), measured on the ventriculogram, and forward stroke volume, measured by indicator dilution or the Fick method (147,151). If both mitral regurgitation and aortic regurgitation are present, this technique cannot measure either leak accurately but only provides the sum of the two leaks (145). In such cases, and in the simpler cases of a leak at only the mitral or aortic valve, quantification of the regurgitation can

be obtained by indicator dilution using the technique of simultaneous upstream and downstream sampling (144,145,157,158).

An alternative approach to the left ventricle is by the transseptal technique. With a second catheter inserted by the retrograde arterial approach into the aortic root, left ventricular and aortic pressures can be recorded simultaneously. In addition, left ventricular volumes can be measured by the indicator-washout technique; indicator (indocyanine green or cold saline) is injected into the left ventricle and blood is sampled from the aorta (149–151). Finally, any aortic regurgitation present can be quantified by indicator dilution using the upstream sampling technique. This can be done either by successive paired dilution curves, one with ventricular injection and aortic sampling and the other with aortic injection and ventricular sampling, or with nonthermal indicators and an additional sampling site through a peripheral arterial needle, by simultaneous recording of the upstream (ventricular) and downstream (arterial) curves with aortic root injection (145).

As has been previously pointed out, in the case of combined valve lesions with both aortic and mitral regurgitation, accurate quantification of the leaks cannot be obtained by quantitative ventriculography coupled with cardiac output measurement, which can measure only the sum of the two leaks. It can, however, where required, be obtained by the dilution method. In such cases, after measurement of aortic regurgitation, the transseptal catheter is withdrawn into the left atrium, the aortic catheter is advanced into the left ventricle, and the curve pairs for mitral regurgitation measurement are obtained either sequentially or, with a downstream arterial sampling site, simultaneously (157,158). As noted earlier, however, semiquantitative estimates of the degree of aortic regurgitation and accurate quantitative estimates of aortic valve area are usually obtained by means of echocardiographic studies.

The transseptal method has advantages in data acquisition, including simultaneity of pressure recordings, availability of upstream–

downstream dilution curves, and aortography and ventriculography with a minimum of catheter repositioning. Its morbidity and mortality, however, exceed those of the retrograde arterial route of entry into the left ventricle. In most laboratories, therefore, it is used only in the small fraction of cases (1% to 5%, depending on the skill of the operator) when an arterial catheter cannot be manipulated into the left ventricle by the retrograde approach.

A third approach to the left ventricle is by direct puncture through the left anterior chest wall at the site of the apex impulse. With systemic arterial pressure obtained through an aortic catheter or a brachial, radial, or femoral needle, the "apical stick" permits recording of the aortic gradient, the left ventricular *dP/dt*, and, perhaps, a left ventricular indicator washout curve but nothing more. The needle is not a suitable conduit for opaque-dye injection or indicator-dilution sampling. In infants with an arterial needle in place, it allows rapid measurement of the outflow tract gradient. For older patients, however, it is not a procedure of choice but a backup when the retrograde arterial or transseptal methods or both fail to secure gradient data.

From gradient, flow, and heart rate, the estimated area of the systolic orifice is calculated by the formula of Gorlin and Gorlin. In the adult, the normal valve has an area of 3 cm^2 (2.6 to 3.6 cm^2), and a gradient becomes detectable at an area of 2 cm^2 or less. Areas of 1.5 to 2.0 cm^2 represent mild stenosis; areas of 1.1 to 1.5 cm^2, moderate stenosis; areas 1.0 cm^2 or less, moderately severe or "surgical" stenosis; and areas less than 0.75 cm^2, severe or "critical" stenosis. The importance of the valve area cannot be overemphasized. Although a large gradient (more than 50 mm Hg) almost invariably indicates a moderately severe or severe stenosis (the exceptions represent conditions such as combination of lesser degrees of stenosis with a high-output state secondary to thyrotoxicosis, anemia, arteriovenous fistula, and Paget's disease), a small gradient (e.g., 15 to 30 mm Hg) may mean either a mild to moderate stenosis or a severe stenosis with low cardiac output. Such

small gradients are to be anticipated in patients with left ventricular failure and in those with coexisting high-grade mitral stenosis.

Unlike the situation in mitral stenosis, the gradient in valvular aortic stenosis does not exhibit a striking increase with exercise, because the tachycardia of exercise occurs principally at the expense of diastolic time, and systolic time per minute increases almost in proportion to the increase in flow. Moreover, in patients with mixed aortic valve lesions, exercise is associated with an increase in net forward flow, a decrease in aortic regurgitant flow, and little or no change in total transvalvular flow, so that the gradient during exercise differs little from that observed at rest (159).

Therapy

Medical Management

No medical therapy is required for the asymptomatic patient with valvular aortic stenosis except for prophylaxis against infective endocarditis in all, prophylaxis against acute rheumatic fever where appropriate, and the interdiction of strenuous physical exertion in those with high-grade lesions. Prophylaxis against infective endocarditis is indicated regardless of the patient's age, the apparent severity of the lesion, and the pathologic anatomy of the valve.

Prophylaxis against rheumatic fever is obviously not indicated in patients with echocardiographic evidence of unicuspid or bicuspid congenital deformities and need not be prescribed in most adults with isolated calcific stenosis, with most due to congenital lesions or to a chronic degenerative process. It should be advised, however, in the adolescent or young adult patient with combined aortic and mitral disease or with isolated valvular aortic stenosis and either a documented history of prior acute rheumatic fever or echocardiographic findings consistent with a three-cusped valve.

Strenuous physical exertion, such as competitive athletics, should be prohibited in patients with lesions of apparent high grade because of the risk of sudden death. The incidence of sudden death in asymptomatic valvular aortic stenosis has been estimated to be 3% to 5% in the adult and perhaps twice that figure in the child (34).

If left ventricular failure; angina pectoris; or dizziness, syncope, or near syncope occurs, arrangements should be made for prompt cardiac catheterization, with an eye to early surgical intervention. Before the catheterization study, left ventricular failure and angina pectoris should be brought under control with conventional therapy. Despite the fixed orifice, reduction of afterload has been helpful in managing failure in valvular aortic stenosis (160,161). In addition, intraaortic balloon counterpulsation has been effective in stabilizing patients with critical and decompensated valvular aortic stenosis before surgery (162). Improvement with counterpulsation was not associated with systolic unloading of the left ventricle and resulted almost entirely from an increase in aortic diastolic pressure and the diastolic coronary filling gradient (162).

The loss of the "booster pump" effect of atrial contraction as a result of atrial fibrillation can seriously impair left ventricular function in aortic stenosis. Paroxysms of this arrhythmia require the use of countershock and antiarrhythmic medication to effect reversion to normal rhythm. Long-term pharmacologic control of atrial fibrillation, however, is an infrequent management problem in valvular aortic stenosis because the atrial arrhythmia most often reflects underlying left ventricular pump failure, which requires that the patient be considered for surgery.

Unlike mitral stenosis, valvular aortic stenosis presents no indications for long-term anticoagulation. Systemic emboli do occur very infrequently in valvular aortic stenosis, and the embolus usually is not a clot but a calcific fleck from the valve, which is a situation not amenable to control by anticoagulant therapy.

Patients not referred for surgical therapy should be followed closely because valvular aortic stenosis, whether congenital, rheu-matic, or degenerative-calcific, tends to be a progressive lesion (22d,22e,163–167). Rates of progression based on serial hemodynamic studies are not uniform or predictable. Serial studies showed no progression in some patients, whereas in others increases in stenosis have ranged from less than $0.1\ cm^2/yr$ to as much as $0.3\ cm^2/yr$ (163–167). Although mild lesions have been reported to progress more rapidly than severe ones and degenerative-calcific lesions more rapidly than those of other causes, it seems prudent to regard any patient with mild or moderate aortic stenosis as a candidate for progression to severe stenosis in as little as 2 to 5 years (163–167). If new symptoms develop, all such patients should be seen immediately and, if asymptomatic, at intervals of not more than 6 months. Increases in QRS voltage, left ventricular mass by echocardiography, and aortic valve gradient by Doppler ultrasound may all provide convenient noninvasive evidence of advances in severity.

Surgical Treatment

The symptomatic patient with valvular aortic stenosis reqires surgical treatment. Operation is indicated when left ventricular failure, angina pectoris, dizziness, syncope, or near syncope occurs in the adult patient in whom the history, physical findings, and noninvasive-study findings are consistent with a high-grade (moderately severe or severe) obstruction and in whom the diagnosis is confirmed by catheterization.

The most ominous of the preceding symptoms is left ventricular failure. With medical therapy alone, approximately 50% of patients with valvular aortic stenosis who have exhibited left ventricular failure die within 2 years. For syncope (and its equivalents) and angina pectoris, the mean life expectancies are 3 and 5 years, respectively (34). Moreover, in the symptomatic patient, there is a 15% to 20% incidence of sudden death. In general, in any symptomatic patient with valvular aortic stenosis, the risk of sudden death is at least equal to that of surgery, and cardiac catheterization and operation should be performed with no unnecessary delay. Indeed, to minimize delay between the advent of symptoms and surgical correction, some cardiologists elect to have catheterization studies performed even before the onset of symptoms in adult patients suspected of having a moderately severe or severe obstruction. Surgery is often recommended in children with severe aortic stenosis in the absence of symptoms, because in this age group the risk of surgery is clearly less than that of sudden death (34). In selected symptomatic patients, especially the gravely ill infant, 2D echocardiography and Doppler ultrasound suffice diagnostically, thus avoiding possible complications of catheterization and angiography and permitting an expeditious operation (168). In many patients, however, cardiac catheterization is advisable to ascertain the presence and severity of coronary disease, other valve lesions, and myocardial deficits (169).

In adult patients, open commissurotomy or valvuloplasty may be possible in a few with noncalcific stenosis; however, in most adults, surgical correction requires valve replacement. This can be performed with any of over 40 artificial valve models or with human (homograft) or porcine (xenograft) tissue valves (170,171). The mechanical prostheses include caged-ball, central-disc, tilting-disc, and twin-disc valves. The aortic valve homograft has been used particularly in Great Britain. The tissue valve used most extensively in this country is the glutaraldehyde-preserved, flexible, stent-mounted, porcine xenograft, but bioprostheses of bovine parietal pericardium are also used (172).

The hemodynamic performance of all these valves is satisfactory, although the artificial valves and the smaller sizes of porcine bioprostheses are inherently slightly stenotic. The principal advantage of the mechanical prostheses is their documented durability and their chief disadvantage is their propensity for thromboembolism (173,174). Over the years, the incidence of thromboembolism has decreased significantly, possibly because of earlier operation, better anticoagulant therapy,

and improved valve design (173–175). A risk of thromboembolism, however, even with satisfactory anticoagulant therapy, continues for at least 15 years after placement of a mechanical prosthesis (176). Currently, it is recommended that all patients with synthetic prostheses are on permanent anticoagulation therapy. In the case of the porcine xenograft, anticoagulant therapy is not regarded as necessary in the aortic position. Indeed, a higher survival rate and event-free survival rate has been reported for patients with bioprostheses and no anticoagulant therapy than for patients with mechanical valves, with or without anticoagulant therapy, or for patients with bioprostheses and anticoagulant therapy (177).

With porcine xenografts, the principal problem is valve dysfunction caused by tissue failure, particularly in children and younger adults (178–183). Deterioration of porcine xenografts due to tissue failure has usually led to regurgitation and occasionally recurrent stenosis. Valve replacement is required. Deterioration is usually associated with calcium deposition in the bioprosthetic valve but can occur without calcification (179,184–191). Such failure is ordinarily not catastrophic, is associated with echocardiographically demonstrable morphologic abnormalities, and can be anticipated on the basis of echocardiographic determinations of increasing cuspal thickness (180,192–194). The association of calcification and valve failure has led to investigations of calcification inhibition by incorporating surfactants into the valve tissue or by steric inhibition of crystal growth by diphosphonate compounds (195,196). Balloon or surgical valvotomy is the operation of choice in children (197–200).

In adults, the glutaraldehyde-preserved porcine valve has a low frequency of deterioration during the first 5 years after implantation; however, there is a significant incidence of tissue failure thereafter (187,201). In several studies, each involving over 1,000 patients, the actuarially determined freedom from primary valve failure for porcine valves in the aortic position was 98% at 5 years, 95% at 6 years, and 91% at 10 years (187,201). Although the tissue-failure rate is less for porcine valves in the aortic position than in the mitral valves, the trend for valves in place more than 5 years is disturbing (187,201,202). Bioprostheses should probably be confined to the elderly, in whom anticoagulant therapy may have a higher risk, and to potentially childbearing postadolescent women, in whom there is risk of embryopathy and a high frequency of fetal death caused by warfarin (203).

Reports of the Ionescu-Shiley bovine pericardial valve and of the unstented antibiotic-sterilized homograft indicate advantages and problems comparable with those of the porcine xenograft (172,204 207). Other problems with valvular prostheses include periprosthetic leaks due to fistulous tracts at the line of valve insertion, swelling or change in the shape of the caged ball ("ball variance"), interference with movement of the poppet (ball or disc) by thrombus, trauma to erythrocytes with possible resultant hemolytic anemia and an associated increase in the incidence of cholelithiasis, strut fracture, and the risk of infective endocarditis (170,208–215).

Despite these problems, the treatment of valvular aortic stenosis by valve replacement is undeniably successful. The early mortality (within 30 days of operation) is less than 5% (173,177,180,182,216,217). Survivors exhibit complete or substantial relief of symptoms, reversal of functional deficits, regression of left ventricular dilatation and hypertrophy, and improvement in longevity (218–223). Long-term survival is not related to gender, incidence of angina or syncope, or electrocardiographic signs of left ventricular hypertrophy. It is related to age, functional status (e.g., radiographic cardiomegaly, New York Heart Association [NYHA] functional classification, congestive heart failure, left atrial and pulmonary artery mean pressures, ejection fraction, and cardiac index), and condition of the coronary arteries (history of recent or remote myocardial infarction, segmental left ventricular wall dysfunction, and coronary stenoses on arteriography) (218). None of

these conditions to which long-term survival is related, however, constitutes a contraindication to surgery. Specifically, reasonable operative risk and satisfactory postoperative rehabilitation have been shown for the elderly, for those with pronounced functional deficits, and even for those operated on emergently because of rapid hemodynamic deterioration (219–221,224–230a). Combined aortic valve replacement and myocardial revascularization, although entailing a risk greater than that for either procedure alone, is usually performed in patients with high-grade narrowing of both the valve and the coronary arteries (180,223). The need for the combined operation, and therefore for routine coronary arteriography before the operation, has been questioned (231). These practices seem prudent, however, because the presence or absence of angina pectoris in valvular aortic stenosis does not reliably coincide with the presence or absence of significant coronary artery disease (40,232). Moreover, the combined surgery has an operative risk of 5% or less based on the last few years of several series (177,233). The combined procedure appreciably reduces the risk of perioperative myocardial infarction, an event that significantly increases immediate and early operative mortality and probably also protects against late attrition (218,223,234). Indeed, failure of left ventricular function to improve postoperatively suggests uncorrected coronary artery disease (219).

The best results are expected with a prosthesis implanted on an elective basis, using hypothermic potassium-induced cardioplegia, in a patient without mitral valve disease, cardiomegaly, symptoms at rest, or physiologic evidence of left ventricular failure (218,220, 223–225). Many of these variables correlate with immediate operative mortality and not with long-term survival. After successful aortic valve replacement, with associated coronary artery bypass grafting where indicated, long-term survival is appreciably better than reported for patients managed without surgery. For example, in the extensive series of Copeland et al.(218), with more than 1,100 patients operated on over a 13-year period and a mean follow-up of 4.4 years, the 5-year survival rate, calculated by the actuarial method, was 69% for all patients and 77% for those discharged from the hospital. Several other studies indicate that the total 5-year survival is probably 74% to 84% (177,180,235). This is in contrast to the 38% and 48% 5-year survival rates without surgery reported by Rapaport (236) and by Frank et al. (237), respectively. Moreover, in a comparison of patients in whom recommended valve replacement was or was not performed, the 3-year survival was 87% with the operation and only 21% in a clinically and hemodynamically comparable group without replacement (238). Even for the elderly, the actuarial probability of survival is good (61% at 5 years) (224,225). Moreover, 90% to 95% of surviving patients, at any age, are in NYHA functional class I or II (218,224,225,238).

Catheter balloon valvuloplasty has been used in a number of older patients with critical calcific aortic stenosis and problematic comorbid conditions that relatively contraindicate surgery (e.g., severe chronic obstructive pulmonary disease). The short-term results with this treatment modality were acceptable but rapid (i.e., 3 to 12 months), and restenosis of the aortic valve was usually observed (238a–238c). The average increase in aortic valve area was only 0.3 cm^2. The 30-day, 1-year, and 3-year mortalities were high for this procedure due to rapid restenosis and modest increases in aortic valve area. Therefore, aortic balloon valvuloplasty is only indicated as a "bridge" procedure for patients with critical aortic stenosis who require emergent noncardiac surgery or who demonstrate refractory heart failure or shock (238a–238c). The long-term management of such patients should include eventual aortic valve replacement. Young patients with critical, noncalcific, congenital aortic stenosis are usually excellent candidates for catheter balloon valvuloplasty. These individuals obtain excellent long-term results from this procedure.

NONVALVULAR AORTIC STENOSIS

The nonvalvular obstructions to left ventricular outflow are all congenital lesions and constitute one fourth of cases of congenital aortic stenosis. These lesions may be grouped in a number of ways: subvalvular versus supravalvular, discrete versus diffuse, and fixed (static) versus variable (dynamic).

Three outflow tract abnormalities are associated with subvalvular obstruction: a membranous diaphragm, a fibromuscular narrowing (tunnel deformity), and a muscular hypertrophy. The supravalvular lesions, all involving the ascending aorta, can also be divided into three types: a fibromembranous lesion, a focal hourglass constriction, and a generalized hypoplasia. The subvalvular and supravalvular membranous lesions and the hourglass constriction are discrete lesions; the tunnel deformity and aortic hypoplasia are diffuse. In muscular subaortic stenosis, the myocardial hypertrophy, especially of the septum (asymmetric septal hypertrophy [ASH]), is diffuse, but the obstruction is probably discrete and due to systolic abutment of the anterior mitral leaflet against the septum. The outflow obstruction in this muscular variety of subvalvular stenosis is dynamic, varying with changes in preload, afterload, and contractility, but the other two types of subvalvular stenosis and all supravalvular stenoses are fixed obstructions.

The pathophysiologic features of all these nonvalvular stenoses are the same as in the valvular lesions: a systolic overload compensated anatomically by left ventricular hypertrophy and physiologically by left ventricular systolic hypertension, by a systolic gradient between the left ventricle and the aorta, and by prolongation of the period of ejection. Clinically, the essential features are, as in valvular lesions, an ejection systolic murmur, a prominent fourth heart sound (S$_4$), an undisplaced but forceful apical impulse, dizziness and syncope, left ventricular hypertrophy, conduction disturbances, freedom from congestive symptoms until left ventricular decompensation occurs, and risk of sudden death. The nonvalvular lesions differ, however, from valvular aortic stenosis and among themselves in the following important respects (Tables 7-3, 7-4, 7-5):

1. The nonvalvular obstructions do not themselves calcify and, unless there is a coexisting lesion of the aortic valve, do not present with visible calcification.
2. In contrast with valvular aortic stenosis, in which an ejection sound is audible in virtually all noncalcific stenosis and approximately one half of those with calcific stenosis, the nonvalvular outflow obstructions are not associated with an audible ejection sound (84,239–242).
3. Although functional compromise of the coronary circulation from abbreviation of diastole and from high intramyocardial tension may be present, coexisting coronary atherosclerosis is uncommon because of the lower age associated with congenital disease. Involvement of the coronary ostia is not seen, because there is no pathologic valve substrate on which deposition of calcium may take place. Although angina and other manifestations of ischemic heart disease occur with these lesions, they are much less frequent than in valvular aortic stenosis.
4. Because the site of obstruction (and the gradient) is between the proximal and distal aorta in supravalvular lesions and between the body of the ventricle and the outflow tract in subvalvular lesions, turbulence in the proximal aorta is absent in supravalvular stenosis and attenuated in the subvalvular lesions. For this reason, supravalvular stenosis never and subvalvular stenosis rarely presents with appreciable dilatation of the ascending aorta (80,82,239). The rare subvalvular lesion that does exhibit conspicuous dilatation of the proximal aorta is usually a discrete membranous obstruction immediately subjacent to the aortic valve.
5. The fixed lesions exhibit the typical pulse retardation and characteristic postextrasystolic increase in pulse pressure seen in the valvular lesion (1,82). In muscular subaortic stenosis, however, the initial arterial upstroke is brisk and pulse pressure in the pulse after an extra systole fails to widen or is reduced. In addition, the systolic murmur increases with sudden squatting and decreases with the Valsalva maneuver in the fixed lesions, whereas the opposite response to these interventions is observed with the dynamic obstruction of muscular stenosis (82).
6. Regurgitant diastolic murmurs are extremely common in fixed subvalvular lesions, uncommon in supravalvular obstructions, and extremely rare in muscular stenosis (82,241,242).
7. The discrete lesions differ from the diffuse in their greater amenability to, and ease of, surgical correction.

Discrete Subaortic Stenosis

Discrete subaortic stenosis (DSS) is due to a dense, crescentic, fibrous membrane or ridge, 1 to 2 mm thick, encircling and narrowing the outflow tract several millimeters to 2 cm (but usually about 1 cm) below the aortic valve. The aortic annulus is normal in diameter and, except for the localized ridge, the outflow tract is not narrow. In isolated DSS, the aortic valve is three cusped and nonstenotic; however, the cusps are almost always thickened and exhibit jet lesions on their ventricular surfaces from the impact of blood ejected through the subjacent obstruction (243,244). Mitral regurgitation may accompany the outflow obstruction, because the membrane or ridge is partly attached to the anterior leaflet of the mitral valve. Other congenital lesions occasionally associated include coarctation of the aorta, ventricular septal defect, valvular stenoses (aortic, pulmonic, or mitral), persistent left superior vena cava, patent ductus arteriosus, incomplete atrioventricular canal, double-outlet right ventricle, supravalvular aortic stenosis, sinus of Valsalva aneurysm, and parachute mitral valve (244–247). Rarely, in the absence of the usual pathology, DSS may be due to a mitral valve anomaly such as attachment of the anterior leaflet to the ventricular septum or accessory mitral tissue with or without parachute deformity (12,240,248–250).

History

As with all congenital lesions obstructing left ventricular outflow, the systolic murmur is frequently detected at birth and is heard in most patients by 1 year of age and in virtually all by the age of 8. There is, however, often a long period of freedom from symptoms, which may not appear until adulthood, and the lesion is compatible with relatively long survival, the mean age of death being 35 (243). Sung et al. (246) reported that 26% of their 138 patients were adults, the oldest being 65 years of age. A familial history of the disease is rare, and there is no history of rheumatic fever.

Physical Findings

The ejection systolic murmur is not distinguishable from that of valvular aortic stenosis. In infants and children, however, the murmur and thrill may be maximal along the left sternal border. Although an ejection sound may occasionally be recorded, most observers agree that, except with other coexisting abnormalities, an audible ejection sound is an extreme rarity (239–242). This is in contrast to congenital valvular stenosis, in which an ejection sound is almost invariably heard before calcification and immobilization have occurred (84,239). The amplitude characteristics of the S_2 complex are not helpful in differential diagnosis (A_2 may be absent, diminished, normal, or increased), but the presence of paradoxical splitting of S_2, although uncommon, signifies (in the absence of left bundle branch block) a severe obstruction (82).

As a result of the cusp thickening and jet lesions that have been described, a high-pitched blowing diastolic murmur reflecting mild aortic regurgitation is heard in addition to an ejection systolic murmur in most patients and in virtually all adults with DSS (242–244). Thus, the absence of a regurgitant diastolic murmur in an adult with outflow obstruction speaks strongly against a diagnosis of DSS. The presence of a regurgitant diastolic murmur strongly favors a fixed rather than a muscular lesion but is otherwise not diagnostically useful. In DSS, the delayed carotid upstroke, a characteristic of fixed lesions, also excludes a muscular stenosis. As for the remaining diagnostic possibilities, the tunnel lesion and the supravalvular stenoses are rare, together constituting no more than 5% of congenital aortic stenosis, whereas DSS constitutes almost 20%. They may signify their presence by their special features (inequality of carotid and brachial pulses in the supravalvular stenoses; accompanying abnormalities, e.g., of facies and mentation, in both the supravalvular and tunnel lesions).

Distinction from ventricular septal defect (suggested by the locus of maximal murmur and thrill in some patients) is usually easy. The murmur of the septal defect is regurgitant and, even when not pansystolic, begins with the S_1. The murmur of fixed outflow obstruction is usually diminished with the Valsalva maneuver and with sudden standing, unchanged with vasopressors, and increased with vasodilators, whereas that of the septal defect is unchanged, increased, and decreased respectively with these interventions. With a large defect, there may be a rumbling mid-diastolic flow murmur at the apex. The small septal defect produces no signs of ventricular overloading, whereas the large one produces biventricular overloading with cardiomegaly, as well as pulmonary plethora, on the chest roentgenograms.

The high incidence of associated cardiac defects is a major problem in diagnosis, especially in younger patients (244,245). In 65% of their pediatric series, Newfeld et al. (245) found the DSS to be initially masked by such associated lesions. In patients who reach adulthood, associated lesions, although frequent (almost 50% in the series of Sung et al. [246]), usually do not conceal the obvious outflow tract obstruction.

Laboratory Findings

The chest roentgenograms exhibit no special diagnostic features in DSS. Aortic valvular calcification is not seen, and dilatation of the ascending aorta is absent or mild. Concentric left ventricular hypertrophy may be noted. Cardiomegaly, as in valvular stenosis, signifies left ventricular failure.

Similarly, the ECG offers no differential diagnostic aid, showing only the features of left ventricular pressure overload and conduction abnormalities when present; however, the ECG is important in evaluating severity.

The echocardiogram may be diagnostic by demonstrating the membrane or ridge (251). In the absence of this specific finding, other useful data include symmetric hypertrophy of the left ventricle (rather than disproportionate septal hypertrophy); fluttering of the aortic leaflets (which occurs with normal valves and in a variety of abnormal conditions, including DSS, but is extremely rare in valvular aortic stenosis); a very early, intrasystolic, partial closure of the aortic valve (intrasystolic closure is also seen with hypertrophic subaortic stenosis but tends to be mid-systolic); and the absence of features of valvular stenosis (leaflet calcification), of the tunnel lesion (narrowed outflow tract), of hypertrophic stenosis (ASH and systolic anterior motion [SAM] of the mitral valve), and of supravalvular lesions (diffuse or discrete nar-

rowing of the aorta or an intraaortic membrane). M-mode echocardiography, by detecting both early systolic and mid-systolic partial aortic valve closure, demonstrates the simultaneous presence of discrete and hypertrophic subaortic stenoses (252). Doppler ultrasound studies have been useful in differentiating DSS from valvular stenosis and in estimating the severity of DSS (127,138).

Cardiac catheterization may show a subvalvular gradient, with no gradient between the distal outflow tract and aorta, and a slow upstroke of the aortic pressure pulse (Fig. 7-17). Often, however, membrane and valve are so close that a subaortic gradient cannot be demonstrated. Particularly in patients in whom a discrete subvalvular or supravalvular obstruction is a possibility, it is essential to use a catheter with a single hole. Otherwise, a hybrid tracing may be obtained by recording with some holes above and some below the obstruction. Even with such a catheter, however, the closeness of the valve to the membranous obstruction may preclude demonstration of the subvalvular or supravalvular chamber. The catheter must be changed for selective cinefluorography, because a single-hole catheter will be thrust out of position during pressure injection of opaque dye.

A left ventriculogram may demonstrate the membrane or ridge as an unopacified line below the aortic valve. This requires that the plane of the lesion be approximately perpen-

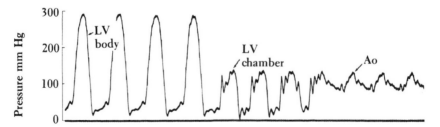

FIG. 7-17. Catheter pullback from the left ventricle (*LV*) to the aorta (*Ao*) in a patient with discrete subvalvular aortic stenosis. Note the marked systolic hypertension in the body of the left ventricle, the abrupt transition to a ventricular pulse with normal systolic pressure, the absence of a gradient between the subvalvular portion of the left ventricle ("LV chamber") and the aorta, and the delayed upstroke distal to the obstruction (in LV as well as Ao) typical of a fixed stenosis. (From ref. 244, with permission.)

dicular to the plane of the film. An aortogram usually shows aortic regurgitation. The subvalvular membrane is occasionally discerned on aortography but not on ventriculography (253). Both the ventriculogram and the aortogram may show a "subaortic jet" in systole due to the subvalvular narrowing of the ejection stream (254). Incomplete opening of the aortic valve is also a recognized angiocardiographic sign of subvalvular stenosis and is a radiographic analogue of the intrasystolic closure of the valve seen echocardiographically (253,254).

Endocarditis

A major feature of DSS is that the traumatized aortic valve is at high risk of infective endocarditis. In two reports of children, adolescents, and young adults, endocarditis occurred in 12% and 14% of patients during an average observation period of only 6 years in each study (255,256). Roberts (243,257) has suggested that DSS may be the cardiac lesion most often complicated by infective endocarditis. In such cases, the infecting organism, because it is on a previously abnormal valve in a young person, is likely to be viridans streptococcus, an organism of low virulence and high sensitivity to penicillin therapy. Delay in diagnosis, however, may permit complete cuspal destruction. Moreover, the latter may be unsuspected, because the subaortic membrane obstructs back flow and forward flow, with the result that decreased systemic diastolic pressure, widened pulse pressure, and left ventricular dilatation may not occur (243).

Therapy

Treatment of DSS consists of operative resection of the membrane. Usually, this results in complete relief of obstruction and is accomplished with low risk (10,197,240,244,246). Injury to the mitral valve may result, because the membrane is partly attached to its anterior leaflet. If the operation is not performed before adulthood, associated aortic cuspal damage

may necessitate aortic valve replacement. This was required in approximately one third of the adults operated on by Sung et al. (246). Another third needed correction of associated congenital cardiac anomalies (almost all involving the left heart). In only one third did membranectomy alone suffice (246).

Like valvular aortic stenosis, DSS is progressive, and there are serial hemodynamic observations indicating that it is more progressive than the valvular lesion (258). In patients not treated with surgery, increases in gradients have been observed in 87% to 100% of those in whom repeat catheterizations have been performed (255,256,258). To prevent sudden death and to anticipate a worsening of obstruction, these patients should be followed closely, should be recommended for operation at smaller gradients (e.g., 30 mm Hg) than used as criteria in valvular lesions, and should have the DSS, however mild, corrected if they undergo an operation for another congenital heart lesion.

After surgery, prophylaxis against infective endocarditis must be lifelong because the risk of infection of the traumatized aortic leaflets is the same after membrane resection as before (256).

Tunnel Subaortic Stenosis

Tunnel subaortic stenosis, a tubular fibromuscular narrowing, is a rare variety of subaortic stenosis that must be differentiated from other left ventricular outflow obstructions because of the difficulties it presents in surgical correction. Although the pathoanatomic features are very variable, the characteristic feature is a diffuse narrowing of the outflow tract, extending about 1 to 3 cm below the aortic annulus, due to a markedly thickened ventricular muscle covered by a thick layer of fibrous tissue extending into the anterior leaflet of the mitral valve. The dimensions of this tunnel-like narrowing remain relatively constant during the cardiac cycle. It is frequently associated with a small aortic annulus. Other abnormalities occasionally observed include a small mitral orifice, a hypoplastic ascending aorta, ASH, coarctation of the aorta, hypertrophic subpulmonic stenosis, valvular pulmonic stenosis, anterior position of the mitral valve, ventricular septal defect, tricuspid mitral valve, incomplete atrioventricular canal, patent ductus arteriosus, Shone's syndrome (supravalvular ring of the left atrium, parachute mitral valve, coarctation of the aorta, and subvalvular aortic stenosis), Noonan's syndrome (congenital heart disease and associated noncardiac abnormalities, including hypertelorism, ptosis, webbed neck, small stature, undescended testes in the male, mild mental retardation, pectus carinatum and excavatum, triangular facies, and low-set ears), and complete transposition of the great vessels (159,259,260).

Some authors have treated the tunnel deformity as a variety of DSS, leading to confusion in the literature (240,251,253). Its pathologic features and the recognized difficulties of surgery indicate that it is more appropriately categorized, according to Reis et al. (244), Sung et al. (246), and Maron et al. (261), as a diffuse lesion, albeit frequently accompanied by a component of discrete obstruction due to the small aortic annulus.

History and Physical Findings

The essential clinical features are the onset of symptoms at any time from infancy to adulthood; a high risk of sudden death, usually during exertion; an ejection systolic murmur noted at birth or in early childhood, loudest at the second to fourth left intercostal spaces, and usually accompanied by a thrill; a regurgitant diastolic murmur in most; a left ventricular heave; the absence of an audible ejection click; prolongation of the carotid upstroke; and anatomic diagnosis usually made by electrocardiography or cardiac catheterization and angiocardiography (although occasionally not until surgery or autopsy).

Laboratory Findings

There may be left ventricular hypertrophy on the ECG. Chest roentgenograms show an undilated or mildly dilated ascending aorta, cardiomegaly in the decompensated patient, and the absence of valvular calcification.

The echocardiographic findings include marked narrowing of the outflow tract; often a separate narrowing of the aortic annulus; left ventricular hypertrophy, usually concentric but occasionally with disproportionate septal thickening; reduced E-F slope of the anterior mitral leaflet; occasionally, an anterior displacement of the mitral leaflets or SAM of the mitral valve, with or without disproportionate septal thickening; and, occasionally, a small mitral orifice, indicated by a fixed and abnormally reduced interleaflet distance during diastole. An adequate precatheterization echocardiogram should alert the hemodynamics-angiocardiography laboratory to the diagnosis and permit confirmation of tunnel lesions before an operation.

At catheterization, the fundamental hemodynamic datum (Fig. 7-17) is a subvalvular pressure gradient. In some patients there is an additional gradient at the valvular level due to the diminutive annulus. In some, as in 3 of 11 patients of Maron et al. (261), there may be yet another subvalvular gradient that reflects the presence of several zones of fibrous, muscular, or fibromuscular narrowing in a lesion shown angiographically, surgically, or at autopsy to be a diffuse tunnel obstruction.

Angiography shows a long tubular narrowing of the left ventricular outflow tract that changes only slightly in diameter during the cardiac cycle; thickened aortic leaflets; no or slight dilatation of the ascending aorta; occasionally, a narrowing of the ascending aorta, representing an associated outflow-obstructive anomaly; and in most patients, aortic regurgitation.

Therapy

Treatment by resection of fibrous tissue or of fibrous tissue and muscle has yielded unsatisfactory results in terms of relief of obstruction (261). Other attempts at repair have used valved conduits connecting the left ventricle to the abdominal aorta or enlargement of the ventricular outflow tract and, if necessary, the annulus, with a patch combined with insertion of an aortic prosthesis (aortoventriculoplasty) (262,263).

The ventricular apicoaortic valved conduit is effective in relieving complex outflow tract obstructions with acceptable operative mortality, significant reduction in ventriculoaortic gradient, and early relief of symptoms (264,265). In follow-up, however, a significant number of patients develop one or more of the following: severe insufficiency of the extracardiac valve, some degree of conduit obstruction, infective endocarditis, recurrence of symptoms, and need for reoperation (265). Certainly, there is no reason to expect the prosthetic valve to behave any better in an extracardiac conduit than in the native valve position. An antibiotically sterilized or fresh sterile homograft may improve the fate of the apicoaortic conduits. The procedure has the advantage that the extracardiac location of the conduit facilitates reoperation for malfunction and permits future surgery, if necessary, on the native outflow tract.

Aortoventriculoplasty is also effective in reducing the gradient and relieving symptoms. Bjornstad et al. (263) reported a 21% mortality in 1979. Mortality has now been reduced to 12.7% (in a series of 47 patients) and 6% (in another series of 18 patients) (266,267). Late deaths in these two series were 0 and 6%, respectively, and the high incidence of right bundle branch block and left anterior hemiblock reported in 1979 has been sharply curtailed (263,266,267). Currently, aortoventriculoplasty seems the procedure of choice for tunnel stenosis, hypoplastic annulus, and stenosis secondary to previously implanted small aortic valve prosthesis (267).

Hypertrophic Cardiomyopathy

Hypertrophic cardiomyopathy, the remaining variety of subvalvular aortic stenosis, is a relatively common autosomal dominant genetic disease (268) with variable phenotypic penetrance. The histologic architecture is disordered with hypertrophied, bizarrely shaped, and disorganized myocardial cells (269,270). There is disproportionate hypertrophy of a hypodynamic interventricular septum, anterior displacement and thickening of the mitral valve leaflets, and, in some cases, a significant functional obstruction of the left ventricular outflow tract as a result of systolic apposition of either mitral leaflet, the anterior in 90%, with the hypertrophied interventricular septum (268,271 277). Although this abnormality has been given a remarkably extensive list of names (muscular subaortic stenosis, idiopathic hypertrophic subaortic stenosis, ASH, familial left ventricular hypertrophy, and others), Maron and Epstein (278) have presented a convincing plea for the adoption of hypertrophic cardiomyopathy as the most comprehensive and least ambiguous term for this disorder.

The disordered histologic picture is not confined to the disproportionately hypertrophied interventricular septum or to the subvalvular myocardium but can be generalized, especially in nonobstructive cases (279). Moreover, although myocardial disorganization can be found to a very limited degree in almost half of normal hearts and those with other congenital or acquired heart diseases, its extent in any tissue section and its widespread distribution throughout septum and free wall in hypertrophic cardiomyopathy indicate that the latter is a diffuse cardiomyopathic process (280). This disorganization is absent in the normal developing heart but characteristic of infants with hypertrophic cardiomyopathy and is probably the fundamental morphologic manifestation of the genetic defect (281). A variety of gene abnormalities in the synthetic pathways for actin and myosin can produce the clinical syndrome of hypertrophic cardiomyopathy (282–285).

Pathophysiologic Features

There are hemodynamic abnormalities in both systole and diastole. Systolic pump function has been described as supernormal, and a hypercontractile state has been posited based

on rapidity of ejection with or without obstruction; in the obstructive variety, on high
ejection fraction and angiographically visualized cavity obliteration; and on the increase in
gradient with inotropic agents and the benefits of negative inotropy (275,286–291). In
nonobstructive cardiomyopathy, however,
there is evidence suggesting that ejection performance is maintained by the left ventricular
hypertrophy and by a reduced afterload,
whereas unit-muscle performance (minute-
work/mass) and end-systolic stress-to-volume
ratio are depressed, consistent with impaired
contractility of myocardial tissue (292). It is
possible that the presence or absence of obstruction in hypertrophic cardiomyopathy depends on the contractile state of the myocardium. In dogs, SAM accompanied by a
left ventricular outflow tract gradient can be
evoked by a pharmacologically induced increase in contractility in a dose-related fashion (293). In humans, provocable gradients
and symptoms have been observed to be ameliorated or abolished after ventricular injury
secondary to myocardial infarction (294–296).
Caplan et al. (296) report that the symptomatic
improvement and abolition of a provocable
gradient were accompanied by prolongation of
isovolumic relaxation, decrease in ejection
fraction, and disappearance of SAM.

In diastole, an increased left ventricular
muscle mass with associated increased stiffness of the myocardium results in diminished left ventricular compliance, which is
manifested by a subnormal rate of atrioventricular filling and a high end-diastolic pressure at a normal end-diastolic volume (297).
The diastolic abnormality, to which the term
inflow obstruction has been applied, can result in elevation of left atrial and pulmonary
venous pressures and therefore in pulmonary
congestive symptoms. These have been referred to as "diastolic left ventricular failure" (298).

It is probably true, as Epstein et al. (299)
have stated, that most patients with this disorder have a predominantly nonobstructive
problem. It is probably also true, however, as

Goodwin (274) has reported, that most patients at some time have an outflow obstruction indicated by a systolic gradient and
murmur. The debate as to whether the gradient and murmur represent true obstruction or
are merely epiphenomena resulting from a
hypercontractile state appears to have been
settled by Maron et al. (300). They showed
that left ventricular ejection dynamics, assessed by pulsed Doppler echocardiography,
are similar in normal subjects and in those
with nonobstructive hypertrophic cardiomyopathy. The patterns of left ventricular emptying are distinctly different in patients with
either a significant subaortic gradient or a
substantial mitral SAM with prolonged mi-
tral-septal apposition. Although left ventricular emptying is accelerated in patients with
evidence of obstruction, systole is not prematurely shortened but significantly prolonged with the ventricle continuing to contract and shorten after the appearance of the
subaortic gradient and the SAM of the mitral
valve (300).

History

The murmur may first be noted at any age
from early childhood to late adulthood
(301,302). As with other outflow obstructions, there is usually a long period of freedom from symptoms. The principal symptoms are anginal pain, presyncope, syncope,
and dyspnea (275). Hardarson et al. (301) reported the mean age at onset of symptoms to
be 28 years, but severe symptoms may be
noted at any age from childhood through
senescence (302). A positive family history
of heart murmur or of heart disease with
sudden death, frequently in childhood, is
common. There is no history of rheumatic
fever. In those with a familial history, there
is no sexual predominance, but in the spo-
radic variety, the male-to-female ratio is 4:1.
Recently, population-based studies have
demonstrated that the cardiac mortality rate
for asymptomatic patients with hypertrophic

cardiomyopathy is very low. Prevailing misconceptions of this entity as an unfavorable condition are probably based on skewed patient referrals to tertiary care centers (302a, 302b).

Physical Findings

The murmur is ejection systolic in type but differs from that of valvular aortic stenosis in being louder at the lower left sternal border or at the apex (1,82,275). In addition, as a result of mitral regurgitation frequently accompanying the abnormal position and motion of the anterior leaflet of the mitral valve, there may be a regurgitant systolic murmur at the apex that may radiate into the axilla (275,303,304). Interventions that increase the afterload and presumably diminish the obstruction by distending the outflow tract, for example, sudden squatting, vasopressors (phenylephrine or methoxamine), isometric exercise (handgrip), deep inspiration, and the Müller maneuver, diminish the intensity of the murmur (299,305). Interventions that diminish afterload, such as amyl nitrite and nitroglycerin, or that cause a decrease in ventricular cavity size by diminishing inflow, such as sudden standing and the Valsalva maneuver, are associated with an increased intensity of the murmur (299). Agents that augment contractility, such as the β-agonist isoproterenol, increase the obstruction and the intensity of the murmur, whereas agents that diminish contractility, such as the beta-blocker propranolol, diminish the obstruction and the intensity of the murmur (299).

An audible ejection sound is rare. The S_2 is frequently single or paradoxically split. When A_2 can be heard, it is usually normal but occasionally diminished in intensity. A regurgitant diastolic murmur is very rare (82).

The arterial pulse differs strikingly from that observed in all other varieties of aortic stenosis (1,82,275). It is characterized by a brisk upstroke and occasionally has a bisferiens character due to a rapid unsustained initial impulse followed by a slow and sustained impulse of lower peak amplitude. The carotid is the arterial pulse at which this is most likely to be appreciated. In most cases, only the initial rapidly rising impulse is palpable. The finding of a brisk carotid upstroke in a patient with signs that suggest aortic stenosis (e.g., ejection systolic murmur, left ventricular hypertrophy, syncope) justifies a presumptive diagnosis of hypertrophic cardiomyopathy. Even in patients in whom the second component of the pulse is not found during physical examination, an indirect carotid pulse tracing usually demonstrates the bifid contour. Occasionally, the same phenomenon is responsible for a double systolic impulse at the cardiac apex, although most instances of apical double impulse in hypertrophic cardiomyopathy are due to the presence of a prominent A wave.

Laboratory Findings

Significant chest roentgenographic findings are left ventricular hypertrophy and, if dilatation has occurred, left ventricular enlargement; the absence of valvular calcification and of poststenotic dilatation of the ascending aorta; and left atrial enlargement, occasionally so great that a primary mitral lesion is suspected (275).

The ECG is abnormal in most patients with hypertrophic cardiomyopathy. Savage et al. (306) reported abnormalities in almost three fourths of their asymptomatic and nonobstructed patients, in over 90% of those without obstruction but with symptoms, and in almost 100% of those with obstruction, whether symptomatic or not. The most common findings were repolarization abnormalities and left ventricular hypertrophy, each occurring in over 70% of their patients. Left atrial abnormalities occurred in about one half, and abnormal Q waves, indistinguishable from those of myocardial infarction, occurred in about one third. Abnormalities that occurred with lesser frequency were right atrial hypertrophy, biatrial hypertrophy, atrial fibrillation, left or right bundle branch block, hemiblocks, intraventricular conduction disturbance, and preexcitation (Wolff-Parkinson-White) pattern. None of the abnormalities is unique to hypertrophic cardiomyopathy; however, the finding of right atrial and left ventricular hypertrophy, occurring in 12%, was notable, because this combination, which had previously been noted by others, is rare in valvular aortic stenosis (307). Moreover, the incidence of atrial fibrillation, of Wolff-Parkinson-White syndrome, and of left atrial or biatrial hypertrophy is higher in hypertrophic cardiomyopathy than in valvular aortic stenosis (308). Although tracings consistent with preexcitation are diagnostically useful, electrophysiologic studies may show no anomalous conduction. Thus, the diagnosis of preexcitation cannot be made reliably from surface

ECGs in hypertrophic cardiomyopathy, and the delta waves may reflect abnormal intraventricular excitation (309).

The M-mode echocardiogram (Figs. 7-18 and 7-19) is extremely valuable and usually permits the diagnosis to be made or a suspected diagnosis to be confirmed before cardiac catheterization. The cardinal echocardiographic features are as follows:

1. Hypertrophy of the interventricular septum, measured both in absolute terms (millimeters of septal thickness) and as a disproportion between septal thickness and that of the left ventricular free wall (ASH) (299);
2. Diminished amplitude of interventricular septal excursions (hypokinesia) (272);
3. Abnormally anterior position of the mitral valve, measured as the septal-mitral valve distance at the onset of systole (276);

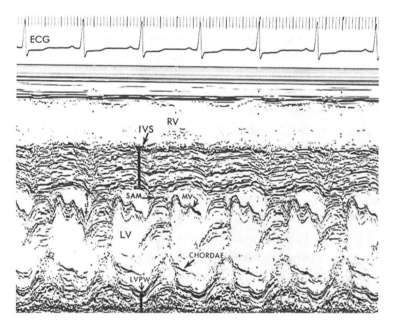

FIG. 7-18. Echocardiogram in hypertrophic obstructive cardiomyopathy. Note the marked thickening of the interventricular septum (*IVS*) in comparison with the posterior wall of the left ventricle (*LVPW*); the small excursions of the IVS compared with those of the LVPW; the anterior position of the mitral valve (*MV*) and its distance from the IVS at the onset of systole (marked *d* beneath the second R wave of the electrocardiogram) being abnormally small; and the systolic anterior motion (*SAM*) of the mitral valve, which here results in sustained abutment of the anterior leaflet against the IVS during systole. *RV*, right ventricle; *LV*, left ventricle.

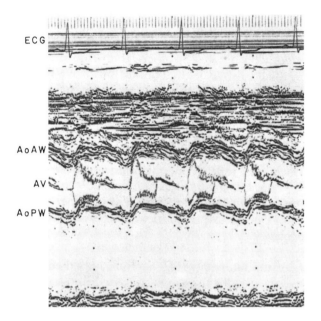

FIG. 7-19. Echocardiogram in hypertrophic obstructive cardiomyopathy. After the aortic valve (*AV*) opens, the leaflets are seen to move away from the anterior and posterior aortic walls (*AoAW* and *AoPW*) to a position of partial intrasystolic closure. The resultant figure of the open valve differs from the parallelograms seen in the normal valve (Fig. 7-7), aortic sclerosis (Fig. 7-8), bicuspid deformity (Fig. 7-9), and calcific stenosis (Fig. 7-10). Note also the fine fluttering of the leaflets; this occurs with normal valves and in all varieties of subvalvular obstruction but is extremely rare in valvular aortic stenosis.

4. SAM of the mitral valve (310);
5. Mid-systolic partial closure of the aortic valve, occurring later than the early intrasystolic closure seen with fixed subvalvular lesions (311,312);
6. A reduced end-systolic volume, seen as a small end-systolic cavity dimension (299,311);
7. A reduced E-F slope, indicating abnormal left ventricular filling.

Features such as septal thickening, reduced E-F slope, septal hypokinesia, and diminutive end-systolic cavity volume can be found in disorders other than hypertrophic cardiomyopathy. Even the features (ASH, SAM, and mid-systolic closure) that are highly characteristic of hypertrophic cardiomyopathy are neither found in all patients with this disorder nor unique to it (313). Actual values for the sensitivity and specificity of these findings depend, as with all quantitative diagnostic signs, on the empirical value arbitrarily used to distinguish between "normal" and "abnormal." It is clear, however, that the most sensitive signs are septal thickness (normal, 11 mm) and ASH, the ratio of septal thickness to that of the posterior wall (normal, less than 1.3); the most specific signs are ASH, SAM, and mid-systolic closure; SAM is found in only 3% of patients with cardiac disorders other than hypertrophic cardiomyopathy (one half of whom have transposition of the great vessels) and, in the absence of ASH, SAM is 99% specific for hypertrophic cardiomyopathy; and SAM and mid-systolic closure are features particularly pointing to the obstructive variety of hypertrophic cardiomyopathy (312,314,316). Although no feature is pathognomonic, various combinations (e.g., ASH and hypokinesia; marked septal thickening with SAM, ASH, and mid-systolic closure) make an alternative diagnosis extremely unlikely. For example, Doi et al. (314) concluded that a septal thickness greater than 13 mm in conjunction with either SAM or mid-systolic closure best differentiates obstructive hypertrophic cardiomyopathy from both the nonobstructive variety and normal subjects. The intimate relation of SAM and septal contact with the severity of obstruction is indicated by the observation that late systolic contact is brief and associated with a small pressure gradient but early contact is prolonged and associated with a large gradient

(317). As noted earlier, the difference in timing of partial intrasystolic aortic valve closure (early with fixed subvalvular lesions, mid-systolic with hypertrophic cardiomyopathy) has permitted echocardiography to detect the coexistence of DSS and hypertrophic obstructive cardiomyopathy (252).

The major problem in echocardiographic diagnosis of hypertrophic cardiomyopathy is associated with ASH alone. Several groups have suggested that because most cases of hypertrophic cardiomyopathy are genetically transmitted, the distinction in cases of ASH alone between hypertrophic cardiomyopathy and other cardiac or systemic diseases is best made by echocardiographic study of family members (315,318). An abnormal septal to free wall ratio in one or more relatives suggests hypertrophic cardiomyopathy in the index case. Conversely, a normal ratio in five or more first-degree adult relatives indicates the absence of a genetically transmitted disease (315). Genetic analyses can also help to distinguish primary hypertrophic cardiomyopathy from secondary ASH.

Two-dimensional Echocardiography

Patients have been described in whom symptoms, an abnormal ECG, and family history were all consistent with hypertrophic cardiomyopathy yet no ventricular hypertrophy could be found on the M-mode echocardiogram because the hypertrophy was localized to areas inaccessible to the M-mode beam. 2D echocardiography can reliably detect these anterior, anterolateral, posteroseptal, and apical zones of left ventricular hypertrophy (319). The ratio of septal-to-free wall thickness is inadequate to depict the complex morphology of the left ventricle in hypertrophic cardiomyopathy, and 2D echocardiographic studies have demonstrated remarkable heterogeneity in the distribution of hypertrophy (319,320–323). What has made M-mode echocardiography so remarkably successful in

detecting or confirming a diagnosis of ASH is the fact that ventricular hypertrophy is asymmetric in hypertrophic cardiomyopathy with the most frequent involvement being the anterobasal portion of the interventricular septum and the least frequent being the posterior free wall (Figs. 7-18 and 7-20). In approximately 5% of patients, however, ventricular hypertrophy may selectively spare the septum and involve only segments of the free wall (319,321). Indeed, several patients have been described in whom dynamic obstructive hypertrophic cardiomyopathy occurred in the absence of anterior and basal ventricular hypertrophy but with substantial thickening confined to the posterobasal left ventricular free wall (324).

Magnetic Resonance Imaging

Observations using gated magnetic resonance imaging are generally entirely consistent with those of 2D echocardiography. Magnetic resonance imaging has the advantages of a larger field of view, sharper discrimination of endocardial and epicardial surfaces, and three-dimensional imaging capability. In contrast, echocardiography has infinite variability in imaging planes, whereas magnetic resonance imaging uses fixed transverse, sagittal, and coronal planes. Both techniques share the advantage over digital subtraction angiography and computed axial tomography with contrast enhancement of being wholly noninvasive (325).

Differential Diagnosis

Differential diagnosis includes ventricular septal defect (suggested by the location of the thrill and loudest murmur), ischemic heart disease (suggested by an anginal syndrome or prominent Q waves or both, with the murmur attributed to papillary muscle dysfunction), rheumatic heart disease, and other causes of left ventricular outflow obstruction (Tables 7-3, 7-4, and 7-5).

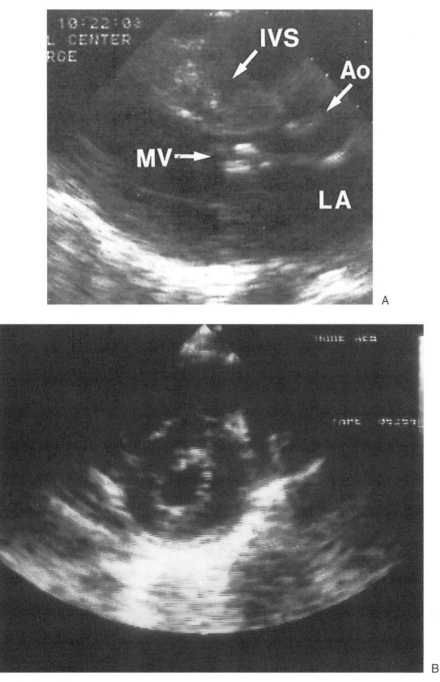

FIG. 7-20. A: Two-dimensional echocardiogram in hypertrophic cardiomyopathy. The tracing, obtained during early systole, shows the thickened anterior leaflet of the mitral valve (*MV*) moving toward the very thickened interventricular septum (*IVS*). *LA*, left atrium; *Ao*, aorta. **B:** Cross-sectional view of marked symmetric left ventricular hypertrophy in a 35-year-old patient with hypertrophic cardiomyopathy.

A small ventricular septal defect does not present with a sustained left ventricular heave, double systolic apical impulse, single or paradoxically split S_2, prominent S_4, left atrial or ventricular enlargement on roentgenograms, or ECG abnormalities. A large defect exhibits pulmonary plethora on chest roentgenograms. The murmur of a septal defect increases, whereas that of obstructive cardiomyopathy decreases, with sudden squatting, vasopressors, and handgrip. The murmur of obstructive cardiomyopathy increases after amyl nitrite, sudden standing, or a Valsalva maneuver, whereas that of a ventricular septal defect decreases after amyl nitrite and is not significantly changed by standing or a Valsalva maneuver.

The murmur of mitral regurgitation from any cause behaves like that of the ventricular septal defect with respect to squatting, vasodilators, and vasopressors; may decrease with sudden standing; and exhibits a biphasic response of decrease with later increase to the Valsalva maneuver. With mitral regurgitation, S_1 may be diminished, there is normal or wide splitting of S_2 but not the single or paradoxically split S_2 often found with obstructive cardiomyopathy, S_3 is commonly present even without left ventricular failure, and an S_4 is not heard except with mitral regurgitation due to ruptured chordae.

Obstructive hypertrophic cardiomyopathy is distinguished from congenital and acquired valvular aortic stenosis by the presence in the cardiomyopathy of a positive family history of sudden childhood deaths and by the presence in the valve lesion of some or all of the following: ejection sound, regurgitant diastolic murmur, delayed arterial upstroke, dilated ascending aorta, and aortic valvular calcification. It is distinguished from the other subvalvular stenoses by the presence in the latter of a regurgitant diastolic murmur and delayed carotid upstroke and from supravalvular stenosis by the location of the murmur.

Differential diagnosis from rheumatic heart disease is based on the criteria described for mitral regurgitation and valvular aortic stenosis. In cases of combined aortic and mitral disease, the incidence of a history of rheumatic fever is very high, whereas the patient with hypertrophic cardiomyopathy masquerading as multivalvular heart disease does not have a history of rheumatic fever.

Distinction from ischemic heart disease may be difficult, especially in nonobstructive cardiomyopathy. Features that should heighten suspicion of the cardiomyopathy are a family history of sudden childhood death, Wolff-Parkinson-White pattern or the combination of left ventricular and right atrial hypertrophy on the ECG, and the elicitation of an ejection systolic murmur by nitrites, sudden standing, or the Valsalva maneuver (326,327). In the obstructive variety, in addition to all of the preceding, the history of a murmur detected in childhood or youth, the characteristic response of the murmur to various physiologic and pharmacologic provocations, the unique arterial pulse, and a bifid systolic apical impulse all point to the outflow obstructive lesion. Hypertrophic cardiomyopathy and ischemic heart disease, however, not infrequently coexist (328). Angiographically demonstrated coronary artery disease has been reported in 15% to 20% of patients with hypertrophic cardiomyopathy and in 25% of those aged 40 years or older (329,330).

Even without angiographically demonstrable coronary artery disease, patients with hypertrophic cardiomyopathy have angina pectoris, suffer myocardial infarction, and exhibit abnormal lactate metabolism with pacing and reversible, regional, perfusion defects with exercise (308,331–333). The evidence of ischemia has been attributed to compression of the septal perforating coronary arteries, limited vasodilatory reserve, intramyocardial small vessel disease due to intimal hyperplasia and medial hypertrophy, and a capillary density not adequately proportional to the increased myocardial mass (331,332,334–336). In addition, a recent report has described that during intensive metabolic stress associated with high pacing rates, there is a marked rise in left ventricular end-diastolic pressure and a concomitant fall in great cardiac vein flow in patients with hypertrophic cardiomyopathy but not in patients with chest pain syndromes and no associated cardiomyopathy (337). The authors speculate that the elevated end-diastolic pressure exceeds the critical closing pressure of the coronary microvasculature and compromises the perfusion pressure across the coronary bed. Such a situation could lead to a self-perpetuating cycle of worsening ischemia. That report also describes a paradoxical and unexplained fall in coronary arteriovenous oxygen difference in the hypertrophic cardiomyopathy patients who were paced to the point of severe angina and metabolic evidence of ischemia. The latter phenomenon, possibly reflecting an abnormal myocellular–capillary relationship, may be unique to hypertrophic cardiomyopathy.

Hypertrophic cardiomyopathy presents two special problems of differential diagnosis at the two extremes of life. In infants, it must be distinguished from a nonfamilial cardiomyopathy described in neonates of diabetic mothers (338). Probably part of the generalized organomegaly in such children, this condition presents with congestive heart failure, an ejection systolic murmur, disproportionate septal thickening, SAM of the anterior mitral leaflet, an outflow tract gradient, exacerbation of symptoms with digitalis, symptomatic improvement with propranolol, and spontaneous regression of the ASH, SAM, gradient, and symptoms within the first few months of life. This clinical course and the absence of positive echocardiographic findings in first-degree family members distinguish this disorder from the genetically transmitted hypertrophic cardiomyopathy.

In the elderly, obstructive cardiomyopathy is a frequently missed diagnosis, in part because its incidence (17% of left ventricular outflow obstruction in patients over the age of 65 [11]) is not appreciated and in part because coexistent disorders of aging alter the presentation. Whiting et al. (339), in a study in which echocardiographic data were apparently not available, reported that a diagnosis of hypertrophic cardiomyopathy was not considered before cardiac catheterization in two thirds of the patients over the age of 60 with this disorder who underwent cardiac catheterization at the Massachusetts General Hospital. Among the misleading signs in the older patients were diastolic blowing murmurs and aortic or mitral valvular calcification. Erroneous diagnoses included mitral regurgitation, valvular aortic stenosis, and coronary artery disease with papillary muscle dysfunction.

At cardiac catheterization, the essential diagnostic finding is a gradient between the body and outflow tract of the left ventricle with a brisk initial upstroke distal to the obstruction (Figs. 7-21 and 7-22). When a gradient is not present at rest, it may be provocable with isoproterenol, amyl nitrite, or the Valsalva maneuver. Except in the elderly with coincidental aortic sclerosis, there is no aortic valvular calcification. Left ventriculography shows an abnormal, banana-shaped, or ballet slipper-shaped left ventricular cavity; massive hypertrophy of the interventricular septum, especially in its superior portion; prominent papillary muscles; stellate projections of opaque dye into the interstices of the columnae carneae; an anterior position of the mitral valve; a high ejection fraction; and, in some cases, mitral regurgitation, an hourglass constriction in the midcavity, and end-systolic obliteration of the cavity. Axial left ventriculography (i.e., a caudocranial left anterior oblique view) has been reported to show all findings detectable on conventional views but also a better profile of the mitral valve, septum, and posterior left ventricular wall and ready identification, not usual in nonangled views, of SAM (340). Coronary arteriography may show systolic narrowing of the septal perforating branches (which is not specific for this disorder) and shows significant atherosclerotic narrowings in a sizable minority of cases (329,330).

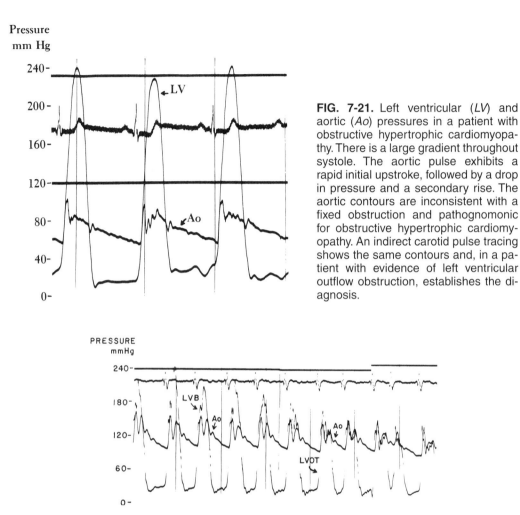

FIG. 7-21. Left ventricular (*LV*) and aortic (*Ao*) pressures in a patient with obstructive hypertrophic cardiomyopathy. There is a large gradient throughout systole. The aortic pulse exhibits a rapid initial upstroke, followed by a drop in pressure and a secondary rise. The aortic contours are inconsistent with a fixed obstruction and pathognomonic for obstructive hypertrophic cardiomyopathy. An indirect carotid pulse tracing shows the same contours and, in a patient with evidence of left ventricular outflow obstruction, establishes the diagnosis.

FIG. 7-22. Pressure tracings recorded at cardiac catheterization in a patient with obstructive hypertrophic cardiomyopathy. One catheter has been inserted by the retrograde arterial approach into the body of the left ventricle (*LVB*). A second catheter has been introduced by the same technique into the root of the aorta (*Ao*). A systolic gradient is evident in the left-hand portion of the recording, which also shows the typical rapid initial upstroke and bifid contour of the aortic pulse and a characteristic notch on the upstroke of the left ventricular pulse. On withdrawal of the LV catheter toward the Ao, there is no gradient between the left ventricular outflow tract (*LVOT*) (i.e., the subvalvular portion of the LV) and the aorta, which excludes a diagnosis of valvular aortic stenosis.

Clinical Course

The natural history of the disease is extremely variable (301,302,308,341–343). The condition of most patients is stable for many years. Deterioration is usually slow but occasionally is rapid, especially with the advent of atrial fibrillation. In such cases, the loss of the atrial booster pump may severely compromise diastolic filling; however, atrial fibrillation may merely signal a critical deterioration in the state of the left ventricular myocardium. A few patients improve spontaneously, perhaps as a result of a decrease in myocardial contractility with aging. Some improve after myocardial infarction with lessening of symptoms, loss of gradient, decrease in ejection fraction, and disappearance of SAM (296).

One sixth die suddenly and unexpectedly (301,302).

The high incidence of sudden and unexpected death in referral populations is the most important feature of the natural history of hypertrophic cardiomyopathy. Such deaths make up most of the annual mortality of 3% to 4% (301,302). Sudden death constituted about five sixths of all cardiac deaths in several series (302,344). In some patients, sudden death is the first manifestation of the disorder (342). It occurs in both the obstructive and nonobstructive varieties and may occur in either sex, at any age, and regardless of the presence or absence of symptoms (345). Many sudden deaths are associated with moderate or severe effort, but in one report, most occurred during sedentary activities (301,302, 345). However, as noted earlier, population-based studies demonstrate a generally benign course for most patients with hypertrophic cardiomyopathy.

The cause of these deaths is presumed to be an arrhythmia. A study using ambulatory electrocardiographic monitoring suggested that threatening arrhythmias are virtually ubiquitous in hypertrophic cardiomyopathy. Specifically, of 30 patients, only 1 had no arrhythmia during monitoring, whereas 14 (46%) had supraventricular tachycardia or paroxysmal atrial fibrillation, 13 (43%) had multiform or paired ventricular extrasystoles, and 8 (26%) had ventricular tachycardia (346). These serious arrhythmias were not predicted by any clinical or laboratory measurement and occurred in patients who were taking propranolol. Supraventricular tachycardia and paroxysmal atrial fibrillation were not significantly associated with sudden death in follow-up periods of 4 years in one study and 1 to 4 years (mean, 2.6 years) in another (347,348). Ventricular arrhythmias, however, which occurred during ambulatory ECG monitoring in most patients in both studies, including ventricular tachycardia in 20% in one study and 28% in the other, did carry a significant risk of subsequent sudden death or of cardiac arrest with successful resuscitation (347,348). Ventricular tachycardia in particular identifies a subgroup at great risk. Twenty-four percent had cardiac arrest during follow-up compared with 3% in patients with ventricular arrhythmias without ventricular tachycardia. The annual mortality rate was 9% in those with ventricular tachycardia compared with 1% for patients with high-grade ventricular arrhythmias without ventricular tachycardia (347).

In patients who do not die suddenly, death usually results from chronic congestive heart failure. Increased inflow resistance with pulmonary congestion, an elevated jugular venous pressure dominated by an A wave, and fluid retention characterize this stage, and the murmur of outflow obstruction may actually diminish (343). A few patients die as a result of systemic emboli, which are a particular risk in the patient with congestive heart failure. There is also a small but definite risk of infective endocarditis, which has occurred in 5% to 9% in various series (308).

Prognosis in this disorder is very variable. Favorable prognostic features are the absence of symptoms at the time of detection of the murmur, the absence of left atrial hypertrophy on the ECG, and the absence of a high end-diastolic pressure at catheterization (308,342). Unfavorable signs are a family history of sudden death; a very thick interventricular septum; left ventricular hypertrophy with ST-T abnormalities and deep Q waves on the ECG; progression of left ventricular hypertrophy; hypertrophy confined to the left ventricular apex; heart failure in infants; syncope, dyspnea, and chest pain in adults; and ventricular tachycardia at any age (344–352).

Therapy

Before left ventricular failure, rational therapy should be directed at relieving symptoms (angina, presyncope, syncope, and nonprogressive dyspnea), alleviating or eliminating outflow obstruction, reducing inflow resistance, preventing and controlling arrhythmias, and preventing infective endocarditis. Beta blockade is the mainstay of therapy at this stage. It relieves symptoms, decreases ventricular stiffness, is antiarrhythmic, and abolishes or diminishes the increased obstruction occurring during hyperadrenergic states (exercise and excitement), although it does not abolish obstruction at rest. Unfortunately, however, at the doses used in most series, beta blockade has not prevented sudden death, symptomatic deterioration, or arrhythmias (301,302,343,345,346). Suboptimal doses were probably given to many subjects. Frank et al. (353), attempting "complete" β-receptor blockade, used an average dose of 462 mg propranolol daily and at least 320 mg/day in all patients, supplemented by the control of arrhythmias with drugs or pacemaker insertion or both. During a follow-up from 2 to 13 years (mean, 5 years), all 22 patients, symptomatic at the onset of therapy, exhibited significant symptomatic improvement in dyspnea, angina, syncope, presyncope, and palpitations, and all were alive.

Recently, calcium-channel blocking agents have been shown to be a useful alternative or additive to beta blockade. Although there are disagreements in published reports, probably reflecting differences in dose size, dosing technique, duration of follow-up, and the specific variables measured, the following conclusions seem well supported. Verapamil depresses inotropy, has no effect on cardiac output, or is associated with an increase in cardiac output; improves diastolic (i.e., relaxation) performance even in doses insufficient to affect systolic function; decreases the outflow tract gradient; decreases left ventricular end-diastolic pressure; alleviates symptoms; and improves exercise capacity (354–359). Nifedipine is beneficial in some patients and has a negative influence in others. Its beneficial effects include improved rates of left ventricular diastolic filling, reduced left ventricular end-diastolic pressure and the pressure-volume relation, indicating increased distensibility; and an improved rate of isovolumic left ventricular relaxation (360).

Verapamil is effective in alleviating symptoms, diminishing the gradient, and increasing exercise capacity in patients who have not responded to propranolol (361). It is therefore indicated in patients in whom beta blockade has been ineffective or is contraindicated (e.g., asthma). Calcium-channel blockade may also be useful in patients who have had a suboptimal response to beta blockade, because nifedipine and propranolol used together have been reported to be more effective than either alone (362). Calcium-channel blockade also may be the first therapeutic choice in patients with bronchospastic disease or symptomatic nonobstructive hypertrophic cardiomyopathy in whom diastolic failure is the principal problem (361). Verapamil, however, has potentially serious side effects secondary to depressions in inotropy, sinus node function, and junctional tissue conduction (363). It should not be used therefore in patients with obstructive hypertrophic cardiomyopathy and an elevated pulmonary capillary wedge pressure or history of pulmonary congestion, in patients with sinus node or junctional tissue abnormalities who do not have a pacemaker in place, or in patients with systemic hypotension or moderate increases in PR interval (361). Adverse hemodynamic or electrophysiologic effects may be encountered in a significant minority of patients despite these precautions (363).

Calcium-channel blocking agents are effective in the majority of patients who continue to be symptomatic after beta blockade, and there may be an alternative to beta blockade in selected patients; however, there is a lack of experience from which one can predicate that it will be any more effective in avoiding sudden death (359). There is evidence that verapamil is inferior to amiodarone in the management of refractory arrhythmias (atrial fibrillation and ventricular tachycardia) (364).

The antiarrhythmic drug, disopyramide, is also a potent negative inotropic agent. Given intravenously during cardiac catheterization, it abolishes the basal outflow tract gradient. Given in a maintenance oral dosage, it reduces SAM, the intensity of the systolic murmur, and the left ventricular ejection time, and is associated with improved exercise tolerance and functional capacity (365).

Two recently employed forms of therapy for hypertrophic cardiomyopathy include dual-chamber pacing and alcohol-induced septal necrosis. A number of investigators have examined the effect of chronic dual-chamber pacing in patients with obstructive hypertrophic cardiomyopathy (365a–365c). Dual-chamber pacing decreases the subaortic gradient and relieves symptoms in many patients. In some individuals, however, symptoms do not change and may even worsen. Occasionally, symptoms improve in the absence of any alteration in the subaortic gradient, suggesting a placebo effect. The mechanism whereby dual-chamber pacing reduces outflow tract obstruction is still debated. It has been suggested that the beneficial effect is the result of pacing-induced paradoxical septal wall motion that increases left ventricular outflow tract diameter, thereby decreasing mitral valve apposition to the septal wall.

Another approach to therapy in patients with symptomatic subaortic muscular obstruction is catheter-induced septal necrosis by means of alcohol injection. In this technique, a balloon catheter is positioned in the first septal perforator branch of the left anterior descending coronary artery. The balloon is inflated, thereby obstructing arterial inflow; alcohol is injected distal to the balloon and is allowed to remain in the territory of the first septal perforator for 5 minutes. This induces a zone of myocardial necrosis in the proximal septum that reduces septal contraction and eventually even septal wall thickness (365d,365e). The outflow tract gradient is reduced immediately after this procedure in most patients. Subsequent follow-up reveals further reduction in the gradient as the zone of myocardial necrosis heals with resultant thinning of the proximal septum. Left ventricular relaxation and compliance are likewise improved. Patients report significant reduction in symptoms, and standardized exercise testing demonstrates significantly increased exercise tolerance. Long-term follow-up for this procedure as compared with surgical results is not yet available.

Several surgical approaches to the alleviation or elimination of obstruction have been used. The most popular (the Morrow procedure) consists of the resection of a wedge of muscle from the superior portion of the interventricular septum and the undercutting of adjacent muscle (left ventricular myectomy and myotomy) (366). Excellent results in terms of symptomatic and hemodynamic improvement follow operation (367). There is symptomatic improvement in approximately 90% of survivors during the first postoperative years, a profound reduction in resting gradient in almost all patients, elimination of the gradient in some, abolition of mitral regurgitation, and reduction in left ventricular end-diastolic pressure (367,368). In addition, there is a postoperative decrease in left atrial size in patients under the age of 40, a decrease in the high ejection fractions prevailing preoperatively, and a reduction in or elimination of SAM (which does not occur with beta-blockers) (369–371). Of considerable importance, because it refutes the speculation that improvement with surgery results merely from intraoperative myocardial damage, is the proof of enhanced cardiac performance, with a great increase in exercise capacity and peak oxygen consumption during intense treadmill exercise in most postoperative patients (372).

Operative mortality has been high, averaging 14% for reports from five major cardiac centers (353). Although recent surgical results have improved, with an overall operative mortality of only 8% for the largest reported series (over 300 patients operated on at the National Heart, Lung, and Blood Institute since 1960) (373), enthusiasm for surgery has been tempered by the continued occurrence of symptomatic deterioration, congestive failure, and sudden death. Of surgical survivors, 12% exhibited persistent or recurrent symptomatic disability and 9% died (about one half suddenly and one half after chronic congestive heart failure) between 7 months and 13 years after the operation (367). The surgical procedure did not alter the overall annual mortality, which, including immediate operative deaths and late deaths due to the cardiac disease, which was 3.5% or approximately the same as the average mortality (about 3%) reported by

Hardarson et al. (301) and Shah et al. (302) for unoperated patients (367). In both the National Institute group and the study of Shah et al., however, there was a lower annual mortality rate (only 1.8%) among patients who survived surgery than in untreated patients and those treated with propranolol. Shah et al. (302) also noted a lower incidence (7%) of sudden death after surgery. Although no properly designed prospective study of medical therapy versus surgical therapy has been reported, these results suggest that myotomy-myectomy does not increase long-term mortality and may actually decrease it.

Thus, both pharmacotherapy and surgery diminish hypercontractility and improve left ventricular distensibility and both are effective in control of angina, presyncope, syncope, and dyspnea. Only surgery and disopyramide (in one small series), however, are effective in attenuating or eliminating SAM of the mitral valve and in profoundly reducing or abolishing obstruction at rest (365). Neither removes the risk of sudden death. Surgery appears to lower it appreciably, and propranolol in daily doses of 320 mg or more, supplemented by drug and pacemaker management of arrhythmias, may do so also. An effect on long-term mortality is unproved for surgery and uncertain for propranolol, because of disagreement about the appropriate dosage and about the desirability of treating asymptomatic patients without obstruction at rest.

Currently, it seems prudent to reserve operation for patients with the obstructive variety of hypertrophic cardiomyopathy who have severe symptoms that do not respond satisfactorily to all medical therapy, have been resuscitated from episodes of apparent sudden death, or have two or more primary relatives who died suddenly of hypertrophic cardiomyopathy (361). Goodwin and Oakley (298) believe that medical therapy is indicated in all patients with hypertrophic cardiomyopathy, whether obstructive or nonobstructive, with or without symptoms. The group at the National Institutes of Health recommends medical therapy in symptomatic patients who have marked ventricular septal thickening and a distinctly abnormal ECG or are members of families with "malignant hypertrophic cardiomyopathy" (341,349).

Other therapy includes interdiction of strenuous or competitive athletics and prophylaxis against infective endocarditis. In the patient with congestive heart failure, digitalis, diuretics, salt restriction, and small rate-controlling doses of propranolol are recommended.

Supravalvular Aortic Stenosis

Lesions in which the narrowing lies distal to the aortic valve are the least common variety of left ventricular outflow obstruction (11). Of the three anatomic types, the hourglass deformity, a circumferential waistlike constriction, is by far the most common, constituting about two thirds of the supravalvular obstructions (374). In addition to the constriction of the aorta in this lesion, there is often a severe medial thickening and a superimposed proliferation of the intima, narrowing the aortic lumen further (11). The fibromembranous variety, in which there is either a diaphragm with a central opening or a crescent-shaped fibrous membrane partially encircling the lumen, is the least common type (13%). Its crescentic semicircumferential form is often not stenotic at all but merely an incidental finding. A hypoplastic variety, in which there is a diffuse narrowing of the ascending aorta, makes up about one fifth of the supravalvular obstructions. Patients with this variety are the least likely to survive to older childhood or adulthood because of its inherent severity and frequent association with other anomalies that constitute a hypoplastic left-heart syndrome (12).

The discrete obstructions are located just above the coronary ostia, at the edge of the sinuses of Valsalva. As a result, the coronary arteries are thought to be perfused mainly in systole and are subjected to the very high pressures prevailing in the left ventricle. Therefore, these arteries exhibit a marked thickening, with extensive medial hypertrophy, and are dilated, elongated, and tortuous (374). Despite their large external dimensions, some of the coronary arteries have focal intimal lesions secondary to either fibrous thickening or premature atherosclerosis with resultant luminal encroachment (12). In addition, the free margin of one or more cusps sometimes adheres to the wall of the aorta at the site of narrowing. This attachment may exclude one sinus of Valsalva and its coronary artery from the aortic lumen. The coronary artery so involved becomes smaller, whereas the opposite coronary artery exhibits the typical dilatation, elongation, thickening, and tortuosity.

Some cases are familial, with an autosomal dominant transmission with incomplete penetrance (375,376). These cases are not associated with abnormalities of appearance or mentation. There is another group, nonfamilial, in which the supravalvular stenosis is part of a syndrome of multiple anomalies, including hypertelorism, convergent strabismus, hypognathism, mental retardation, unusual dental malformations, and multiple stenoses of the peripheral pulmonary arteries (377). Many of these patients have a history of infantile hypercalcemia, which is characterized by high calcium, normal phosphorus, normal or low alkaline phosphatase, mental and growth retardation, irritability, muscular hypotonia, anorexia, vomiting, generalized osteosclerosis, renal dysfunction, hypertension, "elfin" facies, and heart murmur (377–379). Its cause is unknown. The occurrence in the same patient of the infantile hypercalcemia syndrome and the syndrome of supravalvular stenosis with multiple anomalies suggests that both are caused by a metabolic disturbance *in utero*. Experimental vitamin D intoxication in rabbits results in supravalvular aortic stenosis in their offspring (380). A gestational derangement of vitamin D metabolism may be the common basis of the two syndromes. In a third group, the supravalvular stenosis is associated with neither a positive family history nor a history of infantile hypercalcemia.

In addition to stenosis of the peripheral pulmonary arteries, associated cardiac anomalies include hypoplasia of the pulmonary trunk, stenosis of branches of the aortic arch, coarctation of the aorta, and Marfan's syndrome. Cardiac sequelae include infective endocarditis occurring on the intima of the aorta in the area of narrowing and dissecting aneurysm beginning just distal to the stenosis.

History and Physical Findings

The essential features of the clinical presentation are similar to those of congenital valvular aortic stenosis. The symptoms are those of all left ventricular outflow obstruction: angina, presyncope, syncope, and dyspnea. There is commonly a history of familial murmurs, an occasional family history of sudden childhood death, and, in some nonfamilial cases, a history of neonatal hypercalcemia or renal failure. In these nonfamilial patients, the general appearance is likely to be characterized by wide-set eyes, convergent strabismus, broad forehead, heavy cheeks, small chin, large mouth, pouting lips, upturned nose, a general elfin appearance, malformed teeth, dental malocclusion, and a deep metallic voice.

Inspection may reveal a prominent right carotid pulsation, and the right carotid upstroke may be brisk, whereas that of the left carotid is slow (375). The ejection systolic murmur and thrill are usually maximal in the first right intercostal space just below the clavicle, and the murmur sometimes radiates to the medial aspect of the right arm and usually preferentially to the right carotid artery. Occasionally, the murmur is heard better in the neck than in the chest. In cases where there is stenosis of peripheral pulmonary arteries, there may be a prominent systolic murmur in the axillae and in the back (81,377). The S_2 is usually normal, although the A_2 is occasionally diminished (81). An ejection sound is rare and a regurgitant diastolic murmur uncommon (81,375). Blood pressures in the two arms may be unequal, with systolic and pulse pressures higher in the right arm than in the left (81,82,239,375). The prominence of the right carotid pulsation, difference in right and left carotid upstroke, and inequality of brachial pulses have been attributed to the Coanda effect, a special case of the Bernoulli principle, which describes the tendency of a jet stream to adhere to a wall (381). Although the anatomy of supravalvular stenosis favors a right-sided Coanda effect, a left-sided predominance is possible, and in about one sixth of cases, the brisker pulse may be in the left carotid and the left brachial systolic and pulse pressures may exceed those on the right (381).

Laboratory Findings

The ECG shows a left ventricular overload and no other features of note. The chest roentgenogram may be helpful in showing an absent or diminutive aortic knob and a narrow vascular pedicle (377). Indirect pulse tracings may be useful in recording the differences between the right and left carotid arteries. M-mode echocardiography shows generalized hypertrophy of the left ventricle without ASH, SAM, partial intrasystolic valve closure, or subvalvular abnormality and may on occasion show the intraaortic narrowing (382,383). The 2D echocardiogram, because of its enlarged field of view, allowing the narrowed and surrounding normal areas of the aorta to be recorded simultaneously, more frequently detects and characterizes the supravalvular narrowing (384).

Cardiac catheterization should show a gradient between the proximal and distal aorta that may be as large as 200 mm Hg (Fig. 7-23), and aortography may show a locally constricted or diffusely hypoplastic aorta or an intraaortic membrane, prominent coronary arteries, and adherent aortic valvular leaflets (377). In some cases there is severe pulmonary hypertension as a result of pulmonary arterial stenoses, which may be demonstrable on a pulmonary angiogram. In almost all cases there is a marked bulging of the aorta at the site of the ligamentum arteriosum (377).

Clinical Course and Therapy

The most common causes of fatality are sudden unexpected death and congestive heart failure. In the past, the most common cause of fatality was intraoperative and postoperative death. In the 1965 review of Peterson et al. (374), 27 of the 68 cases (40%) had died, with 15 (56%) of the deaths being operative and 50% of the remaining deaths being sudden and unexpected. Infective aortitis occurs, less commonly than does infective endocarditis in other nonvalvular aortic stenoses, with intimal vegetations located at the site of aortic obstruction (11).

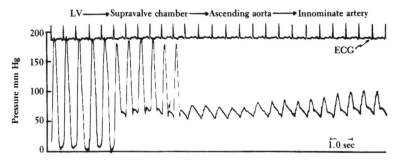

FIG. 7-23. Catheter pullback from left ventricle (*LV*) to innominate artery in a patient with supravalvular aortic stenosis. There is systolic hypertension in the root of the aorta with no gradient between the LV and the proximal aorta and a large gradient between the proximal and distal ascending aorta. The aortic tracing distal to the obstruction also shows the slow finely notched upstroke typical of a fixed obstruction. (From ref. 82, with permission.)

The high operative mortality in the series of Peterson et al. (374) undoubtedly reflected the frequency with which exact diagnosis was made only at the time of surgical exploration. The first correct preoperative diagnosis was made in 1959, 3 years after the first surgical correction was accomplished (385). With accurate preoperative diagnosis in patients without associated anomalies, the results are considerably better, and the operative mortality is satisfactory. In the hourglass type, the correction is accomplished either by longitudinal aortic incision and the insertion of a prosthetic patch or by resection of the involved segment of the aorta and reanastomosis. Some fibromembranous types are amenable to membranectomy, but most are handled in the same way the hourglass lesions are treated. The most difficult is the diffuse hypoplastic variety, which may necessitate graft replacement of the entire ascending aorta.

REFERENCES

1. Levinson GE. Valvular heart disease. In: Gordon BL, ed. *Clinical Cardiopulmonary Physiology*, 3rd ed. New York: Grune & Stratton, 1969:245–258.
1a. Julius BK, Spillmann M, Vassalli G, Villari B, Eberli FR, Hess OM. Angina pectoris in patients with aortic stenosis and normal coronary arteries—mechanisms and pathophysiological concepts. *Circulation* 1997;95: 892–898.
2. Roberts WC. Aortic valve stenosis and the congenitally malformed aortic valve. In: Roberts WC, ed. *Congenital Heart Disease in Adults*. Philadelphia: FA Davis, 1979:416–426.
3. Roberts WC, Virmani R. Aschoff bodies at necropsy in valvular heart disease. Evidence from an analysis of 543 patients over 14 years of age that rheumatic heart disease, at least anatomically, is a disease of the mitral valve. *Circulation* 1978;57:803.
4. Bacon APC, Mathews MB. Congenital bicuspid aortic valves and the aetiology of isolated aortic valvular stenosis. *Q J Med* 1979;28:545.
5. Roberts WC. Anatomically isolated aortic valvular disease. The case against its being of rheumatic etiology. *Am J Med* 1970;49:151.
6. Subramanian R, Olson LJ, Edwards WD. Surgical pathology of pure aortic stenosis: a study of 374 cases. *Mayo Clin Proc* 1984;59:683.
7. Subramanian R, Olson LJ, Edwards WD. Surgical pathology of combined aortic stenosis and insufficiency: a study of 213 cases. *Mayo Clin Proc* 1985;60: 247.
8. Pomerance A. Isolated aortic stenosis. In: Pomerance A, Davies MJ, eds. *The Pathology of the Heart*. London: Blackwell, 1985:327–341.

9. Ellis FH, Kirklin JW. Congenital valvular aortic stenosis: anatomic findings and surgical technique. *J Thorac Cardiovasc Surg* 1962;43:199.
10. Morrow AG, Goldblatt A, Braunwald E. Congenital aortic stenosis. II. Surgical treatment and the result of operation. *Circulation* 1963;27:450.
11. Roberts WC. Valvular, subvalvular, and supravalvular aortic stenosis: morphologic features. *Cardiovasc Clin* 1973;5:97.
12. Edwards JE. Pathology of left ventricular outflow tract obstruction. *Circulation* 1965;31:586.
13. Reeve R Jr, Robinson SJ. Hypoplastic annulus an unusual type of aortic stenosis: a report of 3 cases in children. *Dis Chest* 1964;45:99.
14. Roberts WC. The congenitally bicuspid aortic valve. A study of 85 autopsy cases. *Am J Cardiol* 1970;26:72.
15. Stein PD, Sabbah HN, Pitha JV. Continuing disease process of calcific aortic stenosis: role of microthrombi and turbulent flow. *Am J Cardiol* 1977;39: 159.
16. Fenoglio JJ Jr, et al. Congenital bicuspid aortic valve after age 20. *Am J Cardiol* 1977;39:164.
17. Roberts WC, et al. Congenitally bicuspid aortic valve causing severe, pure aortic regurgitation without superimposed infective endocarditis. Analysis of 13 patients requiring aortic valve replacement. *Am J Cardiol* 1981;47:206.
17a. Sabet HY, Edwards WA, Tazelaar HD, Daly RC. Congenitally bicuspid aortic valves: a surgical pathology study of 542 cases (1991 through 1996) and a literature review of 2,715 additional cases. *Mayo Clin Proc* 1999;74:14–26.
18. Larson EW, Edwards WD. Risk factors for aortic dissection: a necropsy study of 161 cases. *Am J Cardiol* 1984;53:849.
19. Vollebergh FEMG, Becker AE. Minor congenital variations of cusp size in tricuspid aortic valves: Possible link with isolated aortic stenosis. *Br Heart J* 1977; 39:1006.
20. Roberts WC, Perloff JK, Constantino T. Severe valvular aortic stenosis in patients over 65 years of age. A clinicopathologic study. *Am J Cardiol* 1971;27:497.
21. Campbell M. Calcific aortic stenosis and congenital bicuspid aortic valves. *Br Heart J* 1968;30:606.
22. Bruns DL, Van der Hauwaert LG. Aortic systolic murmur developing with increasing age. *Br Heart J* 1958; 20:370.
22a. Stewart BF, Siscovick, D, Lind BK, et al. Clinical factors associated with calcific aortic valve disease. *J Am Coll Cardiol* 1997;29:630–634.
22b. Juvonen J, Juvonen T, Laurila A, et al. Can degenerative aortic valve stenosis be related to persistent *Chlamydia pneumoniae* infection? *Ann Intern Med* 1998;128:741–744.
22c. Juvonen J, Laurila A, Juvonen T, et al. Detection of *Chlamydia pneumoniae* in human nonrheumatic stenotic aortic valves. *J Am Coll Cardiol* 1997;29: 1054–1059.
22d. Lester SJ, Heilbron B, Gin K, Dodek A, Jue J. The natural history and rate of progression of aortic stenosis. *Chest* 1998;113:1109–1114.
22e. Otto CA, Burwash IG, Legget ME, et al. Prospective study of asymptomatic valvular aortic stenosis clinical, electrocardiographic and exercise predictors of outcome. *Circulation* 1997;95:2262–2270.

23. Bulkley BH, Roberts WC. The heart in systemic lupus erythematosus and the changes induced in it by corticosteriod therapy: a study of 36 necropsy patients. *Am J Med* 1975;48:243.
24. Pritzker MR, et al. Acquired aortic stenosis in systemic lupus erythematosus. *Ann Intern Med* 1980;93:434.
25. Lerman BB, et al. Aortic stenosis associated with systemic lupus erythematosus. *Am J Med* 1982;72:707.
26. Silver MD. Obstruction to blood flow related to the aortic valve. In: Silver MD, ed. *Cardiovascular Pathology.* New York: Churchill Livingstone, 2nd ed., 1991;985–1012.
27. Gould L, et al. Cardiac manifestations of ochronoses. *J Thorac Cardiovasc Surg* 1976;72:788.
28. Roberts WC, et al. Cardiovascular pathology in hyperlipoproteinemia: anatomic observations in 42 necropsy patients with normal or abnormal lipoprotein patterns. *Am J Cardiol* 1073;31:557.
29. Dinsmore RE, Lees RS. Vascular calcification in types II and IV hyperlipoproteinemia: radiographic appearance and clinical significance. *AJR Am J Roentgenol* 1985;144:895.
30. Roberts WC, et al. Valvular stenosis produced by active infective endocarditis. *Circulation* 1967;36:449.
31. Arnett EN, Roberts WC. Pathology of active infective endocarditis: a necropsy analysis of 192 patients. *J Thorac Cardiovasc Surg* 1982;30:327.
32. Detrano RC, Yiannikas J, Salcedo EE. Two-dimensional echocardiographic assessment of radiation-induced valvular heart disease. *Am Heart J* 1984;107:584.
33. Wood P. Aortic stenosis. *Am J Cardiol* 1958;1:553.
34. Ross J Jr, Braunwald E. Aortic stenosis. *Circulation* 1968;38[Suppl V]:61.
35. Flamm MD, et al. Mechanism of effort syncope in aortic stenosis. *Circulation* 1967;36[Suppl II]:190.
36. Mark AL, et al. Abnormal vascular response to exercise in patients with aortic stenosis. *J Clin Invest* 1973;52:1138.
37. Johnson AM. Aortic stenosis, sudden death and left ventricular baroreceptors. *Br Heart J* 1971;33:1.
37a. Sorgato A, Faggiano P, Aurigemma GP, Rusconi C, Gaasch WH. Ventricular arrhythmias in adult aortic stenosis—prevalence, mechanisms and clinical relevance. *Chest* 1998;113:482–491.
38. Schwartz LS, et al. Syncope and sudden death in aortic stenosis. *Am J Cardiol* 1969;23:647.
39. Hakki A, et al. Angina pectoris and coronary artery disease in patients with severe aortic valve disease. *Am Heart J* 1980;100:441.
40. Green SJ, et al. Relation of angina pectoris to coronary artery disease in aortic valve stenosis. *Am J Cardiol* 1985;55:1063.
41. Exadactylos N, Sugrue DD, Oakley CM. Prevalence of coronary artery disease in patients with isolated aortic valve stenosis. *Br Heart J* 1984;51:121.
42. Hancock EW. Aortic stenosis, angina pectoris, and coronary artery disease. *Am Heart J* 1977;93:382.
43. Fallen EL, Elliott WC, Gorlin R. Mechanisms of angina in aortic stenosis. *Circulation* 1967;36:480.
44. Trenouth RS, Phelps NC, Neill WA. Determinants of left ventricular hypertrophy and oxygen supply in chronic aortic valve disease. *Circulation* 1976;53:644.
45. Abdulali SA, et al. Coronary artery luminal diameter in aortic stenosis. *Am J Cardiol* 1985;55:450.
46. Bertrand ME, et al. Coronary sinus blood flow at rest and during isometric exercise in patients with aortic valve disease: mechanism of angina pectoris in presence of normal coronary arteries. *Am J Cardiol* 1981;47:199.
47. Neill WA, Fluri-Lundeen JH. Myocardial oxygen supply in left ventricular hypertrophy and coronary heart disease. *Am J Cardiol* 1979;44:747.
48. Thormann J, Schlepper M. Comparison of myocardial flow, hemodynamic changes, and lactate metabolism during isoproterenol stress in patients with coronary heart disease and severe aortic stenosis. *Clin Cardiol* 1979;2:437.
49. Nadell R, et al. Myocardial oxygen supply/demand ratio in aortic stenosis: hemodynamic and echocardiographic evaluation of patients with and without angina pectoris. *J Am Coll Cardiol* 1983;2:258.
50. Swanton RH, Brooksby IAB, Jenkins BS. Determinants of angina in aortic stenosis and the importance of coronary arteriography. *Br Heart J* 1977;39:1347.
51. Hoffman JIE, Buckberg GD. The myocardial supply:demand ratio a critical review. *Am J Cardiol* 1978;41:327.
52. Marcus ML, et al. Decreased coronary reserve: a mechanism for angina pectoris in patients with aortic stenosis and normal coronary arteries. *N Engl J Med* 1982;307:1362.
53. Tauchert M, Hilger HH. Application of the coronary reserve concept to the study of myocardial perfusion. In: Schaper W, ed. *The Pathophysiology of Myocardial Perfusion.* Amsterdam: Elsevier, 1979:141–167.
54. Pichard AD, et al. Coronary flow studies in patients with left ventricular hypertrophy of the hypertensive type: evidence for an impaired coronary vascular reserve. *Am J Cardiol* 1981;47:547.
55. Marcus ML, Mueller TM, Gascho JM, Kerber RE. Effects of cardiac hypertrophy secondary to hypertension on the coronary circulation. *Am J Cardiol* 1979;44:1023–1028.
56. Breisch EA, et al. Myocardial blood flow and capillary density in chronic pressure overload of the feline left ventricle. *Cardiovasc Res* 1980;14:469.
57. Opherk D, et al. Reduction of coronary reserve: a mechanism for angina pectoris in patients with arterial hypertension and normal coronary arteries. *Circulation* 1984;69:1.
58. Kveselis DA, et al. Hemodynamic determinants of exercise-induced ST-segment depression in children with valvar aortic stenosis. *Am J Cardiol* 1985;55:1133.
59. Attarian DE, et al. Characteristics of chronic left ventricular hypertrophy induced by subcoronary valvular aortic stenosis: II. Response to ischemia. *J Thorac Cardiovasc Surg* 1981;81:389.
60. Holley KE, et al. Spontaneous calcific embolization associated with calcific aortic stenosis. *Circulation* 1963;27:197.
61. Soulié P, et al. Les embolies calcaires des orificielles calcifees du coeur gauche. *Arch Mal Coeur* 1969;62:1657.
62. Pleet AB, Massey EW, Vengrow ME. TIA, stroke, and the bicuspid aortic valve. *Neurology* 1981;31:1540.
63. Hollenhurst RW. Significance of bright plaques in the retinal arteries. *JAMA* 1961;178:23.
64. Catelli P. Stenosi aortica valvolare calcifica ed emboli retiniche. *Cardiol Prat* 1968;19:303.

65. Penner R, Font RL. Retinal embolism from calcified vegetations of aortic valve. *Arch Ophthalmology* 1969; 81:565.

66. Brockmeier LB, et al. Calcium emboli to the retinal artery in calcific aortic stenosis. *Am Heart J* 1981;101: 32.

67. Baghdassarian SA, Crawford JB, Rathbun JE. Calcific emboli of the retinal and ciliary arteries. *Am J Ophthalmol* 1970;69:372.

68. Heyde EC. Gastrointestinal bleeding in aortic stenosis [letter]. *N Engl J Med* 1958;259:196.

69. Schwartz BM. Additional note on bleeding in aortic stenosis [letter]. *N Engl J Med* 1958;259:456.

70. Williams RC Jr. Aortic stenosis and unexplained gastrointestinal bleeding. *Arch Intern Med* 1961;108:859.

71. Schoenfeld Y, et al. Aortic stenosis associated with gastrointestinal bleeding: a survey of 612 patients. *Am Heart J* 1980;100:179.

72. Gelfand MW, et al. Gastrointestinal bleeding in aortic stenosis. *Am J Gastroenterol* 1979;71:30.

73. Weaver GA, et al. Gastrointestinal angiodysplasia associated with aortic valve disease: part of a spectrum of angiodysplasia of the gut. *Gastroenterology* 1979; 77:1.

74. Galloway SJ, Casarella WJ, Shimkin PM. Vascular malformation of the right colon as a cause of bleeding in patients with aortic stenosis. *Radiology* 1974; 113:11.

75. McNamara JJ, Austen WG. Gastrointestinal bleeding in patients with acquired valvular heart disease. *Arch Surg* 1968;97:538.

76. Danilewitz D, McKibbin J, Derman D. Cessation of gastrointestinal bleeding after valve replacement of aortic stenosis. *Am Heart J* 1981;101:686.

77. Boyle JM, et al. Severe aortic stenosis in a patient with recurrent gastrointestinal bleeding: replacement of aortic valve with a porcine xenograft. *Am J Gastroenterol* 1981;75:135.

78. Love JW. Syndrome of calcific aortic stenosis and gastrointestinal bleeding: resolution following aortic valve replacement. *J Thorac Cardiovasc Surg* 1982;83: 779.

79. Katznelson G, et al. Combined aortic and mitral stenosis: a clinical and physiological study. *Am J Med* 1960; 29:242.

80. Braunwald E, et al. Congenital aortic stenosis. I. Clinical and hemodynamic findings in 100 patients. *Circulation* 1963;27:426.

81. Perloff JK. Clinical recognition of aortic stenosis. The physical signs and differential diagnosis of the various forms of obstruction to left ventricular outflow. *Prog Cardiovasc Dis* 1968;10:323.

82. Glancy DL, Epstein SE. Differential diagnosis of type and severity of obstruction to left ventricular outflow. *Prog Cardiovasc Dis* 1971;14:153.

83. Effron MK. Aortic stenosis and rupture of mitral chordae tendineae. *J Am Coll Cardiol* 1983;1:1018.

84. Hancock EW. The ejection sound in aortic stenosis. *Am J Med* 1966;40:569.

85. Andersen JA, Hansen BF, Lyngeborg K. Isolated valvular aortic stenosis. *Acta Med Scand* 1975;197:61.

86. Hancock EW, Fleming PR. Aortic stenosis. *Q J Med* 1960;29:209.

87. Frank MJ, et al. The clinical evaluation of aortic regurgitation, with special reference to a neglected sign: the popliteal-brachial pressure gradient. *Arch Intern Med* 1965;116:357.

88. Spodick DH, et al. Rate of rise of the carotid pulse. An investigation of observer error in a common clinical measurement. *Am J Cardiol* 1982;49:159.

89. Alpert JS, Vieweg WVR, Hagan AD. Incidence and morphology of carotid shudders in aortic valve disease. *Am Heart J* 1976;92:435.

90. Chun PKC, Dunn BE. Clinical clue of severe aortic stenosis: simultaneous palpation of the carotid and apical impulses. *Arch Intern Med* 1982;142:2284.

91. Myler RK, Sanders CA. Aortic valve disease and atrial fibrillation: report of 122 patients with electrographic, radiographic, and hemodynamic observations. *Arch Intern Med* 1968;121:530.

92. Eddleman EE Jr, et al. Critical analysis of clinical factors in estimating severity of aortic valve disease. *Am J Cardiol* 1973;31:687.

93. Griffin BP. Valvular heart disease. In: Dale DC, Federman DD, eds. *Scientific American Medicine*. New York: Scientific American, 1998;XI-1–XI-12.

94. Siegel RJ, Roberts WC. Electrocardiographic observations in severe aortic valve stenosis: correlative necropsy study to clinical, hemodynamic, and ECG variables demonstrating relation of 12-lead QRS amplitude to peak systolic transaortic pressure gradient. *Am Heart J* 1982;103:210.

95. Sutnick AI, Soloff LA. P-wave abnormalities as an electrocardiographic index of hemodynamically significant aortic stenosis. *Circulation* 1963;28:814.

96. Contratto AW, Levine SA. Aortic stenosis with special reference to angina pectoris and syncope. *Ann Intern Med* 1937;10:1636.

97. Olshausen KV. Determinants of the incidence and severity of ventricular arrhythmias in aortic valve disease. *Am J Cardiol* 1983;51:1103.

98. Klatte EC, et al. The roentgenographic manifestations of aortic stenosis and aortic valvular insufficiency. *AJR Am J Roentgenol* 1962;88:57.

99. Glancy DL, et al. Calcium in the aortic valve. Roentgenologic and hemodynamic correlations in 148 patients. *Ann Intern Med* 1969;71:245.

100. Reichek N, Devereux RB. Left ventricular hypertrophy: relationship of anatomic, echocardiographic and electrocardiographic findings. *Circulation* 1981;63:1391.

101. Bennett DH, Evans DW, Raj MVJ. Echocardiographic left ventricular dimensions in pressure and volume overload. Their use in assessing aortic stenosis. *Br Heart J* 1975;37:971.

102. Glanz S, et al. Echocardiographic assessment of the severity of aortic stenosis in children and adolescents. *Am J Cardiol* 1976;38:620.

103. Schwartz A, et al. Echocardiographic estimation of aortic-valve gradient in aortic stenosis. *Ann Intern Med* 1978;89:329.

104. Bass JL, et al. Echocardiographic screening to assess the severity of congenital aortic stenosis in children. *Am J Cardiol* 1979;44:82.

105. Massie B. Assessing the severity of aortic stenosis [letter]. *Ann Intern Med* 1979;90:123, 1979.

106. Gewitz MH, et al. Role of echocardiography in aortic stenosis: pre- and post-operative studies. *Am J Cardiol* 1979;43:67.

107. Reichek, N, Devereux RB. Reliable estimation of peak left ventricular systolic pressure by M-mode echocar-

diographic-determined end-diastolic relative wall thickness: identification of severe valvular aortic stenosis in adult patients. *Am Heart J* 1982;103:202.

108. Aziz KU, et al. Echocardiographic assessment of the relation between left ventricular wall and cavity dimensions and peak systolic pressure in children with aortic stenosis. *Am J Cardiol* 1977;40:775.

109. Chin ML, et al. Aortic valve systolic flutter as a screening test for severe aortic stenosis. *Am J Cardiol* 1983;51:981.

110. Williams RG, Tucker CR. *Echocardiographic Diagnosis of Congenital Heart Disease.* Boston: Little, Brown, 1977.

111. Henry WL. Evaluation of older children and adults by M-mode and cross-sectional echocardiography. In: Roberts WC, ed. *Congenital Heart Disease in Adults.* Philadelphia: FA Davis, 1979;139–171.

112. Nanda NC, et al. Echocardiographic recognition of the congenital bicuspid aortic valve. *Circulation* 1974;49:870.

113. Radford DJ, et al. Echocardiographic assessment of bicuspid aortic valves. Angiographic and pathological correlations. *Circulation* 1976;53:80.

114. Yeh H, Winsberg F, Mercer E. Echocardiographic aortic valve orifice dimension: its use in evaluating aortic stenosis and cardiac output. *JCU J Clin Ultrasound* 1973;1:182–189.

115. Chang S, Clements S, Chang J. Aortic stenosis: echocardiographic cusp separation and surgical description of aortic valve in 22 patients. *Am J Cardiol* 1977;39:499.

116. Weyman AE, et al. Cross-sectional echocardiographic assessment of the severity of aortic stenosis in children. *Circulation* 1977;55:773.

117. Weyman AE, et al. Cross-sectional echocardiography in assessing the severity of valvular aortic stenosis. *Circulation* 1975;52:828.

118. Godley RW, et al. Reliability of two-dimensional echocardiography in assessing the severity of valvular aortic stenosis. *Chest* 1981;79:657.

119. Brandenburg RO, et al. Accuracy of 2-dimensional echocardiographic diagnosis of congenitally bicuspid aortic valve: Echocardiographic-anatomic correlation in 115 patients. *Am J Cardiol* 1983;51:1469.

120. Nishimura RA, et al. Doppler echocardiography: theory, instrumentation, technique, and application. *Mayo Clin Proc* 1985;60:321.

121. Richards KL. *Doppler Echocardiography: A Physiologic Approach to Its Use in Adult Cardiology.* New York: Futura Publishing, 1985.

122. Johnson SL, et al. Doppler echocardiography: the localization of cardiac murmurs. *Circulation* 1973;48:810.

123. Baker DW, Rubenstein SA, Lorch GS. Pulsed Doppler echocardiography: principles and applications. *Am J Med* 1977;63:69.

124. Brubakk AO, Angelsen BAJ, Hatle L. Diagnosis of valvular heart disease using transcutaneous Doppler ultrasound. *Cardiovasc Res* 1977;11:461.

125. Richards KL, et al. Noninvasive diagnosis of aortic and mitral valve disease with pulsed-Doppler spectral analysis. *Am J Cardiol* 1983;51:1122.

126. Hatle L, Angelsen B, Tromsdal A. Noninvasive assessment of aortic stenosis by Doppler ultrasound. *Br Heart J* 1980;43:284.

127. Hatle L. Noninvasive assessment and differentiation of

left ventricular outflow obstruction with Doppler ultrasound. *Circulation* 1981;64:381.

128. Stamm R, Martin R. Quantification of pressure gradients across stenotic valves by Doppler ultrasound. *J Am Coll Cardiol* 1983;2:707.

129. Requarth JA, et al. In vitro verification of Doppler prediction of transvalve pressure gradient and orifice area in stenosis. *Am J Cardiol* 1984;53:1364.

130. Colocousis JS, Hutsman LL, Curreri PW. Estimation of stroke volume changes by ultrasonic Doppler. *Circulation* 1977;56:914.

131. Fisher DC, et al. The effect of variations on pulsed Doppler sampling site on calculation of cardiac output: an experimental study in open-chest dogs. *Circulation* 1983;67:370.

132. Huntsman LL, et al. Noninvasive Doppler determination of cardiac output in man: clinical validation. *Circulation* 1983;67:593.

133. Fisher DC, et al. The mitral valve orifice method for noninvasive two-dimensional echo Doppler determinations of cardiac output. *Circulation* 1983;67:872.

134. Nishimura RA, et al. Noninvasive measurement of cardiac output by continuous-wave Doppler echocardiography: initial experience and review of the literature. *Mayo Clin Proc* 1984;59:484.

135. Kosturakis D, et al. Noninvasive quantification of stenotic semilunar valve areas by Doppler echocardiography. *J Am Coll Cardiol* 1984;3:1256.

136. Warth DC, et al. A new method to calculate aortic valve area without left heart catheterization. *Circulation* 1984;70:978.

137. Hatle L, Angelsen B. *Doppler Ultrasound in Cardiology: Physical Principles and Clinical Applications.* Philadelphia: Lea & Febiger, 1982.

138. Lima CO, et al. Prediction of the severity of left ventricular outflow tract obstruction by quantitative two-dimensional echocardiographic Doppler studies. *Circulation* 1983;68:348.

139. Williams GA, et al. Value of multiple echocardiographic views in the evaluation of aortic stenosis in adults by continuous-wave Doppler. *Am J Cardiol* 1985;55:445.

140. Miyatake K, et al. Clinical applications of a new type of real-time two-dimensional Doppler flow imaging system. *Am J Cardiol* 1984;54:857.

140a. Kim CJ, Berglund H, Nishioka T, Luo H, Siegel RJ. Correspondence of aortic valve area determination from transesophageal echocardiography, transthoracic echocardiography, and cardiac catheterization. *Am Heart J* 1996;132:1163–1172.

141. Omoto R. *Color Atlas of Real-Time Two-Dimensional Doppler Echocardiography.* Tokyo: Shindam-to-Chiryo, 1984.

142. Otto CM, et al. Measurement of peak flow velocity in adults with valvular aortic stenosis using high pulse repetition frequency duplex pulsed Doppler echocardiography. *J Am Coll Cardiol* 1984;3:494.

143. Rahimtoola SH. Perspective on valvular heart disease: update II. In: Knoebel S, ed. *Era in Cardiovascular Medicine.* New York: Elsevier, 1991:45–70.

143a. Popovic AD, Thomas JD, Neskovic AN, Cosgrove DM, Stewart WJ, Lauer MS. Time-related trends in the preoperative evaluation of patients with aortic stenosis. *Am J Cardiol* 1997;80:1464–1468.

144. Levinson GE, Cudkowicz L, Abelmann WH. Measure-

ment of regional blood flow by indicator dilution. *Science* 1959;129:840.

145. Frank MJ, et al. Measurement of aortic regurgitation by upstream sampling using continuous infusions of indicator. *Circulation* 1966;33:545.

146. Frank MJ, Casanegra, P, Levinson GE. Accuracy of measurements of aortic regurgitation using continuous dye infusions. *J Appl Physiol* 1966;21:1405.

147. Sandler H, et al. Quantitation of valvular insufficiency in man by angiocardiography. *Am Heart J* 1963;65: 501.

148. Levine HJ, et al. Force-velocity relations in failing and nonfailing hearts of subjects with aortic stenosis. *Am J Med Sci* 1970;259:79.

149. Gorlin R, et al. Left ventricular volume in man measured by thermodilution. *J Clin Invest* 1964;43:1203.

150. Levinson GE, et al. Studies of cardiopulmonary blood volume. Measurement of left ventricular volume by dye dilution. *Circulation* 1967;35:1038.

151. Kennedy JW, et al. Quantitative angiocardiography. III. Relationships of left ventricular pressure, volume, and mass in aortic valve disease. *Circulation* 1968;38: 838.

152. Gault JH, Ross J Jr, Braunwald E. Contractile state of the left ventricle in man. Instantaneous tension-velocity-length relations in patients with and without disease of the left ventricular myocardium. *Circ Res* 1968;22:1451.

153. Frank MJ, Levinson GE. An index of the contractile state of the myocardium in man. *J Clin Invest* 1968;47: 1615.

154. Karliner JS, Peterson KL, Ross J Jr. Myocardial mechanics: assessment of isovolumic and ejection phase indices of left ventricular performance. In: Grossman W, ed. *Cardiac Catheterization and Angiography*. Philadelphia: Lea & Febiger, 2nd ed. 1980;245–267.

155. Levinson GE. The myocardial factor in rheumatic heart disease. In: Bailey C, ed. *Advances in the Management of Clinical Heart Disease*. Mt. Kisco, NY: Futura Publishing, 1976;149–189.

156. Lehman JS, Boyle JJ, Debbas JN. Quantitation of aortic valvular insufficiency by catheter thoracic aortography. *Radiology* 1972;79:361.

157. Levinson GE, et al. Measurement of mitral regurgitation in man from simultaneous atrial and arterial dilution curves after ventricular injection. *Circulation* 1961; 24:720.

158. Frank MJ, et al. Measurement of mitral regurgitation in man by upstream sampling method using continuous indicator infusions. *Circulation* 1967;35:100.

159. Ettinger PO, Frank MJ, Levinson GE. Hemodynamics at rest and during exercise in combined aortic stenosis and regurgitation. *Circulation* 1972;45:267.

160. Greenberg BH, Massie BM. Beneficial effects of afterload reduction therapy in patients with congestive heart failure and moderate aortic stenosis. *Circulation* 1980;61:1212.

161. Awan NA, et al. Beneficial effects of nitroprusside administration on left ventricular dysfunction and myocardial ischemia in severe aortic stenosis. *Am Heart J* 1981;101:386.

162. Folland ED, et al. Intraaortic balloon counterpulsation as a temporary support measure in decompensated critical aortic stenosis. *J Am Coll Cardiol* 1985;5:711.

163. Wagner S, Selzer A. Patterns of progression of aortic stenosis: a longitudinal hemodynamic study. *Circulation* 1982;65:709.

164. Jonasson R, et al. Rate of progression of severity of valvular aortic stenosis. *Acta Med Scand* 1983;213:51.

165. Nestico PF, et al. Progression of isolated aortic stenosis: analysis of 29 patients having more than one cardiac catheterization. *Am J Cardiol* 1983;52:1054.

166. Bogart D, et al. Progression of aortic stenosis. *Chest* 1979;76:391.

167. Cheitlin MD, et al. Rate of progression of severity of valvular aortic stenosis in the adult. *Am Heart J* 1979; 98:689.

168. Huhta JC, et al. Echocardiography in the diagnosis and management of symptomatic aortic valve stenosis in infants. *Circulation* 1984;70:438.

169. Roberts WC. Reasons for cardiac catheterization before cardiac valve replacement. *N Engl J Med* 1982; 306:1291.

170. Lafrak EA, Starr A. *Cardiac Valve Prostheses*. New York: Appleton-Century-Crofts, 1979.

171. Gallucci V, et al. Heart valve replacement with the Hancock bioprosthesis: a 5–11 year follow-up. In: Cohn LH, Gallucci V, eds. *Cardiac Bioprostheses. Proceedings of the Second International Symposium*. New York: Yorke Medical, 1982:9.

172. Gonzalez-Lavin L, et al. Five-year experience with the Ionescu-Shiley bovine pericardial valve in the aortic position. *Ann Thorac Surg* 1983;36:270.

173. Teply JF, et al. The ultimate prognosis after valve replacement: an assessment at twenty years. *Ann Thorac Surg* 1981;32:111.

174. Wain WH, Drury PJ, Ross DN. Aortic valve replacement with Starr-Edwards valves over 14 years. *Ann Thorac Surg* 1982;33:562.

175. Fuster V, et al. Systemic thromboembolism in mitral and aortic Starr-Edwards prostheses: a 10–19 year follow-up. *Circ C V Surg* 1982;66:1157.

176. McGoon MD, et al. Aortic and mitral valve incompetence: long-term follow-up (10 to 19 years) of patients treated with the Starr-Edwards prosthesis. *J Am Coll Cardiol* 1984;3:930.

177. Lytle BW, et al. Replacement of aortic valve combined with myocardial revascularization: determinants of early and late risk for 500 patients, 1967–1981. *Circulation* 1983;68:1149.

178. Curcio CA, et al. Calcification of glutaraldehyde-preserved porcine xenografts in young patients. *J Thorac Cardiovasc Surg* 1981;81:621.

179. Dunn JM. Porcine valve durability in children. *Ann Thorac Surg* 1981;32:357.

180. Craver JM, et al. Porcine cardiac xenograft valves: analysis of survival, valve failure and explanation. *Ann Thorac Surg* 1982;34:16.

181. Geha AS, et al. Factors affecting performance and thromboembolism after porcine xenograft cardiac valve replacement. *J Thorac Cardiovasc Surg* 1982; 83:377.

182. Gardner TJ, et al. Valve replacement in children: a fifteen-year perspective. *J Thorac Cardiovasc Surg* 1982; 83:178.

183. Gallo I, et al. Degeneration in porcine bioprosthetic cardiac valves: incidence of primary tissue failures among 938 bioprostheses at risk. *Am J Cardiol* 1984; 53:1061.

184. Kutsche LM, et al. An important complication of Han-

cock mitral valve replacement in children. *Circulation* 1979;60[Suppl I]:I98.

185. Ferrans VJ, et al. Calcific deposits in porcine bioprostheses: structure and pathogenesis. *Am J Cardiol* 1980; 46:72.

186. Sanders SP, et al. Use of Hancock porcine xenografts in children and adolescents. *Am J Cardiol* 1980;46: 429.

187. Schoen FJ, Collins JJ, Cohn LH. Long-term failure rate and morphologic correlations in porcine bioprosthetic heart valves. *Am J Cardiol* 1983;51:957.

188. Schoen RJ, Levy RJ. Bioprosthetic heart valve failure: pathology and pathogenesis. In: Waller B, ed. *Cardiology Clinics. Cardiac Morphology*. Vol. 2. Philadelphia: W.B. Saunders, 1984:717.

189. Williams JB, et al. Considerations in selection and management of patients undergoing valve replacement with glutaraldehyde-fixed porcine bioprostheses. *Ann Thorac Surg* 1980;30:247.

190. Ishihara T, et al. Structure and classification of cuspal tears and perforations in porcine bioprosthetic cardiac valves implanted in patients. *Am J Cardiol* 1981;48: 665.

191. Stein PD, et al. Relation of calcification to torn leaflets of spontaneously degenerated porcine bioprosthetic valves. *Circulation* 1983;68[Suppl III]:III205(abst).

192. Grenadier E, et al. Detection of deterioration or infection of homograft and porcine xenograft bioprosthetic valves in mitral and aortic positions by two-dimensional echocardiographic examination. *J Am Coll Cardiol* 1983;2:452.

193. Forman MB, et al. Correlation of two-dimensional echocardiography and pathologic findings in porcine valve dysfunction. *J Am Coll Cardiol* 1985;5:224.

194. Alam M, Goldstein S, Lakier JB. Echocardiographic changes in the thickness of porcine valves with time. *Chest* 1981;79:663.

195. Carpentier A, et al. Techniques for prevention of calcification of valvular bioprostheses. *Circulation* 1984; 70[Suppl I]:I165.

196. Levy RJ, et al. Inhibition by diphosphonate compounds of calcification of porcine bioprosthetic heart valve cusps implanted subcutaneously in rats. *Circulation* 1985;71:349.

197. Jones M, Barnhart GR, Morrow AG. Late results after operations for left ventricular outflow tract obstruction. *Am J Cardiol* 1982;50:569.

198. Dobell ARC, et al. Congenital valvular aortic stenosis: surgical management and long-term results. *J Thorac Cardiovasc Surg* 1981;81:916.

199. Presbitero P, et al. Open aortic valvotomy for congenital aortic stenosis: late results. *Br Heart J* 1982;47:26.

200. Ankeney JL, Tzeng TS, Liebman J. Surgical therapy for congenital aortic valvular stenosis: a 23-year experience. *J Thorac Cardiovasc Surg* 1983;85:41.

201. Oyer PE, et al. Clinical durability of the Hancock porcine bioprosthetic valve. *J Thorac Cardiovasc Surg* 1980;80:824.

202. Warnes CA, et al. Comparison of late degenerative changes in porcine bioprostheses in the mitral and aortic valve position in the same patient. *Am J Cardiol* 1983;51:965.

203. Salazar E, et al. The problem of cardiac valve prostheses, anticoagulants, pregnancy. *Circulation* 1984;70 [Suppl I]:I169.

204. Shimon D, et al. Accelerated calcific degeneration of a bovine pericardial valve in an adolescent. *J Thorac Cardiovasc Surg* 1982;83:794.

205. Walker WE, et al. Early experience with the Ionescu-Shiley pericardial xenograft valve: accelerated calcification in children. *J Thorac Cardiovasc Surg* 1983; 86:570.

206. Fiddler GI, et al. Calcification of glutaraldehyde-preserved porcine and bovine xenograft valves in young children. *Ann Thorac Surg* 1983;35:257.

207. Penta A, et al. Patient status 10 or more years after "fresh" homograft replacement of the aortic valve. *Circulation* 70[Suppl I]:I182.

208. Hylen JC, et al. Aortic ball variance: diagnosis and treatment. *Ann Intern Med* 1970;72:1.

209. Sears DA, Crosby WH. Intravascular hemolysis due to intracardiac prosthetic devices. *Am J Med* 1965;39:341.

210. Santinga JT, et al. Hemolysis in the aortic prosthetic valve. *Chest* 1976;69:56.

211. Harrison EC, et al. Cholelithiasis: a frequent complication of artificial valve replacement. *Am Heart J* 1978;95:483.

212. Marshall WG, et al. Early results of valve replacement with the Bjork-Shiley convexoconcave prosthesis. *Ann Thorac Surg* 1984;37:398.

213. Wolfe SM, Greenberg A. Strut fractures with the Bjork-Shiley valve [letter]. *N Engl J Med* 1985;312: 314.

214. Kloster FE. Infective prosthetic valve endocarditis. In: Rahimtoola SH, ed. *Infective Endocarditis*. New York: Grune & Stratton, 1978:291–305.

215. Calderwood SB. Risk factors for the development of prosthetic valve endocarditis. *Circulation* 1985;72:31.

216. Cohn LH, et al. Five-to-eight-year follow-up of patients undergoing porcine heart valve replacement. *N Engl J Med* 1981;304:258.

217. Williams WG, et al. Experience with aortic and mitral valve replacement in children. *J Thorac Cardiovasc Surg* 1981;81:326.

218. Copeland JG, et al. Long-term follow-up after isolated aortic valve replacement. *J Thorac Cardiovasc Surg* 1977;74:875.

219. Thompson R, et al. Influence of preoperative left ventricular function on results of homograft replacement of the aortic valve for aortic stenosis. *Am J Cardiol* 1979;43:929.

220. Stephenson W, MacVaugh H III, Edmunds LH Jr. Surgery using cardiopulmonary bypass in the elderly. *Circulation* 1978;58:250.

220a. Lund O, Jensen FT, Emmertsen K, et al. Left ventricular systolic and diastolic function in aortic stenosis prognostic value after valve replacement and underlying mechanisms. *Eur Heart J* 1997;18:1977–1987.

221. Schwarz F, et al. Impaired left ventricular function in chronic aortic valve disease: survival and function after replacement by Bjork-Shiley prosthesis. *Circulation* 1979;60:48.

222. Kennedy JW, Doces J, Stewart DK. Left ventricular function before and following aortic valve replacement. *Circulation* 1977;56:944.

223. Miller DC, et al. Surgical implications and results of combined aortic valve replacement and myocardial revascularization. *Am J Cardiol* 1979;43:494.

224. Murphy ES, et al. Severe aortic stenosis in patients 60 years of age and older: left ventricular function and

10-year survival after valve replacement. *Circulation* 1981;64:184.

225. Copeland JG, et al. Isolated aortic valve replacement in patients older than 65 years. *JAMA* 1977;237:1578.

226. Smith N, McAnulty JH, Rahimtoola S. Severe aortic stenosis with impaired left ventricular function and clinical heart failure: results of valve replacement. *Circulation* 1978;58:255.

227. Croke RP, et al. Reversal of advanced left ventricular dysfunction following aortic valve replacement for aortic stenosis. *Ann Thorac Surg* 1977;24:38.

228. O'Toole JD, et al. Effect of preoperative ejection fraction on survival and hemodynamic improvement following aortic valve replacement. *Circulation* 1978;58:1175.

229. Ross J Jr. Afterload mismatch in aortic and mitral valve disease: implications for surgical therapy. *J Am Coll Cardiol* 1985;5:811.

230. Sanders JH, et al. Emergency aortic valve replacement. *Am J Surg* 1976;131:495.

230a. Connolly HM, Oh JK, Orszulak TA, et al. Aortic valve replacement for aortic stenosis with severe left ventricular dysfunction. Prognostic indicators. *Circulation* 1997;95:2395–2400.

231. Bonow RO, et al. Aortic valve replacement without myocardial revascularization in patients with combined aortic valvular and coronary artery disease. *Circulation* 1981;63:243.

232. Kirklin JW, Douchoukos NT. Aortic valve replacement without myocardial revascularization [editorial]. *Circulation* 1981;63:252.

233. Nunley DL, Grunkemeier GL, Starr A. Aortic valve replacement with coronary bypass grafting: significant determinants of 10-year survival. *J Thorac Cardiovasc Surg* 1983;85:705.

234. Richardson JV. Combined aortic valve replacement and myocardial revascularization: results in 220 patients. *Circulation* 1979;59:75.

235. Angell WW, Angell JD, Kosek JC. Twelve year experience with glutaraldehyde-preserved porcine xenografts. *J Thorac Cardiovasc Surg* 1982;83:493.

236. Rapaport E. Natural history of aortic and mitral valve disease. *Am J Cardiol* 1975;35:221.

237. Frank S, Johnson A, Ross J Jr. Natural history of valvular aortic stenosis. *Br Heart J* 1973;35:41.

238. Schwarz F, et al. Effect of aortic valve replacement on survival. *Circulation* 1982;66:1105.

238a. Rahimtoola SH. Catheter balloon valvuloplasty for severe calcific aortic stenosis: a limited role. *J Am Coll Cardiol* 1994;23:1076–1078.

238b. Otto CM, Mickel MC, Kennedy JW, et al. Three year outcome after balloon aortic valvuloplasty: insights into prognosis of vavlular aortic stenosis. *Circulation* 1994;89:642–650.

238c. Moreno PR, Jang IK, Newell JB, Block PC, Palacios IF. The role of percutaneous aortic balloon valvuloplasty in patients with cardiogenic shock and critical aortic stenosis. *J Am Coll Cardiol* 1994;23:1071–1075.

239. Hancock EW. Differentiation of valvar, subvalvar and supravalvar aortic stenosis. *Guy's Hosp Rep* 1961;110:1.

240. Kelly DT, Wulfsberg BA, Rowe RD. Discrete subaortic stenosis. *Circulation* 1972;46:309.

241. Vogel JHK, Blount SG Jr. Clinical evaluation in localizing level of obstruction to outflow from left ventri-

cle. Importance of early systolic ejection click. *Am J Cardiol* 1965;15:782.

242. Lees MH, et al. Congenital aortic stenosis. Operative indications and surgical results. *Br Heart J* 1962;24:31.

243. Roberts WC. Discrete subaortic stenosis. In: Roberts WC, ed. *Congenital Heart Disease in Adults.* Philadelphia: FA Davis, 1979:426–429.

244. Reis RL, Peterson LM, Mason DT, Simon AL, Morrow AG. Congenital fixed subvalvular aortic stenosis. An anatomical classification and correlations with operative results. *Circulation* 1971;43[Suppl I]:11.

245. Newfeld EA, et al. Discrete subvalvular aortic stenosis in childhood. Study of 51 patients. *Am J Cardiol* 1976;38:53.

246. Sung CS, Price EC, Cooley DA. Discrete subaortic stenosis in adults. *Am J Cardiol* 1978;42:283.

247. Fontana RS, Edwards JE. *Congenital Cardiac Disease. A Review of 357 Cases Studied Pathologically.* Philadelphia: WB Saunders, 1962.

248. Jue KL, Edwards JE. Anomalous attachment of mitral valve causing subaortic atresia. *Circulation* 1967;35:928.

249. Cooperberg B, Hazell S, Ashmore PG. Parachute accessory anterior mitral valve leaflet causing left ventricular outflow tract obstruction. *Circulation* 1976;53:908.

250. Kuribayashi R, et al. Subaortic stenosis caused by an accessory tissue of the mitral valve. *J Cardiovasc Surg* 1979;20:591.

251. Krueger SK, et al. Echocardiography in discrete subaortic stenosis. *Circulation* 1979;59:506.

252. Hagaman JF, Wolfe C, Craige E. Early aortic valve closure in combined idiopathic hypertrophic subaortic stenosis and discrete subaortic stenosis. *Am J Cardiol* 1980;45:1083.

253. Deutsch V, et al. Subaortic stenosis (discrete form): classification and angiocardiographic features. *Radiology* 1971;101:275.

254. Lundquist CB, Amplatz K. The subvalvular aortic jet. *Radiology* 1965;85:635.

255. Shem-Tov A, et al. Clinical presentation and natural history of mild discrete subaortic stenosis: follow-up of 1–17 years. *Circulation* 1982;66:509.

256. Wright GB, et al. Fixed subaortic stenosis in the young: medical and surgical course in 83 patients. *Am J Cardiol* 1983;52:830.

257. Roberts WC. Characteristics and consequences of infective endocarditis (active or healed or both) learned from morphologic studies. In: Rahimtoola SH, ed. *Infective Endocarditis.* New York: Grune & Stratton, 1978:55–123.

258. Mody MR, Mody GT. Serial hemodynamic observations in congenital valvular and subvalvular stenosis. *Am Heart J* 1975;89:137.

259. Shone MB, et al. The developmental complex of "parachute mitral valve," supravalvular ring of left atrium, subaortic stenosis, and coarctation of aorta. *Am J Cardiol* 1963;11:714.

260. Noonan JA, Ehmke DA. Associated noncardiac malformations in children with congenital heart disease. *J Pediatr* 1963;63:468.

261. Maron BJ, et al. Tunnel subaortic stenosis. *Circulation* 1976;54:403.

262. Reder RF, et al. Left ventricle to aorta valved conduit

for relief of diffuse left ventricular outflow tract obstruction. *Am J Cardiol* 1977;39:1068.

263. Bjornstad PG, et al. Aortoventriculoplasty for tunnel subaortic stenosis and other obstructions of the left ventricular outflow tract. *Circulation* 1979;60:59.

264. Ergin MA, et al. Experience with left ventricular apicoaortic conduits for complicated left ventricular outflow obstruction in children and young adults. *Ann Thorac Surg* 1981;32:369.

265. Rocchini AP, et al. Clinical and hemodynamic follow-up of left ventricular to aortic conduits in patients with aortic stenosis. *J Am Coll Cardiol* 1983;1:1135.

266. de Vivie ER, et al. Aortoventriculoplasty for different types of left ventricular outflow tract obstructions. *J Cardiovasc Surg* 1982;23:6.

267. Misbach GA, et al. Left ventricular outflow enlargement by the Konno procedure. *J Thorac Cardiovasc Surg* 1982;84:696.

268. Clark CE, Henry WL, Epstein SE. Familial prevalence and genetic transmission of idiopathic hypertrophic subaortic stenosis. *N Engl J Med* 1973;289:709.

269. Teare D. Asymmetrical hypertrophy of the heart in young adults. *Br Heart J* 1958;20:1.

270. Maron BJ, Roberts WC. Quantitative analysis of cardiac muscle cell disorganization in the ventricular septum of patients with hypertrophic cardiomyopathy. *Circulation* 1979;59:689.

271. Henry WL, Clark CE, Epstein SE. Asymmetric septal hypertrophy (ASH): echocardiographic identification of the pathognomonic anatomic abnormality of IHSS. *Circulation* 1973;47:225.

272. Rossen RM, et al. Ventricular systolic septal thickening and excursion in idiopathic hypertrophic subaortic stenosis. *N Engl J Med* 1974;291:1317.

273. Fix P, et al. Muscular subvalvular aortic stenosis: abnormal anterior mitral leaflet possibly the primary factor. *Acta Radiol* 1964;2:177.

274. Goodwin JF. IHSS? HOCM? ASH: a plea for unity. *Am Heart J* 1975;89:269–277.

275. Braunwald E, et al. Subaortic stenosis. American Heart Association Monograph Number 10. New York: The American Heart Association, 1964:119.

276. Henry WL, Clark CE, Griffith JM. Mechanism of left ventricular outflow obstruction in patients with obstructive asymmetric septal hypertrophy (idiopathic hypertrophic subaortic stenosis). *Am J Cardiol* 1975;35:337.

277. Maron BJ, et al. Systolic anterior motion of the posterior mitral leaflet: a previously unrecognized cause of dynamic subaortic obstruction in patients with hypertrophic cardiomyopathy. *Circulation* 1983;68:282.

278. Maron BJ, Epstein SE. Hypertrophic cardiomyopathy: a discussion of nomenclature. *Am J Cardiol* 1979;43:1242.

279. Maron BJ, et al. Differences in distribution of myocardial abnormalities in patients with obstructive and nonobstructive asymmetric septal hypertrophy (ASH): light and electron microscopic findings. *Circulation* 1974;50:436.

280. Maron BJ, Anan TJ, Roberts WC. Quantitative analysis of the distribution of cardiac muscle cell disorganization in the left ventricular wall of patients with hypertrophic cardiomyopathy. *Circulation* 1981;63:882.

281. Maron BJ, Roberts WC. Hypertrophic cardiomyopathy and cardiac muscle cell disorganization revisited: relation between the two and significance. *Am Heart J* 1981;101:95.

282. Wigle ED, Rakowski H, Kimball BP, Williams WG. Hypertrophic cardiomyopathy—clinical spectrum and treatment. *Circulation* 1995;92:1680–1692.

283. Marian AJ, Roberts R. Recent advances in the molecular genetics of hypertrophic cardiomyopathy. *Circulation* 1995;92:1336–1347.

284. Nimura H, Bachinski LL, Sangwatanaroj S, et al. Mutations in the gene for cardiac myosin binding protein C and late onset familial hypertrophic cardiomyopathy. *N Engl J Med* 1998;338:1248–1257.

285. Brugada R, Kelsey W, Lechin M, et al. Role of candidate modifier genes on the phenotypic expression of hypertrophy in patients with hypertrophic cardiomyopathy. *J Invest Med* 1997;45:542–551.

286. Canedo MI, Frank MJ. Therapy of hypertrophic cardiomyopathy: medical or surgical? Clinical and pathophysiologic considerations. *Am J Cardiol* 1981;48:383.

287. Murgo JP. Does outflow obstruction exist in hypertrophic cardiomyopathy? *N Engl J Med* 1982;107:1008.

288. Murgo JP, et al. Dynamics of left ventricular ejection in obstructive and nonobstructive hypertrophied cardiomyopathy. *J Clin Invest* 1980;66:1369.

289. Goodwin JF. The frontiers of cardiomyopathy. *Br Heart J* 1982;48:1.

290. Glancy DL, et al. The dynamic nature of left ventricular outflow obstruction in idiopathic hypertrophic subaortic stenosis. *Ann Intern Med* 1971;75:589.

291. Wynne J, Braunwald E. Hypertrophic cardiomyopathy. In: Braunwald E, ed. *Heart Disease. A Textbook of Cardiovascular Medicine.* Philadelphia: WB Saunders, 1980:1447.

292. Hirota Y, et al. Hypertrophic nonobstructive cardiomyopathy: a precise assessment of hemodynamic characteristics and clinical implications. *Am J Cardiol* 1982;50:990.

293. Sakurai S, et al. Production of systolic anterior motion of the mitral valve in dogs. *Circulation* 1985;71:805.

294. Carter WH, Whalen RE, McIntosh HD. Reversal of hemodynamic and phonocardiographic abnormalities in idiopathic hypertrophic subaortic stenosis. *Am J Cardiol* 1971;28:722.

295. Kossowsky WA, et al. Acute myocardial infarction in idiopathic hypertrophic subaortic stenosis. *Chest* 1973;64:529.

296. Caplan J, et al. Clinical improvement in hypertrophic cardiomyopathy after inferior myocardial infarction. *J Am Coll Cardiol* 1985;5:797.

297. Gotsman MS, Lewis BS. Left ventricular volumes and compliance in hypertrophic cardiomyopathy. *Chest* 1974;66:498.

298. Goodwin JF, Oakley CM. The cardiomyopathies. *Br Heart J* 1972;34:545.

299. Epstein SE, et al. Asymmetric septal hypertrophy. *Ann Intern Med* 1974;81:650.

300. Maron BJ, et al. Dynamic subaortic obstruction in hypertrophic cardiomyopathy: analysis by pulsed Doppler echocardiography. *J Am Coll Cardiol* 1985;6:1.

301. Hardarson T, et al. Prognosis and mortality of hypertrophic obstructive cardiomyopathy. *Lancet* 1973;2:1462.

302. Shah PM, et al. The natural and unnatural history of hypertrophic obstructive cardiomyopathy. *Circ Res* 1974; 35[Suppl 2]:179.

302a. Takagi E, Yamakado T, Nakano T. Prognosis of completely asymptomatic adult patients with hypertrophic cardiomyopathy. *J Am Coll Cardiol* 1999;33:206–211.

302b. Maron BJ, Casey SA, Poliac LC, Gohman TE, Almquist A, Aeppli DM. Clinical course of cover hypertrophic cardiomyopathy in a regional United States cohort. *JAMA* 1999;281:650–655.

303. Dinsmore RE, Sanders CA, Harthorne JW. Mitral regurgitation in idiopathic hypertrophic subaortic stenosis. *N Engl J Med* 1966;275:1225.

304. Pridie RB, Oakley CM. Mechanism of mitral regurgitation in hypertrophic obstructive cardiomyopathy. *Br Heart J* 1970;32:203.

305. Buda AJ, Mackenzie GW, Wigle ED. Effect of negative intrathoracic pressure on left ventricular outflow tract obstruction in muscular subaortic stenosis. *Circulation* 1981;63:875.

306. Savage DD, et al. Electrocardiographic findings in patients with obstructive and nonobstructive hypertrophic cardiomyopathy. *Circulation* 1978;48:402.

307. Goodwin JF, et al. Obstructive cardiomyopathy simulating aortic stenosis. *Br Heart J* 1960;22:403.

308. Frank S, Braunwald E. Idiopathic hypertrophic subaortic stenosis. Clinical analysis of 126 patients with emphasis on the natural history. *Circulation* 1968;37:759.

309. Cosio FG, et al. Preexcitation patterns in hypertrophic cardiomyopathy. *Am Heart J* 1981;101:233.

310. Shah PM, Gramiak, R, Kramer DH. Ultrasound location of left ventricular outflow obstruction in hypertrophic obstructive cardiomyopathy. *Circulation* 1969; 40:3.

311. Tajik AJ, Giuliani ER. Echocardiographic observations in idiopathic hypertrophic subaortic stenosis. *Mayo Clin Proc* 1974;49:89.

312. Chahine RA, et al. Mid-systolic closure of aortic valve in hypertrophic cardiomyopathy. *Am J Cardiol* 1979; 43:17.

313. Wei JY, Weiss JL, Bulkley BH. The heterogeneity of hypertrophic cardiomyopathy: an autopsy and one dimensional echocardiographic study. *Am J Cardiol* 1980;45:24.

314. Doi YL, et al. M-mode echocardiography in hypertrophic cardiomyopathy: diagnostic criteria and prediction of obstruction. *Am J Cardiol* 1980;45:6.

315. Maron BJ, Epstein SE. Hypertrophic cardiomyopathy. Recent observations regarding the specificity of three hallmarks of the disease: asymmetric septal hypertrophy, septal disorganization, and systolic anterior motion of the anterior mitral leaflet. *Am J Cardiol* 1980; 45:141.

316. Maron BJ, Gottdiener JS, Lowell WP. Specificity of systolic anterior motion of anterior mitral leaflet for hypertrophic cardiomyopathy. Prevalence in large population of patients with other cardiac diseases. *Br Heart J* 1981;45:206.

317. Pollick C, Rakowski H, Wigle ED. Muscular subaortic stenosis: the quantitative relationship between systolic anterior motion and the pressure gradient. *Circulation* 1984;69:43.

318. ten Cate FJ, et al. Prevalence of diagnostic abnormalities in patients with genetically transmitted asymmetric septal hypertrophy. *Am J Cardiol* 1979;43:731.

319. Maron BJ, et al. Hypertrophic cardiomyopathy with unusual locations of left ventricular hypertrophy undetectable by M-mode echocardiography. *Circulation* 1981;63:409.

320. Maron BJ. Asymmetry in hypertrophic cardiomyopathy: the septal to free wall thickness ratio revisited. *Am J Cardiol* 1985;55:835.

321. Maron BJ, Gottdiener JS, Epstein SE. Patterns and significance of the distribution of left ventricular hypertrophy in hypertrophic cardiomyopathy: a wide-angle, two-dimensional echocardiographic study of 125 patients. *Am J Cardiol* 1981;48:418.

322. Ciro E, Nichols PF III, Maron BJ. Heterogeneous morphologic expression of genetically transmitted hypertrophic cardiomyopathy. Two-dimensional echocardiographic analysis. *Circulation* 1983;67:1227.

323. Maron BJ, et al. Patterns of inheritance in hypertrophic cardiomyopathy. Assessment by M-mode and two-dimensional echocardiography. *Am J Cardiol* 1984;53: 1087.

324. Maron BJ, et al. Unusual distribution of left ventricular hypertrophy in obstructive hypertrophic cardiomyopathy: localized posterobasal free wall thickening in two patients. *J Am Coll Cardiol* 1985;5:1474.

325. Higgins CB, et al. Magnetic resonance imaging in hypertrophic cardiomyopathy. *Am J Cardiol* 1985;55: 1121.

326. Ibrahim M, et al. Systolic time intervals in valvular aortic stenosis and idiopathic hypertrophic subaortic stenosis. *Br Heart J* 1973;35:276.

327. Rothfeld EL, Zucker IR. Vectorcardiographic analysis of the pseudo-infarction pattern in idiopathic hypertrophic subaortic stenosis. *Angiology* 1971;22:609.

328. Lie JT. Hypertrophic cardiomyopathy and coronary heart disease. *Mayo Clin Proc* 1980;55:54.

329. Walston A II, Behar VS. Spectrum of coronary artery disease in idiopathic hypertrophic subaortic stenosis. *Am J Cardiol* 1976;38:12.

330. Lardani, H, Serrano JA, Villamil RJ. Hemodynamics and coronary angiography in idiopathic hypertrophic subaortic stenosis. *Am J Cardiol* 1978;41:476.

331. Maron BJ, Epstein SE, Roberts WC. Hypertrophic cardiomyopathy and transmural myocardial infarction without significant atherosclerosis of the extramural coronary arteries. *Am J Cardiol* 1979;43:1086.

332. Thompson DS, et al. Effects of propranolol on myocardial oxygen consumption, substrate extraction, and hemodynamics in hypertrophic obstructive cardiomyopathy. *Br Heart J* 1980;44:488.

333. Hanrath P, et al. Myocardial thallium-201 imaging in hypertrophic obstructive cardiomyopathy. *Eur Heart J* 1981;2:177.

334. Pichard AD, et al. Septal perforator compression (narrowing) in idiopathic hypertrophic subaortic stenosis. *Am J Cardiol* 1977;40:310.

335. James TH, Marshall TK. De subitaneis mortibus. XII. Asymmetrical hypertrophy of the heart. *Circulation* 1975;51:1149.

336. Pasternac A, et al. Pathophysiology of chest pain in patients with cardiomyopathies and normal coronary arteries. *Circulation* 1982;65:778.

337. Cannon RO III, et al. Myocardial ischemia in patients with hypertrophic cardiomyopathy: contribution of inadequate vasodilator reserve and elevated left ventricular filling pressures. *Circulation* 1985;71:234.

338. Gutgesell HP, et al. Transient hypertrophic subaortic stenosis in infants of diabetic mothers. *J Pediatr* 1976; 89:120.

339. Whiting RB, et al. Idiopathic hypertrophic subaortic stenosis in the elderly. *N Engl J Med* 1971;285:196.

340. Green CE, Elliott LP, Coghlan HC. Improved cineangiographic evaluation of hypertrophic cardiomyopathy by caudocranial left anterior oblique view. *Am Heart J* 1981;102:1015.

341. Maron B, Epstein SE. Clinical course of patients with hypertrophic cardiomyopathy. In: Roberts WC, ed. *Congenital Heart Disease in Adults.* Philadelphia: FA Davis, 1979:253–265.

342. Maron BJ, et al. Sudden death in patients with hypertrophic cardiomyopathy: characterization of 26 patients without functional limitation. *Am J Cardiol* 1978;41:803.

343. Swan DA, et al. Analysis of the symptomatic course and treatment of hypertrophic obstructive cardiomyopathy. *Br Heart J* 1971;33:671.

344. McKenna W, et al. Prognosis in hypertrophic cardiomyopathy: role of age and clinical, electrocardiographic and hemodynamic features. *Am J Cardiol* 1981;47:531.

345. Maron BJ, Roberts WC, Epstein SE. Sudden death in hypertrophic cardiomyopathy: profile of 78 patients. *Circulation* 1982;65:1388.

346. McKenna WJ, et al. Arrhythmia in hypertrophic cardiomyopathy: exercise and 48 hour ambulatory electrocardiographic assessment with and without beta adrenergic blocking therapy. *Am J Cardiol* 1980;45: 1.

347. Maron BJ, et al. Prognostic significance of 24 hour ambulatory electrocardiographic monitoring in patients with hypertrophic cardiomyopathy: a prospective study. *Am J Cardiol* 1981;48:252.

348. McKenna WJ, et al. Arrhythmia in hypertrophic cardiomyopathy. I. Influence on prognosis. *Br Heart J* 1981;46:168.

349. Maron BJ, et al. "Malignant" hypertrophic cardiomyopathy: identification of a subgroup of families with unusually frequent premature death. *Am J Cardiol* 1978;41:1133.

350. McKenna WJ, et al. The natural history of LV hypertrophy in HC: an electrocardiographic study. *Circulation* 1982;66:1233.

351. Maron BJ, et al. Hypertrophic cardiomyopathy with ventricular septal hypertrophy localized to the apical region of the left ventricle (apical hypertrophic cardiomyopathy). *Am J Cardiol* 1982;49:1838.

352. Maron BJ, et al. Hypertrophic cardiomyopathy in infants: clinical and natural history. *Circulation* 1982; 65:7.

353. Frank MJ, et al. Long-term medical management of hypertrophic obstructive cardiomyopathy. *Am J Cardiol* 1978;42:993.

354. Bonow RO, et al. Effects of verapamil on left ventricular systolic and diastolic function in patients with hypertrophic cardiomyopathy: pressure-volume analysis with a nonimaging scintillation probe. *Circulation* 1983;68:1062.

355. Hanrath P, et al. Influence of verapamil therapy on left ventricular performance at rest and during exercise in hypertrophic cardiomyopathy. *Am J Cardiol* 1983;52: 544.

356. Spicer RL, et al. Hemodynamic effects of verapamil in children and adolescents with hypertrophic cardiomyopathy. *Circulation* 1983;67:413.

357. Bonow RO, et al. Atrial systole and left ventricular filling in hypertrophic cardiomyopathy: effect of verapamil. *Am J Cardiol* 1983;51:1386.

358. Bonow RO, et al. Effects of verapamil on left ventricular systolic function and diastolic filling in patients with hypertrophic cardiomyopathy. *Circulation* 1981; 64:787.

359. Rosing DR, et al. Verapamil therapy: new approach to the pharmacologic treatment of hypertrophic cardiomyopathy. Effects of long-term administration. *Am J Cardiol* 1981;48:545.

360. Lorell BH, et al. Modification of abnormal LV diastolic properties by nifedipine in patients with HC. *Circulation* 1982;65:499.

361. Rosing DR, Epstein SE. Verapamil in the treatment of hypertrophic cardiomyopathy. *Ann Intern Med* 1982; 96:670.

362. Landmark D, et al. Hemodynamic effects of nifedipine and propranolol in hypertrophic obstructive cardiomyopathy. *Br Heart J* 1982;48:19.

363. Epstein SE, Rosing DR. Verapamil: its potential for causing serious complications in patients with hypertrophic cardiomyopathy. *Circulation* 1981;64:437.

364. McKenna WJ, et al. Arrhythmia in hypertrophic cardiomyopathy. II. Comparison of amiodarone and verapamil in treatment. *Br Heart J* 1981;46:173.

365. Pollick C. Muscular subaortic stenosis. Hemodynamic and clinical improvement after disopyramide. *N Engl J Med* 1982;307:997.

365a. Kappenberger L, Linde C, Daubert C, et al. Pacing in hypertrophic obstructive cardiomyopathy A randomized crossover study. *Eur Heart J* 1997;18:1249–1256.

365b. Gadler F, Linde C, Juhlin-Dannfelt A, Ribeiro A, Ryden L. Long-term effects of dual chamber pacing in patients with hypertrophic cardiomyopathy without outflow tract obstruction at rest. *Eur Heart J* 1997;18: 636–642.

365c. Nishimura RA, Trusty JM, Hayes DL, et al. Dual chamber pacing for hypertrophic cardiomyopathy: a randomized, double-blind, crossover trial. *J Am Coll Cardiol* 1997;29:435–441.

365d. Nagueh SF, Lakkis NM, Middleton KJ, et al. Changes in left ventricular diastolic function 6 months after nonsurgical septal reduction therapy for hypertrophic obstructive cardiomyopathy. *Circulation* 1999;99: 344–347.

365e. Fabver L, Seggewiss H, Gleichmann U. Percutaneous transluminal septal myocardial ablation in hypertrophic cardiomyopathy. Results with respect to intraprocedural myocardial contrast echocardiography. *Circulation* 1998;98:2415–2421.

366. Morrow AG, et al. Operative treatment in idiopathic subaortic stenosis: techniques and the results of preoperative and postoperative clinical and hemodynamic assessments. *Circulation* 1968;37:589.

367. Maron BJ, et al. Long-term clinical course and symptomatic status of patients after operation for hypertrophic subaortic stenosis. *Circulation* 1978;57:1205.

368. Beahrs MM, et al. Hypertrophic obstructive cardiomyopathy: ten-to-21-year follow-up after partial septal myectomy. *Am J Cardiol* 1983;51:1160.

369. Watson DC, et al. Effects of operation on left atrial size and the occurrence of atrial fibrillation in patients with hypertrophic subaortic stenosis. *Circulation* 1977;55:178.

370. Schapira JN, et al. Single and two-dimensional echocardiographic visualization of the effects of septal myectomy in idiopathic hypertrophic subaortic stenosis. *Circulation* 1978;58:850.

371. Shah PM, Sylvester LT. Echocardiography in the diagnosis of hypertrophic obstructive cardiomyopathy. *Am J Med* 1977;62:830.

372. Redwood DR, et al. Exercise performance after septal myotomy and myectomy in patients with obstructive hypertrophic cardiomyopathy. *Am J Cardiol* 1979;44:215.

373. Maron BJ, et al. Results of surgery for idiopathic hypertrophic subaortic stenosis. *J Cardiovasc Med* 1980; 5:145.

374. Peterson TA, Todd DB, Edwards JE. Supravalvular aortic stenosis. *J Thorac Cardiovasc Surg* 1965;50:734.

375. Logan WFWE, et al. Familial supravalvular aortic stenosis. *Br Heart J* 1965;27:547.

376. Kahler RL, et al. Familial congenital heart disease. *Am J Med* 1966;40:384.

377. Beuren AJ, et al. The syndrome of supravalvular aortic stenosis, peripheral pulmonary stenosis, mental retardation and similar facial appearance. *Am J Cardiol* 1964;13:471.

378. Black JA, Bonham-Carter RE. Association between aortic stenosis and facies of severe infantile hypercalcaemia. *Lancet* 1963;2:745.

379. Garcia RE, et al. Idiopathic hypercalcemia and supravalvular aortic stenosis. *N Engl J Med* 1964;271:117.

380. Friedman WF, Roberts WC. Vitamin D and the supravalvular aortic stenosis syndrome. The transplacental effects of vitamin D on the aorta of the rabbit. *Circulation* 1966;34:77.

381. French JW, Guntheroth WC. An explanation of asymmetric upper extremity blood pressures in supravalvular aortic stenosis. *Circulation* 1970;42:31.

382. Usher BW, Goulden, O, Margo JP. Echocardiographic detection of supravalvular aortic stenosis. *Circulation* 1974;49:1257.

383. Bolen JL, Popp RL, French JW. Echocardiographic features of supravalvular aortic stenosis. *Circulation* 1975;52:817.

384. Weyman AE, et al. Cross-sectional echocardiographic characterization of aortic obstruction. l. Supravalvular aortic stenosis and aortic hypoplasia. *Circulation* 1978; 57:491.

385. McGoon DC, et al. The surgical treatment of supravalvular aortic stenosis. *J Thorac Cardiovasc Surg* 1961;41:125.

8

Chronic Aortic Regurgitation

Robert O. Bonow

Department of Medicine, Division of Cardiology,
Northwestern University Medical School and Memorial Hospital, Chicago, Illinois 60611

Chronic aortic regurgitation (AR) imposes a volume load on the left ventricle, resulting in a number of compensatory processes that serve to maintain normal left ventricular (LV) function despite the increased workload. These processes permit most patients to remain asymptomatic for decades, and in many patients compensatory LV hypertrophy and chamber dilatation successfully balance the regurgitant volume so that a stable equilibrium is achieved, normal LV systolic function is maintained even in the face of severe regurgitation, and symptoms do not develop. In other patients, however, severe AR is an insidious and progressive disease that ultimately leads to symptoms and/or LV systolic dysfunction. These latter patients present diagnostic and therapeutic challenges to the clinician, the most notable and controversial of which is the optimal timing of valve replacement surgery. The decision to proceed with aortic valve replacement (AVR) should be based on a knowledge of the pathophysiology and natural history of chronic AR and the results of AVR. This chapter addresses these important principles.

ETIOLOGY

Chronic AR may be the result of a number of pathologic processes affecting the aortic valve, both common and uncommon. The more common etiologies include idiopathic dilatation, congenital abnormalities of the aortic valve (especially bicuspid valves), calcific degenerative valves, systemic hypertension, rheumatic heart disease, infective endocarditis, myxomatous degeneration, and diseases of the ascending aorta such as dissections and Marfan's syndrome. Among the less common etiologies are traumatic injuries to the aortic valve, ankylosing spondylitis, syphilitic aortitis, rheumatoid arthritis, discrete subaortic stenosis, and ventricular septal defects with prolapse of an aortic cusp. Most of these lesions result in chronic AR with the slow progressive LV dilatation noted above associated with a prolonged asymptomatic phase. However, some lesions produce acute severe AR with the potential for sudden onset of heart failure and/or cardiogenic shock; principal among these are infective endocarditis, aortic dissection, and trauma.

PATHOPHYSIOLOGY

The volume load of chronic AR sets in motion a number of compensatory mechanisms, and the magnitude and progressive nature of these compensatory changes are a manifestation of the severity of the regurgitant volume. The LV end-diastolic volume increases to accommodate the regurgitant volume and does so with an increase in chamber compliance so that the augmented end-diastolic volume is not associated with an increase in diastolic filling pressure. The increased end-diastolic volume translates into an increase in total stroke volume, resulting in forward stroke volume that is maintained within the normal range. In addition, the ventricle adapts to the volume load by producing new sarcomeres and thus the development of eccentric LV hypertrophy (1). As a result, although LV preload is increased, preload at the sarcomere level remains normal or near normal, and the normal contractile performance of each unit along the enlarged circumference contributes to the enhanced total stroke volume (2). Hence, LV preload reserve is maintained, and overall LV ejection performance is normal. In keeping with this concept, measures of LV ejection performance such as ejection fraction and fractional shortening remain in the normal range. However, the augmented LV chamber volume results in an increase in systolic wall stress and afterload, and the heightened afterload is also a stimulus for additional concentric hypertrophy (1,3). Thus, AR represents a condition of combined volume overload and pressure overload, with a combined hypertrophic response of both eccentric and concentric hypertrophy. As the valvular regurgitation evolves with time, progressive increases in chamber volume and afterload are stimuli for continued recruitment of preload reserve and further compensatory hypertrophy, and these mechanisms allow the ventricle to maintain normal ejection performance (4,5). As a result of the maintenance of normal LV systolic function, normal forward stroke volume, and normal diastolic pressures despite the increase in LV diastolic volume, most patients with chronic AR remain asymptomatic, and the duration of this period of hemodynamic compensation may last for decades. In such patients, therapy with afterload-reducing agents has the potential to reduce the degree of regurgitation and its associated hemodynamic burden, thereby reducing the extent of compensatory dilatation and hypertrophy and, in theory, prolonging the duration of this compensated phase.

In many patients, however, the balance between excessive afterload and the combination of preload reserve and compensatory hypertrophy either cannot be achieved or cannot be maintained indefinitely (5,6), and a

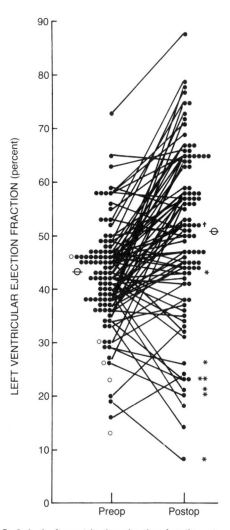

FIG. 8-1. Left ventricular ejection fraction at rest by radionuclide angiography before (*Preop*) and 6 months after (*Postop*) aortic valve replacement in 93 consecutive patients with chronic aortic regurgitation. Open circles indicate patients who died before the 6 month reevaluation, asterisks indicate patients who died from congestive heart failure after the 6-month study, and the cross indicates one patient who died suddenly after the 6-month study. (From ref. 18, with permission.)

condition of afterload mismatch ensues. Any further increase in afterload at this point will result in a reduction in systolic ejection performance and a decrease in ejection fraction (and other ejection phase indexes) into the subnormal range. Although it is possible that LV systolic dysfunction may arise, at least initially, purely on the basis of such afterload mismatch, which is a reversible phenomenon, impaired myocardial contractility also may contribute to this process, and this latter mechanism is often irreversible.

Symptoms of dyspnea or fatigue often develop at this transition point in the natural history as a result of declining systolic function. However, the transition from the compensated to the decompensated state can occur in a silent and insidious manner, and it is possible for patients to remain asymptomatic until severe and irreversible LV dysfunction has occurred.

As noted above, depressed LV systolic function is initially a potentially reversible process related to afterload mismatch, and complete reversal of LV dilatation and systolic dysfunction occurs commonly after successful AVR (7–18), as shown in Fig. 8-1. With time, however, as progressive severe LV chamber enlargement and remodeling develop, depressed myocardial contractility may predominate over excessive loading as the principal mechanism for declining systolic function. At its extreme, this process will progress to the point that the potential benefits of surgical intervention cannot be attained (Fig. 8-1), and patients are at risk of persistent LV dilatation, LV dysfunction, and death after technically successful valve replacement (15,19–28).

NATURAL HISTORY OF ASYMPTOMATIC PATIENTS

Patients with Normal Left Ventricular Systolic Function

The natural history of asymptomatic patients with chronic severe AR and normal LV systolic function is characterized by a very gradual rate of deterioration to symptoms, LV systolic dysfunction, or death (Fig. 8-2), and most such patients have an excellent outcome with conservative nonsurgical management. Although there are no large-scale series evaluating the natural history of asymptomatic patients in whom noninvasive testing documented normal LV systolic function, the American College of Cardiology/American Heart Association guidelines for managing of patients with valvular heart disease (29) analyzed seven relative small series that provided very consistent observations (30–37). The results of these series are tabulated in Table 8-1 (29). The seven series involved 490 patients with significant AR and normal LV function with a mean follow-up period of 6.4 years (range, 3.7 to 14.2 years). The likelihood of patients developing symptoms or LV systolic dysfunction was 4.3% per year. Sudden death occurred in six patients, an average mortality rate less than 0.2% per year. In six of these studies reporting the rate of development of asymptomatic LV dysfunction (31–35), 36 of 463 patients developed LV systolic dysfunction without symptoms during a mean 5.9 year follow-up period, a rate of 1.3% per year.

Thus, the overall outcome of asymptomatic patients with normal LV systolic function is excellent, and most patients develop symptoms before or coincident with the onset of LV dysfunction (Fig. 8-2). These observations indicate that the most important aspect of the baseline and serial evaluation of patients with chronic severe AR is a careful and detailed history, with attention to changes in effort tolerance and onset of symptoms. However, it is noteworthy that roughly 25% of patients who die or develop systolic dysfunction do so before the onset of warning symptoms (31–35), indicating that careful questioning of patients regarding changes in symptomatic status and effort tolerance alone is not sufficient in the serial evaluation of asymptomatic patients. For this reason, noninvasive evaluation of LV function is essential. Such testing is also important clinically because patients at risk of future symptoms, death, or LV dysfunction can

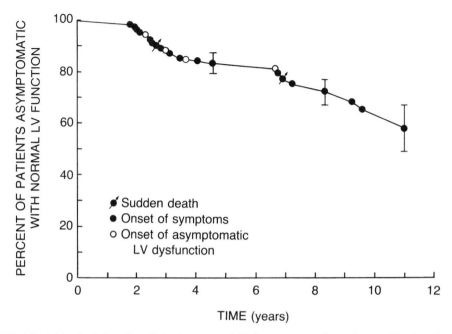

FIG. 8-2. Life table depicting the clinical course of 104 asymptomatic patients with chronic severe aortic regurgitation and normal left ventricular ejection fraction on initial evaluation. Brackets indicate SEE. At 11 years, 58% ± 9% of the patients were alive and asymptomatic with normal left ventricular function, an attrition rate less than 4% per year. (From ref. 33, with permission.)

be identified on the basis of LV size and function. Three of the seven natural history studies (32,33,35) provided concordant information regarding factors that are associated with higher risk: age, LV end-systolic dimension (or volume), and LV end-diastolic dimension (or volume). The LV ejection fraction during exercise was also identified in these studies, but this may not be an independent risk factor, because the direction and magnitude of change in ejection fraction during exercise is related not only to myocardial contractility (38) but also to the severity of the volume overload (33,39–41) and exercise-induced changes in preload and peripheral resistance (42). In a multivariate analysis (33), only age and end-systolic dimension were independent predictors of outcome on initial study, as were the rate of increase in end-systolic dimension and decrease in resting ejection fraction during serial longitudinal studies; the exercise ejection fraction and

change in ejection fraction from rest to exercise were not significant predictors of outcome. During a mean follow-up period of 8 years, patients with initial end-systolic dimensions greater than 50 mm had a 19% likelihood per year of death, symptoms, and/or LV dysfunction; those with end-systolic dimensions of 40 to 50 mm had a likelihood of 6% per year; and those with dimensions less than 40 mm had no likelihood (33).

Patients with Left Ventricular Systolic Dysfunction

Unlike asymptomatic patients with chronic severe AR and normal LV systolic function at rest, patients with LV systolic dysfunction in the setting of chronic severe AR appear to have a much more aggressive natural history with a steeper rate of attrition. The available data from small series (18,43,44) suggest that most such patients do

TABLE 8-1. *Studies of the natural history of asymptomatic patients with aortic regurgitation*

Study	Number of patients	Mean follow-up (yr)	Progression to symptoms, death or LV dysfunction (rate/yr)	Progression to asymptomatic LV dysfunction		Mortality (no. of patients)	Comments
				n	Rate/yr		
Bonow et al. (30,33)	104	8.0	3.8%	4	0.5%	2	Outcome predicted by LV ESD, EDD, change in EF with exercise, and rate of change in ESD and rest EF with time
Scognamiglio et al. (31)[a]	30	4.7	2.1%	3	2.1%	0	Three patients developing asymptomatic LV dysfunction initially had lower PAP/ESV ratios and trend toward higher LV ESD and EDD and lower FS
Siemienczuk et al. (32)	50	3.7	4.0%	1	0.5%	0	Patients included those receiving placebo and medical drop-outs in a randomized drug trial; included some patients with NYHA FC II symptoms; outcome predicted by LV ESV, EDV, change in EF with exercise, and end-systolic wall stress
Tornos et al. (35)	101	4.6	3.0%	6	1.3%	0	Outcome predicted by pulse pressure, LV ESD, EDD, and rest EF
Ishii et al. (36)	27	14.2	3.6%	—	—	0	Development of symptoms predicted by systolic BP, LV ESD, EDD, mass index, and wall thickness
Scognamiglio et al. (34)[a]	74	6.0	5.7%	15	3.4%	0	All patients received digoxin in a randomized drug trial
Borer et al. (37)	104	7.3	6.2%	7	0.9%	4	20% of patients in NYHA FC II; outcome predicted by initial FC II symptoms, change in EF with exercise, LV ESD, and LV FS
Average	490	6.4	4.3%	36	1.3%	(0.19%/year)	

[a]Two studies by same authors involved separate patient groups.

BP, blood pressure; EDD, end-diastolic dimension; EDV, END-diastolic volume, EF, ejection fraction; ESD, end-systolic dimension; ESV, end-systolic volume; FC, functional class; FS, fractional shortening; LV, left ventricular; PAP, pulmonary artery pressure; NYHA,

From ref. 29, with permission.

not remain symptom free for long periods of time but become candidates for operation because of symptomatic indications within only a few years (Fig. 8-3). Although this analysis is limited by small numbers of reported patients, the time course between the demonstration of LV systolic dysfunction at rest and the onset of symptoms is relatively short: Two thirds or more of asymptomatic patients who manifest evidence of ventricular dysfunction develop symptoms requiring operation within only 2 to 3 years (29).

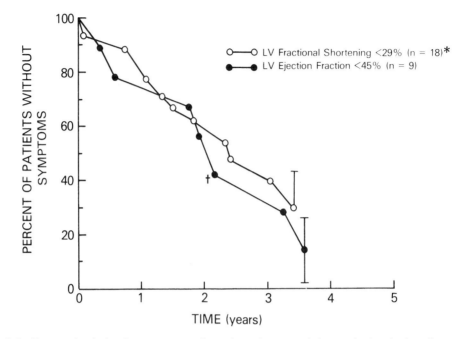

FIG. 8-3. Temporal relation in asymptomatic patients between left ventricular dysfunction and the onset of symptoms, based on echocardiographic data (*open symbols*) combined from two series (43,44) and on radionuclide angiographic data (*closed symbols*) (18). The cross indicates a patient who died suddenly during the follow-up period. (From ref. 18, with permission.)

CLINICAL PRESENTATION

History

In the absence of complications, patients with aortic regurgitation are asymptomatic for decades. Many are not even aware of a heart murmur, because the high-pitched, blowing diastolic murmur of aortic insufficiency is often overlooked. It is not uncommon for patients with aortic regurgitation to engage in athletics and vigorous work-related activities. Some otherwise asymptomatic patients are aware of the increased vigor of contraction of the left ventricle, particularly on lying down. Other patients note forceful pulsations of the neck vessels or audible heart tones. Slight orthostatic dizziness may be reported by otherwise asymptomatic patients with low systemic diastolic blood pressure.

Symptoms in patients with aortic regurgitation usually consist of angina pectoris or heart failure or both. Angina pectoris may be the result of associated coronary atherosclerosis, or it may occur with widely patent coronary arteries. In the latter situation, angina pectoris is the result of low aortic diastolic pressure that leads to decreased myocardial perfusion in the face of increased myocardial oxygen demands secondary to increased left ventricular volume and systolic pressure. Angina is not common in patients with aortic regurgitation.

An unusual form of angina pectoris in patients with aortic insufficiency and normal coronary arteries occurs in paroxysms, usually at night. These attacks are severe, frequently associated with nightmares, dyspnea, forceful and rapid heart action, skin flushing, profuse sweating, and a very wide pulse pressure (up to 200–250 mm Hg). Diffuse abdominal or epigastric pain has also been noted during such paroxysms.

Ostial coronary atherosclerotic narrowings may develop in patients with luetic aortic regurgitation. Such patients are prone to particularly severe attacks of angina pectoris that are often associated with marked dyspnea.

Many patients with aortic regurgitation report chest discomfort that may be described by some observers as angina pectoris. Close questioning, however, reveals that in many, the discomfort is prolonged, mild, and localized to the region of the left breast. Only an occasional patient with aortic regurgitation and normal coronary arteries relates a classic history of effort-induced angina pectoris.

Congestive heart failure is the most common symptom that develops in patients with aortic regurgitation. It usually appears after decades during which the patient reported no symptoms whatsoever. Left ventricular failure precedes right ventricular failure. Symptoms of heart failure may be insidious in onset, with patients initially noting only slightly decreased exercise tolerance. Stable dyspnea on exertion may occur for a short period of time, or it may be present for a number of years before more severe symptoms of left ventricular failure (orthopnea, paroxysmal nocturnal dyspnea) develop. Paroxysmal dyspnea may be severe and is more common in patients with luetic aortic regurgitation, possibly because of the presence of ostial coronary arterial obstruction in the latter group of patients. Death is rare in asymptomatic patients with aortic regurgitation who have been followed for many years.

Dyspnea may be relieved with the eventual onset of right ventricular failure with or without overt tricuspid regurgitation. Patients with left and right ventricular failure secondary to aortic regurgitation are severely incapacitated.

Palpitations are not uncommon in patients with aortic regurgitation. As noted earlier, palpitations are often not the result of arrhythmias. Rather, they represent the patient's awareness of forceful left ventricular contraction. Atrial and ventricular arrhythmias, do occur in patients with aortic regurgitation, usually late in the natural history of this condition when left or right ventricular failure (or both) has supervened. Ventricular arrhythmias are common in patients with aortic regurgitation. Presence and severity correlate directly with the severity of left ventricular dysfunction. In contrast to aortic stenosis, syncope

rarely, if ever, occurs in patients with aortic regurgitation.

Survival of patients with chronic aortic insufficiency resembles that of patients with mitral valve disease. The prognosis is considerably better than in patients with aortic stenosis. Complications that may worsen prognosis in aortic regurgitation include infectious endocarditis, ostial narrowing of one or both coronary arteries in luetic aortic regurgitation, coexisting coronary artery disease, and atrial or ventricular arrhythmias.

Physical Findings

Patients with aortic regurgitation have a number of characteristic physical findings, so that identification of this valvular lesion is often straightforward.

The diastolic blood pressure is frequently low in persons with moderate or severe degrees of aortic insufficiency. In an occasional patient with severe aortic regurgitation, Korotkov sounds may even be heard when pressure in the blood pressure cuff reaches zero. The systolic blood pressure is normal or elevated so that the pulse pressure is usually wide in these patients. The low diastolic blood pressure is the result of the draining of blood into the left ventricle during diastole. The pulse rate is usually normal in patients without heart failure. In the latter situation, sinus tachycardia is the rule.

Inspection and palpation of the heart usually reveal evidence of left ventricular enlargement and hyperactivity unless aortic regurgitation is mild or chronic pulmonary disease with hyperinflation of the lungs makes it difficult to appreciate the left ventricular impulse. In most patients with clinically important aortic regurgitation, the apical impulse is displaced to the left and below its usual location.

The murmur of aortic regurgitation is usually relatively soft (compared, for example, with the systolic murmur of aortic stenosis), high-pitched, and blowing in character. It is best heard early in diastole but may fill almost all of diastole. The murmur is characteristically decrescendo. On occasion, the murmur is loud and musical in quality. This musical murmur of aortic regurgitation has been referred to as the seagull, or cooing-dove, murmur. It is usually the result of eversion or perforation of an aortic cusp. It is most commonly heard in patients whose aortic regurgitation is the result of syphilis, infectious endocarditis, rheumatic fever, or trauma. Systolic musical (seagull) murmurs occur in a number of conditions, including ruptured chordae tendineae and aortic stenosis. The duration of the murmur is related to the severity of aortic regurgitation. In patients with mild disease, the murmur is early diastolic, brief, and often overlooked.

The murmur of aortic regurgitation is best heard at the base of the heart (along the left sternal edge or in the second right intercostal space) with the diaphragm of the stethoscope and with the patient sitting up, leaning forward, and expiring deeply. In 95 % of the patients with rheumatic aortic insufficiency, the murmur is louder in the third left interspace than in the third right interspace adjacent to the sternum. When the reverse is the case (i.e., the murmur is louder in the third right interspace), aortic regurgitation is the result of a different disease process, usually a disease involving the aortic root, with displacement of the aorta to the right (e.g., aortic aneurysm, syphiditis, or trauma). In an occasional elderly patient or patient with a chest deformity, the murmur of aortic regurgitation is best heard at the apex or in the left axilla.

A systolic ejection murmur (aortic stenotic in quality) frequently accompanies the diastolic murmur of aortic regurgitation. The systolic murmur is the result of increased left ventricular stroke volume passing through an abnormal aortic valve or root or both. This systolic murmur usually radiates to the carotids, where it may be so prominent that it is noted as a carotid thrill or shudder. Distinguishing aortic stenosis with minor or moderate aortic regurgitation from severe aortic regurgitation with a systolic "flow" murmur depends on the presence or absence of associated peripheral signs of aortic regurgitation.

In the absence of mitral valve disease, the first heart sound (S_1) is normal or slightly diminished in intensity in patients with aortic regurgitation. Occasionally, aortic regurgitation is so severe that early closure of the mitral valve occurs, with marked softening or even disappearance of the S_1. This occurs more commonly with acute aortic regurgitation. The second heart sound (S_2) may be normal in splitting and intensity, or the aortic component may be increased in intensity (as in syphilis). In calcific aortic valve disease, the valve leaflets are often immobile or nearly so. Such patients may have a soft or inaudible aortic component of the S_2.

Ejection clicks are occasionally heard in early systole in patients with aortic regurgitation and a dilated aortic root. Rarely, a midsystolic sound can be heard in patients with aortic regurgitation. A fourth heart sound (S_4) is heard in patients with prominent left ventricular hypertrophy, and a third heart sound (S_3) is audible in many patients with left ventricular failure.

Occasionally a patient with isolated aortic regurgitation has a soft, low pitched middiastolic to late diastolic rumbling murmur closely resembling that heard in patients with mitral stenosis. This is termed the Austin Flint murmur, and several explanations have been suggested for its origin:

1. Diastolic mitral regurgitation secondary to markedly increased left ventricular filling pressures in late diastole;
2. Relative mitral stenosis resulting from the aortic regurgitation jet pushing the anterior mitral valve leaflet upward, thus impeding the flow of blood from the left atrium; and
3. Low-pitched vibrations of the aortic regurgitant murmur itself, heard best at the apex because of acoustical filtering properties of a particular patient's thorax.

The second and third explanations are probably the true mechanisms for production of the Austin Flint murmur. The Austin Flint murmur can be distinguished from the murmur of true mitral stenosis on clinical grounds (Table 8-2).

TABLE 8-2. *Distinguishing the murmur of mitral stenosis from the Austin Flint murmur*

Clinical or laboratory finding	Mitral stenosis	Austin Flint murmur
Opening snap present	+	−
S_1 increased	+	−
S_3 present	−	+
Left ventricular enlargement and hypertrophy (physical examination, ECG, chest roentgenogram)	−	+
Right ventricular enlargement and hypertrophy (physical examination, ECG, chest roentgenogram)	+	−
Murmur decreases with amyl nitrite	−	+
Echocardiographic evidence of organic mitral stenosis	+	−
Presence of atrial fibrillation	+	−

Peripheral signs of aortic regurgitation are important clues to the presence and severity of aortic regurgitation. The pulse (felt at the wrist or in the neck) has a characteristic quality, striking the finger rapidly and forcefully and then suddenly disappearing (Corrigan's, or water-hammer, pulse). This quality of the pulse is a result of the large, forcefully ejected left ventricular stroke volume in early systole, with subsequent regurgitation of a significant portion of that blood into the left ventricle during early and mid-diastole. Elevating the wrist increases the amplitude of the radial arterial pulsations in patients with aortic regurgitation, presumably because the elevation of the arm decreases intraarterial pressure leading to a shift in the arterial pressure-volume curve with resultant increased arterial compliance. Corrigan's, or water-hammer, pulse may also be present in patients with patent ductus arteriosus, arteriovenous fistula, or marked peripheral vasodilatation secondary to fever, thyrotoxicosis, or anemia.

The carotid pulse may be bisferiens in patients with severe aortic regurgitation. A prominent thrill or shudder may also be present in pure or predominant aortic regurgitation. The thrill is the tactile perception of low-frequency vibrations of the systolic ejection murmur that, as noted, often occurs in patients with pure aortic regurgitation. Although carotid thrills or shudders are more common in patients with pure or predominant aortic stenosis, they occur with sufficient frequency in aortic regurgitation to render this finding of no use in distinguishing aortic stenosis from aortic regurgitation.

Prominent arterial pulsations may be plainly visible in the neck or temporal vessels of patients with aortic regurgitation. The force of arterial pulsation may impart motion to the head or other structure of the body. Prominent arterial pulsations and peripheral signs resembling aortic regurgitation may occur in patients without aortic insufficiency but with high cardiac output (thyrotoxicosis, peripheral arteriovenous fistula, fever, anemia) and reduced peripheral resistance.

The severity of aortic regurgitation may be estimated from a number of clinical findings. For example, in patients with severe aortic regurgitation, the popliteal arterial systolic cuff pressure is greater by 60 mm Hg or more than the corresponding brachial pressure. In patients with lesser degrees of aortic regurgitation, the differences between these two blood pressure measurements are smaller. In normal persons the difference between popliteal and brachial arterial systolic pressure may be as great as 10 to 20 mm Hg because of normal reflecting wave amplification of the systolic pressure in the more distal popliteal artery.

LABORATORY FINDINGS

Electrocardiogram

The electrocardiogram (ECG) usually demonstrates left ventricular preponderance in patients with aortic regurgitation. Left axis deviation and increased ventricular voltage are common. In moderate aortic regurgitation the lateral precordial leads often demonstrate a small Q wave, a tall R wave, an isoelectric

S-T segment, and an upright T wave (so called diastolic overload of the left ventricle). With more severe degrees of aortic regurgitation, the S-T segment may be depressed or down-sloping or both, and the T waves are inverted in the lateral precordial leads (so-called systolic overload of the left ventricle or left ventricular hypertrophy with strain). There are often deep S waves and occasionally poor R wave progression in the right precordial leads in the presence of left ventricular dilatation or hypertrophy or both.

Patients with aortic regurgitation secondary to inflammatory processes may have prolonged P-R intervals, Mobitz type-1 atrioventricular block, or conduction defects (e.g., left bundle branch block). Patients with aortic insufficiency caused by severe calcific aortic valve disease may also demonstrate conduction defects.

Chest Roentgenogram

In the absence of heart failure, patients with mild to moderate aortic regurgitation may have a relatively normal chest roentgenogram. The mild to moderate left ventricular enlargement present in such patients is often not discernable on the routine posteroanterior chest roentgenogram. With more severe degrees of aortic regurgitation, the left ventricular contour enlarges downward and to the left, producing the "boot-shaped" heart silhouette characteristic of this valvular lesion. Massive left ventricular enlargement is sometimes seen in patients with severe and long-standing aortic insufficiency.

The aortic knob and ascending aorta are often prominent in persons with moderate to severe aortic regurgitation. Fluoroscopic examination of the heart reveals hyperdynamic left ventricular and aortic pulsations.

Linear calcification of the ascending aorta (so-called eggshell calcification) is often present in patients with luetic aortic insufficiency. Calcification of the aortic valve may be present in patients whose aortic regurgitation is the result of a bicuspid or unicuspid valve or rheumatic valvular disease. Widening

of the mediastinum is often a clue to the presence of aortic dissection.

When left ventricular failure develops, the chest roentgenogram may reveal pulmonary vascular redistribution and interstitial or alveolar pulmonary edema. The left atrium may become modestly dilated secondary to elevated left ventricular filling pressures with or without concomitant functional mitral regurgitation. With the development of right ventricular failure, the right heart chambers dilate, resulting in a massively enlarged cardiac silhouette. The roentgenographic distinction of aortic stenosis from aortic regurgitation rests on the finding of a marked left ventricular enlargement in patients with aortic insufficiency.

Echocardiography

Echocardiographic findings in patients with aortic regurgitation include abnormalities of the aortic valve, mitral valve, and left ventricle. In the absence of mitral valve disease, patients with aortic regurgitation demonstrate a broad band (3–4 mm wide) of diastolic flutter or vibration (20–70 Hz) of the anterior mitral leaflet. Increasing severity of aortic regurgitation correlates with more prominent and extensive diastolic fluttering of the anterior mitral valve leaflet. Other abnormalities of the mitral valve echo in aortic regurgitation are rapid diastolic closure rate and mitral valve closure occuring prior to the onset of the QRS complex. The latter finding is associated with severe aortic regurgitation, often acute in nature.

Fluttering of the anterior mitral valve leaflet may be associated with similar vibrations of the posterior mitral leaflet and the interventricular septum. There is no correlation between these vibrations and the presence of the Austin Flint murmur. Early closure of the mitral valve does correlate with the presence of the Austin Flint murmur, suggesting that antegrade, transmitral blood flow in the presence of a functionally narrowed mitral orifice does account for the Austin Flint murmur.

The aortic root is often dilated in patients with aortic regurgitation. Coarse diastolic oscillations of the aortic valve leaflet are occasionally noted in patients with a flail aortic leaflet. Such oscillations may even be visible in the region of the left ventricular outflow tract.

Left ventricular end-diastolic dimensions is often increased in patients with aortic regurgitation. The left ventricle frequently demonstrates hyperdynamic wall motion. This combination of enlarged end-diastolic dimension and increased contractility is termed the *volume overload pattern*. It is also seen in patients with other conditions that result in increased volume work for the left ventricle (e.g., mitral regurgitation).

Echocardiographic determination of left ventricular function detects declining myocardial performance in patients with chronic aortic regurgitation.

Doppler ultrasonic techniques are employed to assess the severity of aortic regurgitation. Doppler echocardiagraphic examinations are both highly sensitive and specific in the detection quantitation of aortic regurgitation.

Cardiac Catheterization and Angiography

Hemodynamic measurements in patients with left ventricular dysfunction usually reveal elevated left ventricular filling pressures (left ventricular mean diastolic, left atrial, pulmonary capillary wedge, pulmo-nary arterial diastolic), often with associated depression of cardiac output. Patients may remain clinically stable for many years despite such abnormal hemodynamic findings. Eventually, right ventricular failure supervenes, with resultant elevation in right heart filling pressures (right ventricular mean diastolic, right atrial, central venous). With severe left ventricular decompensation, left ventricular end-diastolic and aortic diastolic pressures equalize. Table 8-3 summarizes the hemodynamic findings in patients with aortic regurgitation.

Younger patients with aortic regurgitation are less likely than older patients to demonstrate abnormal hemodynamics. Such hemodynamic dysfunction is the rule in patients over age 40. Of patients with mild to moderate symptoms (New York Heart Association [NYHA] functional class II), 50% have abnormal resting hemodynamics. Increasing symptoms usually correlate with increasing evidence of hemodynamic deterioration. Symptoms develop in many patients after marked hemodynamic abnormalities are already present.

Left ventriculography in patients with severe and long-standing aortic regurgitation can demonstrate a number of abnormalities:

1. Increased (occasionally markedly so) end-diastolic volume.
2. Abnormal roundness (increased eccentricity).

TABLE 8-3. *Hemodynamic findings in patients with aortic regurgitation*

Cardiac output and pressures	Compensated	Mild to moderate decompensation	Severe decompensation
Cardiac output	Normal	Normal or ↓	↓↓
Pressures			
Right atrial	Normal	Normal	Normal or ↑
Right ventricular end-diastolic	Normal	Normal	Usually ↑
Pulmonary arterial systolic	Normal	Normal or ↑	↑↑
Pulmonary arterial diastolic	Normal	↑	↑↑
Pulmonary capillary wedge	Normal	↑	↑↑
Left atrial	Normal	↑	↑↑
Left ventricular end-diastolic	Normal or ↑	↑↑	↑↑↑

↑, moderately elevated; ↑↑, markedly elevated; ↑↑↑, very markedly elevated; ↓, moderately reduced; ↓↓, markedly reduced.

3. Reduced regional and global systolic contractile function with resultant decreased ejection fraction and abnormal apex-to-base shortening.
4. Abnormally elevated endsystolic volume and abnormal endsystolic pressure-volume relationship.

These abnormalities are uncommon in patients with predominant aortic stenosis in whom concentric left ventricular hypertrophy without dilatation or increased eccentricity is the rule. Changes in left ventricular shape in aortic regurgitation undoubtedly reflect the abnormal wall stress engendered by the volume overload. Regional left ventricular contraction abnormalities involving anterolateral wall segments have been noted in patients with aortic regurgitation.

The severity of aortic regurgitation can be semiquantitatively (1–4+) estimated by means of supravalvular (aortic root) cineangiography. Considerable error is inherent with this technique. A more accurate method of quantitating aortic regurgitation involves the calculation of total left ventricular cardiac output from the left ventriculogram and forward cardiac output by the Fick technique. The difference between these two measurements of cardiac output represents the volume of aortic regurgitant blood flow. This volume divided by the total left ventricular (cineangiographic) output is termed the *regurgitant fraction* (the fraction of the forward left ventricular stroke volume that regurgitates back into the ventricle during diastole). Patients with mild to moderate aortic regurgitation have regurgitant fractions less than 0.50. Severe aortic regurgitation is associated with a regurgitant fraction greater than 0.50 to 0.60.

DIFFERENTIAL DIAGNOSIS OF AORTIC REGURGITATION

The diagnosis of aortic regurgitation is made in patients with the following signs:

1. a high-pitched, blowing diastolic murmur;
2. left ventricular enlargement on physical examination, ECG, or chest roentgenogram;

3. hyperdynamic peripheral arterial pulses;
4. high-frequency vibrations of the anterior mitral valve leaflet and hyperdynamic left ventricular wall motion recorded on an echocardiogram; and
5. aortic regurgitation demonstrated by doppler echocardiography.

Left ventricular enlargement and hyperdynamic peripheral pulses are often absent in patients with mild to moderate aortic regurgitation. A number of conditions that may be confused with aortic regurgitation follow.

Pulmonic Regurgitation

Patients with congenital or pulmonary hypertensive pulmonic regurgitation (Graham Steell murmur) may have a diastolic murmur resembling that of aortic regurgitation. Congenital pulmonic regurgitation usually produces a low-pitched, harsh murmur that is different in character from the murmur of aortic insufficiency. Peripheral circulatory phenomena, left ventricular enlargement, and echocardiographic mitral valve vibrations are absent in patients with pulmonic regurgitation. The Graham Steell murmur occurs with congenital, mitral valvular, or pulmonary heart disease. The pulmonic component of the S_2 is invariably increased in such patients.

Patent Ductus Arteriosus

The murmur of patent ductus arteriosus may resemble that of aortic regurgitation, particularly when pulmonary hypertension supervenes, and the ductus murmur is no longer continuous. Because of increased left ventricular stroke volume and diastolic runoff of blood into the pulmonary artery, patients with patent ductus arteriosus often have hyperdynamic peripheral pulses and evidence of left ventricular enlargement. Differentiating features of patent ductus arteriosus include late systolic accentuation of the ductus murmur, a systolic thrill in the second or third left intercostal space, prominent ("shunt") vascularity and pulmonary arteries in the chest roentgenogram, and demonstration of a left-to-right shunt by radionuclide angiography or right-heart catheterization.

Mitral Regurgitation

Patients with severe mitral regurgitation frequently have a collapsing quality in the arterial pulse. This is the result of decreasing left ventricular stroke output during the latter half of systole. Such persons may actually have associated aortic insufficiency if mitral valve disease is the result of rheumatic activity. In the absence of aortic insufficiency, patients with severe degrees of mitral regurgitation may demonstrate an early diastolic flow rumble that might occasionally be confused with the murmur of aortic insufficiency; however, mitral valvular flow rumbles are low-pitched and usually heard only at the apex. Patients with combined severe mitral regurgitation and mild aortic insufficiency usually require cardiac catheterization and angiography for quantification of severity of the respective valvular lesions.

Reduced Peripheral Resistance

Reduced peripheral resistance secondary to arteriovenous fistula, anemia, hyperthyroidism, or fever may be diagnosed as aortic regurgitation because of hyperdynamic, collapsing arterial pulses. The characteristic murmur of aortic regurgitation and evidence of left ventricular enlargement are usually absent in patients with hyperdynamic circulation secondary to reduced peripheral resistance.

Hyperkinetic Heart Syndrome

Patients with this poorly understood condition appear to have abnormally increased cardiac sympathetic stimulation. This results in a hyperdynamic circulation with bounding peripheral pulses resembling those of aortic regurgitation. The characteristic murmur of aortic insufficiency is absent.

Rarely, a coronary arteriovenous fistula or a high-grade coronary arterial stenosis may produced a high-pitched diastolic murmur that mimics aortic regurgitation. Cardiac catheterization and angiography are often required to identify these unusual entities.

Other Differential Diagnostic Clues

Differential diagnostic procedures also should be directed at identifying the underlying cause of aortic regurgitation. Historical information may aid in the differentiation of rheumatic, rheumatoid, traumatic, or congenital forms of aortic regurgitation (history of rheumatic fever, rheumatoid arthritis, recent chest trauma, childhood or family history of murmur, or hereditary disease associated with aortic regurgitation such as Marfan's syndrome).

Distinctive physical findings are usually present in patients with aortic regurgitation secondary to Marfan's syndrome (arachnodactyly, ectopia lentis, increased arm span), infectious endocarditis (petechiae, Osler's or Janeway lesions or both, splinter hemorrhages, splenomegaly), rheumatoid arthritis (joint deformaties), ankylosing spondylitis (characteristic posture), osteogenesis imperfecta (blue sclerae), and Ehlers-Danlos syndrome (hyperelasticity of the skin).

Laboratory data are frequently useful in patients with syphilis (positive serologic test for syphilis and linear calcification of ascending aorta on the chest roentgenogram), baterial endocarditis (positive blood culture and latex fixation), rheumatoid arthritis (positive latex fixation), and systemic lupus erythematosus (positive antinuclear antibody [ANA] and lupus erythematosus cell preparation). Echocardiographic examination may suggest that aortic regurgitation is due to primary myxomatous degeneration, bacterial endocarditis, or rheumatic valvular disease (presence of associated abnormalities of the mitral valve).

THERAPY: DETERMINANTS OF OUTCOME AFTER AORTIC VALVE REPLACEMENT

Numerous investigations have demonstrated that preoperative LV systolic function in patients with chronic AR is among the most important determinants of postoperative prognosis, in terms of LV function, heart failure symptoms, and survival (7,15–17,22–28, 45–55). Patients may be risk stratified on the basis of the resting LV ejection fraction measured by contrast angiography, echocardiography, or radionuclide angiography or on the basis of echocardiographic fractional shortening and end-systolic dimension (Table 8-4) (29). Symptomatic patients who undergo AVR with ejection fractions below the normal range comprise a high-risk group with reduced postoperative survival, whereas those with normal indices of LV pump function have an excellent prognosis (Fig. 8-4).

However, it is also apparent from numerous studies that patients with impaired LV systolic function do not represent a homogeneous group. An important subset of patients within this otherwise high-risk group will manifest a substantial improvement in LV function after operation (Fig. 8-1). This improvement in LV function resulting from removal of the severe volume overload and reversal of afterload mismatch is associated with an excellent survival outcome (7,16,17,26,45,46). An important factor responsible for postoperative reversal of LV dysfunction and improved prognosis is the early identification of patients with evidence of LV dysfunction who have minimal or no symptoms, leading to earlier operative intervention before severe symptoms develop (22,56).

This concept is supported by data indicating that asymptomatic or mildly symptomatic patients with LV dysfunction have better long-term postoperative prognosis than more severely symptomatic patients with the same degree of preoperative LV dysfunction (22,24,26,57). The likelihood of improvement in LV function and the magnitude of this improvement are also significantly related to the severity of preoperative symptoms and to the duration of preoperative LV dysfunction (13,17,26). Patients with a brief duration of preoperative LV dysfunction demonstrate a significantly greater decrease in LV dilatation and increase in LV ejection fraction after operation compared with patients in whom the duration of preoperative LV dysfunction is more prolonged (Figs. 8-5 and 8-6).

Hence, in patients with AR and LV systolic dysfunction, the risk of developing irreversible LV dysfunction is greater in patients with more severe symptoms, more severe dysfunction, and more prolonged duration of LV dysfunction. These data support the concept that postoperative survival and postoperative LV function will be enhanced favorably if asymptomatic or mildly symptomatic patients with LV dysfunction undergo operation without waiting for the development of more significant symptoms.

ROLE OF VASODILATOR THERAPY

Vasodilating agents in theory may reduce regurgitant volume and improve forward stroke volume in patients with chronic severe AR (58). These effects should translate into reductions in LV end-diastolic volume, wall stress, and afterload, resulting in preserved or enhanced LV systolic function and reduction in LV mass. In keeping with these concepts, sodium nitroprusside, hydralazine, or nifedipine acutely reduce peripheral vascular resistance in patients with AR, with an immediate increase in forward cardiac output and decrease in regurgitant volume (59–66). These acute hemodynamic changes with nitroprusside and hydralazine result in reduction in end-diastolic volume and augmentation in ejection fraction (59–62), although these changes are less consistent with the acute administration of nifedipine (63–66).

Chronic oral therapy with hydralazine and nifedipine produce similar hemodynamic effects in the small numbers of patients that have been studied in relatively short-term trials lasting 1 to 2 years (67,68), with evidence of reduced end-diastolic volume and increased ejection fraction. Nifedipine therapy also produces a reduction in LV mass (34,68). The effects of angiotensin-converting enzyme (ACE) inhibitors have been less consistent, and the hemodynamic effects depend on the magnitude of reduction in systemic arterial pressure and LV end-diastolic volume

TABLE 8-4. *Preoperative predictors of surgical outcome in aortic regurgitation*

Study	Study design	Number of patients	Outcome assessed	Findings
Forman et al., 1980 (23)	Retrospective	90	Survival	High-risk group dentified by preop iangio LV EF <0.50.
Henry et al., 1980 (47)	Prospective	50	Survival	High-risk group identified by preop echo LV FS <0.25 and/or ESD >55 mm.
Cunha et al., 1980 (22)	Retrospective	86	Survival	High-risk group identified by preop echo LV FS <0.30. Mortality also significantly associated with preop ESD. Among patients with FS <0.30, mortality higher in NYHA FC III–IV than in FC I–II.
Greves et al., 1981 (24)	Retrospective	45	Survival	High-risk group identified by preop angio LV EF <0.45 and/or CI <2.5 L/min. Among patients with EF <0.45, mortality higher in NYHA FC III–IV than in FC I–II.
Kumpuris et al., 1982 (49)	Prospective	43	Survival, heart failure,	Persistent LV dilatation after AVR predicted by preop echo LV ESD, LV function radius/thickness mean and end-systolic wall stress. All deaths occurred in patients with persistent LV dilatation.
Gaasch et al., 1983 (25)	Prospective	32	Symptoms, LV function	Persistent LV dilatation after AVR predicted by echo LV ESD >2.6 cm/m^2, EDD >3.8 cm/m^2, and radius/thickness ratio >3.8. Trend toward worse survival in patients with persistent LV dilatation.
Fioretti et al., 1983 (50)	Retrospective	47	LV function	Persistent LV dysfunction predicted by preop EDD ≥75 mm and/or ESD ≥55 mm.
Stone et al., 1984 (51)	Prospective	113	LV function	Normal LV function after AVR predicted by preop LV FS >0.25, ESD <55 mm, and <80 mm. No preop variable predicted postop LV function.
Bonow et al., 1985, 1988 (17,26)	Prospective	80	Survival, LV function	Postop survival and LV function predicted by preop LV EF, FS, ESD. High-risk group identified by subnormal rest EF. Among patients with subnormal EF, poor exercise tolerance and prolonged duration of LV dysfunction identified the highest risk group.
Daniel et al., 1985 (52)	Retrospective	84	Survival, symptoms, LV function	Outcome after AVR predicted by preop LV FS and ESD. Survival at 2.5 yr was 90.5% with FS >0.25 and ESD ≤55 mm but was only 70% with ESD >55 mm and FS ≤25%.
Cormier et al., 1986 (53)	Prospective	73	Survival	High-risk group identified by preop LV EF <0.40 and ESD ≥55 mm.
Sheiban et al., 1986 (54)	Retrospective	84	Survival	High-risk identified by preop LV EF <0.50 and ESD >55 mm.
Carabello et al., 1987 (16)	Retrospective	14	LV function	Postop LV EF predicted by preop ESD, FS, EDD, radius/thickness ratio.
Taniguchi et al., 1987 (15)	Retrospective	62	Survival	High-risk group identified by preop ESV >200 mL/m^2 and/or EF <0.40.
Michel et al., 1995 (28)	Retrospective	286	LV function	Postop LV dysfunction predicted by preop LV EF, FS, ESD, EDD.
Klodas et al., 1996 (55)	Retrospective	219	Survival	High-risk group identified by preop EF <0.50.

EDD, end-diastolic dimension; EF, ejection fraction; ESD, end-systolic dimension; ESV, end-systolic volume; FC, functional class; FS, fractional shortening; LV, left ventricular; NYHA, New York Heart Association; AVR, aortic valve replacement.
From ref. 29, with permission.

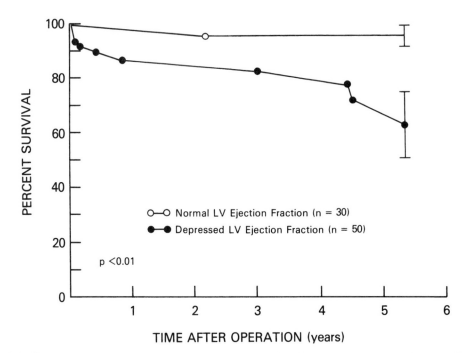

FIG. 8-4. Survival after aortic valve replacement in patients with chronic severe aortic regurgitation. Patients are subgrouped on the basis of preoperative left ventricular ejection fraction. Patients with preoperative left ventricular dysfunction have a significantly greater postoperative risk than those with preserved left ventricular function. (From ref. 26, with permission.)

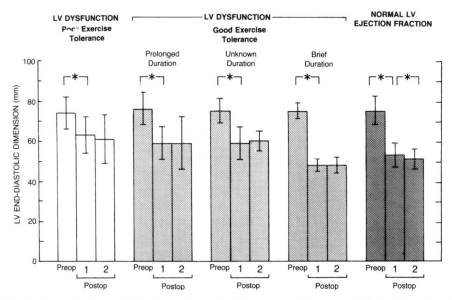

FIG. 8-5. Left ventricular end-diastolic dimension by echocardiography before (*Preop*) and after (*Postop*) operation in patients with normal preoperative ejection fractions and in patients with preoperative ventricular dysfunction subgrouped further on the basis of preoperative exercise tolerance and duration of left ventricular dysfunction. Left ventricular dysfunction is defined as a subnormal ejection fraction at rest by radionuclide angiography. Postoperative data are shown at 6 to 8 months (1) and at 3 to 7 years (2). Asterisks indicate significant differences. (From ref. 17, with permission.)

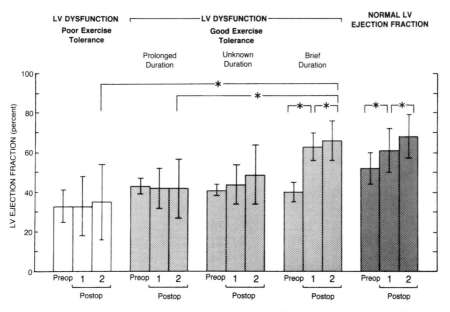

FIG. 8-6. Left ventricular ejection fraction at rest by radionuclide angiography before (*Preop*) and after (*Postop*) operation in the same patients shown in Fig. 8-5. Postoperative data are shown at 6 to 8 months (1) and at 3 to 7 years (2). Asterisks indicate significant differences. (From ref. 17, with permission.)

(69–71). When ACE inhibitors cause significant reduction in systemic blood pressure, these agents reduce LV end-diastolic volume and LV mass, although changes in LV ejection fraction have not been demonstrated consistently (69,71).

The rationale for treating patients with chronic severe AR with vasodilating agents is that the beneficial hemodynamic effects should translate into prolongation of the stable compensated phase in asymptomatic patients who have volume-loaded left ventricles but preserved systolic function. However, it is possible that afterload-reducing therapy may have deleterious effects, as such therapy may result in only a "cosmetic" effect that will mask the early development of significant symptoms or LV dysfunction that would otherwise precede irreversible myocardial dysfunction (3). Thus, patients who develop symptoms or LV dysfunction while receiving effective vasodilator therapy may do so at a more advanced stage in the natural history of the disease than patients reaching the same end points without medical therapy. Only one

study, in which nifedipine was compared with digoxin therapy in 143 patients for a period of 6 years, has examined the effect of vasodilator therapy on the natural history of chronic severe AR (34). The results suggest that such therapy may alter the long-term natural history of chronic asymptomatic AR in a favorable manner, because nifedipine produced a more gradual rate of development of symptoms and/or LV dysfunction than did digoxin (Fig. 8-7). In addition, those patients treated with nifedipine who did undergo AVR because symptoms or LV dysfunction developed had an excellent clinical outcome: All survived operation, and all manifested a reduction in LV diastolic dimension and normalization of LV systolic function after operation (34). These data strongly suggest that the hemodynamic effects of nifedipine represent beneficial changes and do not obscure the development of important signs and symptoms that precede the onset of irreversible LV dysfunction.

Whether similar long-term results may be achieved with ACE inhibitors is uncertain be-

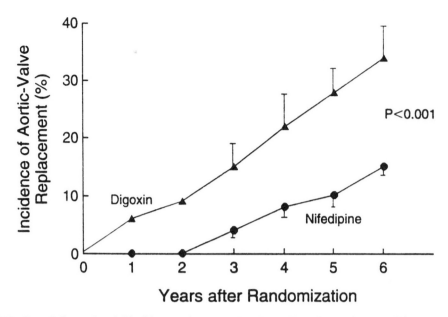

FIG. 8-7. Cumulative actuarial incidence of progression to aortic valve replacement because of development of symptoms or left ventricular dysfunction in initially asymptomatic patients with aortic regurgitation and normal left ventricular systolic function randomized to digoxin or nifedipine. (From ref. 34, with permission.)

cause no long-term studies have investigated the effect of ACE inhibition on the natural history of chronic AR. Because peripheral ACE activity may not be increased in asymptomatic patients with uncomplicated chronic AR, ACE inhibitors may prove to be less effective than more direct acting arterial dilators.

The proposed indications for medical therapy with vasodilating agents are listed in Table 8-5. Chronic therapy with vasodilators should be given only to asymptomatic patients with severe AR (i.e., patients with significantly dilated left ventricles) and normal LV systolic function. Such therapy is not recommended for asymptomatic patients with mild AR and normal LV function because these patients have an excellent outcome with no therapy. In patients with severe AR, vasodilator therapy should not be considered an alternative to AVR in asymptomatic or symptomatic patients with LV systolic dysfunction because such patients should be considered surgical candidates rather than candidates for long-term medical therapy, unless AVR is not recommended because of additional cardiac or noncardiac factors. However, short-term vasodilator therapy is commonly used to improve the hemodynamic profile of patients

TABLE 8-5. *Indications for medical therapy in patients with chronic aortic regurgitation*

Severity of AR	Symptoms	LV function	Management
Mild–Moderate	No	Normal	No medical therapy
Severe	No	Normal	Vasodilator therapy
Severe	No	Depressed	Aortic valve replacement
Severe	Yes	Normal	Aortic valve replacement
Severe	Yes	Depressed	Aortic valve replacement
Severe	Severe	Severely depressed	Medical therapy followed by aortic valve replacement

AR, aortic regurgitation; LV, left ventricle.

with severe heart failure symptoms and severe LV dysfunction before proceeding with AVR.

Whether symptomatic patients with normal LV systolic function can be treated safely with aggressive medical management rather than AVR has not been determined, and there are no data with which to recommend medical therapy for such patients. The standard of care is to proceed with AVR in symptomatic patients rather than to attempt long-term medical therapy (29). The exceptions to this general recommendation are symptomatic patients with AR and normal LV systolic function who are considered to be poor candidates for surgery because of additional cardiac or noncardiac factors.

Although there are sound physiologic principles underlying the use of vasodilator therapy in chronic severe AR, which is supported by a growing body of clinical evidence, there is no compelling information that other drugs have long-term beneficial actions in terms of either hemodynamics or patient outcome. Hence, there are no data with which to recommend the chronic use of digoxin, diuretics, nitrates, or positive inotropic agents in symptomatic or asymptomatic patients with chronic AR.

INDICATIONS FOR AORTIC VALVE REPLACEMENT

Patients with chronic AR should be considered for AVR only if the degree of AR is severe (29), and hence the following discussion applies only to patients with pure severe AR. Whenever there is uncertainty regarding the severity of AR after careful clinical and echocardiographic evaluation, it is important to consider obtaining additional data such as invasive hemodynamic and angiographic information. In patients with only mild AR who have symptoms or LV dysfunction, other etiologies should be considered, such as hypertension, coronary artery disease, and cardiomyopathic processes. On the other hand, patients with mild AR often justifiably require AVR at the time of surgery for coexisting car-

diovascular conditions, such as aortic root repair or coronary artery bypass surgery.

Symptomatic Patients with Normal Left Ventricular Systolic Function

AVR is indicated in patients with normal LV systolic function at rest who have New York Heart Association (NYHA) functional class II to IV symptoms of dyspnea or fatigue or Canadian Heart Association functional class II to IV angina pectoris. In many patients with mild NYHA functional class II dyspnea or fatigue, the etiology of symptoms is unclear, because it is often difficult to differentiate the effects of chronic deconditioning or aging from true cardiac symptoms. In such patients, objective treadmill exercise testing may be valuable to evaluate effort tolerance and symptomatic limitation. If the etiology of these mild symptoms is uncertain and if they do not interfere with the patient's lifestyle, it is reasonable to reevaluate the patient after a period of careful observation. On the other hand, the new development of even mild dyspnea has important implications in patients with severe AR, especially in those patients who also manifest increasing LV cavity dilatation or declining LV systolic function into the low normal range. Thus, the onset of true cardiac symptoms, even if mild, is an indication for AVR in patients with severe AR and preserved systolic function.

Symptomatic Patients with Left Ventricular Systolic Dysfunction

Symptomatic patients with mild to moderate LV systolic dysfunction should undergo AVR. Many have the potential for considerable improvement or normalization of LV function if AVR is performed without undue delay. Although patients with functional class IV symptoms have a low likelihood of recovery of systolic function and have a poor long-term survival compared with patients with less severe symptoms (17,22,23,26), outcome is more favorable with surgical than with medical therapy. In addition, AVR will improve ventricular loading conditions and will expedite subsequent management of LV dysfunction.

Among symptomatic patients with severely depressed LV systolic function (e.g., LV ejection fraction less than 25%), most have developed irreversible myocardial changes, and only a few such patients will manifest a meaningful recovery of LV function after operation (Fig. 8-1). The perioperative mortality associated with AVR may be as high as 10% in these patients, and mortality over the subsequent few years after AVR is very high. However, even in patients with NYHA functional class IV symptoms and ejection fraction less than 25%, the high risks associated with AVR and subsequent medical management of persistent LV dysfunction are usually a better alternative than the even higher risks of long-term medical management alone. In such settings, it is important that the risks of surgical versus medical therapy are discussed in detail with the patient and family.

Asymptomatic Patients

The timing of AVR in asymptomatic patients remains a controversial topic with considerable ongoing debate. However, there is general agreement (5,72–77) that AVR should be indicated in patients with LV systolic dysfunction under resting conditions. An important decision such as valve replacement should not be based on a single noninvasive measurement alone, and it is reasonable to obtain repeat measurements before a recommendation is made to operate on the asymptomatic patient. Echocardiographic assessment of LV ejection fraction is often imprecise, especially in patients with volume-loaded ventricles, and in many patients a separate independent test (such as radionuclide ventriculography or contrast left ventriculography) to confirm echocardiographic evidence of LV systolic dysfunction is warranted.

AVR should also be considered strongly in patients with extreme LV dilatation (end-diastolic dimension greater than 75 mm or end-systolic dimension greater than 55 mm) (29)

even if LV ejection fraction remains in the normal range. Most patients with this degree of LV cavity dilatation will have already developed depressed ejection fraction because of afterload mismatch and will thus be candidates for valve replacement because of LV systolic dysfunction. The elevated end-systolic dimension in this setting is usually a surrogate for systolic dysfunction. However, there is a relatively small number of asymptomatic patients who manifest extreme LV cavity dilatation with preserved systolic function, and these patients should also be considered for surgery because they may be at increased risk of sudden death (33,56). Moreover, the results of surgery are suboptimal when patients with severe LV dilatation undergo AVR after the onset of symptoms and/or LV systolic dysfunction (35). In contrast, the results of AVR in patients with severe LV dilatation have thus far been excellent when LV systolic function is normal (35).

Patients who show progressive LV dilatation on serial noninvasive tests represent a group at higher risk of developing symptoms or LV systolic dysfunction (33), and these patients require more careful monitoring than patients with stable LV dimensions over time. However, patients with enlarging LV dimensions may achieve a new steady state, in which afterload is balanced by LV hypertrophy and recruitment of preload, and may then do well for extended periods of time. Hence, patients manifesting progression in LV cavity size should be observed carefully, but AVR is usually not warranted until the threshold values noted above are reached or until symptoms or LV systolic dysfunction develop.

A decrease in ejection fraction during exercise appears to be a nonspecific finding. The available data would not support this parameter, in and of itself, as an indication for valve replacement in asymptomatic patients with normal systolic function at rest. First, the exercise ejection fraction response to exercise has not been demonstrated to have independent prognostic value in patients undergoing surgery (26). Second, the magnitude of change in ejection fraction with exercise is related to a number of factors, including the severity of the LV volume load (33,39–41) and the exercise-induced changes in both preload and peripheral resistance (42). A decrease in ejection fraction with exercise develops early in the natural history of AR, related to the development of LV dilatation (33).

Evolving Surgical Techniques

There are rapidly expanding surgical options for treating AR, with increasing experience in aortic homografts, pulmonary autografts, unstented tissue valves, and aortic valve repair. If these newer techniques ultimately are demonstrated to improve long-term survival or reduce postoperative valve complications, it is conceivable that the thresholds for recommending operation for AR will be reduced. Until such data are available, however, under most circumstances the indications for operation for AR do not depend on the operative technique to be used.

Concomitant Aortic Root Disease

Diseases of the ascending aorta often are the cause for the onset and progression of AR. The valvular regurgitation itself is often less important, in terms of diagnosis and decision making, than is the primary disease of the aorta. In such patients, diagnostic and management strategies should focus on the underlying aortic root disease and the severity of AR and the effect of AR on LV size and function. In general, patients with severe aortic root dilatation (greater than 50 mm) by echocardiography are considered candidates for combined aortic root reconstruction and AVR, even if the degree of AR is only mild.

SERIAL TESTING OF ASYMPTOMATIC PATIENTS

In most patients with chronic AR, the only procedures required for serial testing during the long-term follow-up period are a careful history, physical examination, and echocar-

diogram. The frequency of repeat echocardiograms depends on the severity of LV dilatation, the level of LV systolic function, and the previous evidence for or against progressive changes in LV size and function. At one extreme, yearly echocardiography is not warranted in asymptomatic patients with mild AR, normal LV systolic function, and evidence of no or mild LV dilatation unless there is a change in symptoms or clinical findings (29). On the other hand, asymptomatic patients with normal systolic function but with moderate to severe AR and moderate to severe LV dilatation require more frequent and more careful reevaluation, with history and physical examination every 6 to 12 months and with yearly echocardiograms. In patients with more advanced LV dilatation (e.g., end-diastolic dimension greater than 70 mm or end-systolic dimension greater than 50 mm) in whom the risk of symptoms or LV dysfunction ranges between 10% and 20% per year (33,35), it is reasonable to perform serial echocardiograms more frequently. Repeat echocardiograms should also be performed under most circumstances when patients first note the onset of symptoms, when there is an equivocal history of changing symptoms or exercise tolerance, or when there are clinical findings suggesting worsening AR or progressive LV dilatation. As noted previously, exercise testing may also be very valuable in assessing functional capacity and symptomatic responses in patients with equivocal changes in symptomatic status.

CONCLUSIONS

AVR is clearly indicated in patients with chronic AR once significant symptoms develop. Lacking important symptoms, operation should also be performed in patients with chronic AR who manifest consistent and reproducible evidence of either LV contractile dysfunction at rest or extreme LV dilatation. Noninvasive imaging techniques should play a pivotal role in this evaluation. An important clinical decision, such as recommending AVR in the asymptomatic patient, should not be based on a single echocardiographic measurement alone. However, when there are consistent indications of impaired contractile function at rest or extreme LV dilatation on repeat measurements, AVR is indicated in the asymptomatic patient. This strategy should reduce the likelihood of irreversible LV dysfunction and enhance long-term postoperative survival of patients with chronic AR.

REFERENCES

1. Grossman W, Jones D, McLaurin LP. Wall stress and patterns of hypertrophy in the human left ventricle. *J Clin Invest* 1975;56:56–64.
2. Ross J Jr, McCullough WH. Nature of enhanced performance of the dilated left ventricle in the dog during chronic volume overloading. *Circ Res* 1972;30:549–556.
3. Weisenbaugh T, Spann JF, Carabello BA. Differences in myocardial performance and load between patients with similar amounts of chronic aortic versus chronic mitral regurgitation. *J Am Coll Cardiol* 1984;3:916–923.
4. Ricci DR. Afterload mismatch and preload reserve in chronic aortic regurgitation. *Circulation* 1982;66:826–834.
5. Ross J Jr. Afterload mismatch in aortic and mitral valve disease: implications for surgical therapy. *J Am Coll Cardiol* 1985;5:811–826.
6. Gaasch WH. Left ventricular radius to wall thickness ratio. *Am J Cardiol* 1979;43:1189–1194.
7. Gaasch WH, Andrias CW, Levine HJ. Chronic aortic regurgitation: the effect of aortic valve replacement on left ventricular volume, mass, and function. *Circulation* 1978;58:825–836.
8. Schwarz F, Flameng W, Langebartels F, Sesto M, Walter P, Schlepper M. Impaired left ventricular function in chronic aortic valve disease: survival and function after replacement by Bjork-Shiley prosthesis. *Circulation* 1979;60:48–58.
9. Borer JS, Rosing DR, Kent KM, et al. Left ventricular function at rest and during exercise after aortic valve replacement in patients with aortic regurgitation. *Am J Cardiol* 1979;44:1297–1305.
10. Clark DG, McAnulty JH, Rahimtoola SH. Valve replacement in aortic insufficiency with left ventricular dysfunction. *Circulation* 1980;61:411–421.
11. Toussaint C, Cribier A, Cazor JL, Sayer R, Letac B. Hemodynamic and angiographic evaluation of aortic regurgitation 7 and 27 months after aortic valve replacement. *Circulation* 1981;64:456–463.
12. Carroll JD, Gaasch WH, Zile MR, Levine HJ. Serial changes in left ventricular function after correction of chronic aortic regurgitation: dependence on early changes in preload and subsequent regression of hypertrophy. *Am J Cardiol* 1983;51:476–482.
13. Bonow RO, Rosing DR, Maron BJ, et al. Reversal of left ventricular dysfunction after valve replacement for chronic aortic regurgitation: influence of duration of preoperative left ventricular dysfunction. *Circulation* 1984;70:570–579.
14. Fioretti P, Roelandt J, Sclavo M, et al. Postoperative regression of left ventricular dimensions in aortic insufficiency: a long-term echocardiography study. *J Am Coll Cardiol* 1985;5:856–861.
15. Taniguchi K, Nakano S, Hirose H, et al. Preoperative left ventricular function: minimal requirement for successful late results of valve replacement for aortic regurgitation. *J Am Coll Cardiol* 1987;10:510–518.
16. Carabello BA, Usher BW, Hendrix GH, Assey ME, Crawford FA, Leman RB. Predictors of outcome for aortic valve replacement in patients with aortic regurgitation and left ventricular dysfunction: a change in the measuring stick. *J Am Coll Cardiol* 1987;10:991–997.
17. Bonow RO, Dodd JT, Maron BJ, et al. Long-term serial changes in left ventricular function and reversal of ventricular dilatation after valve replacement for chronic aortic regurgitation. *Circulation* 1988;78:1108–1120.
18. Bonow RO. Radionuclide angiography in the management of aortic regurgitation. *Circulation* 1991;84[Suppl I]:296–302.
19. Cohn PF, Gorlin R, Cohn LH, Collins JJ Jr. Left ventricular ejection fraction as a prognostic guide in surgical treatment of coronary and valvular heart disease. *Am J Cardiol* 1974;34:136–141.
20. Copeland JG, Griepp RB, Stinson EB, Shumway NE. Long-term follow-up after isolated aortic valve replacement. *J Thorac Cardiovasc Surg* 1977;74:875–889.
21. Herreman F, Ameur A, deVernejoul F, et al. Pre- and postoperative hemodynamic and cineangiographic assessment of left ventricular function in patients with aortic regurgitation. *Am Heart J* 1979;98:63–72.
22. Cunha CLP, Giuliani ER, Fuster V, Seward JB, Brandenburg RO, McGoon DC. Preoperative M-mode echocardiography as a predictor of surgical results in chronic aortic insufficiency. *J Thorac Cardiovasc Surg* 1980;79:256–265.
23. Forman R, Firth BF, Barnard MS. Prognostic significance of preoperative left ventricular ejection fraction and valve lesion in patients with aortic valve replacement. *Am J Cardiol* 1980;45:1120–1125.
24. Greves J, Rahimtoola SH, McAnulty JH, et al. Preoperative criteria predictive of late survival following valve replacement for severe aortic regurgitation. *Am Heart J* 1981;101:300–308.
25. Gaasch WH, Carroll JD, Levine HJ, Criscitiello MG. Chronic aortic regurgitation: prognostic value of left ventricular end-systolic dimension and end-diastolic radius/thickness ratio. *J Am Coll Cardiol* 1983;1:775–782.
26. Bonow RO, Picone AL, McIntosh CL, et al. Survival and functional results after valve replacement for aortic regurgitation from 1976 to 1983: impact of preoperative left ventricular function. *Circulation* 1985;72:1244–1256.
27. Carabello BA, Williams H, Gash AK, et al. Hemodynamic predictors of outcome in patients undergoing valve replacement. *Circulation* 1986;74:1309–1316.
28. Michel PL, Iung B, Jaoude SA, et al. The effect of left ventricular systolic function on long term survival in mitral and aortic regurgitation. *J Heart Valve Dis* 1995;4[Suppl II]:S160–S169.
29. Bonow RO, Carabello B, de Leon AC, et al. ACC/AHA Guidelines for the Management of Patients with Valvular Heart Disease. A Report of the American College of Cardiology/American Heart Association Task Force on Practice Guidelines (Committee on Management of

Patients with Valvular Heart Disease). *J Am Coll Cardiol* (in press).

30. Bonow RO, Rosing DR, McIntosh CL, et al. The natural history of asymptomatic patients with aortic regurgitation and normal left ventricular function. *Circulation* 1983;68:509–517.

31. Scognamiglio R, Fasoli G, Dalla-Volta S. Progression of myocardial dysfunction in asymptomatic patients with severe aortic insufficiency. *Clin Cardiol* 1986;9:151–156.

32. Siemienczuk D, Greenberg B, Morris C, et al. Chronic aortic insufficiency: factors associated with progression to aortic valve replacement. *Ann Intern Med* 1989;110:587–592.

33. Bonow RO, Lakatos E, Maron BJ, Epstein SE. Serial long-term assessment of the natural history of asymptomatic patients with chronic aortic regurgitation and normal left ventricular systolic function. *Circulation* 1991;84:1625–1635.

34. Scognamiglio R, Rahimtoola S, Fasoli G, Nistri S, Dalla-Volta S. Nifedipine in asymptomatic patients with severe aortic regurgitation and normal left ventricular function. *N Engl J Med* 1994;331:689–694.

35. Tornos MP, Olona M, Permanyer-Miralda G, et al. Clinical outcome of severe asymptomatic chronic aortic regurgitation: a long-term prospective follow-up study. *Am Heart J* 1995;130:333–339.

36. Ishii K, Hirota Y, Suwa M, Kita Y, Onaka H, Kawamura K. Natural history and left ventricular response in chronic aortic regurgitation. *Am J Cardiol* 1996;78:357–361.

37. Borer JS, Hochreiter C, Herrold EM, et al. Prediction of indications for valve replacement among asymptomatic or minimally symptomatic patients with chronic aortic regurgitation and normal left ventricular performance. *Circulation* 1998;97:525–534.

38. Shen WF, Roubin GS, Choong CYP, et al. Evaluation of relationship between myocardial contractile state and left ventricular function in patients with aortic regurgitation. *Circulation* 1985;71:31–38.

39. Lewis SM, Riba AL, Berger HJ, et al. Radionuclide angiographic exercise left ventricular performance in chronic aortic regurgitation: relationship to resting echocardiographic ventricular dimensions and systolic wall stress index. *Am Heart J* 1982;103:498–504.

40. Goldman ME, Packer M, Horowitz SF, et al. Relation between exercise-induced changes in ejection fraction and systolic loading conditions at rest in aortic regurgitation. *J Am Coll Cardiol* 1984;3:924–929.

41. Greenberg B, Massie B, Thomas D, et al. Association between the exercise ejection fraction response and systolic wall stress in patients with chronic aortic insufficiency. *Circulation* 1985;71:458–465.

42. Kawanishi DT, McKay CR, Chandraratna AN, et al. Cardiovascular response to dynamic exercise in patients with chronic symptomatic mild-to-moderate and severe aortic regurgitation. *Circulation* 1986;73:62–72.

43. Henry WL, Bonow RO, Rosing DR, Epstein SE. Observations on the optimum time for operative intervention for aortic regurgitation. II. Serial echocardiographic evaluation of asymptomatic patients. *Circulation* 1980;61:484–492.

44. McDonald IG, Jelinek VM. Serial M-mode echocardiography in severe chronic aortic regurgitation. *Circulation* 1980;62:1291–1296.

45. Kennedy JW, Doces J, Stewart DK. Left ventricular function before and following aortic valve replacement. *Circulation* 1977;56:944–950.

46. Pantely G, Morton M, Rahimtoola SH. Effects of successful, uncomplicated valve replacement on ventricular hypertrophy, volume, and performance in aortic stenosis and in aortic incompetence. *J Thorac Cardiovasc Surg* 1978;75:383–391.

47. Henry WL, Bonow RO, Borer JS, et al. Observations on the optimum time for operative intervention for aortic regurgitation. I. Evaluation of the results of aortic valve replacement in symptomatic patients. *Circulation* 1980;61:471–483.

48. Bonow RO, Rosing DR, Kent KM, Epstein SE. Timing of operation for chronic aortic regurgitation. *Am J Cardiol* 1982;50:325–336.

49. Kumpuris AG, Quinones MA, Waggoner AD, Kanon DJ, Nelson JG, Miller RR. Importance of preoperative hypertrophy, wall stress, and end-systolic dimension as predictors of normalization of left ventricular dilatation after valve replacement in chronic aortic insufficiency. *Am J Cardiol* 1982;49:1091–1100.

50. Fioretti P, Roelandt J, Bos RJ, et al. Echocardiography in chronic aortic insufficiency: is valve replacement too late when left ventricular end-systolic dimension reaches 55 mm? *Circulation* 1983;67:216–221.

51. Stone PH, Clark RD, Goldschlager N, Selzer A, Cohn K. Determinants of prognosis of patients with aortic regurgitation who undergo aortic valve replacement. *J Am Coll Cardiol* 1984;3:1118–1126.

52. Daniel WG, Hood WP, Siart A, et al. Chronic aortic regurgitation: reassessment of the prognostic value of preoperative left ventricular end-systolic dimension and fractional shortening. *Circulation* 1985;71:669–680.

53. Cormier B, Vahanian A, Luxereau P, Kassab R, Acar J. Should asymptomatic or mildly symptomatic aortic regurgitation be operated on? *Z Kardiol* 1986;75[Suppl 2]:141–145.

54. Sheiban I, Trevi GP, Casarotto D, et al. Aortic valve replacement in patients with aortic incompetence: preoperative parameters influencing long-term results. *Z Kardiol* 1986;75[Suppl 2]:146–154

55. Klodas E, Enriquez-Sarano M, Tajik AJ, Mullany CJ, Bailey KR, Seward JB. Aortic regurgitation complicated by extreme left ventricular dilation: long-term outcome after surgical correction. *J Am Coll Cardiol* 1996;27:670–677.

56. Turina J, Turina M, Rothlin M, Krayenbuehl HP. Improved late survival in patients with chronic aortic regurgitation by earlier operation. *Circulation* 1984;70 [Suppl I]:147–152.

57. Bonow RO, Borer JS, Rosing DR, et al. Preoperative exercise capacity in symptomatic patients with aortic regurgitation as a predictor of postoperative left ventricular function and long-term prognosis. *Circulation* 1980;62:1280–1290.

58. Levine HJ, Gaasch WH. Vasoactive drugs in chronic regurgitant lesions of the mitral and aortic valves. *J Am Coll Cardiol* 1996;28:1083–1091.

59. Bolen JL, Alderman EL. Hemodynamic consequences of afterload reduction in patients with chronic aortic regurgitation. *Circulation* 1976;53:879–883.

60. Miller RR, Vismara LA, DeMaria AN, Salel AF, Mason DT. Afterload reduction therapy with nitroprusside in severe aortic regurgitation: improved cardiac perfor-

mance and reduced regurgitant volume. *Am J Cardiol* 1976;38:564–567.

61. Greenberg BH, DeMots H, Murphy E, Rahimtoola S. Beneficial effects of hydralazine on rest and exercise hemodynamics in patients with chronic severe aortic insufficiency. *Circulation* 1980;62:49–55.

62. Greenberg BH, DeMots H, Murphy E, Rahimtoola S. Mechanism for improved cardiac performance with arteriolar dilators in aortic insufficiency. *Circulation* 1981;63:263–268.

63. Fioretti P, Benussi B, Scardi S, Klugman S, Brower RW, Camerini F. Afterload reduction with nifedipine in aortic insufficiency. *Am J Cardiol* 1982;49:1728–1732.

64. Shen WF, Roubin GS, Hirasawa K, et al. Noninvasive assessment of acute effects of nifedipine on rest and exercise hemodynamics and cardiac function in patients with aortic regurgitation. *J Am Coll Cardiol* 1984;4:902–907.

65. Scognamiglio R, Fasoli G, Visintin L, Dalla-Volta S. Effects of unloading and positive inotropic interventions on left ventricular function in asymptomatic patients with chronic severe aortic insufficiency. *Clin Cardiol* 1987;10:804–810.

66. Rothlisberger C, Sareli P, Weisenbaugh T. Comparison of single-dose nifedipine and captopril for chronic severe aortic regurgitation. *Am J Cardiol* 1993;72:799–804.

67. Greenberg B, Massie B, Bristow D, et al. Long-term vasodilator therapy of chronic aortic regurgitation: a randomized double-blinded, placebo-controlled clinical trial. *Circulation* 1988;78:92–103.

68. Scognamiglio R, Fasoli G, Ponchia A, Dalla-Volta S. Long-term nifedipine unloading therapy in asymptomatic patients with chronic severe aortic regurgitation. *J Am Coll Cardiol* 1990;16:424–429.

69. Lin M, Chiang HT, Lin SL, et al. Vasodilator therapy in chronic asymptomatic aortic regurgitation: enalapril versus hydralazine therapy. *J Am Coll Cardiol* 1994;24:1046–1053.

70. Weisenbaugh T, Sinovich V, Dullabh A, Sareli P. Six month pilot study of captopril for mildly symptomatic, severe isolated mitral and isolated aortic regurgitation. *J Heart Valve Dis* 1994;3:197–204.

71. Schon HR, Dorn R, Barthel P, Schomig A. Effects of 12 months quinapril therapy in asymptomatic patients with chronic aortic regurgitation. *J Heart Valve Dis* 1994;3:500–509.

72. Rahimtoola SH. Valve replacement should not be performed in all asymptomatic patients with severe aortic incompetence. *J Thorac Cardiovasc Surg* 1980;79:163–172.

73. Nishimura RA, McGoon MD, Schaff HV, Giuliani ER. Chronic aortic regurgitation: indications for operation—1988. *Mayo Clin Proc* 1988;63:270–280.

74. Carabello BA. The changing unnatural history of valvular regurgitation. *Ann Thorac Surg* 1992;53:191–199.

75. Bonow RO. Management of chronic aortic regurgitation. *N Engl J Med* 1994;331;736–737.

76. Bonow RO. Asymptomatic aortic regurgitation: indications for operation. *J Cardiol Surg* 1994;9[Suppl]:170–173.

77. Gaasch WH, Sundaram M, Meyer TE. Managing asymptomatic patients with chronic aortic regurgitation. *Chest* 1997;111:1702–1709.

9

Acute Aortic Insufficiency

Joseph S. Alpert

Department of Medicine, University of Arizona College of Medicine, Tucson, Arizona 85724-5035

Aortic insufficiency (AI) presents in a variety of ways. At one end of the spectrum is the patient with chronic severe AI who may be asymptomatic, with bounding pulses, a heart murmur, and cardiac enlargement secondary to left ventricular dilatation. Such a patient may subsequently develop symptoms of congestive heart failure (CHF). This patient is usually easily recognized because in the absence of CHF, he or she displays the well-known findings associated with chronic severe AI that have been recognized since the time of Corrigan (1,2) (see Chapter 8). At the opposite end of the spectrum is the patient who presents with acute severe AI resulting from destruction or disruption of a previously normal aortic valve. In such patients, acute AI is usually the result of infective endocarditis, dissection of the ascending aorta, trauma, or spontaneous rupture of a myxomatous valve. These patients invariably develop severe CHF that is often refractory to medical therapy; they may require urgent aortic valve replacement (AVR).

Acute severe AI, even in the presence of CHF, can be difficult to identify. In such cases, torrential AI pours into a previously normal left ventricle that lacks the dilatation, hypertrophy, and increased left ventricular compliance present in patients with chronic AI. Because forward stroke output is not increased, the secondary physical signs of chronic severe AI (i.e., increased arterial pulse pressure, bounding pulses, and hyper-

dynamic precordial activity) are usually lacking (3). With the advances in cardiovascular diagnostic techniques, cardiac surgery, and critical care over the past 20 years, the syndrome of acute severe AI has been more frequently recognized and better managed (4).

DEFINITION AND ETIOLOGY OF ACUTE AORTIC INSUFFICIENCY

Acute severe AI is defined as hemodynamically important AI of sudden onset, occurring across a previously competent aortic valve into a left ventricle not previously subjected to volume overload. The causes of acute AI are enumerated in Table 9-1.

Infective Endocarditis

Bacterial or fungal organisms infecting and damaging a native or prosthetic aortic valve are the most common cause of acute severe

TABLE 9-1. *Causes of acute aortic insufficiency*

Infectious endocarditis
Dissection of the ascending aorta
Traumatic disruption of the aortic valve
Spontaneous rupture or prolapse of an aortic valve cusp secondary to degenerative diseases of the valve
After operative or catheter valvuloplasty
Sudden dehiscence of part or all of the sewing ring of a prosthetic aortic valve
Connective tissue disease with inflammation involving the aortic valve, e.g., Takayasu's arteritis

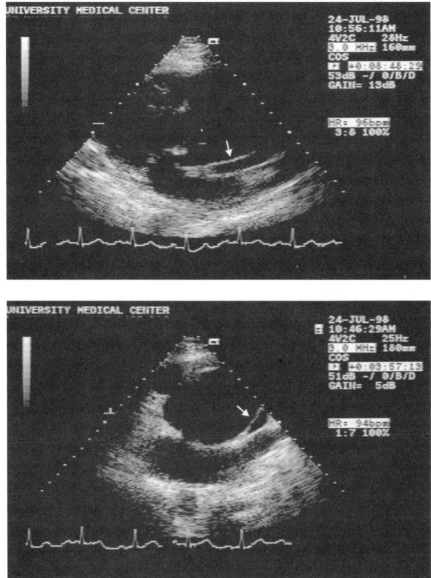

FIG. 9-1. A and B: Echocardiographic images recorded from a 29-year-old man with known Marfan's syndrome with recent onset of tachycardia and shortness of breath. Long-axis and cross-sectional views of the aortic root demonstrate a flap in the posterior portion of the aortic root (*white arrows* in both views), thereby confirming the clinical diagnosis of aortic dissection with acute aortic insufficiency. The aortic root is markedly dilated. Left ventricular function was normal. **C:** Doppler echocardiographic images of the same patient demonstrate a jet of severe aortic insufficiency (*white arrow*).

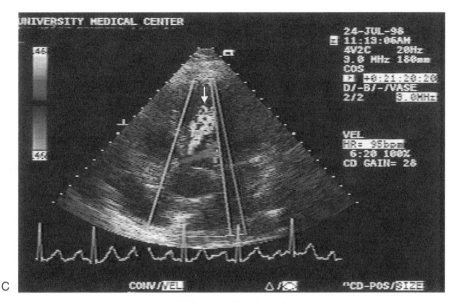

C

FIG. 9-1. *Continued.*

AI. In this setting, bacterial endocarditis is often the result of *Staphylococcus aureus*, which produces necrosis, perforation, and/or detachment of one or more aortic valve leaflets. Infection of the aortic annulus with associated necrosis and abscess formation can further weaken the aortic valve, leading to progressive annular dilation with resultant failure of the aortic valve commissures to coapt properly during diastole. Moreover, annular abscesses can distort the annulus, resulting in failure of one or more aortic cusps to coapt or to prolapse into the left ventricular outflow tract during diastole. Large valvular vegetations may also prevent proper diastolic coaptation of the aortic valve cusps (Fig. 9-2). Although such bulky vegetations are seen in patients with staphylococcal endocarditis, they are more characteristic of fungal endocarditis caused by *Aspergillus, Candida albicans, Histoplasma capsulatum,* or other such species.

Acute endocarditis is often associated with organisms of sufficient virulence to infect a previously normal valve. Such infections are often seen in narcotic addicts as a result of nonsterile intravenous injections or secondary to skin abscess formation that complicates subcutaneous drug use (so-called skin popping). More commonly, infection involves an anatomically bicuspid aortic valve. Often, clinically important aortic stenosis or regurgitation is absent before the onset of infectious endocarditis. Patients with bicuspid aortic valves are at increased risk for aortic valve endocarditis because the bicuspid valve is associated with turbulent flow and abnormal valve thickening, the valve lesion is commonly asymptomatic and has escaped previous detection, and antibiotic prophylaxis has not been prescribed for dental or other surgical procedures (5–9).

Infective endocarditis resulting in acute severe AI is associated with several life-threatening cardiac complications (6,10,11). Annular abscess is nearly always associated with hemodynamically severe AI and may result in gradual or sudden onset of first-, second-, or third-degree atrioventricular block or left bundle branch block secondary to inflammation and necrosis of the atrioventricular node and proximal His-Purkinje portion of the conduction system. The aortic valve infection may erode into the pericardium, resulting in puru-

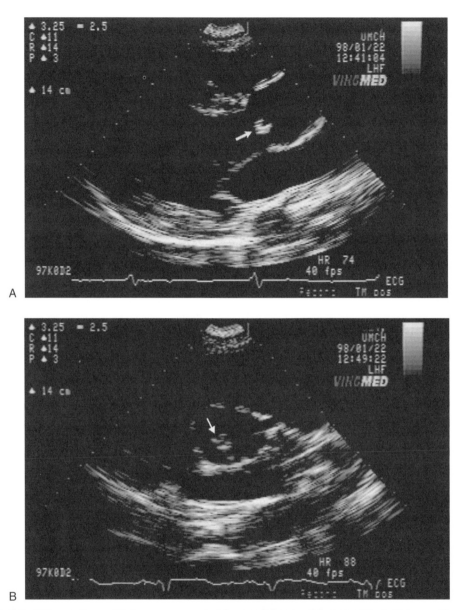

FIG. 9-2. Echocardiographic images recorded from a 34-year-old man with multiple positive blood cultures for enterococcus. The clinical history suggested infectious endocarditis of recent onset. The long-axis **(A)**, cross-sectional **(B)**, and four-chamber **(C)** views demonstrate a vegetation on the right coronary cusp of the aortic valve (*white arrows*). Doppler echocardiography demonstrated severe aortic insufficiency with normal left ventricular function.

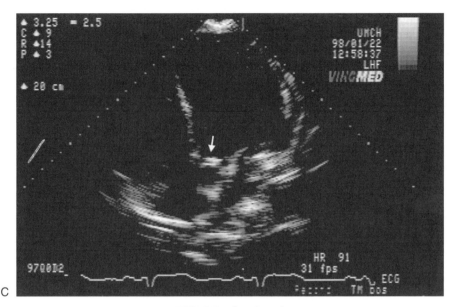

FIG. 9-2. *Continued.*

lent pericarditis, hemopericardium, and cardiac tamponade. Annular abscesses can extend into the membranous intraventricular septum and may lead to septal rupture with a resultant left-to-left shunt. Extension of infection into the muscular septum can also produce ventricular ectopic activity, including ventricular tachycardia together with a variety of infranodal cardiac conduction abnormalities. Infection may extend from the aortic valve and annulus into the contiguous right ventricle or anterolaterally situated right atrium, resulting in an aorta-right ventricular or right atrial fistula. These complications are associated with the development of a continuous machinery-like murmur (related to the substantial left-to-right shunt) and severe CHF. Superior extension of the infection can produce a mycotic aneurysm involving the sinus of Valsalva or proximal ascending aorta. The development of any of these complications in the setting of acute endocarditis mandates urgent consideration of AVR.

Dissection of the Ascending Aorta

Dissection of the ascending aorta with development of a medial hematoma can involve the aortic valve. The hematoma can dissect retrograde and displace the attachments of the aortic valve cusps downward and medially so that one or more aortic valve cusps prolapse into the outflow tract of the left ventricle during diastole, thereby leading to incompetence of the valve. AI is present in approximately 65% of patients with dissection of the ascending aorta (14–17) (Fig. 9-1).

Recognition of aortic dissection complicated by acute severe AI is important, because urgent operative intervention is required (18–20). Suggestive clinical features of aortic dissection include severe chest pain and/or evidence of vascular compromise to the head, upper and/or lower extremities, gut, and/or kidney. Acute AI may be overlooked in patients with dissection who present with other manifestations (e.g., cerebrovascular accident or extremity ischemia).

Patients who develop aortic dissection have often had preexisting chronic hypertension with associated left ventricular hypertrophy and possibly arteriosclerotic heart disease with prior myocardial infarction. These latter conditions lead to decreased left ventricular compliance. In this setting, volume overload of the left ventricle is particularly poorly tolerated: Patients develop severe CHF with markedly decreased forward cardiac output and severe pulmonary congestion.

Connective Tissue Diseases

Some cases of "spontaneous" acute severe AI are related to noninfectious inflammatory processes involving the aortic valve. Acute severe AI can complicate systemic lupus erythematosus as a result of sterile perforation of one or more aortic valve cusps secondary to fibrinoid necrosis of the valve parenchyma (21,22).

Aortitis, with inflammation and furling of the aortic valve leaflets and Whipple's disease, can also result in progressive severe AI (23). In idiopathic giant-cell aortitis (24) and Takayasu's arteritis, the inflammatory process can also lead to severe AI (25). Simultaneous acute aortic and mitral insufficiency have been reported as complications of ankylosing spondylitis (26).

Trauma

Acute disruption of the aortic valve can result from closed-chest or abdominal trauma such as that caused by automobile accidents, crush injuries, or falls (27).

AI is the most common valve lesion observed in patients with closed-chest trauma. Many of these patients do not have signs of chest injury. Initially, there may be no detectable murmur of aortic regurgitation; the murmur and clinical signs associated with acute AI may be first observed several days after the occurrence of chest trauma. Sudden compression of the thoracoabdominal aorta during diastole when the aortic valve is closed can elevate intraaortic pressure, causing aortic cuspal tearing, perforation, or detachment (28). Trauma can damage a previously normal aortic valve; however, valves with myxomatous degeneration are more susceptible to physical injury (29). Although almost always the consequence of high-energy closed-chest or abdominal impact, traumatic AI has also been reported as a result of very strenuous physical activity such as shoveling snow (30) or parturition (31).

The detection of traumatic AI requires careful and thorough cardiovascular evaluation initially when the trauma victim presents to the hospital, after resuscitative and initial therapeutic interventions are complete, and after several weeks of recovery so that delayed manifestations of aortic valve damage are recognized (27).

Spontaneous Aortic Insufficiency Secondary to Myxomatous Degeneration of the Aortic Valve

Sudden eversion or prolapse of an aortic cusp may result in spontaneous acute severe AI. This event is almost invariably associated with a myxomatous valve. Myxomatous valves can also spontaneously perforate (32,33). Spontaneous acute severe AI has also been reported as a result of cuspal eversion occurring in a patient with a bicuspid aortic valve (34). Patients with Marfan's syndrome are particularly prone to develop acute cuspal eversion or prolapse of an aortic valve cusp (33). Rarely, a seemingly normal aortic valve prolapses or ruptures.

Prosthetic Valve Aortic Insufficiency

Sudden partial dehiscence of the sewing ring of a prosthetic valve from the aortic annulus causes acute severe AI. This occasionally occurs after emergency AVR for bacterial endocarditis when the valve is implanted into an infected annulus. It may also occur in the absence of infection (35). Pannus ingrowth, thrombus, or vegetation may impede proper seating of the ball or poppet during diastole, resulting in severe AI. Poppet wear with consequent failure to seat properly may also precipitate AI that is more commonly chronic and progressive in nature and only occasionally acute and catastrophic.

Acute AI is particularly dangerous in patients who have undergone AVR for aortic stenosis. Here, the ventricle is hypertrophied and noncompliant; increased stroke volume in this setting requires marked elevation in ventricular filling pressure with resultant pulmonary congestion (3). Homograft valves and porcine bioprostheses undergo progressive slow degeneration; occasionally, severe acute AI develops in this setting (36). Thus, chronic progressive or acute severe AI may result from gradual or sudden leaflet disruption secondary to degenerative changes in bioprostheses (37–39). Acute severe AI may also result from sudden tearing of a porcine valve leaflet secondary to trauma or endocarditis.

PATHOPHYSIOLOGY

The magnitude of the hemodynamic response that occurs in patients with acute AI is the result of the severity of the volume overload and the rapidity with which the latter develops (40,41).

In *chronic* severe AI, the volume of blood that regurgitates into the left ventricle during diastole increases slowly with time. To accommodate this regurgitant volume, the left ventricle slowly dilates, its walls undergoing minimal thickening, and its compliance increases. This pattern of increased chamber radius with minimal increase in ventricular wall thickness is known as eccentric hypertrophy. It allows the affected ventricle to operate at a larger end-diastolic volume with little or no rise in end-diastolic pressure. As long as systolic function is preserved, such ventricles are capable of ejecting an abnormally large total stroke volume (normal stroke volume plus regurgitant stroke volume). In this manner, systemic perfusion is maintained, left ventricular ejection fraction is preserved (42–44), left ventricular diastolic pressure remains low, and symptoms of heart failure do not develop. In effect, the ventricle is operating at a much greater end-diastolic volume with a normal end-diastolic pressure (i.e., its compliance has increased). Ejection of the large total stroke volume results in a widened arterial pulse pressure.

In sharp contrast to the situation just described in patients with chronic AI is the hemodynamic and clinical scenario seen after acute perforation or destruction of the aortic valve in individuals with previously normal left ventricular volume and function. In these individuals, eccentric hypertrophy is not present and ventricular compliance is normal and remains so despite the sudden regurgitant volume overload (Table 9-2, Fig. 9-3). This overload is poorly tolerated because the left ventricle is now "overfilled" and operating on the steep or noncompliant portion of its diastolic pressure–volume relationship (40). If the volume of acute AI is large, end-diastolic left ventricular pressure is markedly increased, even approaching aortic diastolic pressure. The normal left ventricle, neither hypertro-

TABLE 9-2. *Contrasted hemodynamic responses: chronic vs. acute aortic insufficiency*

Variable	Acute AI	Chronic AI
LV diastolic volume (preload)	Slight increase	Marked increase
LV afterload	Modest increase	Normal or modest decrease
LV diastolic pressure	Marked increase	Normal or modestly increased
LV ejection fraction	Normal	Normal or increased
LV compliance	Normal	Increased
LV ejection velocity (dp/dt)	Normal	Increased
Heart rate	Increased	Normal
Forward or effective stroke volume	Decreased	Normal
Forward or effective cardiac output	Decreased	Normal
Peripheral vascular resistance	Increased	Normal
Arterial pulse pressure	Normal	Marked increase
Aortic systolic pressure	Normal	Increased
Coronary blood flow	Normal or modest decrease	Marked increase
Activation of the SNS	Marked increase	Normal

AI, aortic insufficiency; LV, left ventricular; SNS, sympathetic nervous system.

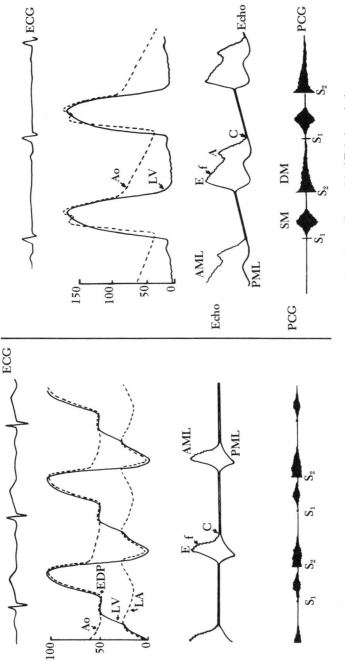

FIG. 9-3. Schematic illustrations comparing the hemodynamic echocardiographic (*Echo*) and phono-cardiographic (*PCG*) manifestations of acute severe **(left)** and chronic severe **(right)** AI. *Ao,* aorta; *LV,* left ventricle; *LA,* left atrium; *EDP,* end-diastolic pressure; *f,* flutter of anterior mitral valve leaflet; *AML,* anterior mitral leaflet; *PML,* posterior mitral leaflet; *SM,* systolic murmur; DM, diastolic murmur; *C,* closure point of mitral valve. (From ref. 4, with permission.)

phied nor dilated, cannot acutely increase its total left ventricular stroke volume sufficiently to maintain forward stroke volume in this setting. There is a resultant precipitous rise in left ventricular end-diastolic pressure without a change in forward cardiac output (40). It is often inaccurately stated that the left ventricle in acute AI is not dilated. Indeed, modest left ventricular dilatation develops but does not exceed a volume 20% to 30% above normal. In patients with marked acute AI, this modest increase in left ventricular volume is insufficient to meet the demands of the large regurgitant volume of blood, and, as already noted, marked elevation in left ventricular diastolic pressure ensues (4). Because left ventricular stroke volume is not markedly increased, arterial pulse pressure remains unchanged, and the bounding arterial pulses of chronic AI are absent. Silvestry et al. (45) recently evaluated ventricular and myocardial efficiency in a dog model of acute aortic regurgitation. They observed that left ventricular compensation during the volume overload of acute aortic regurgitation occurred at the expense of myocardial efficiency. Subsequently, global left ventricular dysfunction developed characterized by depressed systolic mechanics and mechanical, coupling, and contractile inefficiencies (45).

The noncompliant left ventricle and the pericardium limit the increase in left ventricular volume in patients with acute severe AI (41). Cardiac output usually declines as left ventricular failure develops; systemic arterial blood pressure is maintained by a reflex increase in peripheral vascular resistance (Table 9-2) (40).

Regurgitation of aortic blood into the relatively noncompliant left ventricle has several consequences. The rise in left ventricular diastolic pressure can lead to increasing left atrial and pulmonary capillary pressures of sufficient magnitude to produce pulmonary edema. Furthermore, augmentation of early diastolic, left ventricular pressure causes the mitral leaflets to drift toward the closed position. Blood entering the left ventricle from the left atrium flows through these relatively coapted mitral leaflets often giving rise to a low-pitched mid-to-late-diastolic (Austin-Flint) rumbling murmur. Severe acute AI may elevate left ventricular diastolic pressure to such a degree that the latter exceeds left atrial pressure and actually causes premature closure of the mitral valve (32) (Fig. 9-4). Downes et al. (52), using Doppler echocardiographic sampling in the left

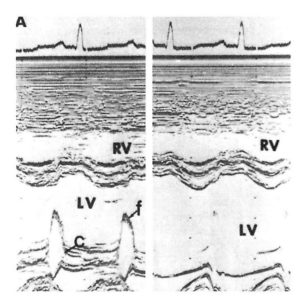

FIG. 9-4. Representative M-mode echocardiogram showing the features of acute severe aortic insufficiency. The features demonstrated include slight left ventricular dilatation, normal to mildly reduced septal and posterior wall excursion, diastolic fluttering, and premature closure of the mitral valve. *RV*, right ventricle; *LV*, left ventricle; *f*, flutter of anterior mitral valve leaflet; *C*, closure point of mitral valve.

atrium, demonstrated late diastolic mitral regurgitation in all patients with acute severe AI and none in patients with chronic AI. Diastolic mitral regurgitation occurred coincident with mitral valve preclosure, regardless of the position of the valve leaflets at the time of initiation of closure. The authors concluded that normal nonregurgitant mitral valve closure apparently requires prepositioning of the mitral valve by a properly timed atrial systole followed by an active ventricular contraction, a situation not present in patients with acute AI. Finally, the often present compensatory tachycardia shortens diastole. These factors taken together appreciably reduce the time during which the mitral valve is open during diastole (47–50). Premature mitral valve closure results in absence or marked softening of the first heart sound.

The patient with acute severe AI and reduced cardiac output often has impaired regional arterial blood flow, manifested as oliguria, pallor and coolness of the skin, deranged temperature regulation secondary to reduced cutaneous blood flow, and gastrointestinal and hepatic dysfunction. With extreme reduction in tissue perfusion, cardiogenic shock and lactic acidosis may be present. Coronary blood flow reserve is decreased in animals with experimental severe acute AI. In patients, retrograde coronary flow develops during diastole in response to severe acute AI; myocardial perfusion is therefore only present during systole in this condition (51,52). Table 9-2 contains a summary of the pathophysiologic differences between acute and chronic severe AI.

CLINICAL PRESENTATION

History

The patient with acute severe AI presents with symptoms of rapid onset due to the precipitous rise in left atrial pressure (pulmonary congestion) and the abrupt reduction in forward cardiac output. Progressive symptoms attributable to pulmonary congestion include dyspnea on exertion, orthopnea and/or a dry minimally productive cough aggravated by re-

cumbency, paroxysmal nocturnal dyspnea, and dyspnea at rest even while sitting upright. Symptoms reflecting the reduction in cardiac output are more subtle and are often overshadowed by those due to pulmonary congestion. The former may include fatigue on exertion, apathy, agitation, and/or a deterioration in intellectual function reflecting impaired cerebral perfusion.

Heart failure of a greater or lesser degree is almost invariably present in patients with acute AI. Heart failure is usually progressive, severe, and eventually fatal in the absence of effective therapy. Milder degrees of heart failure are associated with lesser quantities of acute AI. However, an apparently stable patient may suddenly develop rapidly progressive symptoms and signs of left ventricular decompensation (4,11,14,29). Symptoms of right ventricular failure (abdominal distension secondary to ascites and peripheral edema) are not commonly encountered in patients with acute AI. The clinical picture is usually dominated by the symptoms of acute left ventricular failure (3).

A number of other symptoms relate to the etiology of acute AI. Severe chest and/or back pain, abrupt and severe in onset, is characteristic of aortic dissection. Fever, chills, and malaise with or without evidence of peripheral arterial macro- or microembolism suggest the diagnosis of infective endocarditis. The most common cause of acute AI is infectious endocarditis on a bicuspid aortic valve. This entity is more common in males than in females. A history of recent chest and/or abdominal trauma raises the likelihood of traumatic disruption of the aortic valve. The abrupt onset of cardiac decompensation in the absence of ancillary symptoms or known heart disease suggests sudden disruption or perforation of an aortic valve intrinsically weakened by myxomatous degeneration.

Physical Examination

Physical findings in the patient with acute severe AI reflect the severity of pulmonary congestion and impairment in forward cardiac output with resultant decreased tissue perfusion. A variety of signs relate to the underlying etiology of acute AI.

An understanding of the pathophysiology of acute severe AI, as previously outlined, is mandatory to recognize and interpret the physical findings, particularly with respect to their prognostic and therapeutic implications. As noted earlier, the most prominent features (in contradistinction to chronic, severe, compensated AI) are the manifestations of pulmonary congestion and reduced cardiac output and the relative paucity of findings suggestive of left ventricular volume overload with augmented stroke output. Because of the acute nature of the AI, the left ventricle has not undergone eccentric hypertrophy; widened arterial pulse pressure and dramatic peripheral arterial findings characteristic of chronic compensated AI are absent.

In acute severe AI, forward ventricular stroke output is reduced. The pulse pressure is not appreciably widened, systolic blood pressure is normal or only slightly elevated, and diastolic arterial pressure is usually slightly elevated (40,41). Tachycardia is the rule. The precordium is relatively quiet; conspicuously absent is the laterally displaced, heaving, apical impulse reflecting left ventricular volume overload and eccentric hypertrophy of chronic compensated AI. The first heart sound is usually soft as the regurgitant volume rapidly fills the ventricle and pushes the mitral leaflets toward the closed position before left ventricular activation. With severe acute AI, left ventricular diastolic pressure exceeds left atrial pressure before ventricular activation. Mitral valve closure occurs late in diastole, actually preceding ventricular and even atrial systole. Occasionally, the first heart sound is completely absent.

The second heart sound is also soft and may be absent if one or more aortic valve leaflets have been damaged to the point of little or no diastolic coaptation. An ejection-type murmur of variable intensity is often heard, localized to the base. This reflects turbulent flow across the aortic valve resulting from augmented stroke output through the damaged valve. The diastolic murmur characteristic of chronic severe AI (high-pitched, decrescendo, and lasting throughout most of diastole) is usually absent. Instead, one hears a nondescript short early diastolic murmur of mixed frequencies in patients with acute severe AI. The murmur is often soft. A flail aortic cusp may evoke a musical (narrow frequency band) and very intense diastolic murmur (29). If there is free AI with rapid diastolic equilibration of aortic and left ventricular pressures, the murmur ends well before the end of diastole. An Austin-Flint (mid-diastolic rumble) murmur is often present in acute severe AI (53). A third heart sound is also frequently present, reflecting rapid early diastolic ventricular filling. The cacophony of sounds and murmurs may mimic the two- or three-component rub of pericarditis. A fourth heart sound is usually absent. Rising pulmonary pressures lead to an increase in right ventricular afterload with resultant acute right ventricular failure. Therefore, jugular venous distension with a prominent A wave may be present. Occasionally, tricuspid regurgitation is present accompanied by jugular CV waves and the characteristic systolic murmur. In contradistinction to chronic severe AI, prominent neck pulsations in acute AI are venous in origin (CV waves secondary to tricuspid regurgitation) rather than arterial (bounding carotid arteries secondary to wide pulse pressure). Pulsus alternans is often present in patients with acute AI.

The precordium is usually quiet in acute AI because the left ventricle is neither dilated nor hyperdynamic as in chronic severe AI. The distal extremities are usually pale and cool, reflecting systemic anteriolar vasoconstriction. The physical findings in acute AI and the important differences between chronic and acute AI with respect to clinical manifestations are presented in Table 9-3.

Important ancillary physical findings often provide clues to the cause of the aortic valve dysfunction leading to acute severe AI. Fever, petechiae, purpura, and/or small or large arterial embolic events implicate infective endocarditis. Excruciating chest or back discom-

TABLE 9-3. *Clinical manifestations of severe, acute, aortic insufficiency*

Clinical finding	Acute	Chronic
Congestive heart failure	Early and sudden	Late and insidious
Arterial pulse		
Rate per minute	Increased	Normal
Rate of rise	Not increased	Increased
Systolic pressure	Normal to decreased	Increased
Diastolic pressure	Normal to decreased	Decreased
Pulse pressure	Near normal	Increased
Contour of peak	Single	Bisferiens
Pulsus alternans	Common	Uncommon
Left ventricular impulse	Near normal; minimal lateral displacement; not hyperdynamic	Laterally displaced, hyperdynamic
Auscultation		
First heart sound	Soft to absent	Normal
Aortic component of the second sound	Soft	Normal or decreased
Pulmonic component of the second sound	Normal or increased	Normal
Fourth heart sound	Consistently absent	Usually absent
Third heart sound	Common	Uncommon
Aortic systolic murmur	Grade 3 or less	Grade 3 or more
Aortic regurgitant murmur	Short, medium-pitched	Long, high-pitched
Austin Flint murmur	Mid-diastolic	Presystolic, mid-diastolic, or both
Peripheral arterial auscultatory signs	Absent	Present
Electrocardiogram	Sinus tachycardia, normal left ventricular voltage with minor repolarization abnormalities	Increased left ventricular voltage with major repolarization abnormalities
Chest roentgenogram		
Left ventricle	Normal or modestly increased	Markedly increased
Aortic root and arch	Usually normal	Prominent
Pulmonary venous pattern	Redistributed to upper lobes	Normal

fort and/or an inequality of pulses in the neck, upper, or lower extremities suggest aortic dissection. AI in a tall, thin patient with a long arm span, hyperextensile joints, and/or ectopia lentis points to the diagnosis of annuloaortic ectasia and/or aortic dissection, complicating Marfan's syndrome (54). Table 9-4 is an algorithm that directs the clinician to the etiology of AI as a function of associated ancillary clinical information.

LABORATORY FINDINGS

Chest Roentgenogram

The chest x-ray in patients with acute AI usually reveals bilateral patchy interstitial in-

TABLE 9-4. *Acute aortic insufficiency*

Infectious endocarditis	Aortic dissection	Traumatic AI	Marfan's syndrome with aortic dissection and/or AI	Rupture of a normal or myxomatous aortic valve
Fever Petechiae Purpura Large or small arterial emboli	Severe chest or back pain Inequality of arterial pulses	History of trauma	Tall, thin patient Long arm span Hyperextensile joints Ectopia lentis	No associated findings

AI, aortic insufficiency.

filtrates that progress to confluent alveolar infiltrates emanating from the hilar regions as pulmonary congestion progresses to fulminant pulmonary edema. The lung fields may be reasonably clear if the hemodynamic insult is so acute that there has been insufficient time for the accumulation of extravascular lung water. There is usually apical redistribution of flow in the pulmonary veins. The cardiac silhouette is not enlarged unless there is preexisting chronic valvular, myocardial, or pericardial dysfunction. The absence of cardiomegaly and a dilated ascending aorta essentially rules out the presence of clinically important chronic AI. However, patients with severe acute AI secondary to ascending aortic dissection usually demonstrate a widened transverse mediastinal shadow on the chest x-ray; medial displacement of the aortic knob calcification by greater than 1.0 cm from the outer edge of the aortic shadow is also strongly suggestive of dissection (14,53). Table 9-3 lists the chest roentgenographic findings in acute AI. If there is a suspicion of aortic dissection, it is imperative to obtain a good quality posteroanterior chest film. This study facilitates the detection of true mediastinal widening and/or displacement of calcium in the wall of the aortic knob aorta (14,55).

Electrocardiogram

The electrocardiographic findings in acute severe AI are neither sensitive nor specific. Sinus tachycardia is the rule but is only indicative of the severity of cardiac decompensation. Left ventricular hypertrophy is absent unless there has been a preexisting cardiac condition resulting in chronic volume and/or pressure overload. Acute severe AI does evoke compensatory ventricular dilatation and an increase in myocardial muscle mass such that electrocardiographic criteria for left ventricular hypertrophy can be detected as early as 2 weeks after the onset of severe AI (56). The electrocardiogram may demonstrate nonspecific ST segment and T wave abnormalities related to subendocardial ischemia, hypoxe-

mia, acidosis, and/or other metabolic or electrolyte abnormalities. The pattern of left ventricular hypertrophy and prominent upright left precordial T waves (diastolic-volume overload pattern), characteristic of chronic AI, is absent in acute severe AI (Table 9-3).

Echocardiogram

M-mode, two-dimensional, and Doppler echocardiography are essential in the evaluation of the patient with acute severe AI (48,49,57) (Figs. 9-1, 9-2, 9-5, and 9-6). These studies should be performed at the time of initial presentation and at regular intervals during the acute course of the illness. The initial echocardiogram and Doppler study provide information concerning the hemodynamic severity of the regurgitation, the involvement of other valves, the state of left ventricular function, and the presence of other cardiac abnormalities (e.g., pericardial effusion). The echocardiogram often provides information concerning the cause of AI (e.g., infective endocarditis, aortic dissection). During treatment, serial evaluations assess the patient's therapeutic response and permit prompt detection of valvular or left ventricular deterioration. Echocardiographic findings suggestive of acute severe AI are, for the most part, nonspecific. Systolic wall motion is usually normal, unless there is such a profound degree of afterload mismatch that contractile function is depressed. The pattern of well-compensated left ventricular volume overload (increased end-diastolic dimension, augmented ventricular wall-shortening velocity, and a near-normal end-systolic dimension) suggestive of chronic AI is not present in the patient with acute AI unless there is preexisting chronic aortic and/or mitral insufficiency. In acute AI, the end-diastolic and end-systolic dimensions are normal or only slightly increased. The left atrial dimension is normal or slightly increased unless there is chronic disease of the mitral valve, aortic valve, or myocardium. The right ventricular end-diastolic and end-systolic dimensions are normal or slightly increased.

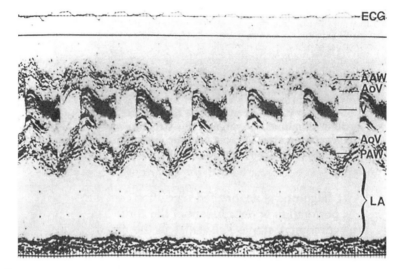

FIG. 9-5. M-mode aortic valve echocardiogram in a patient with acute severe aortic insufficiency secondary to bacterial endocarditis. It demonstrates a dense bacterial vegetation on a leaflet of the aortic valve, which vibrates with a high frequency in diastole as it is buffeted by the high-velocity regurgitant jet. *AAW*, anterior wall of aorta; *AoV*, aortic valve leaflet in systole; *V*, vegetation; *PAW*, posterior wall of aorta; *LA*, left atrium.

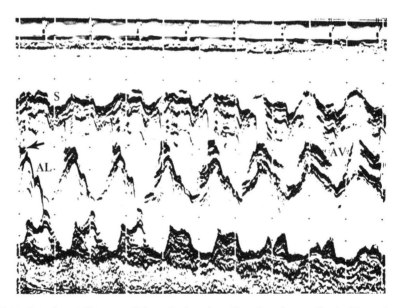

FIG. 9-6. M-mode echocardiogram of the mitral and aortic valves in a patient with acute severe aortic insufficiency secondary to bacterial endocarditis. It demonstrates an abnormally thickened structure contiguous with the aortic valve prolapsing into the left ventricular outflow tract at the onset of diastole (*arrow*) and displaying high-frequency diastolic vibrations. At surgery, this structure was identified as a staphylococcal vegetation attached to a necrotic and partially dehisced aortic valve leaflet. *S*, ventricular septum; *AL*, anterior leaflet of mitral valve; *AV*, aortic valve.

The mitral valve echocardiogram usually reveals anterior and posterior leaflets of normal thickness and mobility unless there is preexisting mitral valvular disease. Large redundant mitral leaflets with exaggerated opening and closing motion and/or the identification of mitral valve prolapse implicate myxomatous degeneration of the mitral valve. This may be present in cases of acute severe AI resulting from annuloaortic ectasia, Marfan's syndrome (Fig. 9-1), and/or spontaneous perforation of an apparently "normal" but probably myxomatous aortic valve. There is usually a reduction in the diastolic rate of mitral valve closure because the overloaded ventricle is relatively noncompliant.

If acute AI is very severe, the mitral valve may close before the onset of the electrocardiogram QRS complex (48–50) (Fig. 9-4). Premature closure of the mitral valve in conjunction with tachycardia results in profound abbreviation of the diastolic filling period. On the echocardiogram, this is evident as shortening of the interval during which the anterior and posterior mitral valve leaflets are separated during diastole. Premature closure of the mitral valve and appreciable shortening of the interval of diastolic flow across the mitral valve are important diagnostic and prognostic echocardiographic findings. They are associated with severe acute AI and left ventricular diastolic hypertension. Under such circumstances, procrastination delays potentially life-saving AVR. Figure 9-4 (left) is an M-mode mitral valve echogram depicting premature closure of the mitral valve, diastolic mitral-valve fluttering, and shortening of the diastolic filling period in a patient with acute severe AI. The right-hand panel of Fig. 9-4 depicts the left ventricular echogram in the same patient. It demonstrates slight left ventricular dilatation and normal to mildly reduced septal and posterior wall excursion characteristic of acute severe AI. The aortic valve echogram may demonstrate opening of the aortic valve in late diastole. As ventricular pressure rises and aortic pressure falls late in diastole, the aortic cusps may float open. Late diastolic recoil of the acutely overdistended

ventricular myocardium together with atrial systole further elevate ventricular pressure and may facilitate this late diastolic opening of the aortic valve (58). Table 9-5 summarizes and contrasts the echocardiographic manifestations of acute and chronic AI.

The echocardiogram of the aortic valve and proximal aortic root can provide specific information regarding the etiology of acute AI (59–66). Shaggy, large, irregular, echo-dense masses in association with the aortic valve leaflets are virtually diagnostic of vegetations resulting from infective endocarditis. Figures 2, 5, and 6 illustrate aortic valve bacterial vegetations of varying echo density and mobility in three patients with acute AI and infective endocarditis. Valvular vegetations are more accurately identified with transesophageal as compared with transthoracic echocardiography (63,64).

Chronic nonspecific thickening of one or more aortic valve leaflets due to rheumatic disease, acquired degenerative changes involving a bicuspid valve, calcification and fibrosis of a normal valve, or an organized sterile vegetation secondary to previous infectious or Libman-Sacks endocarditis may sometimes mimic vegetations of active infective endocarditis.

A fine linear structure, moving in a to-and-fro fashion—in the aortic root during systole and in the left ventricular outflow tract during diastole—suggests bland perforation or de-

TABLE 9-5. *Echo/Doppler manifestations of severe aortic regurgitation*

Echo/Doppler variable	Acute	Chronic
Mitral valve		
Closure	Early	Normal
Opening	Late	Normal
Diastolic mitral regurgitation	Present	Absent
Anterior leaflet E-F slope	Reduced	Normal
Diastolic fluttering	Yes	Yes
Left ventricle		
Systolic wall motion	Normal	
Hyperkinetic		
End-diastolic dimension	Normal	Increased
End-systolic dimension	Normal	Normal
Shortening fraction	Normal	Increased

tachment of an aortic valve cusp. This may be related to trauma, myxomatous degeneration, or congenital malformation of the valve. The echogram of the aortic root may demonstrate dilatation and the characteristic "spadelike" deformity of Marfan's syndrome.

The echocardiographic diagnosis of dissection is suggested by the identification of a redundant echo-dense band located centrally or eccentrically in the proximal aortic root, originating at or just above the aortic annulus and partitioning the aorta into two channels of equal or unequal size (67,68). Figure 9-1 illustrates an echogram of the aortic root in a patient with dissection of the ascending aorta. The intimal flap that has partitioned the aortic root into a true and false lumen is clearly seen in this figure. Transesophageal echocardiography is more accurate then transthoracic echo for the diagnosis of dissection of the aorta (68). Indeed, transesophageal echocardiography is now the preferred diagnostic test when dissection is being considered.

Doppler echocardiography is highly accurate in identifying and quantitating AI (57). This technique yields a semiquantitative estimate of the severity of the aortic regurgitant hemodynamic burden. Indeed, good correlation with angiographic estimation of aortic regurgitant severity has been demonstrated (57). Color-flow Doppler studies are of particular valve in identifying and quantifying aortic regurgitation.

Cardiac Catheterization

In many instances where high-quality Doppler and two-dimensional echocardiograms are obtained and interpreted by experienced cardiologists, cardiac catheterization is not required to confirm the diagnosis of acute severe AI. If there is clearcut Doppler and two-dimensional echocardiographic evidence of aortic valve leaflet destruction, severe AI, and premature closure of the mitral valve in a patient previously free of cardiac disease and presenting with shock and/or pulmonary edema refractory to inotropic and afterload reduction therapy, urgent AVR without prior

catheterization may be life saving. Here, the inevitable delay and the hemodynamic stress associated with cardiac catheterization and angiography put the patient at added risk and may reduce the likelihood of a successful surgical outcome. However, cardiac catheterization, left ventricular angiography, and coronary arteriography are often required in patients with clinical and/or echocardiographic evidence of preexisting heart disease. Specific questions may relate to the presence of mitral insufficiency, prior myocardial infarction, or evidence of coronary artery disease.

In patients with AI and suspected aortic dissection, angiographic (cine or cut film) assessment of the ascending thoracic aorta may be required to confirm the presence and extent of the dissection and the presence and severity of AI.

In the end, the decision to catheterize the patient or not depends on a careful assessment of the clinical situation. If the patient's condition is unstable or deteriorating, cardiac catheterization should be avoided to hasten surgical intervention. On the other hand, if the patient is reasonably stable and important therapeutic information can be gained (e.g., the presence or absence of obstructive coronary artery disease), then cardiac catheterization/angiography should be undertaken.

Hemodynamic findings associated with acute severe AI include an arterial pulse pressure that is slightly increased or of normal amplitude, equilibration of left ventricular and aortic pressures late in diastole, and marked elevation in left ventricular diastolic pressure that may exceed left atrial (pulmonary artery wedge) pressure in late diastole (4). Other hemodynamic findings not specific for acute AI but indicative of the resultant left ventricular failure include elevation in the pulmonary artery wedge pressure to a level often exceeding 25 to 30 mm Hg, mild to modest elevation in mean pulmonary artery pressure such that the pressure gradient across the lungs (pulmonary artery mean minus pulmonary capillary wedge) does not usually exceed 10 to 12 mm Hg, and mild elevation in mean right atrial pressure (8 to 10 mm Hg) with pulmonary arterial and right ventricular systolic pressure in excess of 35 to 45 mm Hg. The hemodynamic findings in acute severe AI are summarized in Table 9-3.

Ventriculographic findings in acute severe AI include normal or near-normal systolic function (ejection fraction at least 0.50) with normal left ventricular systolic wall motion; slight increase in left ventricular end-diastolic and end-systolic volumes; thickening of one or more aortic leaflets or a filling defect at the level of the aortic valve suggestive of a vegetation in patients with acute endocarditis; thickening of the anterior mitral valve leaflet and mitral insufficiency of variable severity if infective endocarditis of the aortic valve causes septic involvement of the anterior leaflet of the mitral valve; high-frequency vibrations of the anterior mitral leaflet as it is pushed toward the closed position in late diastole by the aortic regurgitant stream; and abnormal "filling defects" projecting into the left ventricular outflow tract at the level of the aortic annulus, membranous, or muscular ventricular septum, suggesting vegetations and/or abscess formation in patients with infective endocarditis.

The risk of cardiac catheterization and angiography relate to additional hemodynamic stresses imposed by the procedure and the administration of angiographic contrast medium in a critically ill patient. Concern is often expressed regarding the risk of arterial embolization secondary to catheter-induced traumatic disruption of one or more friable aortic valve vegetations as the catheter crosses the aortic valve during retrograde left ventricular catheterization in patients with infective endocarditis. Although this has not been reported to be a problem for a large number of patients with infective endocarditis, it remains a source of major concern (66).

TREATMENT

The treatment of patients with acute severe AI may be categorized as general supportive cardiovascular measures, pharmacologic (medical) management, and surgical management. These measures are often carried out simultaneously to ensure a satisfactory outcome by stabilizing the patient promptly. It must be emphasized that medical and surgical therapeutic modalities, rather than mutually exclusive, are mutually complementary in the total management of these critically ill patients.

General supportive cardiovascular measures include supplementary inspired oxygen to maintain the arterial Po_2 in excess of 65 mm Hg and/or the arterial oxygen saturation in excess of 95%. If pulmonary congestion progresses to pulmonary edema and acidosis, intubation, assisted mechanical ventilation, and even bicarbonate administration may be required. Pulmonary edema is also managed by the intravenous administration of a potent loop diuretic (furosemide, 20 to 40 mg i.v., or ethacrynic acid, 25 to 50 mg i.v.), intravenous morphine sulfate (serial doses of 2 to 4 mg i.v.), and positioning the patient with the head and thorax elevated at least 45 degrees above the horizontal plane (69).

Acute pulmonary edema often improves dramatically after 1 to 4 mg of morphine administered intravenously. This can be repeated at 10- to 15-minute intervals to reduce preload, afterload, and respiratory muscle work and to allay anxiety. Significant hypotension and alveolar hypoventilation may complicate morphine administration and may require the use of fluids, pressor agents, intubation, and assisted ventilation. Nonetheless, fear of respiratory depression should not prevent the physician from using morphine in the management of acute pulmonary edema.

Evidence of peripheral organ hypoperfusion in the setting of acute AI may mandate pulmonary artery catheterization and intraarterial cannulation so that right and left heart filling pressures, cardiac output, and arterial blood pressure can be monitored continuously. A cardiac index less than 2.0 $L/min/m^2$, a mean pulmonary artery wedge pressure greater than 20 mm Hg, an arterial systolic pressure less than 90 mm Hg; oliguria (urine output less than 30 mL/hr); and other indirect evidence of impaired tissue perfusion (e.g., decreased mental acuity, cool moist skin, pallor) confirm the presence of cardiogenic shock. Bedside hemodynamic assessment not only confirms the presence of cardiogenic shock but also provides a means to monitor the administration of appropriate vasopressors, diuretics, and vasodilators (69–75).

Vasodilator therapy may stabilize and improve the patient's tenuous clinical and hemodynamic status. Nitroprusside in a total dose of 3 to 6 µg/kg/min (starting at 0.5 µg/kg/min) with titration may produce as much as a 30% to 50% increase in cardiac output and a decline in pulmonary artery wedge pressure of similar magnitude with only a modest reduction in arterial pressure. This direct arteriolar and venous smooth-muscle relaxant reduces the impedance to left ventricular ejection (afterload) and left ventricular end-diastolic volume (preload). Nitroprusside reduces the regurgitant volume per beat, improves forward cardiac output, and lowers left ventricular filling pressure, thereby promoting resolution of pulmonary edema. It has been shown that the use of nitroprusside in patients with acute severe AI is associated with a greater than 50% reduction in left ventricular filling pressure, a 20% increase in forward cardiac index, and a 36% decline in systemic vascular resistance. There is also a small but clinically insignificant increase in heart rate (73,74). Intravenous nitroglycerin administration may also be tried as a therapeutic adjunct in these patients, leading to a reduction in aortic regurgitant flow, left ventricular dilatation, and ventricular filling pressure (76).

If the cardiac index is not maintained above 2.0 to 2.2 L/min/m^2 in response to nitroprusside or nitroglycerin infusion despite doses sufficient to lower systolic blood pressure to 90 mm Hg or reduce mean arterial blood pressure by at least 15 mm Hg, a sympathomimetic agent (e.g., dobutamine) should be added. This is necessary to increase cardiac output and to establish arterial blood pressure at a level sufficient to maintain adequate coronary and cerebral perfusion. Dobutamine, a relatively pure β$_1$ myocardial stimulant, augments myocardial contractility and

raises cardiac output with little or no increase in heart rate. Dobutamine, unlike dopamine, lacks intrinsic α-adrenergic agonist activity (75). Therefore, dobutamine elevates neither arterial resistance (increased afterload) nor venous tone (increased preload). Dobutamine infusion is instituted at 3 to 5 µg/kg/min and is increased by 2 to 4 µg/kg/min every 15 to 30 minutes to maintain the cardiac index above 2.0 to 2.2 L/min/m^2 and the systolic arterial pressure in excess of 90 mm Hg. The pulmonary capillary wedge pressure should be held below 20 to 22 mm Hg. Side effects at high doses (more than 15 to 20 µg/kg/min) include tachycardia, ventricular premature contractions, nervousness, anxiety, nausea, and vomiting. Patients with acute severe AI who require parenteral inotropic and vasodilator therapy to reverse cardiogenic shock require prompt AVR. Intraaortic balloon counterpulsation is contraindicated in patients with AI, acute or chronic, because the augmented diastolic blood pressure that results from intraaortic balloon counterpulsation increases the volume of aortic regurgitant blood flow.

Patients with acute AI are critically ill and should be admitted to an intensive care unit. These patients require frequent monitoring of renal function, serum electrolytes, and arterial blood gases. Hypoxemia, initially related to ventilation-perfusion imbalance secondary to pulmonary congestion, may be paradoxically worsened by vasodilator therapy with nitroprusside or nitroglycerin despite a substantial decline in the pulmonary capillary wedge pressure. This paradoxical effect is probably the result of improved perfusion of nonventilated alveoli. Additionally, thiocyanate levels must be monitored in the patient with low cardiac output, impaired hepatic perfusion, and impaired renal function if nitroprusside is administered. Dosage adjustments should be made to avoid toxicity from accumulation of this nitroprusside metabolite.

Definitive management of acute AI resulting from any etiology often requires early AVR. Aortic valvular insufficiency with CHF complicating infective endocarditis can be particularly challenging to manage because it may carry a mortality rate as high as 50% to 90%. Patients with severe heart failure from aortic valve endocarditis have a higher mortality rate than patients with heart failure from mitral valve endocarditis. Although it is desirable to delay AVR until antibiotic therapy is completed, this may not be possible because of the patient's tenuous clinical status in which precipitous deterioration may occur.

The risk of early AVR before completion of antibiotic therapy relates to the possibility of residual infection: AVR may be complicated by infection of the prosthetic valve or by mycotic aneurysm. Fortunately, valve replacement can usually be performed emergently or after only a few days of antibiotic therapy with an acceptably low risk of reinfection (usually less than 10%). When a patient with infectious endocarditis develops cardiogenic shock from acute AI, AVR should be undertaken immediately even though there has been little or no time for antibiotic administration. All patients then receive 4 to 6 weeks of parenteral antibiotic therapy after AVR.

The major risk of valve replacement in these patients relates to the severity of heart failure at the time of surgery. In patients with active endocarditis complicated by severe heart failure, surgery should not be delayed. The increased operative risk consequent to delaying surgery exceeds the potential benefit of completing a full course of antibiotic therapy before valve replacement (77–79).

Other indications for surgery in acute AI secondary to infectious endocarditis include infection of a mechanical prosthetic valve, infection with a fungus or an organism refractory to antibiotic therapy, continued sepsis despite appropriate antimicrobial therapy, recurrent large-vessel emboli, and myocardial abscess as manifested by the development of high-grade atrioventricular block and/or inability to sterilize the blood with appropriate antibiotics.

Aortic Dissection

Hypertension and severe chest pain in these individuals mandate analgesia and rapid control of blood pressure with at least one agent that depresses shear force in the ascending aorta (left ventricular dp/dt). Morphine (3 to 6 mg i.v.) is administered every 5 to 10 minutes and is titrated carefully to produce analgesia while avoiding respiratory depression and/or excessive hypotension (systolic blood pressure below 85 to 90 mm Hg). Intravenous beta blockade (e.g., proprandol, metoprolol, or atendol) is effective in lowering aortic shear force by reducing heart rate and left ventricular dp/dt. Beta blockade is probably contraindicated in patients with decompensated heart failure and in individuals with reactive airways disease. Beta-blockers are administered repetitively as slow intravenous boluses or continuous intravenous infusions using heart rate and blood pressure response to titrate therapeutic efficacy. It is desirable to slow the heart rate to 60 to 90 beats/min or less and to lower the systolic arterial blood pressure to 90 to 110 mm Hg over 45 minutes to 1 hour. Intermittent doses of beta-blockers can be repeated every 4 to 6 hours. Some patients may be partially refractory to beta blockade (because of very high levels of sympathetic tone and circulating catecholamines) unless effective pain control is achieved. Furthermore, satisfactory analgesia cannot be obtained in the patient with active aortic dissection unless control of blood pressure terminates propagation of the dissecting medial hematoma. Achieving this goal invariably requires administration of potent antihypertensive agents (e.g., nitroprusside or the ganglionic blocking agent trimethaphan). Trimethaphan (Arfonad) has generally been replaced by nitroprusside as the preferred hypotensive agent in the treatment of aortic dissection. Nitroprusside lowers arterial blood pressure by reducing systemic vascular resistance and by increasing venous capacitance. This agent has a very rapid onset of action and a very short half-life. Nitroprusside must be administered intravenously; the starting dose is 0.5 to 1 µg/kg/min. The infusion rate should be increased by 0.5 µg/kg/min every 5 minutes. When administered at a precise rate by a constant infusion pump, prompt blood pressure control with minimal overshoot can be achieved. Because of variable and unpredictable individual sensitivity to nitroprusside, this agent requires continuous monitoring of the arterial pressure through an indwelling arterial cannula. Nitroprusside should always be used in conjunction with a β-adrenergic blocking agent to prevent reflex tachycardia and an increase in aortic shear rate.

Proximal aortic dissection with or without AI usually requires immediate surgical repair unless the patient has a serious unrelated illness (e.g., metastatic cancer, severe chronic obstructive lung disease, dementia) that precludes surgical intervention.

REFERENCES

1. Willis FA, Keys TE. *Classics of Cardiology*. New York: Dover Publications, 1941:422.
2. Alpert JS. Chronic aortic regurgitation. In: Alpert JS, Dalen JE, eds. *Valvular Heart Disease*. Boston: Little, Brown, 1980.
3. Benotti JR. Acute aortic insufficiency. In: Alpert JS, Dalen JE, eds. *Valvular Heart Disease*, 2nd ed. Boston: Little, Brown, 1987.
4. Morganroth J, Perloff JK, Zeldis SM, et al. Acute, severe aortic regurgitation. *Ann Intern Med* 1977;87:223.
5. Cohen L, Friedman LR. Damage to aortic valve as a cause of death in bacterial endocarditis. *Ann Intern Med* 1961;55:562.
6. Weinstein L, Rubin RH. Infective endocarditis. *Prog Cardiovasc Dis* 1973;16:239.
7. Robinson MJ, Rendy J. Sequellae of bacterial endocarditis. *Am J Med* 1962;32:922.
8. Roberts WC. The congenitally bicuspid aortic valve. *Am J Cardiol* 1970;26:72.
9. Perloff JK. Innocent or normal murmurs. In: Russek HI, ed. *Cardiovascular Problems*. Baltimore: University Park Press, 1976:27.
10. Dinuble MJ. Surgery in active endocarditis. *Ann Intern Med* 1982;96:650.
11. Braniff BA, Shumway NE, Harrison DC. Valve replacement in active bacterial endocarditis. *N Engl J Med* 1967;276:1464.
12. Durack DT. Infective and noninfective endocarditis. In: Schlant RC, Alexander RW, O'Rourke R, Sonnerblick E, et al., eds. *The Heart*. New York: McGraw-Hill, 1994:1681.
13. Korzeniowski OM, Kaye D. Infective endocarditis. In: Braunwald E, ed. *Heart Disease, A Textbook of Cardiovascular Medicine*. Philadelphia: WB Saunders, 1992:078.
14. Dalen JE, Pape LA, Cohn LH, et al. Dissection of the aorta: pathogenesis, diagnosis and treatment. *Prog Cardiovasc Dis* 1980;23:237.
15. Koster JK, Cohn LH, Meer BB, et al. Late results of operation for acute aortic dissection producing aortic insufficiency. *Ann Thorac Surg* 1978;26:461.
16. Anagnostopoulos CE, Prabhaker MJS, Kittle CF. Aortic dissections and dissecting aneurysms. *Am J Cardiol* 1972;30:263.
17. Cipriano PR, Greipp RB. Acute retrograde dissection of the ascending thoracic aorta. *Am J Cardiol* 1978;43:520.
18. Liddicoat JE, Bekassy SM, Rubio PA, et al. Ascending aortic aneurysms—review of 100 cases. *Circulation* 1975;51[Suppl I]:1202.
19. Dalen JE, Alpert JS, Cohen LH, et al. Dissection of the thoracic aorta, medical or surgical therapy? *Am J Cardiol* 1974;34:803.
20. Kainuma Y, Sakamoto T, Shimakuna T, et al. Successful surgical management of a dissecting aneurysm of the ascending and transverse aorta with heart failure due to sudden, severe aortic valve insufficiency. *J Cardiovasc Surg* 1978;19:387.
21. Thandroyen FT, Matisonn RE, Weir EK. Severe aortic incompetence caused by systemic lupus erythematosus. *S Afr Med J* 1978;54:166.
22. Rawsthorne L, Ptacin MJ, Choi H, et al. Lupus valvulitis necessitating double valve replacement. *Arthritis Rheum* 1981;24:561.
23. Wright CB, Hiratzka LF, Crosslands, et al. Aortic insufficiency requiring valve replacement in Whipple's disease. *Ann Thorac Surg* 1978;25:466.
24. Honig HS, Weintraub AN, Gomes MN, et al. Severe aortic regurgitation secondary to idiopathic aortitis. *Am J Med* 1977;63:623.
25. Soorae AS, McKeown F, Cleland J. Aortic valve replacement for severe aortic regurgitation caused by idiopathic giant cell aortitis. *Thorax* 1980;35:60.
26. Stewart SR, Robbins DL, Castles JJ. Acute fulminant aortic and mitral insufficiency in ankylosing spondylitis. *N Engl J Med* 1978;299:1448.
27. Levene RJ, Roberts WC, Morrow AG. Traumatic aortic regurgitation. *Am J Cardiol* 1962;10:752.
28. Parmley LF, Manion WC, Mattingly TW. Non-penetrating injury to aorta. *Circulation* 1958;17:1086.
29. O'Brien KP, Hitchcock GC, Banat-Boges BG, et al. Spontaneous aortic cusp rupture associated with valvular myxomatous transformation. *Circulation* 1968;37:273.
30. Howard CP. Aortic insufficiency due to rupture by strain of a normal aortic valve. *Can Med J* 1920;18:12.
31. Sainani GS, Szatkowski J. Rupture of a normal aortic valve after physical strain. *Br Heart J* 1969;31:653.
32. Esteves CM, Dillon JC, Walker JD, et al. Echocardiographic manifestations of aortic cusp rupture in a myxomatous aortic valve. *Chest* 1976;69:685.
33. Olenger GN, Korus ME, Bonchek LI. Acute aortic valvular insufficiency due to isolated myxomatous degeneration. *Ann Intern Med* 1978;88:807.
34. Becker AE, Duren DR. Spontaneous rupture of a bicuspid aortic valve. *Chest* 1977;72:361.
35. Salem, BI, Pechacek LW, Leachman RD. Major dehiscence of a prosthetic aortic valve. *Chest* 1979;75:513.
36. Cohn LH, Mudge GH, Pratter F, et al. Five to eight year followup of patients undergoing porcine heart valve replacement. *N Engl J Med* 1981;304:258.
37. Housman LB, Pitt WA, Mazur JH, et al. Mechanical failure (leaflet disruption) of a porcine aortic heterograft. *J Thorac Cardiovasc Surg* 1978;76:212.
38. Cohn LH. Durability of mechanical and biologic prosthetic valves for aortic valve replacement. In: Davila JC, ed. *The Second Henry Ford Hospital International Symposium on Cardiac Surgery*. New York: Appleton-Century-Crofts, 1977:380.
39. Gore JM, Haffajee CI, Collins JJ, et al. Acute sponta-

neous failure of a porcine aortic valve. *Arch Intern Med* 1982;142:1553.

40. Welch GH, Braunwald E, Sarnoff SJ. Hemodynamic effects of quantitatively varied experimental aortic regurgitation. *Circ Res* 1957;5:546.

41. Miller GA, Kirklin JW, Swan JH. Myocardial function and left ventricular volumes in acquired valvular insufficiency. *Circulation* 1965;31:374.

42. Engloff E. Aortic incompetence: Clinical, hemodynamic and angiographic evaluation. *Acta Med Scand* 1972;193[Suppl 538]:3.

43. Grant C, Greene DG, Bunnell IL. Left ventricular enlargement and hypertrophy. *Am J Med* 1965;39:895.

44. Parke TO, Case RB. Normal left ventricular function. *Circulation* 1979;60:4.

45. Silvestry SC, Lilly RE, Atkins BZ, et al. Ventricular and myocardial efficiencies during acute aortic regurgitation in conscious dogs. *Circulation* 1997;96[Suppl II]:II108–II114.

46. Ardehali A, Segal J, Cheitlin MD. Coronary blood flow reserve in acute aortic regurgitation. *J Am Coll Cardiol* 1995;25:1387.

47. Wise JR, Cleland WP, Hallidie-Smith KA, et al. Urgent aortic valve replacement for acute aortic regurgitation due to infective endocarditis. *Lancet* 1971;2:115.

48. Mann T, McLaurin L, Grossman W, et al. Assessing the hemodynamic severity of acute aortic regurgitation due to infective endocarditis. *Lancet* 1971;2:115.

49. Sareli P, Klein HO, Schamroth CL, et al. Contribution of echocardiography and immediate surgery to the management of severe aortic regurgitation from active infective endocarditis. *Am J Cardiol* 1986;57:413–418.

50. Meyer T, Sareli P, Pocock WA, Dean H, Epstein M, Barlow J. Echocardiographic and hemodynamic correlates of diastolic closure of mitral valve and diastolic opening of aortic valve in severe aortic regurgitation. *Am J Cardiol* 1987;59:1144–1148.

51. Nakao S, Nagatomo T, Kiyonaga K, et al. Influences of localized aortic valve damage on coronary artery blood flow in acute aortic regurgitation. An experimental study. *Circulation* 1987;76:201.

52. Downes TR, Nomeir AM, Hackshaw BT, et al. Diastolic mitral regurgitation in acute but not chronic aortic regurgitation: implications regarding the mechanism of mitral closure. *Am Heart J* 1989;117:1106.

53. Fortuin NJ, Craige E. On the mechanism of the Austin Flint murmur. *Circulation* 1972;45:558.

54. Freiden J, Hurwitt ES, Leader E. Ruptured aortic cusp associated with a heritable disorder of connective tissue. *Am J Med* 1962;33:615.

55. Baron MG. Dissecting aneurysm of the aorta. *Circulation* 1971;43:933.

56. Goldschlager N, Pfeifer J, Cohn K, et al. The natural history of aortic regurgitation, a clinical and hemodynamic study. *Am J Med* 1973;54:577.

57. Otto CM, Pearlman AS. *Textbook of Clinical Echocardiography*, Philadelphia: WB Saunders, 1995.

58. Weaver W, Wilson CS, Rourke T, et al. Mid-diastolic aortic valve opening in severe acute aortic regurgitation. *Chest* 1977;55:145.

59. Jackson DH, Murphy GW, Stewart S, et al. Delayed appearance of left-to-right shunt following aortic valvular replacement. *Chest* 1979;75:184.

60. Wann LS, Dillon JC, Weyman AE, et al. Echocardiog-

raphy in bacterial endocarditis. *N Engl J Med* 1976;295:135.

61. Roy P, Tajik AJ, Giuliani ER, et al. Spectrum of echocardiographic findings in bacterial endocarditis. *Circulation* 1976;53:474.

62. Alann LS, Hallam CC, Dillon JC, et al. Comparison of M-mode and cross-sectional echocardiography in infective endocarditis. *Circulation* 1979;60:728.

63. Castello R, Fagan L, Lenzen P, Pearson AC, Labovitz AJ. Comparison of transthoracic and transesophageal echocardiography for assessment of left-sided valvular regurgitation. *Am J Cardiol* 1991;68:1677–1680.

64. Mugge A, Daniel WG, Frank G, Lichtlen PR. Echocardiography in infective endocarditis: reassessment of prognostic implications of vegetation size determined by the transthoracic and the transesophageal approach. *J Am Coll Cardiol* 1989;14:631–638.

65. Melver ET, Berger M, Lutzker LG. Noninvasive methods for detection of valve regurgitations in infective endocarditis. *Am J Cardiol* 1981;47:271.

66. Welton DE, Young JB, Raizner AE, et al. Value and safety of cardiac catheterization during active endocarditis. *Am J Cardiol* 1978;44:1306.

67. Moothart RW, Spangler RD, Blount SG. Echocardiography in aortic root dissection and dilation. *Am J Cardiol* 1975;36:17.

68. Chan KL. Impact of transesophageal echocardiography on the treatment of patients with aortic dissection. *Chest* 1992;101:406–410.

69. Biddle TL, Yu PN. Effect of furosemide on hemodynamics and lung water in acute pulmonary edema secondary to myocardial infarction. *Am J Cardiol* 1979;43:86.

70. Hutter AM Jr, DeSanctis RW, Nathan MJ, et al. Aortic valve surgery as an emergency procedure. *Circulation* 1970;41:623.

71. Cohn JN, Franciosa JA. Vasodilator therapy of cardiac failure. *N Engl J Med* 1977;297:27.

72. Miller RR, Awan NA, Joye JA, et al. Combined dopamine and nitroprusside therapy in congestive heart failure. *Circulation* 1977;55:881.

73. Miller RR, Vismara LA, DeMara AN, et al. Afterload reduction therapy with nitroprusside in severe aortic regurgitation: improved cardiac performance and reduced regurgitant volume. *Am J Cardiol* 1976;38:564.

74. Warner RA, Bowser M, Zuehlhe S, et al. Treatment of acute aortic insufficiency with sodium nitroferricyanide. *Chest* 1977;72:375.

75. Goldberg LI. Dopamine—clinical use of an endogenous catecholamine. *N Engl J Med* 1974;291:707.

76. Klepzig HH, Warner KG, Siouffi SY, et al. Hemodynamic effects of nitroglycerin in an experimental model of acute aortic regurgitation. *J Am Coll Cardiol* 1989;13:927–935.

77. Wilson WR, Danielson GK, Giuliani ER, et al. Cardiac valve replacement in congestive heart failure due to infective endocarditis. *Mayo Clin Proc* 1979;54:223.

78. Larbalestier RI, Kinchla NM, Aranki SF, Couper GS, Collins JJ Jr, Cohn LH. Acute bacterial endocarditis—optimizing surgical results. *Circulation* 1992;86[Suppl 2]:II-68–II-74.

79. Krishnaswami V, Sudhaker PR, Curtis EI, et al. Surgical treatment of acute aortic regurgitation in infective endocarditis. *Ann Thorac Surg* 1976;22:464.

10

Combined Valvular Disease

John A. Paraskos

*Department of Medicine, Cardiology, University of Massachusetts Medical School
and Memorial Health Care, Worcester, Massachusetts 01655*

Serious stenotic and regurgitant lesions often occur at a single valve, and multiple valves may be the site of serious disease. Rheumatic heart disease is still the most likely cause of multiple valvular lesions. The most common combination is mitral stenosis with aortic regurgitation or stenosis. Tricuspid stenosis occurs in combinations with mitral stenosis in a small percentage of patients, and a few of these patients also have aortic stenosis. Important stenosis of all four valves is rare. Functional tricuspid regurgitation is very common in the late stages of mitral disease. Other combinations of valvular lesions are distinctly unusual; they are more likely to result from nonrheumatic causes or from the combined effect of both congenital and rheumatic causes. Significant regurgitation at multiple valves (usually mitral and tricuspid, occasionally accompanied by aortic regurgitation) may be caused by connective tissue abnormalities with myxomatous degeneration of valve tissue. Systemic lupus (1,2) and the use of drugs such as ergotamine (3) or fenfluramine (4) may also cause combined valve lesions. In the ensuing discussion, each possible combination of lesions will be explored separately. However, it must be kept in mind that a small degree of regurgitation of the atrioventricular valves is commonly found by Doppler examination and may be physiologic (5). Trivial regurgitation is also recorded somewhat less frequently at the semilunar valves. In these cases there is no audible murmur and no hemodynamic consequences.

The clinical presentation and natural history of combined lesions is determined by the relative severity of each individual lesion and by the chronicity and order of development. Each of these lesions can be expected to produce its characteristic effects on the heart and circulation. Physical findings and roentgenographic and electrocardiographic changes ordinarily follow the major hemodynamic stresses; therefore, the individual lesions of greatest severity often remain recognizable just as described in the previous chapters. There are important exceptions, however, as when one valvular lesion protects a chamber from the full effects of a concurrent lesion. Mitral stenosis, for example, may protect the left ventricle from the stress of aortic valve disease. Tricuspid stenosis may protect the right ventricle and pulmonary circuit from full effects of mitral stenosis. These neutralizing hemodynamic effects ameliorate and often confuse the clinical presentation: Symptoms, murmurs, and other physical findings may be changed. In these cases, it is the deviation from the expected clinical presentation of the more obvious lesion that alerts the astute physician to the presence of additional valve pathology.

Factors other than combined valvular lesions may also complicate the clinical presentation. The physician must remain alert to the potential complications caused by myocardial damage from the rheumatic process, chronic pressure overload, volume overload, or ischemia; myocardial restriction or diastolic dysfunction brought about by ventricular hypertrophy or coronary artery disease; concurrent infective endocarditis; and the hemodynamic effects of various arrhythmias, particularly those that decrease or eliminate the atrial contribution to ventricular filling.

Medical, interventional, and surgical management of the patient with combined valvular disease is guided by the relative severity of each individual lesion and by the severity of nonvalvular myocardial factors. If the myocardial factors are not excessive, the decision to intervene surgically is prompted by the most symptomatic or life-threatening lesion. Yet, it must be emphasized that the severity of all concurrent lesions must be fully appreciated before deciding for or against a specific form of therapy. In particular, coexisting lesions may seriously complicate cardiac surgery or prevent the expected postoperative improvement.

The need to replace more than one valve should be known in advance, and the decision to proceed should be based on a reasonable estimate of the risk of surgery and the potential benefit to be gained. Although single-valve replacement can usually be performed with an acceptable mortality of less than 5%, simultaneous replacement of aortic and mitral valves carried a mortality of 10% (6), and in one series, triple valve replacement carried an in-hospital mortality of 19% (7). In many cases, a valve, particularly mitral or tricuspid, may be reconstructed rather than replaced. It is not yet known how valve reconstruction affects the operative mortality of multiple valve surgery.

COMBINED AORTIC STENOSIS AND AORTIC REGURGITATION

The combination of aortic stenosis and regurgitation is very common. Approximately two thirds of patients with calcific aortic stenosis have some degree of aortic regurgitation. In a study of congenital aortic stenosis,

Hohn et al. (8) found concurrent aortic regurgitation in 31% of the patients. Aortic regurgitation occurred in similar proportions (20% to 30%) in supravalvular, valvular, and discrete subvalvular stenosis. Frank and Braunwald (9), however, found a murmur of aortic regurgitation in only 7% of patients with hypertrophic obstructive cardiomyopathy (HOCM). When considering the combination of these two lesions, it should be kept in mind that in patients with severe aortic regurgitation, a small pressure gradient is to be expected across the aortic valve even in the absence of stenosis. When either the stenosis or the regurgitation is mild, the case presentation in all important respects is similar to that of the isolated lesion. Very often in predominant stenosis, mild or even moderate aortic regurgitation is missed unless it is demonstrated by aortography or Doppler echocardiography, although the routine use of squatting or handgrip during auscultation usually brings out the short, high-pitched, early diastolic murmur. The likely causes of predominant aortic regurgitation with minor degrees of stenosis are rheumatic valvular disease or congenital bicuspid valve. In such patients with severe aortic regurgitation, the presence of a systolic ejection murmur, even when associated with a thrill, does not confirm significant coexisting stenosis. Other evidence for stenosis may be present, however, such as a delayed carotid upstroke with an anacrotic notch, paradoxical splitting of the second heart sound (S_2), or a single S_2. The systolic murmur itself may be harsher and longer than the flow murmur heard in pure aortic regurgitation (10).

Often, aortic stenosis and regurgitation coexist to a more balanced degree. An immobile and rigid valve, usually heavily calcified, may be both stenotic and regurgitant. Alternatively, infective endocarditis may impose acute severe regurgitation on a congenitally stenotic valve. An aortic orifice fixed at 0.5 cm^2 through systole and diastole is the site of severe stenosis and moderately severe regurgitation. The pressure overload of the aortic stenosis and the volume overload of the aortic regurgitation both contribute significantly to the hemodynamic

TABLE 10-1. *Findings in combined aortic stenosis and aortic regurgitation*

Clinical and laboratory findings	Predominant stenosis	Balanced lesions	Predominant regurgitation
Presenting symptoms			
Syncope	+	±	−
Angina	+	+	+
Effort intolerance	±	+	+
Dyspnea at rest	−	±	+
Physical findings			
Delayed carotid upstroke	+	±	−
Prolonged systolic murmur	+	+	±
Prolonged diastolic murmur	−	±	+
S_3	Late in course	±	Early in course
Chest roentgenogram			
Left ventricle dilated	−	±	++
Echocardiogram			
Aortic cusp thickening	+	+	+
Small aortic "orifice"	+	+	±
Concentric left ventricular hypertrophy	+	+	+
Dilated hyperkinetic left ventricle	−	±	+
Doppler findings			
High-velocity systolic jet	+	+	−
Diastolic subvalvular turbulence	±	+	++
Cardiac catheterization			
Aortic valvular pressure gradient	+	+	±
Aortic regurgitation	0–1+	2–3+	3–4+

consequences (11). The capacity to compensate for the regurgitation may be impaired as the stenosis prevents adequate augmentation of stroke volume. In these relatively balanced lesions, one or the other tends to predominate, but the clinical presentation and physiologic features of the one may be markedly altered by the other. Most often, the clinical features of aortic regurgitation are modified so that its severity is underestimated.

The clinical course is similar to that of the predominant lesion. In more balanced cases, it appears to be that of aortic stenosis. In these situations, the development of angina pectoris, syncope, or left ventricular failure remains a poor prognostic indicator (Table 10-1).

Physical Findings

The physical findings in most patients with combined aortic valve disease include the typical systolic and diastolic murmurs, often with a diastolic inflow rumble at the apex (Austin Flint murmur). Cases have been described, however, in which the diastolic murmur of aortic regurgitation was absent (12). The systolic ejection murmur is expected to be harsher, peak later, occupy more of systole, and radiate more widely than the systolic flow murmur of isolated aortic regurgitation. In a younger patient with a congenital aortic lesion, an ejection click may precede the systolic murmur. The S_2 may be paradoxically split, and the aortic component is diminished or absent. A prominent fourth heart sound (S_4) is common to both severe stenosis and regurgitation. A third heart sound (S_3), however, is not present in predominant stenosis unless severe myocardial failure has supervened. When it is present, therefore, it should alert the clinician to the possibility of severe myopathy or of considerable coexisting regurgitation.

The carotid pulse may be relatively normal, but in patients with a slow upstroke and an anacrotic "shoulder" or notch on the upstroke, the severity of the stenosis is likely to be severe (Fig. 10-1). Alternatively, in patients with important regurgitation but with

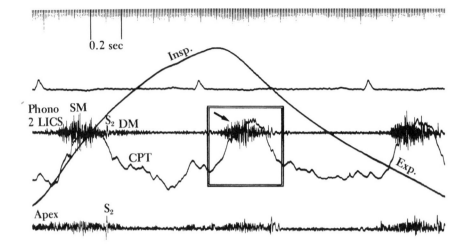

FIG. 10-1. Carotid pulse tracing and phonocardiogram of a patient with predominant aortic stenosis. Note the delay in carotid upstroke. The prominent shudder on the carotid upstroke (*arrow*) is a manifestation of the transmission of the prolonged systolic murmur (*SM*) into the carotid vessels. The higher pitched diastolic murmur (*DM*) is not well recorded. The intensity of the S_2 is diminished (Fig. 10-5). *2LICS*, left intercostal space.

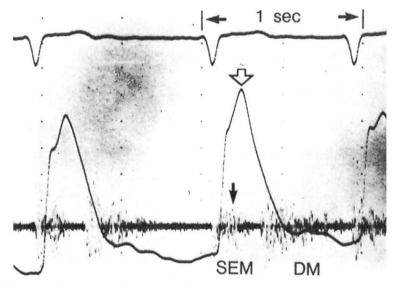

FIG. 10-2. Carotid pulse tracing and phonocardiogram of a patient with predominant aortic regurgitation and minimal aortic stenosis. Note the rapid initial upstroke with a moderate delay in the tidal wave (open arrow). The systolic ejection murmur peaks early in systole (*black arrow*) (Fig. 10-3). *SEM*, systolic ejection murmur; *DM*, diastolic murmur.

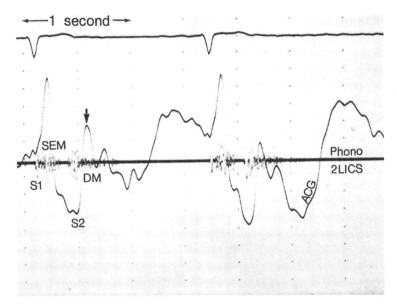

FIG. 10-3. Apexcardiogram of the patient in Fig. 10-2. Note the prominent early diastolic forward thrust (*arrow*), suggesting marked diastolic overload of the left ventricle. *SEM*, systolic ejection murmur; *DM*, diastolic murmur; *2 LICS*, second left intercostal space.

an absent or "trivial" diastolic murmur, a brisk carotid upstroke and widened pulse pressure may reveal the severity of the regurgitation (Fig. 10-2). The presence or absence of a systolic shudder in the carotid pulse is not a helpful diagnostic clue. Its presence simply marks the transmission of the systolic murmur to the neck (13). The character of the apical impulse may be of value. In predominant stenosis the apical impulse may be normal or it may be diffuse and sustained in systole. A palpable presystolic impulse may occur but is not dramatic. If the apical impulse is displaced laterally or inferiorly or if there is a palpable early diastolic shock (Fig. 10-3), the severity of the coexisting regurgitation is likely to be considerable. Such a displaced apical impulse, however, also may be due to myocardial dysfunction with dilatation of the left ventricle.

Laboratory Findings

Electrocardiogram

Left ventricular hypertrophy with ST segments and T waves displaced away from the QRS is common to both lesions. Left atrial abnormality with broad P waves and a prominent terminal negative deflection in V_1 and V_2 is also to be expected. In younger patients with predominant aortic regurgitation, the electrocardiogram (ECG) may display left ventricular hypertrophy by voltage with prominant septal q waves and ST segments and T waves in the same direction as the QRS (volume overload pattern). This pattern is less common in the older patient. The ECG, therefore, is not likely to be helpful in determining the severity of each lesion.

Roentgenogram

The chest roentgenogram is likely to reveal more left ventricular enlargement with the combined lesions than that seen in isolated aortic stenosis (Figs. 10-4 and 10-5). Aortic valve calcification is usually evident with the combined lesion or with isolated stenosis; calcification is unusual in pure regurgitation. Dilatation of the proximal aorta causes a characteristic rightward bulge of the mediastinal shadow, but it is common to both lesions.

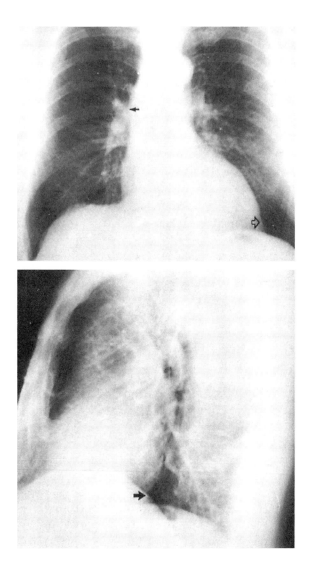

FIG. 10-4. Chest roentgenogram of a patient with balanced aortic stenosis and regurgitation. In the posteroanterior view **(top)**, note the fullness to the right of the aortic root consistent with post-stenotic aortic dilatation (*black arrow*). The left ventricle is rounded and prominent, although the appearance is exaggerated by an apical fat pad (*open arrow*). Mild left ventricular dilatation is suggested on the lateral view **(bottom)** by extension of the left ventricular shadow beyond the shadow of the inferior vena cava by several centimeters.

Echocardiogram

With aortic stenosis, concentric left ventricular hypertrophy is expected without left ventricular dilatation. An increased end-diastolic dimension of the left ventricle with a normal end-systolic dimension suggests that aortic regurgitation with volume overload is present. The severity of the aortic regurgitation can be estimated by Doppler analysis (14). If the systolic dimension of the left ventricle is also increased and the ejection fraction diminished, the muscle is failing. The presence of regional wall motion abnormalities will alert the clinician to associated coronary artery disease with ischemia or infarction. Radionuclide ventriculography and myocardial perfusion scintigraphy are also useful in documenting associated myopathy or coronary disease.

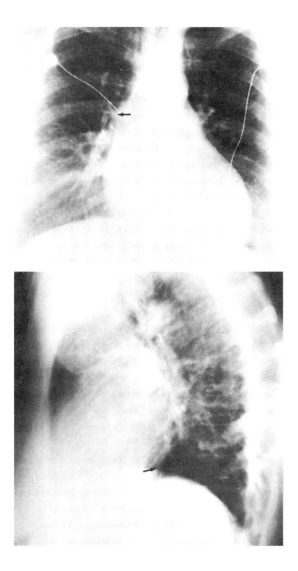

FIG. 10-5. Chest roentgenogram of the patient with predominant aortic stenosis (pulse tracing displayed in Fig. 10-1). **Top:** Posteroanterior view. Note the rounded left ventricular configuration and evidence for poststenotic dilatation of the proximal aorta (*arrow*). **Bottom:** Lateral view shows evidence for mild left ventricular enlargement, because the left ventricular shadow (*arrow*) extends beyond the inferior vena cava shadow.

Other Noninvasive Studies

External pulse-wave recordings of the carotid pulse are largely of academic interest and may be used to document physical findings such as a prolonged (Fig. 10-1) or brisk upstroke time (Fig. 10-2), prolonged ejection time (Fig. 10-1 and 10-6), or a dicrotic wave (Fig. 10-7). The apexcardiogram may reveal a prominent A wave or a sustained systolic bulge. The phonocardiogram is of academic value in documenting that a systolic murmur is particularly prolonged or delayed (Fig 10-1). It is not likely, however, that a phonocardiogram will record a diastolic murmur of aortic regurgitation that is heard only with difficulty on physical examination. The diminished aortic closure sound or paradoxically split S_2 may be displayed, as may be an S_3 or S_4. The usefulness of any of these graphic techniques is largely in improving the physical diagnostic skills of physicians and other health care professionals.

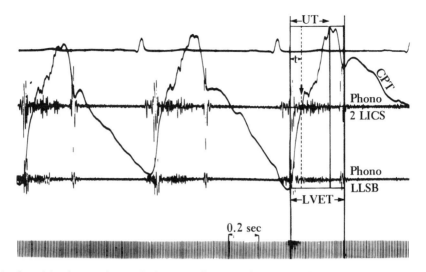

FIG. 10-6. Carotid pulse tracing and phonocardiogram of patient with balanced aortic stenosis and regurgitation. The systolic murmur peaks in early systole, and the diastolic murmur is not well recorded. Note the marked delay in carotid upstroke (*UT*). The time to half-amplitude (*t time*), however, is only minimally prolonged. The carotid pulse in this patient, therefore, did not feel significantly delayed to the clinician's palpating fingers. *LVET*, left ventricular ejection time; *2 LICS*, second left intercostal space; *LLSB*, lower left sternal border.

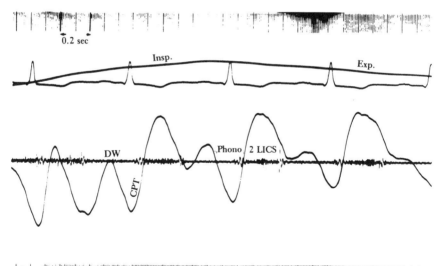

FIG. 10-7. Carotid pulse tracing of a 67-year-old woman with a 90 mm Hg transvalvular aortic gradient and moderate aortic regurgitation (2+) demonstrated on the aortogram. Note the marked dicrotic wave (*DW*), which is more pronounced at onset of inspiration. The upstroke time is delayed. A prominent dicrotic wave is a less common cause of a double-beating (or bisferiens) pulse than is the prominent percussion and tidal wave seen in severe aortic regurgitation or hypertrophic obstructive cardiomyopathy. *2 LICS*, second left intercostal space.

Cardiac Catheterization

Before sending a patient for surgical correction, cardiac catheterization is necessary to assess the status of the coronary arteries and for additional confirmation of the clinical and noninvasive findings. A transvalvular gradient of 25 mm Hg or more is strong evidence of serious aortic stenosis (Figs. 10-8 and 10-9). The cardiac output is normal unless significant left ventricular failure is also present. In the presence of critical aortic stenosis, the aortic valve orifice as estimated by the Gorlin formula is 0.7 cm^2 or less. In the presence of more than trivial aortic regurgitation, however, the Gorlin hydraulic formula underestimates the anatomic systolic orifice. At cardiac catheterization the severity of aortic regurgitation is best estimated from a supravalvular aortogram and the status of left ventricular systolic function from a ventriculogram. However, in the interest of sparing the patient the nephrotoxicity of a large volume of radiographic contrast material, good-quality echocardiography may be relied on to assess these lesions.

Therapy

Once symptoms appear, aortic valve replacement is in order. The appearance of angina, syncope, or left ventricular failure indicates a poor prognosis with either lesion. According to the series of Rotman et al. (11), the long-term survival after aortic valve replacement is better in combined stenosis and regurgitation than in aortic stenosis alone. One possible explanation is that the addition of significant volume overload leads to earlier symptoms and earlier valve replacement.

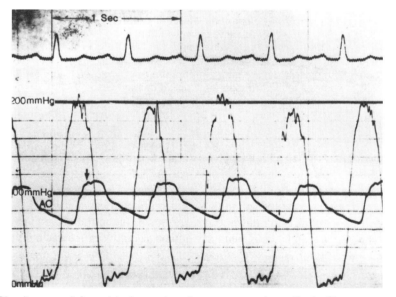

FIG. 10-8. Simultaneous left ventricular and aortic pressures of a patient with murmurs of both aortic stenosis and regurgitation. A transvalvular aortic mean systolic gradient was 66 mm Hg. The cardiac output by the Fick method was 3.5 L/min, and the calculated aortic valve area was 0.3 cm^2. Supravalvular aortography revealed moderately severe regurgitation (3+), so 0.3 cm^2 is an underestimation of the true aortic orifice in this patient with balanced stenosis and regurgitation. Note the relatively normal upstroke in the aortic pressure wave (*arrow*) (Fig. 10-19). *AO,* aorta; *LV,* left ventricle.

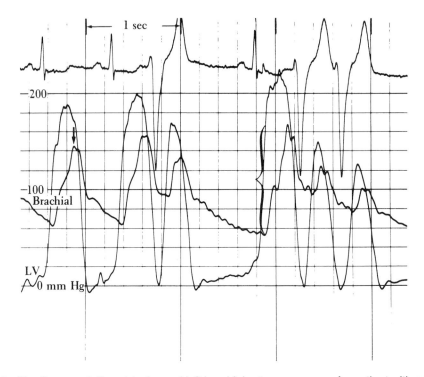

FIG. 10-9. Simultaneous left ventricular and left brachial artery pressure of a patient with mixed aortic stenosis and regurgitation. The patient complained of exertional light-headedness and angina. The mean systolic gradient across the aortic valve was 50 mm Hg, with a cardiac output of 5.1 L/min by the Fick method. An aortic valve area was calculated at 0.7 cm². Moderate (2+) aortic regurgitation was observed on the supravalvular aortogram. This patient has an abnormal upstroke time (*arrow*). The widening of the pulse pressure after a premature beat (*bracket*) is to be expected in valvular aortic stenosis, in contrast to hypertrophic obstructive cardiomyopathy.

COMBINED MITRAL STENOSIS AND MITRAL REGURGITATION

Commissural fusion and loss of tissue often occur together in rheumatic mitral valvulitis; therefore, it is very common for the mitral valve in rheumatic disease to be both stenotic and regurgitant. Although most mixed mitral lesions are of rheumatic origin, congenital lesions, mitral valve dysfunction due to mitral annular calcification, and left atrial tumors must be considered in the differential diagnosis. Infective endocarditis may occur in pure mitral regurgitation or in the combined lesion, and infective endocarditis most commonly makes a valve more regurgitant. It is distinctly unusual for infective endocarditis to develop on a purely stenotic valve; therefore, a left atrial tumor may be a surprise echocardiographic finding when apparent endocarditis and mitral regurgitation develop in a patient with previously suspected mitral stenosis. Another rare circumstance is for fungal endocarditis of the mitral valve to convert a regurgitant lesion to an increasingly more stenotic one because of an enlarging vegetation. This may occur rapidly over the course of weeks.

In most cases of combined mitral stenosis and regurgitation, it is possible to classify the lesion as predominantly one or the other. When the mitral orifice is smaller than 1.5 cm², the stenosis is predominant and determines the clinical presentation and management. When the mitral orifice is greater than 2.0 cm², mitral regurgitation is the dominant lesion, and volume overload of the left ventricle dominates

TABLE 10-2. *Findings in combined mitral stenosis and mitral regurgitation*

Clinical and laboratory findings	Predominant stenosis	Balanced lesions	Predominant regurgitation
Presenting symptoms			
Pulmonary symptoms	+	+	−
Easy fatigability	−	±	+
Physical findings			
Parasternal lift	+	+	Peaks at end-systole
Prominent apical impulse	−	±	+
Prolonged diastolic murmur	+	+	−
S_3	−	-	+
Electrocardiogram			
Right ventricular hypertrophy	±	±	−
Left ventricular hypertrophy	−	±	+
Chest roentgenogram			
Left atrium dilated	±	+	++
Left ventricle dilated	−	±	++
Mitral calcium	±	±	+
Echocardiogram			
Mitral leaflet thickening	+	+	+
Concentric left ventricular hypertrophy	−	±	+
Hyperkinetic left ventricle	−	±	+
Doppler findings			
High-velocity inflow jet	++	++	±
Systolic left atrial turbulance	±	+	++
Cardiac catheterization			
Diastolic valvular gradient	+	+	±
Mitral regurgitation	0–1+	2–3+	3–4+

the clinical picture (15). In some cases the valves are narrowed to a degree that by itself does not produce significant obstruction to left ventricular filling (1.5 to 2.0 cm^2). This type of valve is usually rigid and immobile and often allows considerable regurgitant flow in systole. Thus, the left atrial volume is augmented during systole so that this degree of stenosis is capable of producing hemodynamically significant hindrance to left ventricular filling (16). When left ventricular volume overload and inflow obstruction contribute equally to the hemodynamic abnormalities, balanced mitral stenosis and regurgitation occur. Atrial fibrillation or a rapid ventricular rate (with shortened diastolic filling period) enhances the effect of inflow obstruction.

The clinical course in the patient with predominant stenosis or regurgitation does not differ strikingly from that of the patient with one or the other lesion in isolation. Both mitral stenosis and mitral regurgitation produce symptoms related to pulmonary venous hypertension and to reduced cardiac output. The early development of cough, hemoptysis, and pulmonary edema, however, is more characteristic of stenosis, whereas chronic disability characterized by easy fatigability is more often the primary complaint in the chronic form of mitral regurgitation. When the two lesions are physiologically important, pulmonary symptoms are apt to dominate the clinical presentation. The more severe the mitral regurgitation, the more likely fatigue plays a dominant role (17) (Table 10-2).

Physical Findings

The presence of both an apical holosystolic murmur and an apical diastolic murmur on physical examination suggests the diagnosis of combined mitral regurgitation and stenosis. The intensity of the systolic murmur is of limited value in assessing the severity of the regurgitation. Nevertheless, it is rare for a patient with mild to moderate mitral regurgitation to have a mitral systolic murmur greater than 3/6. In contrast, most patients with severe mitral regurgitation have murmurs of grade 3/6 or louder (17). Patients with combined lesions, however, have had severe but silent mitral regurgitation (18). It is obviously important in these patients not to confuse the murmur of tricuspid regurgitation with that of mitral regurgitation.

Attention to the characteristics of the apical diastolic murmur is of considerable value in determining the relative severity of the two lesions. Although an apical diastolic murmur may be heard in isolated mitral regurgitation, it is usually restricted to early and mid-diastole (Fig. 10-10); it does not extend to end-diastole unless tachycardia is present (16). Presystolic accentuation of this flow murmur may occur but is distinctly unusual. With severe organic mitral stenosis, the diastolic rumbling murmur is usually prolonged. The patients with mitral stenosis due to mitral annular calcification are a dis-

tinct group who are unlikely to have a diastolic rumble or an opening snap (19,20). Although severe silent mitral stenosis does exist in patients with rheumatic disease, it occurs most often in patients with severe pulmonary hypertension and low cardiac output. It is very unlikely to occur in the patient with serious coexisting mitral regurgitation. The presence of an accentuated first heart sound (S_1) or an opening snap favors serious stenosis but does not exclude predominant regurgitation (Fig. 10-11). In contrast, a diminished S_1 and absent opening snap favors predominant regurgitation but does not exclude a significant element of stenosis with a rigid and immobile valve. The presence of a left ventricular S_3 introducing the diastolic rumble excludes severe stenosis. Acute mitral regurgitation grafted on previously mild stenosis (as in the unusual stenosis with endocarditis) may pro-

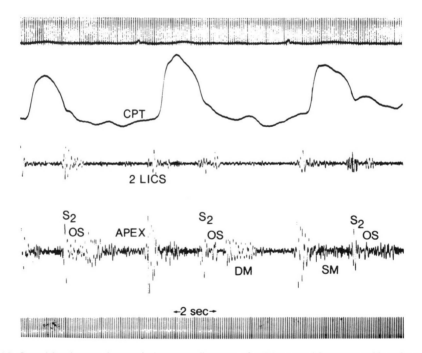

FIG. 10-10. Carotid pulse tracing and phonocardiogram of a 64-year-old woman with pulmonary congestion and easy fatigability. A grade 2/6 high-pitched holosystolic murmur (*SM*) was audible at the apex, as well as a grade 2/4 diastolic rumbling murmur preceded by an opening snap (*OS*). A left ventriculogram demonstrated predominant mitral regurgitation (3+). Note the short diastolic murmur (*DM*). The OS occurs 70 to 80 ms after the S_2. These findings are consistent with the mild nature of the mitral obstruction (Figs. 10-15 and 10-20).

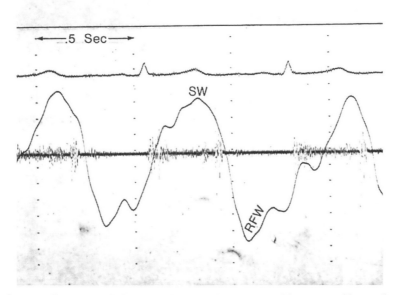

FIG. 10-11. Apexcardiogram and phonocardiogram of a 55-year-old woman with exertional dyspnea and pulmonary congestion. She had murmurs of both mitral stenosis and regurgitation. Predominant mitral regurgitation (3+) was found at catheterization. Note the late systolic expansion wave of the apexcardiogram (*SW*) and the well-preserved rapid filling wave (*RFW*) (Fig. 10-18).

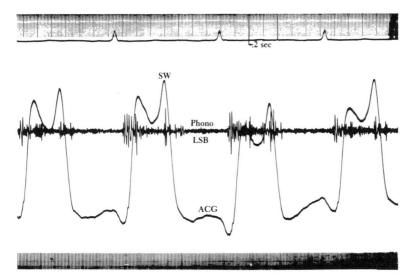

FIG. 10-12. Apexcardiogram of a 53-year-old woman with murmurs of mitral stenosis and regurgitation. The diastolic events are not well recorded. The prominent late systolic bulge (*SW*) was palpable throughout the precordium and sternal edge. This bulge may represent the forward thrust caused by the atrial expansion of severe mitral regurgitation (Fig. 10-25). *LSB*, left sternal border.

duce a prominent S_4. Either an S_3 or S_4 of left ventricular origin, therefore, essentially excludes important mitral stenosis. If these sounds are of left ventricular origin, they should be heard best at the apex and diminish on inspiration. If they are right ventricular in origin, they should be heard at the lower left sternal border and are apt to become louder on inspiration.

Evidence for left ventricular enlargement greatly favors predominant mitral regurgitation, although the evidence may be subtle, especially in the more balanced lesions (17,18). When the apical impulse is diffuse and sustained in systole (Fig. 10-11) or an early diastolic "shock" is appreciated, predominant and severe mitral regurgitation is present, unless of course significant associated aortic disease, myocardial disease, or hypertension is a complicating factor. If a left parasternal lift is present, it may be confused with a prominent apical impulse. A parasternal lift peaking early in systole is usually due to right ventricular strain and is secondary to pulmonary hypertension. Although this may develop in either lesion, it is likely to be most prominent in mitral stenosis. A left parasternal lift that rises more slowly and peaks at end-systole is likely to be caused by severe mitral regurgitation and is due to the anterior thrust of systolic left atrial expansion (Fig. 10-12).

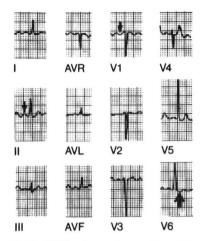

FIG. 10-13. ECG of a patient with evidence of mixed mitral stenosis and regurgitation. Left atrial abnormality is evident by the wide P wave (0.12 s) in lead 2 and the prominent terminal negative deflection in lead V_1 (*small arrows*). The precordial voltage suggests left ventricular hypertrophy and is evidence against isolated or predominant mitral stenosis. ST sagging is seen in leads V_5 and V_6 (*large arrow*) and may be due to early left ventricular strain. This patient was not taking cardiac glycosides; otherwise the ST abnormality may have been attributed to digitalis effect.

Laboratory Findings

Electrocardiogram

The ECG can be expected to demonstrate left atrial abnormality in a patient with a significant mitral lesion, whether predominant stenosis, regurgitation, or a balanced lesion. Atrial fibrillation is also common in any of these situations. Left ventricular hypertrophy, however, is not seen in isolated mitral stenosis. Its presence strongly favors serious associated regurgitation or associated aortic, hypertensive, or myocardial disease (Fig. 10-13). It was only electrocardiographic evidence of left ventricular hypertrophy that revealed silent mitral regurgitation in three of four cases described by Aravanis (18). In contrast, electrocardiographic evidence of left ventricular hypertrophy was not helpful in the series described by Janton et al. (17). The demonstration of right ventricular hypertrophy by ECG is uncommon in chronic mitral regurgitation, even when other evidence of right ventricular stress is present (21). An ECG that demonstrates only right ventricular hypertrophy favors predominant stenosis. Nevertheless, when stenosis and regurgitation are both severe, the ECG may demonstrate combined ventricular hypertrophy, apparent absence of ventricular hypertrophy (Fig. 10-14), or hypertrophy of either ventricle in isolation (22).

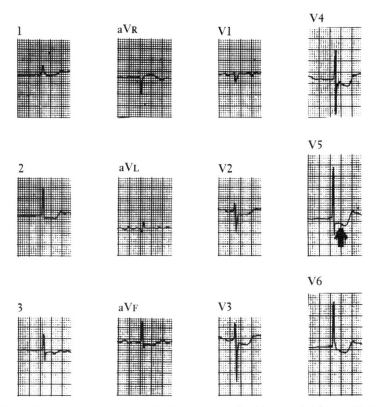

FIG. 10-14. ECG of a patient with mixed mitral disease and evidence of right ventricular failure with peripheral edema and a murmur of tricuspid regurgitation. The chest roentgenogram showed considerable right ventricular dilatation. The ECG fails to demonstrate right ventricular hypertrophy. This finding speaks strongly against mitral stenosis as the predominant left-sided lesion. The marked ST depression in V₂–V₆ (*arrow*) suggests left ventricular strain but may be due in part to digitalis effect or even to unsuspected coronary artery disease.

Roentgenogram

The chest roentgenogram may be useful in identifying the predominant lesion. Marked stenosis with mild or trivial regurgitation displays the most dramatic changes in pulmonary vasculature with varying degrees of right ventricular dilatation and modest left atrial enlargement without left ventricular enlargement. Unfortunately, the distinction between right and left ventricular dilatation may be difficult on the chest roentgenogram (Figs. 10-15 and 10-16). Indeed, an enlarged cardiac silhouette with severe pulmonary vascular changes may occur with pure mitral stenosis as a result of pulmonary venous hypertension and marked right ventricular enlargement. A giant left atrium is far more likely to be associated with chronic predominant mitral regurgitation. Calcification of the mitral valve implies a rheumatic origin, and in one series, calcification was twice as likely to be present when there was an important degree of associated regurgitation rather than with isolated stenosis (65% vs. 32%) (17,23). A C- or J-shaped opacity in the inferoposterior region of the cardiac silhouette is characteristic of mitral annular calcification and suggests a degenerative nonrheumatic etiology.

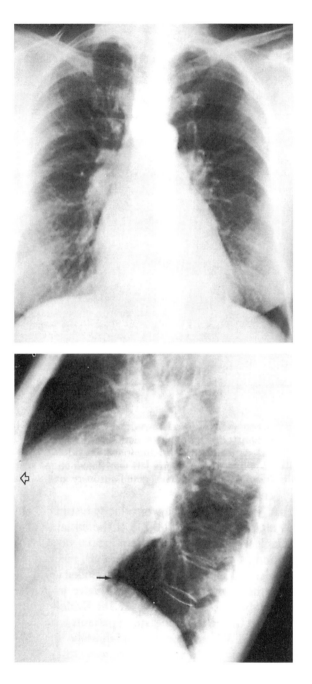

FIG. 10-15. Chest roentgenogram of the 64-year-old woman whose carotid pulse tracing and phonocardiogram are displayed in Fig. 10-10. **Top:** Posteroanterior view. **Bottom:** Lateral view. Moderately severe (3+) mitral regurgitation was seen on left ventriculography, and the left ventricle was hypokinetic and dilated on echocardiography. The evidence for left ventricular enlargement is minimal on this film. Encroachment of the left ventricular shadow (*black arrow*) on the inferior vena cava is seen on the lateral film. Right ventricular dilatation is suggested by the encroachment of the cardiac shadow on the retrosternal space (*open arrow*). Nevertheless, the echocardiogram revealed a normally sized right ventricle.

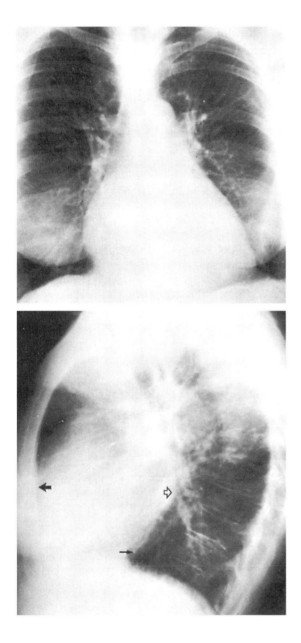

FIG. 10-16. Chest roentgenogram of the 48-year-old woman with murmurs of mitral stenosis and regurgitation whose apexcardiogram and phonocardiogram are displayed in Fig. 10-17. **Top:** Note the generalized cardiomegaly on the posteroanterior view. The cardiothoracic ratio is greater than 50%. **Bottom:** The lateral view also suggests left atrial enlargement (*open arrow*), minimal left ventricular enlargement (*small black arrow*), and considerable right ventricular enlargement (*large black arrow*). The echocardiogram, however, demonstrated the reverse: considerable left ventricular dilatation and no significant right ventricular dilatation.

Echocardiogram

Assessment of the degree of stenosis at the mitral valve has been found to be both reliable and reproducible. Evidence for volume overload may be present in the echocardiogram of patients with significant mitral regurgitation. Concentric left ventricular hypertrophy suggests that serious regurgitation or coexisting aortic valvular disease, hypertension, or myocardial disease is present. Doppler echocardiography has proven useful in the detection and quantification of both mitral stenosis and regurgitation (24,25). Radionuclide ventriculography may also be useful by giving evidence for volume overload (26,27).

Apexcardiogram

The apexcardiogram is of academic interest in documenting abnormalities of the apex impulse. A prominent sustained systolic expansion wave with a prominent rapid filling wave is expected with significant or predominant mitral regurgitation (Fig. 10-11). Timing of apical sounds with combined phonocardiography and apexcardiography may help determine whether an early diastolic sound is an opening snap or an S_3 (Fig. 10-17). A presystolic expansion wave (A wave) on the apexcardiogram makes important mitral stenosis unlikely.

Cardiac Catheterization

Cardiac catheterization in predominant mitral stenosis documents normal left ventricular pressures in diastole and a transvalvular pressure gradient throughout diastole (except for longer cycle lengths in atrial fibrillation or bradycardias) (Fig. 10-18). The pressure gradient recorded in isolated or predominant mitral regurgitation is greatest in early diastole and disappears in mid-diastole to late diastole (28) (Figs. 10-19 and 10-20). Persistence of the gradient throughout diastole, therefore, favors severe coexisting stenosis. The Gorlin hydraulic formula underestimates the mitral

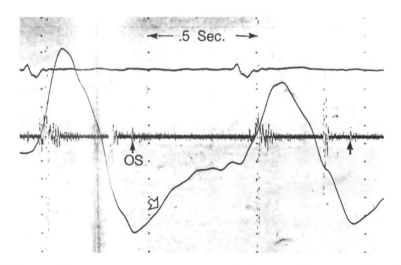

FIG. 10-17. Apexcardiogram and phonocardiogram of a 48-year-old woman with pulmonary congestion whose chest roentgenogram is shown in Fig. 10-16. She had murmurs of both mitral stenosis and regurgitation. Mild mitral regurgitation (1+) was observed on left ventriculogram. Note the absence of a rapid filling wave (*open arrow*) suggesting predominant mitral stenosis. The opening snap (*OS, black arrow*) was recorded 100 ms after the S_2. In this patient, the relatively long interval between the S_2 and the OS is explained by a small mitral gradient of only 10 mm Hg at rest. The cardiac index was diminished at 2.0 L/min/m².

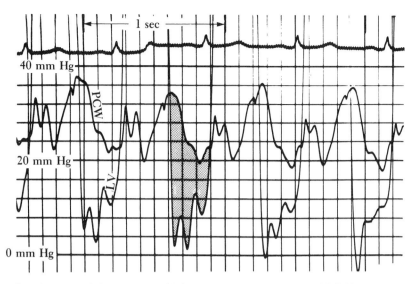

FIG. 10-18. Simultaneous left ventricular (*LV*) and pulmonary capillary (*PCW*) pressures in the 55-year-old woman with pulmonary congestion and exertional dyspnea whose apexcardiogram is displayed in Fig. 10-11. She had murmurs of both mitral stenosis and regurgitation but without evidence of left ventricular abnormality on either physical examination or ECG. Note the sustained diastolic gradient (*stippled area*). A mean diastolic gradient of 17 mm Hg was recorded across the mitral valve with a cardiac output of 4 L/min/m^2 by the Fick method. The mitral valve area was calculated to be 0.7 cm^2. The left ventriculogram revealed moderately severe (3+) mitral regurgitation. The calculated area of 0.7 cm^2 therefore underestimates the anatomic area. These data confirm balanced mitral stenosis and regurgitation.

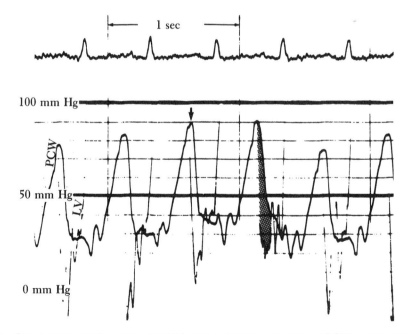

FIG. 10-19. Simultaneous left ventricular (*LV*) and pulmonary capillary (*PCW*) pressures in the patient whose aortic gradient is depicted in Fig. 10-8. This patient showed evidence not only of mixed aortic disease but also of mixed mitral disease; however, note the absence of a sustained diastolic gradient (*stippled area*). The exaggerated systolic regurgitant wave (*arrow*) in the pulmonary capillary pressure, with a rapid diastolic fall, is characteristic of severe mitral regurgitation and is strong evidence against significant diastolic obstruction at the mitral valve. The left ventriculogram demonstrated severe (4+) mitral regurgitation.

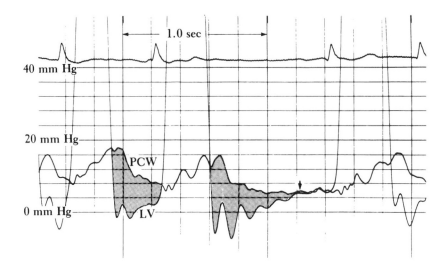

FIG. 10-20. Simultaneous left ventricular (*LV*) and pulmonary capillary (*PCW*) pressures in a 64-year-old woman with mixed mitral disease and pulmonary symptoms (also see Figs. 10-10 and 10-15). Note the sustained mitral diastolic gradient in shorter cycles and effacement of the diastolic gradient in longer cycles (*stippled areas*). The mean diastolic gradient was 11 mm Hg and the cardiac output was 3.4 L/min. The calculated mitral valve area of 0.8 cm² underestimated the anatomic area because moderately severe mitral regurgitation (3+) was observed on left ventriculography. The left ventricular ejection fraction was calculated at 73%.

anatomic orifice when mitral regurgitation coexists. The severity of mitral regurgitation is best estimated from contrast left ventriculography or Doppler echocardiography.

Therapy

In rheumatic mitral stenosis, the coexistence of serious mitral regurgitation negates the possibility of conventional mitral valvuloplasty or commissurotomy. In these patients, a prosthetic valve is usually required if symptoms of left ventricular failure mandate surgical intervention. Rheumatic patients with a pliable noncalcified valve and with no more than mild mitral regurgitation may be considered for valvuloplasty either open or by balloon valvotomy (29,30). In a similar way, the presence of severe mitral scarring in a patient with predominant mitral regurgitation makes effective valve reconstruction difficult. In one study, mild to moderate stenosis did not prevent adequate reconstruction (31).

COMBINED AORTIC STENOSIS AND MITRAL STENOSIS

When both the aortic and mitral valves are diseased, the cause is most commonly rheumatic. In rheumatic valvular disease the mitral valve is always involved to some extent; the aortic valve is also usually involved. Accordingly, combined aortic and mitral disease is very common. Nevertheless, the combination of severe stenosis of both valves without significant regurgitation at either valve is uncommon. In a series of 150 patients with combined aortic and mitral disease, only 10 were found to have essentially pure stenosis of both valves (32). Isolated aortic valve disease is seldom rheumatic. Shone's anomaly is a rare congenital lesion involving aortic stenosis, multiple left heart obstructions, and often mitral stenosis as well (33).

In isolated aortic stenosis, the basal cardiac output remains normal or even mildly increased until left ventricular failure supervenes (34). When an important degree of mitral stenosis is also present, cardiac output is lowered (32). This is probably due to the inability of left atrial systole to contribute to left ventricular filling. Because of the lower cardiac output, the clinical presentation of either lesion may be modified, with aortic stenosis more apt to be overlooked than mitral stenosis.

The symptoms of the mitral stenosis usually predominate, with early dyspnea, cough, hemoptysis, or pulmonary edema. Reactive pulmonary hypertension may lead to symptoms of right ventricular failure. Systemic emboli are also much more common than with isolated aortic stenosis (35,36). On the other hand, angina or syncope is more likely than with isolated mitral stenosis (32,36–39) (Table 10-3).

Physical Findings

When both these lesions are severe, the physical findings are usually more suggestive of severe mitral stenosis. Aortic stenosis may be suggested by a systolic ejection murmur or other evidence of aortic valvular disease (Table 10-4). Nevertheless, in an unusual patient, the typical findings of aortic stenosis may be present whereas the characteristic apical diastolic murmur of mitral stenosis is absent. The accentuated S_1 and opening snap of mitral stenosis may also be attenuated (36). The aortic systolic murmur is likely to be less intense than in isolated aortic stenosis (40). The carotid upstroke is less apt to feel delayed and the apex impulse less apt to be diffuse or sustained than in isolated aortic stenosis (Figs. 10-21 and 10-22) If, however, any of

TABLE 10-3. *Findings in combined aortic stenosis and mitral stenosis*

Clinical and laboratory findings	Predominant aortic stenosis	Both severe	Predominant mitral stenosis
Presenting symptoms			
Syncope	+	+	–
Angina	+	±	–
Pulmonary symptoms	–	+	+
Systemic emboli	–	+	+
Physical findings			
Delayed carotid upstroke	+	±	–
Prominent apical impulse	+	±	–
Prolonged systolic murmur	+	±	–
Prolonged diastolic murmur	–	+	+
Electrocardiogram			
Right ventricular hypertrophy	–	±	±
Left ventricular hypertrophy	+	±	–
Atrial fibrillation	–	+	+
Chest roentgenogram			
Aortic valve calcium	+	±	–
Poststenotic aortic dilatation	+	±	–
Left atrium dilated	±	+	+
Left ventricular hypertrophy	–	+	+
Echocardiogram			
Aortic cusps thickened	+	+	±
Mitral leaflets thickened	±	+	+
Left ventricular hypertrophy	+	±	–
Doppler findings			
High-velocity systolic jet	++	+	–
High-velocity inflow jet	–	+	++
Cardiac catheterization			
Systolic aortic gradient	+	±	–
Diastolic mitral gradient	–	+	+

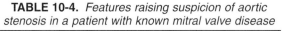
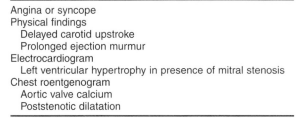

TABLE 10-4. *Features raising suspicion of aortic stenosis in a patient with known mitral valve disease*

Angina or syncope
Physical findings
    Delayed carotid upstroke
    Prolonged ejection murmur
Electrocardiogram
    Left ventricular hypertrophy in presence of mitral stenosis
Chest roentgenogram
    Aortic valve calcium
    Poststenotic dilatation

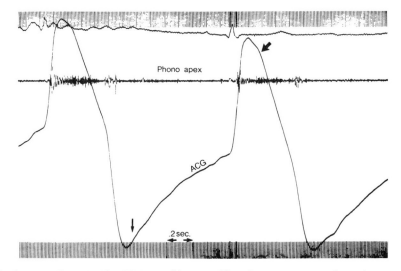

FIG. 10-21. Apexcardiogram of a 66-year-old man with pulmonary congestion whose carotid pulse tracing is displayed in Fig. 10-22. Note the absence of a rapid filling wave (*small arrow*), suggesting mitral stenosis. The systolic expansion wave appears normal (*large arrow*) and is consistent with the finding that the apex impulse was unremarkable on palpation.

these findings are present in a patient thought to have isolated mitral stenosis, coexisting aortic stenosis must be considered.

Laboratory Findings

In this combination of lesions, the ECG may fail to demonstrate left ventricular hypertrophy; however, as in isolated mitral stenosis, left atrial abnormality or atrial fibrillation is very common (32,35,36). Right ventricular hypertrophy may or may not be seen on the ECG. Obviously, if left ventricular hypertrophy is present on the ECG of a patient thought

to have isolated mitral stenosis, associated mitral regurgitation or aortic valve disease must be given strong consideration.

The chest roentgenogram in patients with both aortic and mitral stenosis is usually similar to that of patients with isolated mitral stenosis; evidence for left ventricular enlargement is unusual. Calcium in the aortic valve and poststenotic dilatation of the proximal aorta may occur but are less likely than in isolated aortic stenosis.

The echocardiogram can be very useful in demonstrating disease of both the aortic and mitral valves. The appearance of mitral stenosis on the echocardiogram is not likely to be affected by coexisting aortic stenosis. Concentric left ventricular hypertrophy is often lacking when aortic stenosis is accompanied by severe mitral stenosis. The estimation of the transmitral and transaortic gradient by Doppler echocardiograph is likely to be decreased because of the diminished cardiac output in this combination of lesions. The echocardiographic assessment of the severity of aortic stenosis may be influenced by the associated mitral stenosis: The planimetered aortic valve area may also be lessened due to the low cardiac output. The continuity equation, however, should give a reasonable estimate of the associated aortic stenosis.

Carotid pulse tracings may be of academic interest in allowing precise measurement of carotid upstroke time and left ventricular ejection time (Fig. 10-22). Although a normal carotid pulse tracing may be present in combined aortic and mitral stenosis, an abnormal tracing is the rule (34).

At cardiac catheterization, both the transmitral and transaortic gradients are likely to be small because of the diminished cardiac output (32,35–38). It has also been observed that the transvalvular aortic gradient and the aortic valve calculation may be decreased in patients with left ventricular failure and low cardiac output (41). In such patients, inotropes have been used to augment cardiac output in an attempt to better evaluate the severity of the aortic stenosis (42). If the aortic gradient is not augmented along with the cardiac output, it is assumed that the aortic stenosis is less severe and that valve replacement would be of no value. It is not known whether such testing would be of use in patients with combined aortic and mitral stenoses in whom the severity of the aortic stenosis is in question.

Angiography is helpful in ruling out silent regurgitation of either valve. It is also often useful in demonstrating the immobility and rigidity of each valve and the jet of radiolu-

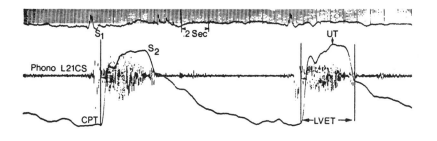

FIG. 10-22. Carotid pulse tracing and phonocardiogram of a 66-year-old man with pulmonary congestion, severe mitral stenosis, and aortic stenosis. Note the delayed upstroke time (*UT*) and left ventricular ejection time (*LVET*), yet the initial half of the upstroke is normal at 40 ms (*small arrows*). The carotid pulses felt normal to examiners; however, the prolonged crescendo-decrescendo murmur led to the suspicion of significant coexisting aortic stenosis. The diastolic murmur with presystolic accentuation is poorly recorded (Fig. 10-21). *2 LICS*, second left intercostal space.

cent bloodstreaming across a narrowed orifice.

Therapy

In patients with mitral and aortic stenosis, the signs and symptoms of mitral stenosis predominate, and the aortic stenosis may be overlooked. If only the mitral lesion is corrected, severe aortic stenosis becomes manifest promptly in the postoperative period. In patients with both mitral stenosis in whom the severity of the aortic stenosis is in question, transcutaneous balloon valvotomy may prove invaluable (43).

COMBINED AORTIC REGURGITATION AND MITRAL STENOSIS

The combination of severe mitral stenosis with severe aortic regurgitation is uncommon. As many as two thirds of patients with severe mitral stenosis have an early blowing diastolic murmur along the left sternal border. Although in the past this murmur was often thought to be Graham Steell's murmur of pulmonic regurgitation, it has been shown that most subjects with such a murmur have some degree of aortic regurgitation (44). The murmur is more likely to be a true Graham Steell's murmur of pulmonic regurgitation if there is evidence of severe pulmonary hypertension without the widened pulse pressure or peripheral signs of aortic regurgitation (45). If the diastolic murmur of semilunar valve regurgitation increases during handgrip and squatting and decreases during inhalation of amyl nitrite, it is more likely to be a murmur of aortic regurgitation (46). Most patients with severe aortic regurgitation who are suspected of having coexisting mitral stenosis actually have Austin Flint diastolic murmurs.

Symptoms alone are not likely to be helpful in the recognition of this combination of lesions. If a patient with obvious aortic regurgi-

TABLE 10-5. *Findings in combined aortic regurgitation and mitral stenosis*

Clinical and laboratory findings	Predominant aortic regurgitation	Both severe	Predominant mitral stenosis
Presenting symptoms			
Angina	+	+	−
Effort intolerance	±	+	+
Pulmonary symptoms	−	+	+
Systemic emboli	−	+	+
Physical findings			
Widened pulse pressure	+	±	−
Parasternal lift	−	±	+
Prominent apical impulse	+	±	−
Loud S_1	−	±	+
S_3 or S_4	+	±	−
Effect of squatting or handgrip on diastolic murmur	↑	↑ or ↓	↓
Electrocardiogram			
Right ventricular hypertrophy	−	±	±
Left ventricular hypertrophy	+	±	−
Atrial fibrillation	−	+	+
Chest roentgenogram			
Left ventricle dilated	+	±	−
Right ventricle dilated	−	±	+
Echocardiogram			
Left ventricular hypertrophy and hyperkinetic left ventricle	+	±	−
Doppler findings			
High-velocity inflow jet	−	+	++
Subaortic diastolic turbulence	++	+	±
Cardiac catheterization			
Diastolic mitral gradient	−	+	+
Aortic regurgitation	3–4+	2–4+	0–1+

↑, increased; ↓, decreased.

tation presents with apparently early dyspnea, pulmonary edema, hemoptysis, or systemic emboli, the astute clinician may suspect coexisting mitral stenosis (Tables 10-5
and 10-6).

Even severe aortic regurgitation is occasionally silent when accompanied by severe
mitral disease (12). In the presence of severe
mitral stenosis, the widened pulse pressure
and peripheral signs of aortic regurgitation
may be absent (47). In this combination the
apical diastolic rumble is usually present
along with an accentuated S_1 and an opening
snap. Differentiation between aortic regurgitation and Graham Steell's murmur, and between organic mitral stenosis and an Austin
Flint murmur can usually be made at the
bedside by using various maneuvers. Squatting or isometric handgrip elevates peripheral vascular resistance and intensifies the
murmur of aortic regurgitation and the
Austin Flint murmur. When the patient suddenly returns to the upright position, both
these murmurs decrease in intensity. Exercise or amyl nitrite inhalation intensifies the
murmur of organic mitral stenosis while diminishing the murmur of aortic regurgitation
and the Austin Flint murmur. A rapidly collapsing and prominent apical impulse displaced leftward or inferiorly is characteristic
of aortic regurgitation and is inconsistent
with isolated mitral stenosis.

TABLE 10-6. *Features raising suspicion of
mitral stenosis in a patient with known
aortic valve disease*

Prominent pulmonary symptoms
  Cough
  Dyspnea
  Hemoptysis
  Systemic emboli
Physical findings
  Parasternal lift
  Loud S_1 and/or opening snap
  Diastolic murmur
Electrocardiogram
  Presence of right ventricular hypertrophy
  Absence of left ventricular hypertrophy
Chest roentgenogram
  Prominent pulmonary vascular markings
  Right ventricular dilatation

Laboratory Findings

The ECG may show evidence of left ventricular hypertrophy to alert the clinician to
the severity of concurrent aortic regurgitation.
Although left atrial abnormality on the ECG
is apt to occur with either lesion, atrial fibrillation suggests associated mitral stenosis
(48). Right ventricular hypertrophy in the
ECG is also suggestive of mitral stenosis, because it is uncommon even in advanced aortic
regurgitation.

The chest roentgenogram may be typical of
isolated mitral stenosis but often provides
some evidence of left ventricular enlargement. Calcium in the aortic valve and dilatation of the proximal aorta are less likely than
in isolated aortic disease (Fig. 10-23)

The echocardiogram readily reveals this
combination of lesions. Aortic cusp thickening with or without aortic root dilatation
points to the aortic valve as the site of disease.
Left ventricular hypertrophy and volume
overload of the left ventricle suggests severe
aortic regurgitation. Severe aortic regurgitation is apt to cause premature closure of the
mitral valve, mimicking some of the features
of mitral stenosis. An important degree of mitral stenosis, however, is marked by thickened
mitral leaflets with diastolic doming. Doppler
analysis can be expected to demonstrate turbulent flow under the aortic valve at the same
time the left ventricular inflow velocity characteristics unmask a significant mitral gradient and prolonged pressure half-time. Separation of the diastolic turbulence of aortic
regurgitation from the inflow turbulence
caused by mitral stenosis may require careful
searching by the ultrasonographer. Radionuclide ventriculography may also demonstrate
volume overload of the left ventricle inconsistent with isolated mitral stenosis (27).

Cardiac catheterization may prove misleading in combined aortic regurgitation and mitral stenosis: The left ventricular diastolic
pressure is often elevated and the transmitral
gradient at rest may be small. It is often helpful in this circumstance to repeat pressure
measurements and cardiac output determina-

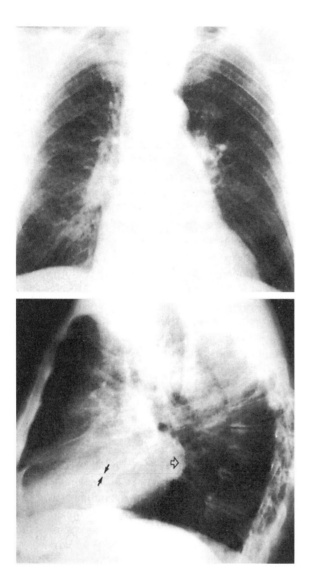

FIG. 10-23. Chest roentgenogram of the 66-year-old man with aortic regurgitation and mitral stenosis whose graphic recordings are displayed in Figs. 10-21 and 10-22. **Top:** Posteroanterior view. **Bottom:** Lateral view. The patient presented with pulmonary congestion and murmurs of mitral and aortic stenosis. Mitral valve calcification was seen on lateral view (*black arrows*), but no aortic valve calcification was observed. Poststenotic dilatation of the proximal aorta is not evident. Note the left atrial enlargement (*open arrow*), pulmonary venous engorgement, pulmonary artery dilatation, and fluid in the fissure. The left ventricular enlargement makes isolated mitral stenosis unlikely. This enlargement could have been caused by myopathy or by significant regurgitation at either the aortic or mitral valve. This patient's supravalvular aortogram showed moderate (3+) aortic regurgitation.

tions during exercise or a pharmacologically induced increase in cardiac output. Supravalvular aortography may be used in assessing the severity of concurrent aortic regurgitation or as additional corroboration of the Doppler echocardiographic findings.

Therapy

If a patient with severe mitral stenosis has moderate to severe aortic regurgitation, aortic valve replacement will most probably be re-quired during cardiac surgery. If the mitral valve is amenable to transcutaneous balloon valvotomy, symptoms may be ameliorated enough to delay the need for valve surgery (49).

COMBINED AORTIC REGURGITATION AND MITRAL REGURGITATION

Perhaps the most common combination of rheumatic valvular lesions is aortic regurgita-

TABLE 10-7. *Findings in combined aortic regurgitation and mitral regurgitation*

Clinical and laboratory findings	Predominant aortic regurgitation	Both severe	Predominant mitral regurgitation
Presenting symptoms			
Angina	+	+	±
Easy fatigability	+	+	+
Pulmonary symptoms	–	+	+
Physical findings			
Widened pulse pressure	+	+	–
Parasternal lift	–	±	+
Prolonged diastolic murmur	+	+	–
Prolonged systolic murmur	±	+	+
S$_4$	+	–	–
Electrocardiogram			
Left ventricular hypertrophy and left atrial abnormality	+	+	+
Atrial fibrillation	-	+	+
Chest roentgenogram			
Left ventricle dilated	+	+	+
Left atrium dilated	±	+	+
Echocardiogram			
Left ventricular hypertrophy and hyperkinesis	+	+	+
Doppler findings			
Diastolic subaortic turbulence	++	++	±
Systolic left atrial turbulence	±	++	++
Cardiac catheterization			
Valvular gradients	±	±	±
Aortic regurgitation	3–4+	2–4+	1–2+
Mitral regurgitation	1–2+	2–4+	3–4+

tion and mitral regurgitation, with or without coexisting stenoses (50). Combined mitral and aortic regurgitation may also be caused by mucopolysaccharidoses (51) or by connective tissue abnormalities with myxomatous degeneration of valve tissue (52). In this circumstance, coexisting tricuspid regurgitation is often present as well. Of course, chordal rupture or infective endocarditis may supervene to produce regurgitation in previously diseased valves, whether the original disease was congenital or rheumatic.

Mild to moderate aortic regurgitation is well tolerated when the major lesion is significant mitral regurgitation (53). In contrast, when the major lesion is severe aortic regurgitation, any degree of mitral regurgitation can be expected to worsen as the left ventricle dilates and its distorted geometry affects papillary muscle function. In the presence of free aortic regurgitation, a competent mitral valve is important, because it protects the left atrium and lungs from the effects of aortic re-

gurgitation. An incompetent mitral valve may even allow the lower resistance of the left atrium and pulmonary veins to augment aortic regurgitation through end-diastolic mitral regurgitation (54). As a result, a serious amount of mitral regurgitation is not tolerated for long in the presence of severe aortic regurgitation. This is borne out by the observation that the left ventricular systolic function is likely to be lower than with either lesion in isolation; also their prognosis and surgical results are poorer (55).

The presenting symptoms are not likely to aid in the recognition of this combination. Certainly, pulmonary symptoms may be more pronounced and earlier than with either lesion in isolation (Table 10-7).

Physical Findings

The physical findings are likely to suggest the concurrence of both lesions by the presence of the characteristic systolic and diastolic murmurs. An occasional patient has been described in whom either the aortic regurgitation or the mitral regurgitation has been silent. An S_3 is common to either lesion as are apical diastolic murmurs. An S_4, however, suggests predominant aortic regurgitation or the recent onset of mitral regurgitation. It should also be kept in mind that severe aortic regurgitation may cause sufficient enlargement of the left ventricle and distortion of its geometry to produce significant mitral regurgitation and a holosystolic apical murmur. A widened pulse pressure and peripheral signs of aortic regurgitation are helpful in suggesting the importance of the associated aortic regurgitation; however, severe mitral regurgitation itself may produce a brisk carotid upstroke. The apical impulse is likely to be diffuse and sustained, and a diastolic shock may be palpable with either lesion.

Laboratory Findings

The ECG demonstrates left ventricular hypertrophy with either or both lesions. Left atrial abnormality is also common to both, although atrial fibrillation early in the course suggests coexisting mitral valve disease. Right ventricular hypertrophy would be unlikely unless considerable mitral stenosis was also present.

The chest roentgenogram demonstrates left ventricular enlargement with either lesion; however, considerable left atrial dilatation is not likely with aortic regurgitation alone. Calcification may be present in both valves when the cause is rheumatic. On fluoroscopy, systolic expansion of the left atrium may be present and testifies to the hemodynamic significance of an apical holosystolic murmur.

The echocardiogram is useful in demonstrating the rheumatic or myxomatous nature of the disease. In the former, marked thickening of aortic and mitral cusps and leaflets with limited excursion or doming is likely. In the latter, reduplicated valve echoes with increased valvular excursion and mitral systolic prolapse point to myxomatous degeneration (52). Volume overload from either lesion should be evident by echocardiography or radionuclide ventriculopathy. A reliable assessment of the severity of each lesion should be readily available by Doppler analysis or by cardiac catheterization with angiographic studies. In one study of 44 patients who underwent double-valve replacement for this combination of lesions, increased end-systolic left ventricular diameter and depressed ejection fraction were independent predictors of operative risk and postoperative systolic performance (56).

COMBINED AORTIC STENOSIS AND MITRAL REGURGITATION

Severe aortic stenosis combined with serious mitral regurgitation is the least common of the left-sided rheumatic combinations. In the elderly, this combination may be due to severe calcific aortic stenosis and mitral annular calcification (57), although usually one or the other predominates.

When both lesions are significant, this combination causes a very undesirable set of hemodynamic circumstances. The elevated systolic pressure (afterload) in the left ventricle augments the severity of the mitral regurgitation. Simultaneously, mitral regurgitation diminishes the end-systolic volume and reduces the beneficial effect of increased preload on left ventricular performance. These factors result in a low cardiac output combined with severe pulmonary venous hypertension. In patients with critical aortic stenosis, a holosystolic murmur at the apex often represents papillary muscle dysfunction secondary to left ventricular dilatation. This occurs late in the course of aortic stenosis and indicates a poor prognosis.

If both lesions are severe, the symptoms are apt to include angina, syncope, easy fatigability, early dyspnea, pulmonary congestion, and possibly systemic emboli (Table 10-8).

TABLE 10-8. *Findings in combined aortic stenosis and mitral regurgitation*

Clinical and laboratory findings	Predominant aortic stenosis	Both severe	Predominant mitral regurgitation
Presenting symptoms			
Syncope	+	+	−
Angina	+	+	−
Easy fatigability	−	+	+
Pulmonary symptoms	-	±	±
Physical findings			
Delayed carotid upstroke	+	±	−
Effect of squatting or handgrip on systolic murmur	Decreased or unchanged	Increased	Increased
S_3	−	+	+
S_4	+	±	−
Electrocardiogram			
Left ventricular hypertrophy and left atrial abnormality	+	+	+
Atrial fabrillation	−	±	±
Chest roentgenogram			
Left ventricular and left atrial dilatation	±	+	+
Aortic valve calcium	+	+	±
Poststenotic dilatation of aorta	+	+	±
Echocardiogram			
Left ventricular hypertrophy	+	+	+
Dilated left ventricle	±	±	+
Hyperkinetic left ventricle	−	+	+
Doppler findings			
High systolic aortic jet	++	+	−
Left atrial systolic turbulence	±	++	++
Cardiac catheterization			
Aortic valvular gradient	+	+	-
Mitral regurgitation	0–2+	2–4+	3–4+

Physical Findings

On physical examination, the two systolic murmurs may be difficult to distinguish. The murmur of aortic stenosis is harsh and loudest in the second right intercostal space, but it is also heard well at the apex (Gallivardin's phenomenon), where it may be of higher frequency. The S_2 is usually diminished, and a prolonged ejection murmur of aortic stenosis may closely simulate a holosystolic murmur at the apex. The murmur of severe mitral regurgitation, on the other hand, may radiate toward the base, particularly when due to chordal rupture. It may also take on a crescendo-decrescendo pattern more closely simulating an ejection murmur. Radiation of such mitral regurgitant murmurs to the dorsal spine may help to differentiate them from a murmur of aortic stenosis, but occasionally the latter also radiates posteriorly.

Physiologic or pharmacologic maneuvers, such as squatting, handgrip, or amyl nitrite administration, are apt to influence a mitral regurgitant murmur substantially while not causing significant alterations in the murmur of valvular aortic stenosis. Amyl nitrite or exercise can augment the murmur of aortic stenosis while decreasing the murmur of mitral regurgitation. HOCM often mimics this combination of lesions. A Valsalva maneuver, however, augments the systolic murmurs of this entity while diminishing the murmurs of valvular aortic stenosis and mitral regurgitation. In combined aortic stenosis and mitral regurgitation, the murmur of mitral regurgitation is not likely to be silent, even though it may be masked by the aortic murmur. The aortic stenosis murmur, however, may indeed become inaudible, especially when left ventricular function deteriorates

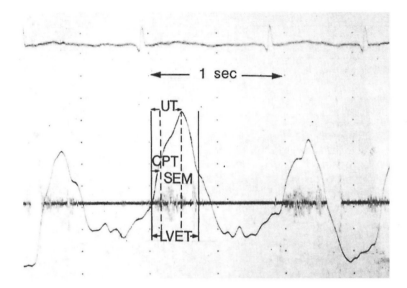

FIG. 10-24. Carotid pulse tracing and phonocardiogram recorded at the second left intercostal space of a 60-year-old woman with murmurs of stenosis and regurgitation at both the aortic and mitral valves. This patient had symptoms of both pulmonary congestion and right ventricular failure for the previous 18 months. Note the delay in upstroke time (*UT*) and left ventricular ejection time (*LVET*) and the delayed peaking of the systolic ejection murmur (*SEM*). These findings point to severe aortic stenosis.

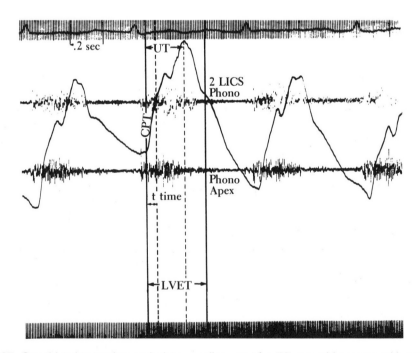

FIG. 10-25. Carotid pulse tracing and phonocardiogram of a 53-year-old woman with murmurs of stenosis and regurgitation at both the aortic and mitral valves. She had pulmonary congestion of recent onset. Both the time to half-amplitude (*t time*) and left ventricular ejection time (*LVET*) are relatively normal, but the upstroke time (*UT*) remained markedly abnormal, suggesting important aortic stenosis (Fig. 10-12). *2 LICS*, second left intercostal space.

and cardiac output falls significantly. An S_3 is likely to be heard if mitral regurgitation is severe or if the left ventricle has begun to fail. A prominent S_4, however, is unlikely in the presence of a significant degree of chronic mitral regurgitation.

The carotid pulse is usually delayed and characteristic of aortic stenosis (Fig. 10-24). It is possible, however, for coexisting mitral regurgitation to "normalize" the carotid upstroke and left ventricular ejection time (Fig. 10-25). The apical impulse is diffuse and sustained. A prominent diastolic shock points strongly to associated severe mitral regurgitation.

Laboratory Findings

The ECG is usually of little value in distinguishing these two lesions. Both lesions produce left ventricular hypertrophy and left atrial enlargement. Atrial fibrillation, however, should raise the suspicion of associated mitral disease because this rhythm is uncommon in isolated aortic stenosis until late in the course when left ventricular failure has supervened.

Because isolated aortic stenosis is not likely to cause left ventricular enlargement except late in the course, a chest roentgenogram that demonstrates left ventricular and left atrial enlargement may be caused by associated mitral regurgitation. Poststenotic dilatation of the ascending aorta may be a clue to unsuspected aortic stenosis. Finally, calcium may be expected in the aortic valve and is also commonly seen in the mitral valve.

The echocardiogram with Doppler studies will readily demonstrate both lesions. Indirect evidence for considerable mitral regurgitation may be found in volume overload of the left ventricle by echocardiography or radionuclide ventriculography.

Cardiac catheterization is necessary for the measurement of the transaortic pressure gradient, cardiac output, and valve area. Left ventriculography is useful for further assessment of the severity of mitral regurgitation and estimation of left ventricular systolic function.

Therapy

If mitral regurgitation is mild to moderate and pulmonary congestion is not a prominent part of the patient's symptoms, aortic valve replacement may suffice or the mitral valve may be reconstructed. Even without mitral valve replacement, considerable improvement in mitral regurgitation can be expected after successful aortic valve replacement. This improvement is due not only to decreased intraventricular pressure but also to favorable changes in ventricular morphology (58). In many cases, however, either the mitral valve must be reconstructed or both valves must be replaced.

BALANCED STENOSIS AND REGURGITATION OF AORTIC AND MITRAL VALVES

Although balanced stenosis and regurgitation of the aortic and mitral valves is an uncommon combination, it is far from rare. Rigid immobile leaflets of both valves can result from rheumatic valvulitis. The clinical presentation is likely to be dominated by pulmonary congestion. Physical examination may reveal murmurs of all four hemodynamic lesions.

Left ventricular enlargement and volume overload, as determined by various methods, suggest that severe aortic or mitral regurgitation (or both) is present. One or the other of these lesions may be apparent on physical examination; however, the possibility of "masked" or "silent" lesions must be kept in mind. Nonexistent lesions may be mimicked by Austin Flint, Graham Steell's, or even tricuspid murmurs. The unusual patient who falls into this category is most probably recognized only after careful analysis of echocardiography with Doppler studies, cardiac catheterization, and angiographic data (Figs. 10-8, 10-9, and 10-18 to 10-20).

TRICUSPID STENOSIS IN COMBINED VALVULAR DISEASE

Tricuspid stenosis is very unusual as an isolated lesion. When isolated tricuspid stenosis is found, it may represent a rare congenital lesion or an obstructing right atrial mass. Tricuspid stenosis may also be caused by carcinoid heart disease, endomyocardial fibrosis or fibroelastosis, and, more rarely, by systemic lupus erythematosus (59) or Loeffler's endocarditis (60–62). In most patients, tricuspid stenosis is due to rheumatic valvulitis and is associated with coexisting disease of the mitral and aortic valves (63). Indeed, rheumatic tricuspid stenosis almost always coexists with mitral stenosis and only rarely with predominant mitral regurgitation (64). When the aortic valve is significantly involved, the aortic valve may be stenotic, regurgitant, or balanced.

Some degree of rheumatic scarring of the tricuspid valve was found at autopsy in 30% of patients with rheumatic heart disease, but usually the lesion is of no hemodynamic significance (60). Tricuspid stenosis of varying degree has been found in 10% to 23% of such autopsies (60,65). Tricuspid stenosis was clinically undetected in all but a few of these patients (63,66). Tricuspid stenosis is, therefore, a lesion that easily escapes detection. Furthermore, it may cause incorrect assessment of the severity of other coexisting lesions. Failure to detect it can explain the lack of improvement in a patient who undergoes mitral or aortic valve surgery.

TABLE 10-9. *Findings in tricuspid stenosis combined with mitral valve disease*

Clinical and laboratory findings	Mitral disease with tricuspid stenosis	Mitral disease without tricuspid stenosis
Presenting symptoms		
Dyspnea	+	+
Orthopnea	+	+
Paroxysmal nocturnal dyspnea	−	+
Pulmonary edema	−	+
Hemoptysis	−	+
Easy fatigability	+	+
Neck fluttering	+	−
Physical findings		
Jugular veins		
Giant A waves	+	−
Slow Y descent	+	−
Split S_1	+	−
Parasternal lift	−	+
High-pitched short diastolic murmur, lower left sternal border	+	−
Electrocardiogram		
Prolonged PR interval	+	−
Atrial fibrillation	+	+
Right ventricular hypertrophy	±	+
P waves taller than QRS in V_1	+	±
Chest roentgenogram		
Pulmonary vascular engorgement	±	+
Right atrial dilatation	+	−
Echocardiogram		
Tricuspid leaflet thickening with restricted diastolic velocity	±	−
Right ventricular dilatation	±	+
Doppler findings		
Respiratory variation of right ventricular inflow velocity	++	±
Tricuspid valve pressure half-time	+	−
Cardiac catheterization		
Tricuspid diastolic gradient	+	−

The patient with rheumatic tricuspid stenosis is usually a woman with coexisting mitral stenosis. Gibson and Wood (62) emphasized the relative paucity of pulmonary symptoms. Perloff and Harvey (63), however, found effort dyspnea and orthopnea in most of their patients, yet they commented on the lack of acute paroxysmal symptoms such as paroxysmal nocturnal dyspnea, severe pulmonary edema, and sudden massive hemoptysis.

Symptoms usually attributed to tricuspid stenosis are easy fatigability and effort intolerance resulting from restriction of cardiac output (Table 10-9). Perceptible fluttering in the neck due to the giant jugular venous A waves has been described (63). Hepatomegaly with right upper quadrant pain, peripheral edema, and ascites represents late disease and usually occurs only after atrial fibrillation has developed (66).

Physical Findings

Characteristic physical findings are most helpful in alerting the physician to coexisting tricuspid stenosis. In patients with sinus rhythm, the jugular veins demonstrate a "giant" presystolic pulsation with a gentle Y descent in early diastole. In atrial fibrillation, the presystolic wave disappears, but the slow Y descent persists and may be noticeable on careful inspection. Large presystolic jugular pulsations may also be caused by pulmonic stenosis or pulmonary hypertension. In the latter situations, a parasternal "right ventricular" lift is expected. In tricuspid stenosis, such a lift is absent (62).

Auscultatory examination of patients with combined tricuspid and mitral stenosis may provide several important clues. The S_1 may be split because of concomitant delay in both the mitral and tricuspid components of the first heart sound. This delayed tricuspid closure sound should not be mistaken for a pulmonic ejection click. The pulmonic ejection click is most audible at the upper left sternal border, diminishing in intensity with inspiration. In contrast, the tricuspid closure sound is best heard at the lower left sternal border and changes little or may increase in intensity with inspiration. Inspiratory splitting of the S_2 is unusual in tricuspid stenosis, perhaps because inspiratory augmentation of right ventricular stroke volume is inhibited (63). A tricuspid opening snap is likely to be present but is difficult to distinguish from the coexisting mitral opening snap (62,63).

The most helpful auscultatory sign is the diastolic murmur of tricuspid stenosis. It is best heard at the lower left sternal edge, in contrast to the murmur of mitral stenosis, which is best heard nearer the apex. A coexisting tricuspid murmur is often heard better at the lower left sternal edge, where it becomes louder and may be higher pitched. In patients with sinus rhythm, the murmur is predominantly presystolic with little or no mid-diastolic component. With atrial fibrillation, the murmur is early to mid-diastolic and fades toward the subsequent S_2. The most reliable feature of the tricuspid stenosis murmur is its inspiratory augmentation, as emphasized by Rivero-Carvallo (67). When murmurs of both tricuspid stenosis and regurgitation are present, inspiratory augmentation of the diastolic murmur and reduction of the systolic murmur indicate that the dominant lesion is tricuspid stenosis (60,66).

Laboratory Findings

If the patient is in sinus rhythm, tall peaked P waves ("p pulmonale") without associated right ventricular hypertrophy is suggestive electrocardiographic evidence for tricuspid stenosis (62,63,68). A prolonged PR interval is frequently present and may represent a delay in intraatrial conduction time. Many patients are in atrial fibrillation, however, and some demonstrate right ventricular hypertrophy (60). An electrocardiographic pattern reported to be highly suggestive of tricuspid stenosis is a diminutive rsr' complex in V_1 and V_2 associated with P waves of greater amplitude than the QRS (68).

The chest roentgenogram of patients with combined tricuspid and mitral stenosis characteristically demonstrates right atrial enlargement without much enlargement of the pulmonary arteries (62,63–68).

The echocardiogram is most useful. In patients with organic tricuspid disease, the tricuspid valve is thickened. Restriction in diastolic velocity and associated inflow turbulence is seen, similar to that recorded for the stenotic mitral valve. The echocardiogram also demonstrates the coexisting mitral stenosis and normal right ventricular cavity size. Unusual causes of tricuspid valve obstruction, such as right atrial tumor, thrombus, or large tricuspid vegetation, may be discovered by echocardiography. In addition, echocardiography allows more adequate visualization of the tricuspid valve, right atrium, and right ventricle (69,70). Doppler measurements of tricuspid flow velocity are lower than those recorded across stenotic mitral valves. Hatle and colleagues (71,72) noted greater respiratory variation in velocity than in normal subjects. They also recorded delays in the pressure half-time similar to those recorded across the stenotic mitral valve.

The jugular venous pulse tracing is most dramatic in patients in sinus rhythm who demonstrate very large peaked presystolic (A) waves. A gentle Y descent is recorded from a diminutive V wave, even when atrial fibrillation is present.

Cardiac catheterization confirms the diagnosis of tricuspid stenosis if a transvalvular diastolic gradient of over 3 mm Hg is recorded. The gradient is usually small, and respiratory variation in right atrial pressure may render a gradient inapparent on pulling the catheter from the right ventricle into the right atrium. Exercise or the use of amyl nitrite may be very helpful in widening the diastolic gradient and allowing the calculation of the tricuspid orifice area (73,74). Exercise also widens the transmitral gradient (which is usually decreased with coexisting tricuspid stenosis) and allows a more reliable calculation of the mitral orifice area.

Therapy

Management of the patient usually focuses on the more severe lesion, mitral stenosis. Accompanying tricuspid stenosis can result in underestimation of the severity of mitral stenosis (due to the paucity of paroxysmal pulmonary symptoms). Diuretic therapy is not apt to be affected by coexisting tricuspid disease. When the patient is operated on for coexisting mitral or aortic disease, simultaneous tricuspid valvuloplasty or replacement is necessary if the expected improvement in cardiac output is to occur. Percutaneous balloon valvotomy of the tricuspid valve has been performed in conjunction with aortic valvotomy (75) and mitral valvotomy (76).

TRICUSPID REGURGITATION IN COMBINED VALVULAR DISEASE

Tricuspid regurgitation may be the result of organic derangement of the tricuspid valve apparatus, or it may be functional and secondary to pulmonary hypertension with resultant right ventricular and tricuspid annular dilatation. Severe organic tricuspid regurgitation is often caused by rheumatic disease; but as with tricuspid stenosis, rheumatic tricuspid regurgitation is never an isolated lesion. When rheumatic scarring of the tricuspid valve is present, there is associated anatomic evidence of mitral and aortic disease as well (60). Clinically isolated tricuspid regurgitation is, therefore, most likely to be of nonrheumatic origin, that is, it may be congenital (endocardial cushion defects or Ebstein's anomaly) or the result of carcinoid heart disease, infective endocarditis, myxomatous degeneration, ischemia, infarction, or trauma (52,77–80). Functional tricuspid regurgitation occurs more frequently than organic tricuspid regurgitation. It may be associated with either primary or secondary pulmonary hypertension. The symptoms and physical findings that may be attributed to the associated tricuspid regurgitation are described in Chapter 12. In general, patients with combined valvular disease and tricuspid regurgitation are less apt to have paroxysmal pulmonary symptoms than those without it (81,82).

The classic murmur of tricuspid regurgitation is a holosystolic murmur at the lower left sternal border; however, it may be silent or, when present, may masquerade as associated mitral regurgitation (82). When present, inspiratory augmentation of the murmur's intensity indicates its tricuspid origin (Rivero-Carvallo's sign) (83). The absence of inspiratory augmentation, however, does not exclude tricuspid regurgitation. When mitral valve disease coexists, the two systolic murmurs may simply be observed to have a wider range than that noted with isolated mitral regurgitation. A short diastolic rumble at the lower sternal border may be heard in severe tricuspid regurgitation because of increased flow across the tricuspid valve. In rheumatic disease, however, a diastolic rumble is more likely to be due to associated mitral stenosis or, occasionally, to both mitral and tricuspid stenoses. The presence of an opening snap makes organic stenosis more likely. On the other hand, an S_3 at the apex that is increased on expiration excludes important mitral stenosis, whereas an S_3 at the lower sternal border that increases on inspiration should exclude important tricuspid stenosis. When murmurs of tricuspid stenosis and regurgitation coexist, it is suggested that inspiratory augmentation of the systolic murmur indicates predominant regurgitation (60,66).

Laboratory Findings

The ECG demonstrates atrial fibrillation in 80% to 96% of patients with severe tricuspid regurgitation (81,84,85). If left ventricular hypertrophy is present, the presence of coexisting important mitral regurgitation or aortic valvular disease should be suspected. The chest roentgenogram may be expected to show right atrial and ventricular dilatation. Isolated right-sided lesions should spare the left atrium and ventricle. In rheumatic disease, the left atrium should be moderately enlarged secondary to coexisting mitral stenosis. Associated left-sided regurgitant lesions can result in generalized cardiac dilatation, often with associated calcification of the mitral and aortic valves. The tricuspid valve is unlikely to show calcification on fluoroscopy. Functional tricuspid regurgitation due to pulmonary disease or primary pulmonary hypertension may be indicated by roentgenographically demonstrated involvement of the lung parenchyma or marked dilatation of the proximal pulmonary arteries with narrowed distal vessels. Functional tricuspid regurgitation due to mitral stenosis should be accompanied by impressive pulmonary vascular redistribution. Estimation of the right atrial enlargement is difficult by chest roentgenography. It should be remembered that marked enlargement of the right ventricle may cause an overall enlargement of the cardiac silhouette, which mimics associated left ventricular enlargement. It is also true that left ventricular dilatation alone may cause anterior displacement of the cardiac silhouette, mimicking right ventricular dilatation by filling in the retrosternal area on the lateral chest roentgenogram (Figs. 10-26 and 10-27). Right atrial dilatation is suggested by marked protrusion of the cardiac silhouette to the right on the posteroanterior roentgenographic view. A distance greater than 4 cm from the midline of the thorax to the right atrial border is suggestive of at least moderate enlargement of this chamber (81).

The echocardiogram gives a more reliable measure of comparative left and right ventricular size than does the chest roentgenogram. Echocardiography often allows demonstration of tricuspid valve abnormalities when the valve is the site of congenital or rheumatic disease. Tricuspid regurgitation is easily demonstrated by color Doppler analysis. If the regurgitation complicates tricuspid stenosis, the right ventricular inflow velocity is apt to be higher with a more rapid pressure falloff (72). The tricuspid annulus size may also be estimated by echocardiography (86).

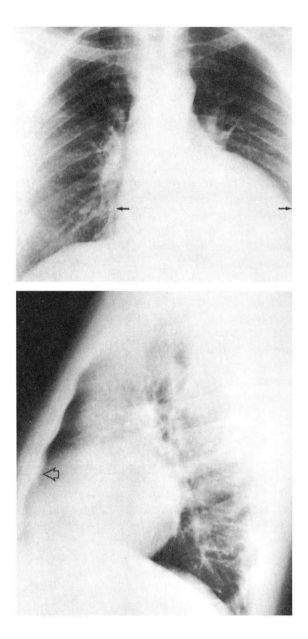

FIG. 10-26. Chest roentgenogram of a 40-year-old man with pulmonary congestion, fatigue, murmurs of aortic and mitral regurgitation, and possibly tricuspid regurgitation. The possibility of tricuspid regurgitation was strengthened by the apparent enlargement of the right ventricle seen on the lateral view **(bottom)** with filling of the lower half of the retrosternal space by the cardiac silhouette (*open arrow*). On the posteroanterior view **(top)**, the enlarged cardiac silhouette (*arrows*) was thought to be partly caused by right ventricular dilatation (Fig. 10-27).

Therapy

The management of tricuspid regurgitation in combined valvular disease depends on its organic or functional nature. Whether medical management or surgical intervention is decided on depends largely on the associated mitral or aortic lesions. Symptoms of fatigue, dyspnea, or severe peripheral edema are initially controlled with conventional methods. If the patient's symptoms are refractory to medical therapy or if the patient has other lesions requiring surgical intervention, the surgeon must decide how to manage the tricuspid lesion (86). If the preoperative pulmonary artery systolic pressure is greater than 60 mm Hg (suggesting functional regurgitation) and the valve leaflet and annulus appear adequate

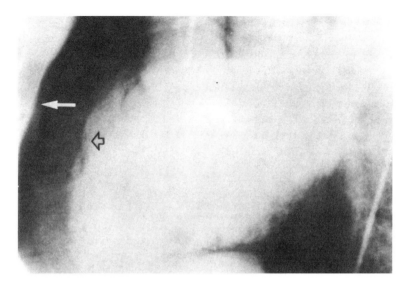

FIG. 10-27. Left ventriculogram in the lateral projection of the same patient whose chest roentgenograms are displayed in Fig. 10-26. Left ventricular dilatation has caused anterior displacement of the right ventricle with resultant filling of the retrosternal space (*white arrow*). The anterior extent of the left ventricle is indicated by the open arrow.

on intraoperative inspection, the valve may be left untouched. If the annulus is dilated, tricuspid annuloplasty can be performed (87–89). If severe organic disease is found, the tricuspid valve must be replaced (89,90). The echocardiogram has been found useful in determining these parameters preoperatively (86,91).

PULMONIC VALVULAR LESIONS IN COMBINED VALVULAR DISEASE

Etiology

Pulmonic valvular disease is usually a congenital lesion, more often stenosis than regurgitation. Congenital pulmonic valvular disease is often isolated but may be associated with other lesions.

Acquired disease of the pulmonic valve is distinctly unusual. Any of the diseases that may cause lesions of other valves rarely attacks the pulmonic valve. Significant rheumatic involvement of the pulmonic valve is distinctly unusual; when it occurs it is usually in patients with quadrivalvular in-

volvement (91). Carcinoid heart disease is one condition in which there is a predilection for the pulmonic valve; it must always be considered when acquired lesions are seen in the pulmonic valve, especially if combined with simultaneously acquired tricuspid valve lesions (80,92,93). The symptoms of metastatic carcinoid or argentaffin tumors are caused by the elaboration of serotonin (5-hydroxytryptamine) from the tumor. Serotonin has a stimulating effect on smooth muscle in various organ systems, including the blood vessels, bronchi, and gastrointestinal tract. Cutaneous flushes with apparent cyanosis and telangiectases, bronchoconstriction, and increased intestinal motility with diarrhea should increase the suspicion of malignant carcinoid. Palpitations and stiffness or swelling of the face are also described. The blood pressure is usually reduced during the flush in contrast to the hypertension usually seen in pheochromocytoma. The endocardium of the right ventricle and right-sided valves is involved in most patients with hepatic metastases. Inactivation of serotonin by the lungs explains the relative sparing of the left ventricle. Although severe involvement of the left-sided endocardium and valves is rare, it may presumably occur with a rare functioning carcinoid tumor of the bronchi, rare metastatic carcinoid to the lung, or hepatic metastases with a right-to-left shunt (92). Similar lesions affecting left-sided valves have been attributed to the use of fenfluramine and dexfenfluramine (4).

The scarring caused by malignant carcinoid is frequently seen in the right ventricular outflow tract and pulmonic valve. Pulmonic stenosis, regurgitation, or a combination of both may ensue. Pulmonic stenosis is the most common hemodynamically significant lesion and may require surgical management with valvuloplasty or replacement. The tricuspid valve may also be involved to varying degrees. Surgery is often warranted, because the malignant tumor is usually slow growing and may be kept under control for decades. Indeed, heart involvement is the leading cause of death in the syndrome of metastatic carcinoid (94).

Infective endocarditis may attack the pulmonic valve along with the tricuspid or other valves. Tuberculosis and gonococcal infection are unusual forms of infective endocarditis with a predilection for the pulmonic valve (95). Myxomatous degeneration may cause pulmonic regurgitation in conjunction with varying degrees of coexisting regurgitation in other valves, especially in patients with Marfan's syndrome. It may be expected that a rare patient will be found with serious simultaneous quadrivalvular regurgitation. Multivalvular myxomatous degeneration has rarely been observed as an X-linked inherited disorder (96).

Rheumatic disease may involve the pulmonic valve, but it is distinctly unusual. Rheumatic pulmonic valvular involvement is observed at autopsy in a small percentage of patients with rheumatic heart disease (97–100). Simultaneous involvement of all four valves is more likely to be the result of a combination of causes, such as congenital, rheumatic, infective, or degenerative disease.

A unitary cause for quadrivalvular disease would be either rheumatic heart disease or myxomatous degeneration. Only one case of quadrivalvular disease occurred in 585 patients with rheumatic heart disease and in only 1 of 400 patients undergoing cardiac catheterization at The New York Hospital (97,98). These patients, as well as a few others whose cases have been reported, had stenosis of all four valves (99).

The symptoms caused by the pulmonic lesion in combined valvular disease cannot be separated from those caused by the other valvular lesions. Certainly, patients with severe pulmonic stenosis may have any of the signs or symptoms of right ventricular failure. Organic pulmonic regurgitation, however, is well tolerated unless complicated by pulmonary hypertension or associated tricuspid regurgitation. In these latter instances, significant pulmonic regurgitation will contribute to the symptoms of right ventricular failure.

Physical Findings

The murmur of pulmonic stenosis is typically crescendo-decrescendo and may last beyond the aortic closure sound. An ejection click that becomes fainter on inspiration is often heard in mild or moderate congenital pulmonic stenosis but is not expected in rheumatic pulmonic stenosis. When it accompanies aortic stenosis, the murmur of pulmonic stenosis is usually obscured. In patients with quadrivalvular disease, large venous A waves are more likely to be ascribed to associated tricuspid stenosis than to pulmonic stenosis.

Associated pulmonic regurgitation is also difficult to recognize in the presence of associated aortic or mitral disease. In the absence of pulmonary hypertension, the moderately pitched crescendo-decrescendo mid-diastolic murmur of organic pulmonic regurgitation is best heard at the fourth or fifth intercostal space along the left sternal border. This murmur may be obscured by or confused with the diastolic rumble of tricuspid or mitral stenosis or the Austin Flint murmur of aortic regurgitation. In the presence of pulmonary hypertension, this murmur is higher pitched and may be mistaken for the murmur of the more common lesion of aortic regurgitation.

The carotid pulse tends to be low in amplitude in pulmonic stenosis, but the character of the upstroke is affected by associated left-sided lesions (e.g., aortic regurgitation or stenosis). A parasternal lift is likely to be sustained with pulmonic stenosis, collapsing with pulmonic regurgitation. These findings could be attributed to other lesions: the sustained impulse to pulmonary hypertension or mitral regurgitation and the collapsing impulse to tricuspid regurgitation. Briefly, neither the history nor physical findings can be expected to lead to the recognition of rheumatic pulmonic involvement in combination with other valvular disease.

Laboratory Findings

The ECG does not uncover associated pulmonic valvular lesions. In quadrivalvular disease the ECG is indistinguishable from that of triple valvular disease with significant tricuspid involvement. In the rare case of acquired tricuspid stenosis, the coexistence of pulmonic stenosis resulting from carcinoid might be suggested by electrocardiographic evidence of right ventricular hypertrophy. Neither chest roentgenograms nor fluoroscopy are helpful except in the rare instance of pulmonic valve calcification.

The first indication of combined pulmonic valvular disease is likely to be found on echocardiography. At cardiac catheterization, pulmonic stenosis is revealed by demonstrating a significant systolic gradient across the pulmonic valve. Severe pulmonic regurgitation causes equalization of pressures in the right ventricle and pulmonary artery in diastole. Pulmonic regurgitation is readily seen by echocardiography and also may be demonstrated angiographically. In the absence of pulmonary hypertension, significant pulmonic regurgitation must represent an organic lesion.

Therapy

Recognizing the rare case of important pulmonic valvular involvement allows one to alert the surgeon. Valvuloplasty of the stenotic pulmonic valve may be required as part of a multivalvular procedure. Pulmonic valve replacement should rarely be necessary, because pulmonic regurgitation is well tolerated if associated tricuspid regurgitation and pulmonary hypertension are absent or relieved.

SPECIFIC NONRHEUMATIC FORMS OF COMBINED VALVULAR DISEASE

Discrete Subaortic Stenosis

A discrete fibrous or fibromuscular ring located below the aortic valve may cause obstruction to left ventricular outflow. This lesion is not rare, occurring approximately one fifth as often as valvular stenosis (101,102). Van Praagh et al. (103) theorized that the lesion represents a developmental abnormality of endocardial cushion tissue that is involved in forming the mitral valve. The subvalvular stenosis may range from a thin discrete fibrous membrane to a fibromuscular stenosis involving muscular hypertrophy and narrowing of the outflow tract (104). The fibromuscular type occurs lower in the outflow tract and is apt to involve the anterior leaflet of the mitral valve.

Aortic regurgitation often coexists with discrete subvalvular stenosis (105). Aortic incompetence is the result of turbulent blood flow distal to the stenotic lesion. Thickening of the valve due to long-standing turbulent flow produces actual aortic valve damage (106). In rare cases of a discrete subaortic fibrous ring, strands may be attached to the aortic cusps themselves (104). Infective endocarditis of the aortic valve may develop in discrete subaortic stenosis (107). In one study, the murmur of aortic regurgitation was heard in 9 of 25 patients with discrete subvalvular aortic stenosis (104). In all these patients, the regurgitation was mild and did not contribute to the clinical picture or complicate the surgical intervention. An apical mid-diastolic murmur was heard in 7 of 25 patients (104). These seven patients were from a group of 12 persons in whom subvalvular stenosis was the result of fibromuscular narrowing of the outflow tract with considerable secondary myocardial hypertrophy. The fibromuscular membrane was attached to the anterior leaflet of the mitral valve, and accessory mitral valve tissue was also present in some of these patients. The apical mid-diastolic murmur is most likely the result of encroachment and interference by the fibromuscular membrane on the mitral valve leaflet. In several cases, surgery resulted in relief of the subvalvular obstruction and disappearance of the mid-diastolic rumble. In 1 of the 12 patients with a fibromuscular ring, mild mitral regurgitation due to involvement of the anterior mitral leaflet in the obstructing ring was present. It is interesting that this patient required mitral valve replacement because surgical correction of the subaortic obstruction could not be accomplished successfully without sacrificing the mitral valve (104).

The most helpful techniques for differentiating discrete subaortic stenosis from valvular stenosis are the echocardiogram and cardiac catheterization with angiography. Rarely, congenital valvular aortic stenosis is associated with discrete subaortic stenosis. This association may be diagnosed by careful echocardiography or cardiac catheterization (108).

In patients with discrete subaortic stenosis, the echocardiogram demonstrates normal aortic valve cusps, unless a bicuspid aortic valve coexists. Aortic valve opening may be interrupted by early systolic closure, whereas the mitral valve appears normal. Occasionally, the subaortic membrane or a constricted left ventricular outflow tract is demonstrated (109).

Cardiac catheterization with careful pullback pressure measurements usually demonstrates that the level of the obstruction is below the aortic valve. Unfortunately, the discrete membrane may be so close to the aortic valve that one cannot distinguish valvular from subvalvular stenosis either by pressure measurements or by left ventriculography. Mitral stenosis can be excluded at catheterization and by a precatheterization echocardiogram. Although mild aortic or even mitral regurgitation may be seen on angiography, the valve leaflets themselves should appear thin, pliable, and of normal amplitude. The anterior mitral leaflet, however, may be restricted in motion when it is attached to a fibromuscular ring.

Therapeutic interventions are dictated almost entirely by the severity of left ventricular outflow obstruction. The degree of aortic regurgitation is usually of no therapeutic significance unless the valve has been damaged by infective endocarditis. The rare need for mitral replacement has already been mentioned.

Hypertrophic Obstructive Cardiomyopathy (Idiopathic Hypertrophic Subaortic Stenosis)

HOCM is a form of cardiomyopathy with massive hypertrophy of the left ventricle. This lesion is discussed in this chapter because of its mimicry of combined valvular heart disease, particularly aortic stenosis with mitral regurgitation. Mitral stenosis, aortic regurgitation, and other nonvalvular lesions may also be simulated by some of the symptoms and physical findings (110). The ventricular hypertrophy is not distributed concentrically (as in valvular aortic stenosis) but tends to involve the interventricular septum and outflow tract in an asymmetric fashion (111). Marked distortion of the left ventricle is caused by this hypertrophy and by abnormal tethering of the mitral valve because of malpositioned and hypertrophied papillary muscles. The mitral valve is displaced anteriorly, close to the interventricular septum (111,112). Abnormal anterior motion of the anterior mitral leaflet may occur in systole and has been thought to contribute to left ventricular outflow obstruction. Moderately severe mitral regurgitation often coexists. The degree of left ventricular outflow obstruction is variable, of questionable significance, and may change in a single patient over the course of years or from moment to moment under the influence of physiologic or pharmacologic stimuli (111,113). The feature that most patients have in common is an asymmetrically hypertrophied interventricular septum. The area of the left ventricle involved in the asymmetric hypertrophy is variable, however (114,115). This condition may be genetically transmitted as a non–sex-linked autosomal dominant character (116). The disease is most often first discovered in young adults but may become manifest during childhood or late adult life.

The most frequently encountered symptoms are exertional dyspnea, light-headedness or "graying-out spells," and angina pectoris. Syncope is not as common as with valvular aortic stenosis and does not carry the same ominous prognosis. Palpitations due to ventricular arrhythmias are frequent. Pulmonary edema and even right ventricular failure may develop, and the clinical picture may be similar to that of congestive cardiomyopathy (9,111).

Physical Findings

The characteristic features of HOCM observed on physical examination include a prominent double apical impulse with an abnormally prominent presystolic expansion wave (A wave). Occasionally, there are two systolic expansion waves so that a triple outward impulse is noted. Although a systolic thrill may be present at the apex or lower left sternal border, it is not felt in the carotids or jugular notch. The carotids and peripheral pulses are unusually brisk in upstroke and may be bifid (bisferiens). This characteristic pulse differentiates HOCM from valvular aortic stenosis, but it mimics the pulse of predominant aortic regurgitation. Most patients have an audible S_4 and often an S_3 as well.

The characteristic systolic murmur is crescendo-decrescendo, loudest at the left sternal border and apex, and not radiating well to the neck. The murmur may be soft or absent in cases of hypertrophic cardiomyopathy without significant obstruction.

A Valsalva maneuver or the assumption of the upright position provokes or increases left ventricular obstruction and augments the systolic ejection murmur. Assuming the supine position, with legs elevated, reduces both the obstruction and the murmur. A variety of vasoactive drugs, diuretics, and inotropic agents can influence the obstruction by affecting one or more of the determinants of obstruction: the systolic volume of the left ventricle, the inotropic force of ventricular contraction, resistance to left ventricular ejection (afterload), or resistance to left ventricular relaxation. The influence of left ventricular contractility on the obstruction is well illustrated by the effect of postextrasystolic inotropic potentiation on the arterial pulse pressure.

The beat after a premature beat is characterized by an increased force of contraction. This increased inotropy is in excess of what can be accounted for by the compensatory pause with its expected increased ventricular filling. The increased inotropy usually causes a widening of the atrial pulse pressure in normal subjects or in patients with other forms of heart disease. Patients with HOCM are unique in that they exhibit a postextrasystolic pulse pressure that is no greater than and usually narrower than the preextrasystolic pulse pressure (111).

In HOCM, an additional holosystolic murmur can be heard in approximately half the patients (9,111). This condition may therefore be mistaken for combined rheumatic aortic stenosis and mitral regurgitation. The symptoms of exertional dyspnea coupled with brisk carotid pulses may further suggest that the diagnosis is mild aortic stenosis with severe mitral regurgitation (Table 10-10). The systolic (outflow tract and mitral regurgitation) murmurs of HOCM both increase

TABLE 10-10. *Features distinguishing HOCM from combined aortic stenosis and mitral regurgitation*

Clinical and laboratory findings	HOCM	Aortic stenosis and mitral regurgitation
Presenting symptoms		
Syncope	±	+
Angina	+	+
Easy fatigability	±	+
Pulmonary symptoms	±	+
Physical findings		
Delayed carotid upstroke	−	+
Effect of Valsalva maneuver on systolic murmur	↑	↓
S_3	+	+
S_4	+	±
Electrocardiogram		
Left ventricular hypertrophy	+	+
Septal Q	+	−
Chest roentgenogram		
Left ventricular dilatation	±	+
Aortic valve calcium	−	+
Echocardiogram		
Left ventricular hypertrophy	+	+
Asymmetric septal hypertrophy	++	−
Systolic anterior motion of mitral valve	+	−
Doppler findings		
High systolic aortic velocity	±	++
High subaortic early systolic velocity	±	+
Left atrial systolic turbulence	±	++
Cardiac catheterization		
Aortic valvular gradient	−	+
Subaortic gradient	±	−
Mitral regurgitation	0–3+	1–4+

HOCM, hypertrophic obstructive cardiomyopathy; ++, emphasis of marked degree and highly correlated; ↑, increased; ↓, decreased.

with a Valsalva maneuver and diminish with squatting or handgrip. On the other hand, the murmur of mitral regurgitation of other etiologies diminishes with a Valsalva maneuver and increases with the elevated afterload brought about by either squatting or handgrip (Table 10-11).

Laboratory Findings

In either rheumatic disease or HOCM, the ECG demonstrates left ventricular hypertrophy with associated ST and T abnormalities (strain) and left atrial enlargement. In HOCM, however, large septal Q waves may be present,

TABLE 10-11. *Effect of various interventions on systolic murmurs*

Intervention	HOCM	Aortic stenosis	Mitral regurgitation	Mitral prolapse
Valsalva	↑	↓	↓	↑ or ↓
Standing	↑	↑ or unchanged	↓	↑
Handgrip or squatting	↓	↓ or unchanged	↑	↓
Supine position with legs elevated	↓	↑ or unchanged	Unchanged	↓
Exercise	↑	↑ or unchanged	↓	↑
Amyl nitrite	↑↑	↑	↓	↑
Isoproterenol	↑↑	↑	↓	↑

HOCM, hypertrophic obstructive cardiomyopathy; ↑, increased; ↓, decreased; ↑↑, markedly increased.

simulating a previous infarction (111). The chest roentgenogram often demonstrates cardiomegaly without valvular calcification in HOCM. No single echocardiographic feature of HOCM is pathognomonic. The overall echocardiographic appearance, however, is distinctive and allows easy differentiation of this condition from combined rheumatic disease (117). Rarely, a patient with a single papillary muscle (parachute mitral valve) displays echocardiographic and even angiographic abnormalities closely resembling HOCM (118). The characteristic subaortic gradient of HOCM may be observed by Doppler findings of a high velocity of flow in the left ventricular outflow tract (72).

In the presence of left ventricular outflow obstruction, cardiac catheterization demonstrates a gradient within the body of the left ventricle itself. Left ventriculography demonstrates moderately severe mitral regurgitation in up to 50% of patients. The characteristic contraction abnormalities and distinctive geometry of the hypertrophied left ventricular cavity help to distinguish this lesion from rheumatic or degenerative valvular disease.

Differential Diagnosis

Uncommonly, patients with HOCM have an early diastolic murmur of aortic regurgitation. Of 126 patients whose cases were reported by Frank and Braunwald (9), nine had such a murmur. On Doppler echocardiography, 22% of 86 patients revealed some degree of aortic regurgitation (119). This diastolic incompetence may be caused by valve distortion brought about by turbulent blood flow in a way similar to that observed in discrete subaortic stenosis. Alternatively, infective endocarditis may develop on such a valve. The bisferiens pulse with brisk carotid upstroke is apt to mislead the clinician into considering aortic regurgitation to be the dominant lesion. Bedside maneuvers, however, should lead to the correct diagnosis. The ECG may help if it demonstrates the large septal Q waves of asymmetric septal hypertrophy. A chest roentgenogram or fluoroscopy does not demonstrate poststenotic dilatation of the ascending aorta or aortic valve calcification in patients with HOCM. Echocardiography and cardiac catheterization will reveal the distinctive features of HOCM. In a rare patient with aortic valvular endocarditis, severe aortic regurgitation may develop. In such a patient, the left ventricle often dilates enough to eliminate the outflow obstruction. In our experience, the echocardiographic and catheterization findings are usually effaced by this process.

The exuberant muscular hypertrophy in HOCM causes a marked decrease in left ventricular distensibility. In severe forms, left ventricular filling may be so impaired as to produce symptoms and signs mimicking mitral stenosis. More often, the combination of mitral stenosis and aortic stenosis is suggested. An apical diastolic rumble may be noted, and the S_1 may be loud, with an S_3 mistaken for an opening snap; however, the diastolic murmur is usually short and is not accompanied by presystolic accentuation (120). A prominent left ventricular apical impulse is incompatible with predominant mitral stenosis and suggests combined valvular disease or a cardiomyopathy such as HOCM. Electrocardiographic evidence of left ventricular hypertrophy also points away from predominant mitral stenosis. If aortic disease or mitral regurgitation is suspected because of associated systolic murmurs, diagnostic bedside maneuvers should allow correct identification of the lesion. Also, the chest roentgenogram and fluoroscopy fail to demonstrate poststenotic aortic dilatation or valvular calcification in patients with HOCM. Although phonocardiography with simultaneous apexcardiography will distinguish an S_3 from an opening snap, this exercise is unnecessary, except as an academic exercise, becasue echocardiography readily distinguishes HOCM from rheumatic mitral stenosis. The echocardiographic evidence for HOCM (asymmetric septal hypertrophy with systolic anterior excursion of the mitral valve and Doppler evidence for outflow obstruction) is usually so distinctive that cardiac catheterization is rarely required to make the diagnosis. If cardiac catheterization is performed, a dynamic outflow gradient may be recorded, no significant transmitral gradient is observed, and ventriculography demonstrates the marked left ventricular hypertrophy and the peculiar ventricular geometry of HOCM.

Therapy

Treatment of HOCM should be both prophylactic and symptomatic. The risk of life-threatening arrhythmias exists even in asymptomatic patients with this disease; therefore, strenuous physical activity should be restricted. Long-term monitoring and exercise testing is advisable even in the asymptomatic subject, so that those with either ventricular tachycardia or paroxysms of supraventricular tachycardia can be identified and treated appropriately (121). Whether or not antiarrhythmic therapy prolongs life remains to be demonstrated. Patients with life-threatening ventricular arrhythmias should be considered for implantable defibrillators.

Digitalis should be avoided unless atrial fibrillation with a rapid ventricular response develops. Diuretics, afterload reduction, and inotropic drugs such as isoproterenol should also be avoided unless consideration has been given to the possibly deleterious hemodynamic effects of these agents. The mainstay of medical therapy is beta-blockade and calcium channel blockade. Aninotropic agents such as disopyramide and amiodarone have been used with some success. Atrioventricular pacing also seems to provide some patients with relief. If patients remain severely symptomatic despite maximal medical therapy, catheter ablation or surgical intervention may be considered.

Surgical myotomy or myectomy has been performed on the "obstructing" muscular ridge (122,123). The operation can be done with approximately a 5% mortality. Major complications, such as complete heart block, ventricular septal defect, or mitral regurgitation, occur in an additional 5%. Many patients obtain a beneficial result (122–124). Despite successful surgery, continuing annual mortal-

ity can be expected, especially in patients with atrial fibrillation (124). Catheter ablation of obstructing septum has been performed using intracoronary ethanol instalation (125). The long-term success of this procedure has yet to be established. If the aortic or mitral valve has been severely damaged by infective endocarditis or by scarring due to turbulent flow, valve replacement may be required.

REFERENCES

1. Libman E, Sacks B. A hitherto undescribed form of valvular and mural endocarditis. *Arch Intern Med* 1924;33:701.
2. Straaton KV, et al. Clinically significant valvular disease in systemic lupus erythematosis. *Am J Med* 1988; 85:645.
3. Horowitz JD. Drugs that induce heart problems. Which agents? What effects? *J Cardiovasc Med* 1983; 8:308.
4. Connoly HM, et al. Valvular heart disease associated with fenfluramine-phentermine. *N Engl J Med* 1997; 337:581.
5. Mishiro Y, et al. Echocardiographic characteristics and causal mechanisms of physiologic mitral regurgitation in young normal subjects. *Clin Cardiol* 1997;20:850.
6. Mueller XM, et al. Perioperative morbidity and mortality in combined aortic and mitral valve surgery. *J Heart Valve Dis* 1997;6:387.
7. Kirklin JW, Pacifico AD. Surgery for acquired valvular heart disease. *N Engl J Med* 1973;288:133.
8. Hohn AR, et al. Aortic stenosis. *Circulation* 1965; 32[Suppl 111]:4.
9. Frank S, Braunwald E. Idiopathic hypertrophic subaortic stenosis. Clinical analysis of 126 patients with emphasis on natural history. *Circulation* 1968;37:759.
10. Gemelli A, et al. Systolic ejection murmur in the differential diagnosis of isolated aortic insufficiency and its association with stenosis (in Italian). *Min Med* 1984;75:1701.
11. Rotman M, et al. Aortic valvular disease: comparison of types and their medical and surgical management. *Am J Med* 1971;51:241.
12. Segal BL, Likoff W, Kaspar AJ. "Silent" rheumatic aortic regurgitation. *Am J Cardiol* 1964;14:628.
13. Alpert JS, Viewag WVR, Hagan AD. Incidence and morphology of carotid shudders in aortic valve disease. *Am Heart J* 1976;92:435.
14. Aurigemma G, et al. Color Doppler mapping of aortic regurgitation with aortic stenosis: comparison with angiography. *Cardiology* 1992;81:251.
15. Nixon PGF, Wooler GH. Clinical assessment of mitral orifice in patients with regurgitation. *Br Med J* 1960; 2:1122.
16. Nixon PGF, Wooler GH. Phases of diastole in mitral valvular disease. *Br Heart J* 1963;25:393.
17. Janton 0H, et al. The clinical determination of mitral insufficiency when associated with mitral stenosis. *Circulation* 1954;10:207.

18. Aravanis C. Silent mitral insufficiency. *Am Heart J* 1965;70:620.

19. Osterberger LE, et al. Functional mitral stenosis in patients with massive mitral annular calcification. *Circulation* 1981;64:472.

20. Labovitz AJ, et al. Frequency of mitral valve dysfunction from mitral anular calcium as detected by Doppler echocardiography. *Am J Cardiol* 1985;55:133.

21. Rios JC, Goo W. Electrocardiographic correlates of rheumatic valvular disease. *Cardiovasc Clin* 1973;5:247.

22. McDonald L, et al. Clinical physiological findings in mitral stenosis and regurgitation. *Medicine (Baltimore)* 1957;36:237.

23. Levy MJ, Edwards JE. Anatomy of mitral insufficiency. *Prog Cardiovasc Dis* 1963;5:119.

24. Patel AK, et al. Detection and estimation of rheumatic mitral regurgitation in the presence of mitral stenosis by pulsed Doppler echocardiography. *Am J Cardiol* 1983;51:986.

25. Dujardin KS, et al. Grading of mitral regurgitation by quantitative Doppler echocardiographic calibration by left ventricular angiography in routine clinical practice. *Circulation* 1997;96:3409.

26. Rigo P, et al. Measurement of aortic and mitral regurgitation by gated cardiac blood pool scans. *Circulation* 1979;60:306.

27. Hurwitz RA, et al. Quantification of aortic and mitral regurgitation in the pediatric population: evaluation by radionuclide angiography. *Am J Cardiol* 1983;51:252.

28. Nixon PGF, Wooler GH. Left ventricular filling pressure gradient in mitral incompetence. *Br Heart J* 1963;25:382.

29. Zhang HP, et al. Comparison of late results of balloon valvotomy in mitral stenosis with versus without mitral regurgitation. *Am J Cardiol* 1998;81:1.

30. Rittoo D, et al. A prospective echocardiographic study of the effects of balloon mitral commissurotomy on pre-existing mitral regurgitation in patients with mitral stenosis. *Cardiology* 1998;89:202.

31. Kumar AS, Rao RN. Mitral valve reconstruction: intermediate term results in rheumatic mitral regurgitation. *J Heart Valve Dis* 1994;3:161.

32. Zitnik RS, et al. The masking of aortic stenosis by mitral stenosis. *Am Heart J* 1965;69:22.

33. Brauner RA, et al. Multiple left heart obstruction (Shone's anomaly) with mitral valve involvement: long-term surgical outcome. *Ann Thorac Surg* 1997;64:721.

34. Dexter L, et al. Aortic stenosis. *Arch Intern Med* 1958;101:254.

35. Uricchio JF, et al. Combined mitral and aortic stenosis: clinical and physiologic features and results of surgery. *Am J Cardiol* 1959;4:479.

36. Uricchio JF, et al. A study of combined mitral and aortic stenosis. *Ann Intern Med* 1959;51:668.

37. Honey M. Clinical haemodynamic observations on combined mitral and aortic stenosis. *Br Heart J* 1961;23:545.

38. Katznelson G, et al. Combined aortic and mitral stenosis: a clinical and physiological study. *Am J Med* 1960;29:242.

39. Schattenberg TT, Titus JL, Parkin TW. Clinical findings in acquired aortic valve stenosis: effect of disease of other valves. *Am Heart J* 1967;73:322.

40. Reid JM, et al. Combined aortic and mitral stenosis. *Br Heart J* 1962;24:509.

41. Cannon JD, et al. Aortic valve resistance as an adjunct to the Gorlin formula in assessing the severity of aortic stenosi in symptomatic patients. *J Am Coll Cardiol* 1992;20:1517.

42. deFilippi CR, et al. Usefulness of dobutamine echocardiography in distinguishing severe from nonsevere valvular aortic stenosis in patients with depressed left ventricular function and low transvalvular gradients. *Am J Cardiol* 1995;75:191.

43. Lee TM, et al. Percutaneous transvenous mitral balloon valvuloplasty alone in patients with combined aortic and mitral stenosis. *Angiology* 1997;48:445.

44. Brest AN, Udhoji V, Likoff W. A re-evaluation of the Graham Steell murmur. *N Engl J Med* 1960;263:1229.

45. Cohn KE, Hultgren HN. The Graham Steell murmur re-evaluated. *N Engl J Med* 1966;274:486.

46. Runco V, et al. Graham Steell murmur versus aortic regurgitation in rheumatic heart disease:Results of aortic valvulography. *Am J Med* 1961;31:71.

47. Cohn LH, et al. Pre-operative assessment of aortic regurgitation in patients with mitral valve disease. *Am J Cardiol* 1967;19:177.

48. Diker E, et al. Prevalence and predictors of atrial fibrillation in rheumatic valvular heart disease. *Am J Cardiol* 1996;77:96.

49. Chen CR, et al. Percutaneous balloon mitral valvuloplasty for mitral stenosis with and without associated aortic regurgitation. *Am Heart J* 1993;125:128.

50. Melvin DB, et al. Computer-based analysis of preoperative and postoperative prognostic factors in 100 patients with combined aortic and mitral valve replacement. *Circulation* 1972;48[Suppl III]:56.

51. Wippermann CF, et al. Mitral and aortic regurgitation in 84 patients with mucopolysaccharidoses. *Eur J Pediatr* 1995;154:98.

52. Rippe JM, et al. Multiple floppy valves: an echocardiographic syndrome. *Am J Med* 1979;66:817.

53. Shine KI, et al. Combined aortic and mitral incompetence: clinical features in surgical management. *Am Heart J* 1968;76:728.

54. Welch GH Jr, Braunwald E, Sarnoff SJ. Hemodynamic effects of quantitatively varied experimental aortic regurgitation. *Circ Res* 1957;5:546.

55. Niles N, et al. Preoperative left and right ventricular performance in combined aortic and mitral regurgitation and comparison with isolated aortic and mitral regurgitation. *Am J Cardiol* 1990;65:1372.

56. Skudicky D, et al. Time-related changes in left ventricular function after double valve replacement for combined aortic and mitral regurgitation in a young rheumatic population: predictors of postoperative left ventricular performance and role of chordal preservation. *Circulation* 1997;95:4.

57. Leibovitch ER. Cardiac valve disorders: growing significance in the elderly. *Geriatrics* 1989;44:91.

58. Harris KM, et al. Improvement in mitral regurgitation after aortic valve replacement. *Am J Cardiol* 1997;80:741.

59. Morelli S, et al. Tricuspid valve steno-insufficiency in systemic lupus erythemoatosus. *Lupus* 1995;4:318.

60. Kitchin A, Turner R. Diagnosis and treatment of tricuspid stenosis. *Br Heart J* 1964;26:354.

61. Weyman AE, Rankin R, King H. Loeffler's endocardi-

tis presenting as mitral and tricuspid stenosis. *Am J Cardiol* 1977;40:438.

62. Gibson R, Wood P. The diagnosis of tricuspid stenosis. *Br Heart J* 1955;17:552.
63. Perloff JK, Harvey WP. Clinical recognition of tricuspid stenosis. *Circulation* 1960;22:346.
64. Morgan JR, et al. Isolated tricuspid stenosis. *Circulation* 1971;44:729.
65. Smith JA, Levine SA. The clinical features of tricuspid stenosis. *Am Heart J* 1942;23:739.
66. El-Sherif N. Rheumatic tricuspid stenosis: A haemodynamic correlation. *Br Heart J* 1971;33:16.
67. Rivero-Carvallo JM. El diagnostico de la estenosis tricuspidea. *Arch Inst Cardiol Mex* 1950;20:1.
68. Killip T, Lukas DS. Tricuspid stenosis: clinical features in twelve cases. *Am J Med* 1958;24:836.
69. Kushner FG, Lam W, Morganroth J. Apex sector echocardiography in evaluation of the right atrium in patients with mitral stenosis and atrial septal defect. *Am J Cardiol* 1978;42:733.
70. Bommer W, et al. Determination of right atrial and right ventricular size by two-dimensional echocardiography. *Circulation* 1979;60:91.
71. Hatle L, Angelsen B, Tromsdal A. Noninvasive assessment of atrioventricular pressure half-time by Doppler ultrasound. *Circulation* 1979;60:1096.
72. Hatle L, Angelsen B. *Doppler Ultrasound in Cardiology. Physical Principles and Clinical Applications.* Philadelphia: Lea & Febiger, 1982.
73. Killip, T, Lukas, DS. Tricuspid stenosis: physiologic criteria for diagnosis and hemodynamic abnormalities. *Circulation* 1957;16:3.
74. Sanders CA, et al. Tricuspid stenosis. A difficult diagnosis in the presence of atrial fibrillation. *Circulation* 1966;33:26.
75. Shrivastava S, et al. Concurrent percutaneous balloon valvotomy for combined rheumatic tricuspid and aortic stenosis. *Intern J Cardiol* 1993;38:183.
76. Bahl VK, et al. Combined dilatation of rheumatic mitral and tricuspid stenosis with Inoue balloon catheter. *Int J Cardiol* 1993;42:178.
77. Glancy DL, et al. Isolated organic tricuspid valvular regurgitation. *Am J Med* 1969;46:989.
78. Sbar S, et al. Chronic tricuspid insufficiency. *South Med J* 1973;66:917.
79. Bain RC, et al. Right-sided bacterial endocarditis and endarteritis: a clinical and pathological study. *Am J Med* 1958;24:98.
80. Roberts WC, Sjoerdsma A. The cardiac disease associated with the carcinoid syndrome (carcinoid heart disease). *Am J Med* 1964;36:5.
81. Sepulveda G, Lukas DS. The diagnosis of tricuspid insufficiency: clinical features in 60 cases with associated mitral valve disease. *Circulation* 1955;11:552.
82. Uricchio JF, et al. Tricuspid regurgitation masquerading as mitral regurgitation in patients with pure mitral stenosis. *Am J Med* 1958;25:224.
83. Rivero-Carvallo JM. Signo para el diagnostico de las insuficiencias tricuspides. *Arch Inst Cardiol Mex* 1946;16:531.
84. Salazar E, Levine HD. Rheumatic tricuspid regurgitation: the clinical spectrum. *Am J Med* 1962;33:111.
85. Muller O, Shillingford J. Tricuspid incompetence. *Br Heart J* 1954;16:195.
86. Tager R, et al. Long-term follow-up of rheumatic patients undergoing left-sided valve replacement with tricuspid annuloplasty; validity of preoperative echocardiographic criteria in the decision to perform tricuspid annuloplasty. *Am J Cardiol* 1998;81:1013.
87. Braunwald NS, Ross J Jr, Morrow AG. Conservative management of tricuspid regurgitation in patients undergoing mitral valve replacement. *Circulation* 1966;35[Suppl I]:63.
88. Wei J, et al. DeVeg's semicircular annuloplasty for tricuspid valve regurgitation. *Ann Thoracic Surg* 1993;55:482.
89. Cohn LH. Tricuspid regurgitation secondary to mitral valve disease: when and how to repair. *J Cardiac Surg* 1994;92[Suppl 2]:237.
90. Prabhakar G, et al. Triple-valve operation in the young rheumatic patient. *Ann Thoracic Surg* 1993;55:482.
91. Kumar N, et al. Rheumatic involvement of all four heart valves—preoperative echocardiographic diagnosis and successful surgical management. *Eur J Cardiothoracic Surg* 1995;9:713.
92. McKusick VA. Carcinoid cardiovascular disease. *Bull Johns Hopkins Hosp* 1956;98:13.
93. Anderson AS, et al. Cardiovascular complications of malignant carcinoid disease. *Am Heart J* 1997;134:4.
94. Konstantinov IE, Peterffy A. Tricuspid and pulmonary valve replacement in carcinoid heart disease: two case reports and a review of the literature. *J Heart Valve Dis* 1997;6:193.
95. Thayer WS. On the cardiac complications of gonorrhea. *Bull Johns Hopkins Hosp* 1922;33:361.
96. Kyndt F, et al. Mapping of X-linked myxomatous valvular dystrophy to chromosome Xq28. *Am J Hum Genet* 1998;62:627.
97. Clawson BJ. Rheumatic heart disease. *Am J Med* 1940; 20:454.
98. Ayres SM, et al. Quadrivalvular rheumatic heart disease: report of a case with marked stenosis of all valves. *Am J Med* 1962;32:467.
99. Gialloreto O, Aerichide N, Allard PP. Stenotic involvement of all four heart valves. Report of three cases. *Am J Cardiol* 1961;7:865.
100. Espino-Vela J, Contreras R, Rustrian Sosa F. Rheumatic pulmonary valve disease. *Am J Cardiol* 1969;23:12.
101. Braunwald E, et al. Congenital aortic stenosis. *Circulation* 1963;27:426.
102. Campbell A. The natural history of congenital aortic stenosis. *Br Heart J* 1968;30:514.
103. Van Praagh R, et al. Tetralogy of Fallot with severe left ventricular outflow tract obstruction due to anomalous attachment of the mitral valve to the ventricular septum. *Am J Cardiol* 1970;26:93.
104. Kelley DT, Wulfsberg BA, Rowe RD. Discrete subaortic stenosis. *Circulation* 1972;46:309.
105. Hancock EW. Differentiation of valvar, subvalvar, and supravalvar aortic stenosis. *Circulation* 1961;24:1311.
106. Edwards JE, Burchell HB. Endocardial and intimal lesions. *Circulation* 1958;18:946.
107. Morrow AG, et al. Discrete subaortic stenosis complicated by aortic valvular regurgitation. *Circulation* 1965;31:163.
108. Schneeweis A, et al. Discrete subaortic stenosis associated with congenital valvular aortic stenosis—a diagnostic challenge. *Am Heart J* 1983;106:55.
109. Popp RL, et al. Echocardiographic findings in discrete subvalvular aortic stenosis. *Circulation* 1974;49:226.

110. Maron BJ, et al. Hypertrophic cardiomyopathy: the great masquerader. Clinical conference from the cardiology branch of the National Heart, Lung and Blood Institute, Bethesda, MD. *Chest* 1978;74:659.

111. Braunwald E, et al. Idiopathic hypertrophic subaortic stenosis: description of the disease based upon an analysis of 64 patients. *Circulation* 1964;29[Suppl IV]:1.

112. Simon AL, Ross J Jr, Gault JH. Angiographic anatomy of the left ventricle and mitral valve in idiopathic hypertrophic subaortic stenosis. *Circulation* 1967;36: 852.

113. Murgo JP, et al. Dynamics of left ventricular ejection in obstructive and nonobstructive hypertrophic cardiomyopathy. *J Clin Invest* 1980;66:1369.

114. Ciro E, Nichols PF III, Maron BJ. Heterogeneous morphologic expression of genetically transmitted hypertrophic cardiomyopathy, two-dimensional echocardiographic analysis. *Circulation* 1983;67:1227.

115. Keren G, et al. Apical hypertrophic cardiornyopathy evaluation by noninvasive and invasive techniques in 12 patients. *Circulation* 1985;71:45.

116. Epstein SE, Henry WL, Clark CE, et al. Asymmetric septal hypertrophy. *Ann Intern Med* 1974;81:650.

117. Henry WL, Clark CE, Epstein SE. Asymmetric septal hypertrophy: Echocardiographic identification of the pathognomonic anatomic abnormality of IHSS. *Circulation* 1973;47:225.

118. Boughner DR, Persand JA. Parachute mitral valve: Echocardiographic findings resembling idiopathic hypertrophic subaortic stenosis. *J Clin Ultrasound* 1976;4:213.

119. Shiota T, et al. Aortic regurgitation in hypertrophic cardiomyopathy as detected by color Doppler echocardiography (in Japanese). *J Cardiol* 1987;17:759.

120. Shabetai R, Davidson S. Asymmetrical hypertrophic cardiomyopathy simulating mitral stenosis. *Circulation* 1972;45:37.

121. Savage DD, et al. Prevalence of arrhythmias during 24-hour electrocardiographic monitoring and exercise testing in patients with obstructive and non-obstructive hypertrophic cardiomyopathy. *Circulation* 1979;59: 866.

122. Morrow AG, et al. Operative treatment in hypertrophic subaortic stenosis. Techniques and results of pre- and post-operative assessment of 83 patients. *Circulation* 1975;52:88.

123. Tajik AJ, et al. Idiopathic hypertrophic subaortic stenosis. Long-term surgical follow-up. *Am J Cardiol* 1974; 34:813.

124. Maron BJ, et al. Long-term clinical course and symptomatic status of patients after operation for hypertrophic subaortic stenosis. *Circulation* 1978;57:1205.

125. Sigwart U. Non-surgical myocardial reduction for hypertrophic obstructive cardiomyopathy. *Lancet* 1995; 346:211.

11

Pulmonic Valve Disease

P. Syamasundar Rao

Division of Pediatric Cardiology, Saint Louis University School of Medicine;
Cardinal Glennon Children's Hospital, St. Louis, Missouri 63104-1095

Diseases of the pulmonary valve are more often congenital in origin and only rarely do acquired disorders such as carcinoid and rheumatic fever affect the pulmonary valve. The pulmonary valve may be stenotic, atretic, or the valve leaflets may be absent. Subvalvar, supravalvar, or branch pulmonary artery stenosis simulate valvar obstruction and have to be considered in the differential diagnosis. Therefore, in this chapter all the above right ventricular outflow tract obstructions are discussed with the major emphasis on pulmonary valve stenosis. Other abnormalities of the pulmonary valve, causing pulmonary regurgitation, both congenital and acquired, are also briefly reviewed.

This condition was first described in 1761 by Morgagni (3), and the pathologic features were enumerated by Meckel (4). In pediatric populations, the prevalence of valvar pulmonary stenosis is 7.5% to 9% of all congenital heart defects (5,6). However, in adult subjects, the prevalence is slightly higher, around 15% (7–9). Gender distribution is nearly equal (8). Although familial forms of pulmonary stenosis have been described (10,11), in general, it is considered to be multifactorial in origin. Recurrence in siblings is in the order of 2% to 3% (12,13). The prevalence in the offspring of a parent with pulmonary stenosis is 3.6% (14). Pulmonary valve stenosis is the most common cardiac lesion in Noonan's syndrome (pheno-

ISOLATED PULMONARY VALVE STENOSIS

Stenotic pulmonary valve may occur without associated congenital abnormalities, although it is more often associated with other structural abnormalities of the heart (Table 11-1). To distinguish the former from the latter, terms such as pulmonary stenosis with normal aortic root or with intact ventricular septum have been used. However, some workers (1), including myself (2), prefer the term isolated pulmonary valve stenosis. The term "isolated" may be used even in the presence of a patent foramen ovale or a small atrial septal defect. The term "congenital" does not need to be used because most are congenital in origin.

TABLE 11-1. *Cardiac lesions and syndromes associated with valvar pulmonary stenosis*

Defects
Atrial septal defect
Ventricular septal defect
Tetralogy of Fallot
Hypoplastic right ventricle
Transposition of the great arteries
Double-outlet right ventricle
Double-inlet left ventricle (single ventricle)
Corrected transposition of the great arteries
Tricuspid atresia
Syndromes
Asplenia syndrome
Rubella syndrome
Noonan's syndrome
Cardiofacial syndrome
Williams syndrome

typically Turner's and genotypically normal [XX or XY]). It is also seen in patients with rubella syndrome. Valvar and supravalvar pulmonary stenosis may also be seen in patients with Williams syndrome (supravalvar aortic stenosis, infantile hypercalcemia, and elfin facies with or without mental retardation).

Pathology

The pathologic features of the stenotic pulmonary valve vary (15–17); the most commonly observed pathology is what is described as a "dome-shaped" pulmonary valve. The fused pulmonary valve leaflets protrude from their attachment into the pulmonary artery as a conical windsocklike structure. The size of the pulmonary valve orifice varies from a pinhole to several millimeters, most usually central in location but can be eccentric. Raphae, presumably fused valve commissures, extend from the stenotic orifice to a variable distance down into the base of the dome-shaped valve. The number of the raphae may vary from zero to seven. Less common variants are unicommissural, bicuspid, and tricuspid valves (Table 11-2). Thickening of the valve leaflets is seen, which may be due to an increase in valve spongeosa or due to excessive fibrous, collagenous, myxomatous, and elastic tissue. Unlike the aortic valve, calcification of the pulmonary valve is rare. Patients with severe pulmonary stenosis who survive into adulthood may demonstrate pulmonary valve calcification (18,19). The valve annulus is abnormal in most cases (17) with partial or complete lack of fibrous back bone; thus, a "true" annulus may not be present.

Pulmonary valve ring hypoplasia and dysplastic pulmonary valves may be present in a small percentage of patients. Pulmonary valve dysplasia is characterized by thickened, nodular, and redundant valve leaflets with minimal or no commissural fusion; valve ring hypoplasia; and lack of poststenotic dilatation of the pulmonary artery (20,21). The obstruction is mainly related to thickened, myxomatous, immobile pulmonary valve cusps and valve ring hypoplasia. Although more common with familial types of pulmonary stenosis, often associated with abnormal facies and developmental delay (22), dysplastic pulmonary valves can be seen in nonfamilial cases and in most patients with Noonan's syndrome (23).

Changes secondary to pulmonary valve obstruction occur in the right ventricle and pulmonary artery. The right ventricular muscle hypertrophy is proportional to the degree (and perhaps duration) of obstruction. Muscle hypertrophy is particularly prominent in the infundibular region and may become physiologically important; this appears to be related to the degree and duration of obstruction (24). There is mild dilatation of the right ventricular cavity. In extremely severe or critical obstruction, the right ventricular cavity may be markedly dilated. In rare cases, the right ventricle may be hypoplastic. The main pulmonary artery is dilated in almost all cases and is independent of the severity of the pulmonary valve obstruction. Sometimes, the dilatation extends into the left pulmonary artery. The dilatation is presumably related to a high-velocity jet across the stenotic valve (25,26). As noted above, such poststenotic dilatation is remarkably absent in subjects with dysplastic pulmonary valves. An interatrial communication, a patent foramen ovale, or an atrial septal defect may be present and may be the seat for right-to-left shunt in patients with severe or long-standing pulmonary stenosis.

Pathophysiology

With significant narrowing of a valve or a blood vessel, there is higher pressure proximal to the obstruction, compared with distal

TABLE 11-2. *Pathology of pulmonary stenosis (17)*

Pathologic anatomy	Percent prevalence
Dome-shaped valve	42
Unicommissural	16
Bicuspid	10
Tricuspid	6
Dysplastic	19
Annulus hypoplasia	6

pressure; this pressure gradient is necessary to maintain flow across the stenotic site. In pulmonic stenosis, hypertrophy of the right ventricle ensues and maintains this forward flow. The magnitude of right ventricular pressure and the pressure gradient across the pulmonary valve are generally proportional to the degree of obstruction. Under usual circumstances, proportional right ventricular hypertrophy maintains normal pulmonary blood flow. If the normal output is not maintained, right heart failure ensues. This occurs in two groups of patients: in neonates with critical pulmonary stenosis and in patients with severe obstruction later in childhood or adulthood.

Changes in left ventricular geometry and decreased left ventricular function can also occur, and these are proportional to the degree of right ventricular hypertrophy (27,28); however, these changes revert to normal after relief of right ventricular outflow tract obstruction.

With increasing right ventricular hypertrophy, right ventricular compliance decreases with resultant increase in end-diastolic pressure and prominent A waves in the right atrium. With an increase in right atrial pressure, a right-to-left shunt may occur if the foramen ovale is patent or an atrial septal defect is present; this will result in systemic arterial desaturation and clinically discernible cyanosis. Such a right-to-left shunt can also occur in patients with an underdeveloped (hypoplastic) right ventricle (29).

Natural History

The natural history depends on the degree of pulmonary valve obstruction. In the U.S. natural history study (30), the severity of pulmonary valve obstruction has been categorized, based on peak-to-peak catheter-measured pulmonary valvar gradient, as follows: trivial, gradient less than 25 mm Hg; mild, gradient 25 to 49 mm Hg; moderate, gradient 50 to 79 mm Hg; and severe, gradient at least 80 mm Hg. A large number of single institutional and multiinstitutional natural history studies (9,30–40) have been published. Although there are some differences in the results or in the interpretation of results, there is a general consensus. Patients with trivial and mild (gradients less than 50 mm Hg) pulmonary stenosis generally remain mild at follow-up. This is particularly true in older children in whom the pulmonary valve area appears to increase in proportion to body size and cardiac output (31,34,38). Indeed, some reports suggested evidence for regression of pulmonary valve obstruction (38,40). In the natural history study (30), only 3 (1.1%) of 261 patients with mild pulmonary stenosis followed for 4 to 8 years developed gradients greater than 60 mm Hg. Patients with moderate stenosis (gradients of 50 to 79 mm Hg), in contradistinction to trivial and mild stenosis, had progressive increase in gradient (30,36,40). The rate of increase in gradient was 8.6 mm Hg/yr in patients with moderate obstruction, whereas the rate of change was –0.6 mm Hg/yr in children with trivial and mild obstruction (40). The increase in gradient in moderate obstructions is related to decrease in pulmonary valve area with increasing age (35). The children with severe obstruction (gradients at least 80 mm Hg) underwent surgical relief of obstruction, and therefore serial catheterization data are not available. Clinical and electrocardiographic data, however, suggest progressive increase in obstruction.

In contradistinction to the above studies (30–40) in children, one study in adults (9) demonstrated a lack of development of symptoms and complications during a follow-up for a mean of 15 years; this was irrespective of degree of obstruction. These findings led the authors to question the need for intervention in asymptomatic patients (9), although the wisdom of such recommendation has been questioned (41). Furthermore, development of myocardial dysfunction and fibrosis with severe obstruction (42) and lower cardiac indices at rest and during exercise in adult subjects with severe stenosis (43) suggest that intervention is indicated with severe obstruction irrespective of age and symptoms.

Clinical Features

Symptoms

Most children with pulmonic stenosis present with asymptomatic cardiac murmurs detected on routine examination; this is particularly true with trivial and mild pulmonary stenosis. Patients with moderate and severe pulmonary stenosis may exhibit mild exertional dyspnea. Adult subjects may not be symptomatic irrespective of severity of obstruction (9). Patients with severe or critical obstruction may present with signs of systemic venous congestion, usually interpreted as congestive heart failure, because of severe right ventricular dysfunction or cyanosis, secondary to right-to-left across a patent foramen ovale or an atrial septal defect. Light-headedness, syncope, and chest pain resembling angina pectoris may be present rarely even in patients without severe obstruction. It is remarkable that a significant number of patients with moderate or severe pulmonary stenosis remain asymptomatic (9,44).

Physical Findings

Clinical findings also depend on the degree of obstruction. Most patients with pulmonary stenosis appear healthy and are well developed. Indeed, chubby rounded faces, described as "moon facies" (6,7,45), was initially thought to be characteristic for this anomaly but is not a helpful diagnostic tool (46). Most patients with trivial, mild, and moderate stenosis and many with severe stenosis are acyanotic; however, some may exhibit cyanosis secondary to interatrial right-to-left shunt. The jugular venous pulse is normal, but in patients with decreased right ventricular compliance, a prominent A wave may be visualized in the neck pulsation. There may be concomitant presystolic pulsation in the liver as well.

In patients with trivial or mild obstruction, the right ventricular impulse is normal. When pulmonary stenosis is moderate to severe, a sustained forceful right ventricular impulse, called a right ventricular heave, is felt. A thrill may be felt in the suprasternal notch and at the left upper sternal border (pulmonic area). The precordial thrill is more likely to be associated with more severe obstruction, although there is no consistent relationship between the thrill and degree of obstruction.

On auscultation, the first heart sound may be normal in intensity or it may be loud. The second heart sound is split widely. The width of the split increases with increasing severity of stenosis. The intensity of pulmonary component of the second heart sound may be loud (in mild stenosis) or soft, diminished, or absent, depending on the severity of obstruction (see below). A fourth heart sound may be heard at the left lower sternal border in patients with severe obstruction and is usually associated with a prominent A wave in the jugular pulse, as alluded to in a preceding paragraph. An ejection systolic click is heard along the left sternal border and varies with respiration (decreases or disappears during inspiration). With increasing severity, the click comes closer to the first heart sound (see below). An ejection systolic murmur of grade II/VI to V/VI is heard best at the left upper sternal border with radiation into infraclavicular regions, axillae and back. The intensity of the murmur is not necessarily related to the severity of pulmonary valve obstruction, but the duration and timing of peaking of the murmur have a good relationship with the severity of stenosis, as detailed in the next section.

An early diastolic decrescendo murmur of pulmonary regurgitation is not usually heard in an average case of pulmonary stenosis. Prior surgical or balloon intervention or valvar calcification (47) may result in such a murmur. Holosystolic murmur at the left lower sternal border indicative of tricuspid regurgitation may be audible in some patients with extremely severe pulmonary stenosis.

Clinical Assessment of Severity

The severity of the pulmonary valve obstruction can often be estimated by careful analysis of auscultatory findings (48,49). The timing of the ejection click, the extent of splitting of the second heart sound, the intensity of the pulmonary component of the second sound, the length (duration) of the systolic murmur, and timing of the peaking of the ejection murmur are usually indicative of the severity of pulmonary valve stenosis (Fig. 11-1). With trivial and mild cases of pulmonary valve obstruction, the click is clearly separated from the first heart sound, almost normal splitting of the second heart sound with normal or slightly increased pulmonary component of the second heart sound is heard, and an ejection systolic diamond-shaped murmur that peaks early in systole and ends way before the aortic component of the second heart sound is appreciated. The findings in moderate pulmonary valve stenosis are an ejection systolic click that is much closer to the first heart sound than in milder forms, widely split second sound with diminished pulmonary component, and an ejection systolic murmur that peaks in mid-to-late systole and ends just before the aortic component of the second heart sound. In severe cases of pulmonary valve narrowing, the auscultatory features are an ejection systolic click, which is either absent or falls so close to the first heart sound that it becomes inseparable from it, markedly increased splitting with a soft or inaudible pulmonary component of the second heart sound and a long ejection systolic murmur, which peaks late in systole and extends beyond the aortic component of the second

Valvular Pulmonic Stenosis

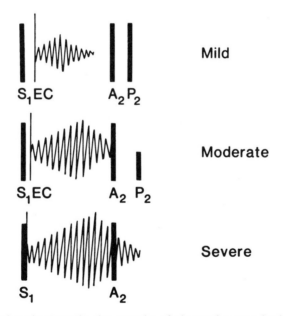

FIG. 11-1. In valvar pulmonic stenosis, the severity of obstruction may be judged by auscultatory findings. In mild stenosis, the ejection click is clearly separated from the first heart sound (S_1), the murmur starts with the click, peaks in early systole, and ends well before the aortic component of the second heart sound (A_2), and the pulmonary component of the second heart sound (P_2) is normal to increased in intensity. In moderate pulmonic stenosis, the click is closer to the first heart sound, the ejection murmur peaks later in the systole and the murmur reaches the A_2, and the second heart sound is widely split with soft pulmonary component. In severe valvar obstruction, the click is either absent or occurs so close to S_1 that it cannot be heard separately and the murmur peaks late in systole and extends beyond the A_2. The second heart sound is widely split with an extremely soft or inaudible P_2. (From ref. 49, with permission.)

heart sound so that the latter cannot be heard. The intensity of the ejection systolic murmur does not, as stated earlier, indicate the severity of obstruction but rather its duration and time of peaking; the longer the murmur and the later it peaks, the more severe is the degree of pulmonary valve obstruction. Similarly, the shorter the time interval between the first heart sound and the ejection click, the wider the splitting of the second heart sound, and the softer the pulmonary component, the more severe is the pulmonary valve stenosis.

Noninvasive Evaluation

Chest Roentgenogram

Chest x-ray, in most patients, shows a normal-sized heart with dilated pulmonary artery segment, representing poststenotic dilatation (Fig. 11-2). In moderate to severe pulmonary valve stenosis, roentgenographic signs of right ventricular enlargement may be present, but cardiomegaly may be seen only in patients with extreme obstruction and right ventricular failure. In such cases, cardiomegaly is secondary to right ventricular and right atrial dilatation. Dilated pulmonary artery may be seen in 80% to 90% of cases (1) and is *not* proportional to the degree of obstruction. Although this poststenotic dilatation is generally not problematic, it may rarely become large and present as a hilar mass simulating neoplasm (50,51). Lack of pulmonary artery dilatation may either be related to posteriorly oriented enlargement of the pulmonary artery or lack of pulmonary artery dilatation in cases

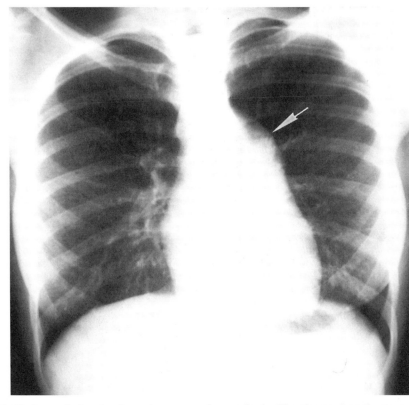

FIG. 11-2. Posteroanterior chest roentgenogram in a patient with valvar pulmonic stenosis showing a normal-sized heart with normal pulmonary vascular markings. Note the prominent main pulmonary artery (*arrow*).

with dysplastic pulmonary valves or in association with supravalvar pulmonary artery stenosis.

Pulmonary vascular markings are usually normal because the pulmonary blood flow is indeed normal in most patients with pulmonary stenosis, although this normal flow is maintained at the expense of high right ventricular pressure and hypertrophy. The pulmonary blood flow is decreased only when there is severe right ventricular failure or right-to-left interatrial shunting takes place, causing pulmonary oligemia.

Electrocardiogram

The electrocardiogram is a useful noninvasive tool in the evaluation of severity of pulmonary stenosis, although it is now surpassed by Doppler evaluation. In trivial and mild pulmonary stenosis, the electrocardiogram may be normal in nearly 50% of patients (7,52). A rightward shift of mean frontal plane vector (right axis deviation) may be all that is seen. The R waves in right chest leads may not exceed the 95th percentile for normal values. Interventricular conduction delay, manifested as rSR' or rSr', may be seen in right chest leads. The P and T waves are normal.

In moderate pulmonary valve stenosis, the electrocardiogram is usually abnormal with rightward shift of the mean frontal plane vector (right axis deviation of +90 to +130 degrees); prominent R waves in the right chest leads, exceeding 95th percentile for age; and deep S waves in left chest leads (S greater than 15 mm in V_5 or greater than 10 mm in V_6). T waves may be normal, although in children less than 10 years of age, the T waves, which are usually inverted in leads V_4 R and V_1, become upright. P waves are normal.

In severe pulmonary stenosis, the electrocardiogram is abnormal with an occasional exception (1). A rightward shift of mean frontal plane vector (right axis deviation more than +110 degrees) and a pure R wave or qR pattern in right chest leads may be seen. The S waves in leads V_5 and V_6 are also increased. The R wave in V_1 usually exceeds 20 mm. In some studies, a good correlation between the height of the R wave in lead V_1 and right ventricular peak systolic pressure was found (53). The height of the R wave in V_1 in mm multiplied by 5 is predictive of right ventricular peak systolic pressure. However, because of variability of this relationship and the availability of Doppler echocardiography, these criteria may not be useful at the present time.

Tall P waves (greater than 2.5 mm) in leads II, aVF, and right precordial leads may be present in severe stenosis. Abnormal orientation of the T waves in right precordial leads and occasional ST changes suggestive of ischemia may be seen.

In patients with pulmonary stenosis and right ventricular hypoplasia, the mean frontal plane vector (QRS axis) may be normal (+30 to +70 degrees) in contradistinction to the rightward shift seen without right ventricular hypoplasia. Superior orientation of the mean QRS vector (left axis) may rarely be seen, which may be related to an abnormality of the left anterior bundle with or without Noonan's syndrome.

Echo-Doppler Studies

M-mode Echocardiogram

Despite demonstration of the usefulness of M-mode tracings, showing deep A waves, of the pulmonary valve in quantitating the degree of obstruction (54), more recent studies (55) and other limitations suggest that M-mode evaluation of the pulmonary valve is not a useful tool.

Two-dimensional Echocardiogram

Precordial short- and long-axis and subcostal views are most useful in the evaluation of the pulmonary valve leaflets. Thickening and doming of the pulmonary valve leaflets can often be visualized (56). Markedly thickened, nodular, and immobile pulmonary valve leaflets, suggestive of dysplastic pulmonary valves, may also be recognized easily. The pulmonary valve annulus can also be visualized and measured;

the latter can be compared with normal values to determine if the annulus is hypoplastic. Such measurements are also useful in the selection of balloon diameter during balloon valvuloplasty. It should be noted, however, that prospective diagnosis of pulmonary stenosis with two-dimensional study (without Doppler echocardiography) was possible in only 64% to 76% of the cases (56,57). However, poststenotic dilatation of the pulmonary artery can be imaged and the right ventricular size, wall thickness, and function can be evaluated by the two-dimensional technique.

Doppler Echocardiogram

Recent advances in understanding of Doppler technology and ready availability of Doppler transducers on echocardiographs have made this technique accessible and superior to other noninvasive modalities of evaluation of pulmonary valve stenosis. Pulsed, continuous-wave, and color Doppler evaluation in conjunction with two-dimensional echocardiography is most useful in confirming the clinical diagnosis and in quantitating the degree of obstruction.

Pulsed Doppler interrogation of the right ventricular outflow tract with sample volume moved across the pulmonary valve demonstrates an abrupt increase in peak Doppler flow velocity, suggesting pulmonary valve obstruction. In addition, the flow pattern in the main pulmonary artery is turbulent instead of being laminar. Color Doppler imaging will also show smooth laminar subpulmonary flow (blue) with some flow acceleration (red) immediately beneath the pulmonary valve and turbulent (mosaic) flow beginning immediately distal to the pulmonary valve leaflets. Furthermore, a narrow jet of color-flow disturbance can be visualized that should be used to align the continuous-wave ultrasound beam to record maximum velocity. The angle of incidence between ultrasound beam and color jet should be kept to a minimum. Two-dimensional and color-flow–directed continuous-wave Doppler recordings from multiple transducer positions, including the precordial short

axis, high parasternal, and subcostal, should be performed for documenting the maximum velocity. Finally, a nonimaging Doppler probe with a wide ultrasound beam should also be used to record the peak velocity across the pulmonary valve.

Several studies (58–61) have demonstrated the usefulness of peak Doppler velocities in predicting the catheter-measured peak-to-peak gradients across the pulmonary valve. The peak instantaneous Doppler gradient may be calculated using a modified Bernoulli equation (62):

$$\Delta P = 4V^2$$

where ΔP is pressure gradient and V is peak Doppler flow velocity in the main pulmonary artery.

When the right ventricular outflow tract velocity, especially when it is high, is incorporated into the Bernoulli equation, Doppler prediction of gradient is even more accurate:

$$\Delta P = 4\ (V_2{}^2 - V_1{}^2)$$

where V_1 and V_2 are peak Doppler flow velocities in the right ventricular outflow tract and the main pulmonary artery, respectively.

Continuous-wave and color Doppler interrogation for tricuspid regurgitant jet is important to further confirm high right ventricular pressure. The right ventricular peak systolic pressure (RVP) may be estimated by using a modified Bernoulli equation:

$$RVP = 4V^2 - ERAP$$

where V is peak tricuspid regurgitant jet velocity and ERAP is estimated right atrial pressure (5 to 10 mm Hg).

It is important that the Doppler study is performed when the patient is quiet and in a resting state; young children and patients who are extremely anxious may have to be mildly sedated. The need for two-dimensional and color-directed Doppler measurement from multiple precordial locations has already been alluded to. It should be remembered that Doppler measurements represent peak instantaneous gradients, whereas catheterization gradients are peak-to-peak gradients, although recognition of this concept is of less importance in the pulmonary valve gradients than in aortic valve gradients.

Infundibular gradients secondary to severe right ventricular hypertrophy may be present, but these are not usually manifested because severe distal pulmonary valve obstruction masks infundibular gradients (63,64). However, the in-fundibular gradients do appear after balloon pulmonary valvuloplasty (24). Triangular pattern (Fig. 11-3) of Doppler signal, similar to that described in subaortic obstruction, is characteristic of infundibular obstruction.

Pulmonary insufficiency can easily be seen by pulsed (Fig. 11-4), continuous-wave (Fig. 11-5), and color Doppler but is unlikely to be

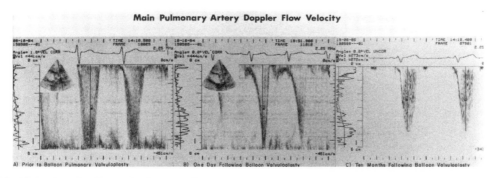

FIG. 11-3. Doppler flow velocity recordings from the main pulmonary artery before (**left**) and 1 day (**center**) and 10 months (**right**) after successful balloon pulmonary valvuloplasty. Note that there is no significant fall in the peak flow velocity on the day after balloon procedure, but there is a characteristic triangular pattern, indicative of infundibular obstruction. At 10-month follow-up, the flow velocity decreased, suggesting resolution of infundibular obstruction. (From ref. 24, with permission.)

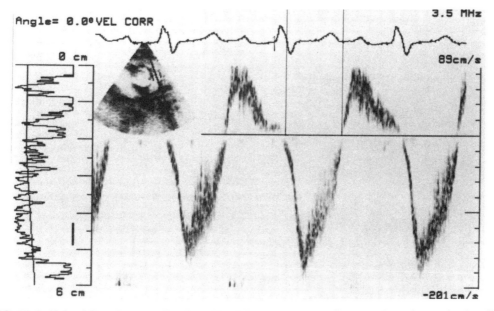

FIG. 11-4. Pulsed Doppler recording from the right ventricular outflow tract in a short-axis view (*inset*) demonstrating mildly increased forward (positive) flow in systole followed by backward (negative) flow indicative of pulmonary insufficiency. This patient had successful surgical pulmonary valvotomy several years before this recording.

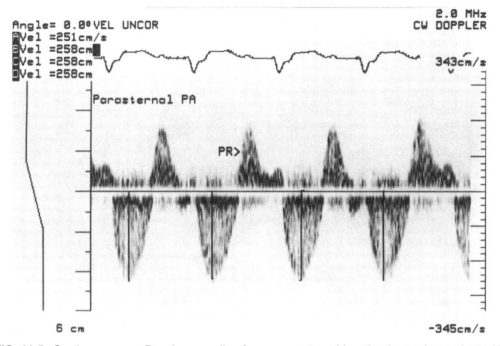

FIG. 11-5. Continuous-wave Doppler recording from a parasternal location in another patient with previous surgical valvotomy demonstrating mild residual pulmonary stenosis with approximately 25 mm Hg peak instantaneous Doppler gradient and mild pulmonary regurgitation (*PR*).

present without prior surgical or balloon pulmonary valvuloplasty. Color Doppler and pulsed Doppler interrogation of the atrial septum is useful and may reveal left-to-right or right-to-left shunt. Because of high sensitivity of color Doppler, contrast echocardiography to document right-to-left shunt (65) is not routinely used.

Other Noninvasive Studies

Computed tomography and magnetic resonance imaging may demonstrate pulmonary valve stenosis, but the current state-of-the-art echo-Doppler studies are more useful in diagnosing and quantitating pulmonary valve obstruction. Myocardial energy demands and perfusion may be evaluated by magnetic resonance spectroscopy and positron emission tomography, but at this time the clinical utility of these techniques in the management of pulmonic stenosis has not been established.

Cardiac Catheterization and Selective Cineangiography

Cardiac catheterization is not essential to establish the diagnosis, although it is an integral part of balloon dilatation. Once the clinical, electrocardiographic, and echocardiographic findings indicate moderate to severe pulmonary valve stenosis (gradient at least 50 mm Hg), cardiac catheterization should be undertaken to confirm the diagnosis and severity of obstruction, to exclude other associated cardiac abnormalities, and to consider balloon pulmonary valvuloplasty.

Oxygen Saturations

Systemic venous oxygen saturations are usually normal. They may be decreased if there is right ventricular failure, indicating low cardiac output and increased peripheral oxygen extraction. Step-up in oxygen saturation in the right atrium may be found if an atrial septal defect is present. If the right heart catheter can be advanced into the left atrium across the interatrial septum, it is important to measure oxygen saturations in the pulmonary veins, left atrium, left ventricle, and a systemic artery to demonstrate right-to-left atrial shunting. Normal pulmonary venous saturations (approximately equal to 96%) with decreased left atrial, left ventricular, and aortic saturations indicate right-to-left shunting. The degree of systemic arterial desaturation depends on the magnitude of right-to-left shunting and is related to decreased right ventricular compliance and consequent elevation of right atrial pressure.

Pressures

Right atrial pressures may be normal in mild to moderate stenosis. In severe pulmonary valve obstruction, a higher than normal right atrial mean pressure with a prominent tall A wave may be recorded. Prominent V waves suggestive of tricuspid regurgitation may be present in extremely severe pulmonary stenosis cases.

The right ventricular peak systolic pressures are increased, and the magnitude of these values is proportional to degree of obstruction. A pressure of 30 to 35 mm Hg or less is generally considered normal, and pressure less than 50 mm Hg may indicate mild stenosis. Right ventricular peak systolic pressure between 50 mm Hg and left ventricular or aortic peak systolic pressures may be present in moderate obstruction. In severe narrowing, the right ventricular systolic pressure exceeds left ventricular or aortic peak systolic pressures. However, the severity of pulmonic stenosis may be better graded by the pulmonary valve gradients, as detailed in Natural History, earlier. The right ventricular end-diastolic pressures are normal in trivial and mild obstructions and may be elevated in moderate to severe stenosis. The right ventricular pressure curve in patients with moderate and severe pulmonary stenosis with intact ventricular septum exhibits a triangular pattern in contradistinction to the flat top trace seen with pulmonary stenosis with a large ventricular septal defect (or tetralogy of Fallot).

Pulmonary arterial pressures are normal in trivial and mild stenosis, whereas in moderate to severe stenosis they are decreased and the pulse pressure is low.

Careful pressure pullback tracings from the pulmonary artery to the right ventricular inflow or right atrium with an end-hole catheter are necessary to document the gradient across the pulmonary valve and infundibulum. Pulmonary valvar gradients less than 25 mm Hg indicate trivial narrowing; 25 to 49 mm Hg, mild; 50 to 79 mm Hg, moderate; and at least 80 mm Hg, severe (30). In some cases, two pressure gradients, one across the valve and another across the infundibulum, may be recorded, indicating both valvar and infundibular stenosis. However, the infundibular gradients may be masked in the presence of more severe valvar obstruction (63,64). Whereas recording of pressure pullbacks is considered important, sometimes, when it is extremely difficult to cross the pulmonic valve, it may not be prudent to perform such a pullback tracing but instead perform balloon dilatation by over-the-wire exchange with a balloon dilatation catheter. In such instances, the decision is based on the separately recorded right ventricular and pulmonary arterial pressures.

Cardiac Index and Valve Area

Cardiac output and index should be measured either by a thermodilution technique or by the Fick principle with measured oxygen consumption. This is done to ensure that the cardiac index is within normal range, so that the recorded pressure gradient is a true reflection of the hemodynamic status of the patient's pulmonary valve abnormality. Calculation of the pulmonary valve area by the Gorlin formula (66) has been advocated by some workers, but because of multiple assumptions that must be made during calculation and because of limitations in applying this formula to calculate the pulmonary valve area (67), we do not routinely calculate it. Instead, we use peak-to-peak pulmonary valve gradients to assess the severity of obstruction after ensuring that the cardiac index is within normal range.

Exercise Response

Several investigators have examined the exercise response of patients with pulmonary stenosis (42,43,68–74), and some workers used isoproterenol infusion to simulate exercise (73–75). An increase in the cardiac index along with an increase in right ventricular pressure and pulmonary valve gradient occurs in children with mild to moderate pulmonary stenosis after exercise or isoproterenol administration. Because the stroke volume increases only slightly, the increase in cardiac output is mostly due to the increase in stroke rate. In children with severe stenosis, there is not a significant increase in cardiac index, and the right ventricular pressure and pulmonary valve gradient may be stable or fall. The stroke volume may remain unchanged or fall. The lack of normal response to exercise in severe stenosis appears to be related to decreased diastolic filling time and increased diastolic filling resistance. In contradistinction to these findings in children, adult subjects with mild to moderate stenosis do not increase cardiac index, have mild increase in heart rate, and do not increase right ventricular pressure or systolic gradients across the pulmonic valve. With severe stenosis, the exercise response is similar to that seen in children, although the cardiac and stroke indices are lower in adults than in children, both at rest and during exercise. Given these data, the indications for intervention are reasonably clear and are based on the severity of obstruction, and therefore routine exercise testing or isoproterenol infusion during catheterization is not necessary.

Angiography

Biplane right ventriculogram in sitting-up (anteroposterior camera tilted to 15 degrees left anterior oblique and 40 degrees cranial) and lateral views (Figs. 11-6 and 11-7) should be performed to confirm the site of obstruction, to evaluate the size and function of the right ventricle, and to measure pulmonary valve annulus, preparatory to balloon pulmonary valvuloplasty. Additional cineangiograms from other locations are not necessary unless the echocardiographic and hemodynamic data suggest other abnormalities. Selective left ventricular angiography and coronary arteriography may be performed in patients older than 50 years, depending on the institutional policy, or in patients with suspected coronary artery disease.

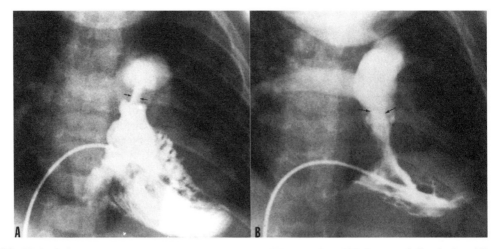

FIG. 11-6. Selected cineangiographic frames from a sitting-up view (15 degrees left anterior oblique and 40 degrees cranial) of a right ventricular angiogram before **(A)** and 15 minutes after **(B)** balloon pulmonary valvuloplasty. Note the thin jet of contrast material passing through the narrowed pulmonary valve (*arrows* in A) that has a marked increase after valvuloplasty (*arrows* in B). (From ref. 2, with permission.)

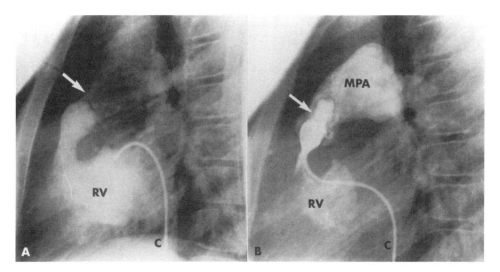

FIG. 11-7. Selected frames from lateral views of right ventricular (*RV*) cineangiograms before **(A)** and after **(B)** balloon pulmonary valvuloplasty. Note the extremely thin jet (*arrow*) before balloon dilatation **(A)** that increased to a much wider jet (*arrow*) after valvuloplasty **(B)**, opacifying the main pulmonary artery (*MPA*). *C*, catheter. (From ref. 105, with permission.)

The right ventricle is either normal in size or is slightly enlarged, contracts well, and exhibits heavy trabeculation and hypertrophy. Marked enlargement of the right ventricular cavity with poor function is seen only with extremely severe or critical obstruction. Infundibular hypertrophy of varying degree may be seen with marked narrowing during mid-to-late systole, which opens up during diastole. With severe infundibular hypertrophy (often seen with severe valvar obstruction), almost complete obliteration of the infundibular cavity (Fig. 11-8A) may

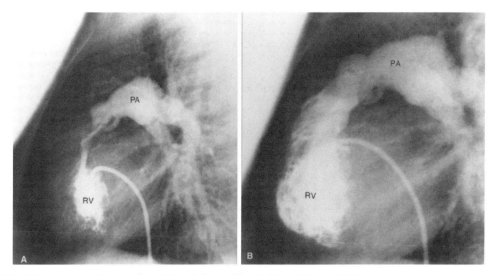

FIG. 11-8. Selected frames from lateral view of the right ventricular (*RV*) cineangiogram showing severe infundibular stenosis **(A)** immediately after balloon valvuloplasty (corresponding to Fig. 11-3, center). At 10 months after balloon valvuloplasty, the right ventricular outflow tract **(B)** is wide open (corresponds to Fig. 11-3, right). Peak-to-peak pulmonary valve gradient was 20 mm Hg, and there was no infundibular gradient. *PA*, pulmonary artery. (From ref. 24, with permission.)

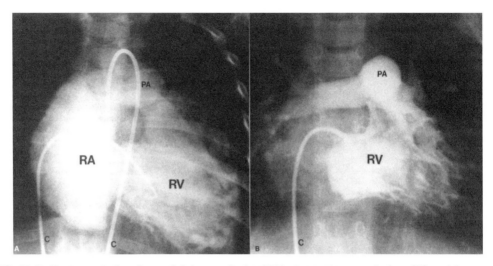

FIG. 11-9. Posteroanterior views of right ventricular (*RV*) cineangiograms before **(A)** and 1 year after **(B)** balloon pulmonary valvuloplasty. Note marked improvement in tricuspid insufficiency at follow-up (B). (From ref. 2, with permission.)

occur. Tricuspid regurgitation (Fig. 11-9A), if present, may be visualized. Hypoplastic right ventricle may also be identified (29,76). Quantitation of right ventricular volumes is feasible (77), and such studies have shown that the right and left ventricular function are preserved in most patients with pulmonary stenosis.

The pulmonary valve leaflets are mild to moderately thickened and dome during systole (Fig. 11-10A), and the pulmonary valve

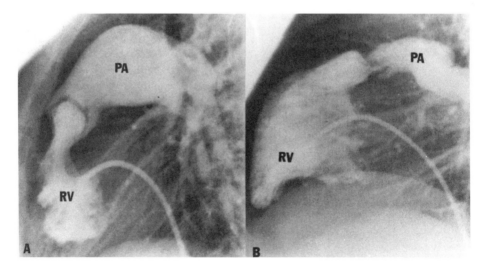

FIG. 11-10. Selected frames from right ventricular cineangiograms of patients without **(A)** and with **(B)** dysplastic pulmonary valves. **A:** Thickened and domed pulmonary valve leaflets are seen. Note poststenotic dilatation of the pulmonary artery (*PA*). **B:** Pulmonary valve leaflets are markedly and unevenly thickened without doming. There was no jet formation and no poststenotic dilatation of the PA. The pulmonary valve ring is smaller than normal. (From ref. 121, with permission.)

orifice is visualized as a jet of the contrast material (Fig. 11-6A). The size of the pulmonary valve annulus is normal in most cases, although it can be hypoplastic in neonates and young infants and in patients with dysplastic pulmonary valves. The main pulmonary artery and sometimes left pulmonary artery are dilated, the so-called post-stenotic dilatation (Figs. 11-7B and 11-10A), and, as stated earlier, the degree of post-stenotic dilatation has no bearing on the severity of the pulmonary valve stenosis. In contrast, patients with dysplastic pulmonary valves exhibit nodular, thickened, immobile pulmonary valve leaflets with annular hypoplasia and do not exhibit poststenotic dilatation (Fig. 11-10B).

The levoangiographic phase should be recorded to evaluate the pulmonary venous return and the left atrium, left ventricle, and aorta. These are usually normal in patients with pulmonary stenosis. If evidence for left-to-right shunt is present, further selective angiography should be performed to define such issues.

Therapy

Patients with trivial (gradient less than 25 mm Hg) and mild (gradient less than 50 mm Hg) pulmonary stenosis do not need intervention to relieve the pulmonary valve obstruction. They should be clinically followed at periodic intervals, perhaps on a yearly basis. During the period of rapid growth, namely infancy and adolescence, more frequent follow-up may be indicated. Routine well-person care, including immunizations as per the primary physician, should be provided. Pulmonary stenosis patients are candidates for infective endocarditis prophylaxis before any bacteremia-producing procedures and surgery, as per the recommendations of the American Heart Association (78). There is no need to limit their exercise or activity level.

Patients with signs of right ventricular failure should be promptly treated with anticongestive measures, including digitalis and diuretics. However, it should be recognized that the problem will not be resolved until the obstruction is relieved, and therefore prompt balloon or surgical intervention should be undertaken. Right ventricular function may not recover completely if intervention is withheld for too long and myocardial damage sets in (79). Discussion of management of neonates with critical pulmonary stenosis is beyond the scope of this chapter and is detailed elsewhere (80–83).

Patients with moderate (gradient 50 to 79 mm Hg) and severe (gradient at least 80 mm Hg) obstruction should, in the opinion of the author, undergo intervention to relieve the pulmonary valve stenosis. There is consensus with this approach in children; however, in adults, there is some controversy because of reported lack of progression and no complication in a group of adults followed for 5 to 24 years (9). Based on the potential for development of myocardial damage, associated with long-term pressure overload of the right ventricle and generally lower cardiac indices, both before and after exercise in adults compared with children and exercise-induced hemodynamic abnormalities in adults, it is prudent that the pulmonary valve obstruction is relieved in adults with moderate to severe pulmonary stenosis, irrespective of symptoms. After relief of obstruction, the recommendations pertaining to routine care, endocarditis prophylaxis, and exercise limitations are the same as those described for trivial and mild stenosis.

Surgical Intervention

Since the first description of surgical relief of pulmonary stenosis by closed pulmonary valvotomy (84,85), a variety of techniques has been developed: valvotomy with inflow occlusion, hypothermia, and by use of cardiopulmonary bypass. Currently, the preferred approach is transpulmonary arterial valvotomy under cardiopulmonary bypass. The results of surgery are generally good with low mortality, 3% to 7% (30,86–89), and decreased right ventricular pressures and pulmonary valve gradients. In the U.S. natural history study, only 3% of 294 patients had gradients greater than 50 mm Hg 4 to 8 years after surgery. The incidence of pulmonary insufficiency at follow-up was between 60% and 90% (30,89). Despite these good results, surgical pulmonary valvotomy has been replaced with transluminal balloon pulmonary valvuloplasty, discussed in the next section. Surgery is reserved for cases in which balloon valvuloplasty is not feasible or has not been successful. One such example is dysplastic pulmonary valve with valve ring hypoplasia. The treatment of this disorder is to excise the obstructive valve leaflets and enlarge the annulus by a transannular patch. Another example is fixed infundibular or supravalvar stenosis after successful balloon valvuloplasty (90).

Balloon Pulmonary Valvuloplasty

The first attempt to relieve pulmonary valve obstruction by transcatheter methodology, to the best of my knowledge, was in the early 1950s by Rubio-Alverez et al. (91,92); they used a ureteral catheter with a wire to cut open the stenotic pulmonary valve. In 1979, Semb et al. (93) used a balloon-tipped angiographic (Berman) catheter to rupture the pulmonary valve commissures by rapidly withdrawing the inflated balloon across the pulmonary valve. More recently, Kan et al. (94) applied the technique of Dotter and Judkins (95) and Gruntzig et al. (96) to relieve pulmonary valve obstruction by the radial forces of balloon inflation of a balloon catheter positioned across the pulmonic valve. This static balloon dilatation technique is currently used throughout the world to relieve pulmonary valve obstruction.

Based on the currently available data, it is the general consensus that balloon valvuloplasty is the treatment option of choice in the management of isolated pulmonary valve stenosis.

Indications

It is generally believed that indications for balloon pulmonary valvuloplasty are similar to those used for surgical pulmonary valvotomy, that is, a moderate degree of pulmonary valve stenosis with a peak-to-peak gradient at least 50 mm Hg with normal cardiac index (97). Some workers use lesser gradients (gradient of 40 mm Hg or right ventricular pressure of 50 mm Hg) for intervention. Careful examination of the available studies (97) suggested that there is only marginal reduction of right ventricular pressure if mild stenoses are dilated, natural history studies revealed trivial and mild stenoses (less than 50 mm Hg gradient) that are likely to remain mild at follow-up (30), and increase in gradient can easily be quantitated by echo-Doppler studies (58–61) at follow-up examination and if an increase in gradient is documented, the patient could then undergo balloon dilatation. Based on these observations, I continue to advocate that balloon dilatation should be performed only in patients with peak-to-peak gradient greater than 50 mm Hg (98).

In adult subjects with moderate to severe stenosis without symptoms, some authors were hesitant to recommend intervention (9). But based on poor response to exercise (43) and potential for development of myocardial fibrosis, I believe it is prudent to provide catheter-directed relief of the obstruction in all patients, including adults, with moderate to severe stenosis, irrespective of the symptoms.

Technique

The technique of balloon pulmonary valvuloplasty involves positioning of a balloon catheter (Fig. 11-11) across the stenotic valve, usually over an extra-stiff exchange-length guidewire, and inflating the balloon, thus producing valvotomy. The recommended balloon/annulus ratio is 1.2 to 1.4 (99–101). When the pulmonary valve annulus is too large to dilate with a single balloon (approximately equal to 20 mm), valvuloplasty with simultaneous inflation of two balloons across the pulmonary valve (Fig. 11-12) may be performed. When two balloons are used, the following formula may be used to calculate the effective balloon size (99):

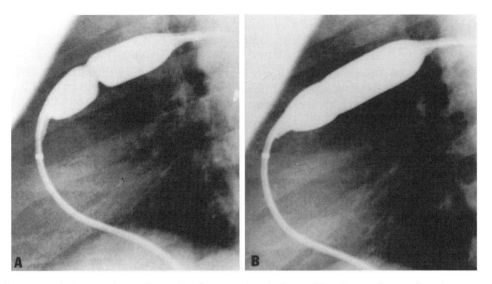

FIG. 11-11. Selected cineradiographic frames of a balloon dilatation catheter placed across a stenotic pulmonary valve. Note "waisting" of the balloon during the initial phases of the balloon inflation **(A)** that was almost completely abolished during the later phases of balloon inflation **(B)**. (From ref. 2, with permission.)

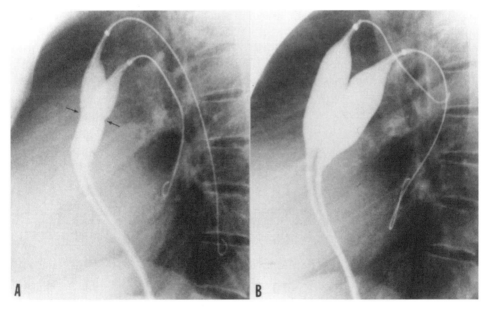

FIG. 11-12. Selected cine frames of two balloon catheters placed across the pulmonary valve showing "waisting" of the balloons (*arrows* in **A**) during the initial phases of balloon inflation that was completely abolished after complete inflation of the balloons **(B)**. (From ref. 2, with permission.)

$$\frac{D_1 + D_2 - \pi \left(\frac{D_1}{2} + \frac{D_2}{2}\right)}{\pi}$$

where D_1 and D_2 are diameters of the balloons used. For further details of the technique, the reader is referred to other publications (2,102,103).

Mechanism of Valvuloplasty

Inflation of a balloon placed across an obstructive lesion exerts radial forces on the stenotic lesion without any axial component (104,105). The mechanism of valvuloplasty has been assessed by direct visual observation of the valve mechanism at surgery (106) or during postmortem examination (107) and by indirect observations of angiographic (105, 108) and echocardiographic (109) studies. Valve commissural splitting, tearing of valve leaflets, and avulsion of the valve leaflets have been observed and are conceivably the mechanism by which pulmonary valve obstruction is relieved by balloon dilatation. The circumferential dilating force exerted by balloon inflation is likely to rupture (tear) the weakest part of the valve mechanism. It is likely that the fused commissures are the weakest links that can be broken with balloon dilatation. However, in a given patient, when the fused commissures are strong and cannot be torn, tears of the valve cusps or avulsion of valve leaflet can occur. The latter events are likely to cause more severe pulmonary insufficiency. Pulmonary valve dysplasia, if severe, may preclude successful balloon valvuloplasty unless there is associated commissural fusion.

Immediate and Intermediate-term Results

Immediate reduction in peak-to-peak gradient and right ventricle-to-left ventricular pressure ratio and increase in pulmonary artery pressure (Fig. 11-13), increase in jet width (Figs. 11-6 and 11-7), and free motion of the pulmonary valve leaflets with less doming have been observed after balloon valvuloplasty (2,90,102,103). Improvement of right ventricular function, tricuspid insufficiency (Fig. 11-9), and right-to-left shunt (110), if such are present before dilatation, has been documented.

At intermediate-term follow-up (usually defined as 2 years or less), both catheterization-measured peak-to-peak (Fig. 11-14) and

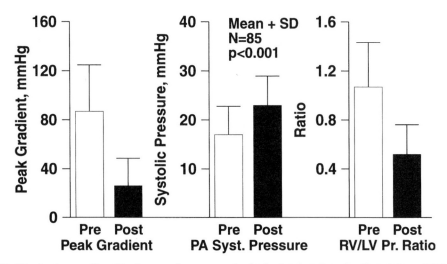

FIG. 11-13. Acute results of balloon pulmonary valvuloplasty showing significant ($p < 0.001$) decrease in peak-to-peak systolic pressure gradient and right ventricle-to-left ventricle peak systolic pressure ratio and increase ($p < 0.001$) in peak pulmonary artery pressure.

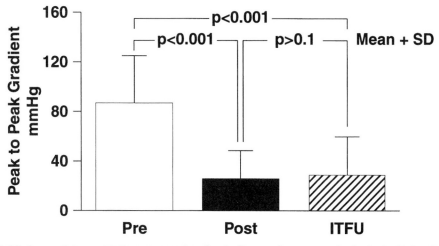

FIG. 11-14. Immediate and follow-up results after balloon pulmonary valvuloplasty. Note significant decrease ($p < 0.0001$) in peak-to-peak systolic pressure gradients measured at cardiac catheterization before (*Pre*) and immediately after (*Post*) balloon dilatation. The gradient measured during repeat catheterization in 47 patients at intermediate-term follow-up (*ITFU*) remains unchanged ($p > 0.1$) compared with the gradients immediately after balloon dilatation and continue to be lower ($p < 0.001$) than those before balloon valvuloplasty. (From ref. 90, with permission.)

Doppler-measured peak instantaneous (Fig. 11-15) gradients remain improved for the group as a whole. However, restenosis, defined as gradient of 50 mm Hg or more, has been observed in nearly 10% of patients. Predictors of restenosis include balloon/annulus ratio less than 1.2 and immediate postvalvulo-plasty gradient at least 30 mm Hg (111). Balloon/annulus ratio and immediate post-valvuloplasty gradients were also identified as predictors of restenosis in a large multiinstitutional valvuloplasty and angioplasty of congenital anomalies (VACA) Registry study (112). In addition, earlier study year, small

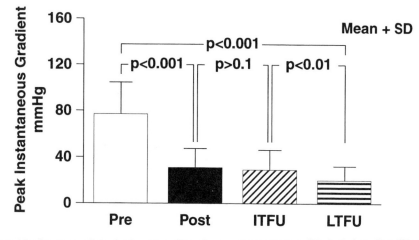

FIG. 11-15. Maximum peak instantaneous Doppler gradients before (*Pre*), 1 day after (*Post*) balloon pulmonary valvuloplasty, and at intermediate-term (*ITFU*) and late (*LTFU*) follow-up. Note significant reduction ($p < 0.001$) after valvuloplasty that remains unchanged ($p > 0.1$) at ITFU. However, at LTFU there was further fall ($p < 0.01$) in the Doppler gradients.

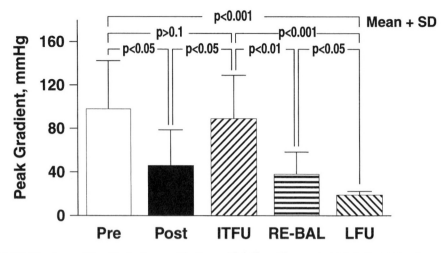

FIG. 11-16. The favorable effect of repeat balloon dilatation after recurrent pulmonary stenosis after previous balloon pulmonary valvuloplasty. In this group of nine patients, the peak-to-peak gradient fell ($p < 0.05$) after balloon dilatation that increased ($p < 0.05$) at intermediate-term follow-up (*ITFU*). Repeat balloon dilatation (*RE-BAL*) reduced ($p < 0.01$) the gradient, which decreased further ($p < 0.05$) at late follow-up (*LFU*). *Pre*, before balloon valvuloplasty; *Post*, immediately after valvuloplasty; *SD*, standard deviation.

valve annulus, and postsurgical/complex pulmonary stenosis were also found to be predictive of restenosis. Patients with restenosis have been successfully treated by performing redilatation (Fig. 11-16) with balloons larger than those used at the time of initial balloon valvuloplasty (113). Redilatation is the procedure of choice in the management of restenosis after previous balloon dilatation.

Infundibular Stenosis

Infundibular gradients occur in nearly 30% of patients; the older the age and higher the severity of obstruction, the greater the prevalence of infundibular reaction (24). When residual infundibular gradient is at least 50 mm Hg beta-blockade, therapy is generally recommended (24,114). Infundibular obstruction regresses to a great degree at follow-up (Figs. 11-3 and 11-8), just as has been demonstrated for infundibular reactions after surgical valvotomy (87,115–117), with a rare patient requiring surgical intervention (90). Issues related to the significance of infundibular obstruction and its management are discussed in greater detail elsewhere (2,24,118).

Follow-up Evaluation

Clinical, electrocardiographic, and echo-Doppler evaluation at 1, 6, and 12 months after the procedure and yearly thereafter is generally recommended. Regression of right ventricular hypertrophy on the electrocardiogram after balloon dilatation has been well documented (119), and the electrocardiogram is a useful adjunct in the evaluation of follow-up results. However, electrocardiographic evidence for hemodynamic improvement does not become apparent until 6 months after valvuloplasty. Doppler gradient is generally reflective of the residual obstruction and is a useful and reliable noninvasive monitoring tool (2,120).

Dysplastic Pulmonary Valves

There is some controversy with regard to the use of balloon dilatation in patients with dysplastic pulmonary valves. Based on our own observations (121) and those of Marantz et al. (122), the results of balloon valvuloplasty with dysplastic valves are comparable with those without. Dysplastic valves did not seem to be responsible for recurrence (111,121). Balloons large enough to produce a balloon/annulus ratio of 1.4 to 1.5 may be needed to produce satisfactory results (121). The reason for differences in opinion and results may, in part, be related to how one classifies morphology of a given valve. There also appears to be variations in degree of fusion of dysplastic valve leaflets in some patients. Those dysplastic valves that have commissural fusion as a part of the pathology are likely to respond to balloon dilatation. Given the marked variation in expression of pulmonary valve dysplasia in clinical practice and given favorable results in some studies (121,122), patients with dysplastic valves should not be excluded from an attempt at balloon dilatation. It seems reasonable to use larger balloons than are recommended for nondysplastic valves; we suggest use of balloons large enough to produce balloon/annulus ratios of 1.4 to 1.5 but avoid using ratios greater than 1.5 for fear of injury to the right ventricular outflow tract (123). If there is an inadequate result after balloon dilations, surgical excision of the obstructive valve leaflets along with transannular patch relief of annular obstruction should be considered.

Comparison with Surgery

Comparison of balloon therapy with surgical valvotomy has limitations (2,90), but there is generally higher mortality and morbidity after surgery. However, greater reduction of gradient is observed after surgery, but the degree and frequency of pulmonary insufficiency may be higher after surgery than after balloon therapy (2,124).

Results in Adult Subjects

Since the initial application of balloon pulmonary valvuloplasty in an adult by Pepine et al. (125), several other groups have used this technique (2,126–130). Because of physical size of the pulmonary valve annulus, many adults may require balloon valvuloplasty using two balloons (126,127). However, as alluded to elsewhere (131,132), the double-balloon technique is comparable with but not superior to the single-balloon technique when equivalent balloon/annulus ratios are compared. More recently, however, the Inoue balloon has been used in adults (128,133,134) with success. The major advantage of the Inoue balloon over the conventional balloons is the adjustable nature of balloon diameter, making stepwise dilatation possible.

Although it is generally recommended that balloon diameter should be 1.2 to 1.4 times larger than that of pulmonary valve annulus for successful dilatation in children (99–101,111), balloon sizes similar to or 1 mm larger than pulmonary valve annulus seem to be effective in adults (129,130,134). However, systematic studies to evaluate the influence of balloon/annulus ratios in adults have not been documented. Based on the available data, I would recommend a balloon/annulus ratio in the range of 1.2 in adults.

Acute results of balloon valvuloplasty in adults (2,126–130,133,134) are excellent and are similar to those reported in children. Success has been documented even in sixth and seventh decades of life (135–137). Based on our experience with teenagers (24,138) and on that of others in adult patients (126,130), infundibular obstruction after balloon dilatation appears to be more common in older patients than in younger patients. The reason for this is probably long-standing right ventricular hypertension and consequent right ventricular infundibular hypertrophy in older patients. However, the infundibular obstruction resolves with time.

Follow-up results, though documented in a few studies, do indicate persistent relief at follow-up. In summary, it appears that successful balloon pulmonary valvuloplasty is feasible in adults.

Long-term Follow-up Results

Whereas immediate and short-term results have been documented, referenced extensively elsewhere (2,102,103), data are scant on long-term follow-up results (90,124, 129,130,139). These studies reveal generally low residual peak instantaneous Doppler gradients (Fig. 11-15) with minimal (1% to 2%) late recurrence of pulmonary stenosis (beyond what was seen at intermediate-term follow-up), need for surgical intervention in approximately 5% of patients to relieve fixed subvalvar or supravalvar stenosis, and actuarial freedom for reintervention in 88% and 84%, respectively, at 5 and 10 years (90). However, pulmonary valve insufficiency is noted in 80% to 90% of patients (90,124,139), but right ventricular volume overloading did not develop nor require surgical intervention because of pulmonary insufficiency. Based on these data, it may be concluded that balloon pulmonary valvuloplasty continues to be the treatment of choice in the management of valvar pulmonary stenosis of moderate to severe degree. Further, longer term (10 to 20 years) follow-up studies to evaluate the significance of residual pulmonary insufficiency should be undertaken.

INTRACAVITARY RIGHT VENTRICULAR OBSTRUCTION

There are several types of right ventricular intracavitary obstructions, and some of these are discussed.

Infundibular Pulmonary Stenosis

Infundibular pulmonary stenosis is more commonly associated with other lesions, namely, tetralogy of Fallot and valvar pulmonary stenosis. In tetralogy of Fallot, infundibular obstruction with or without valvar stenosis is present in two thirds of the tetralogy cases and is related to anterior deviation of infundibular septum and hypertrophy of the components of the crista supraventricularis. Tetralogy of Fallot patients usually present with symptoms in infancy, and discussion of this lesion is beyond the scope of this chapter. Infundibular stenosis associated with valvar pulmonary stenosis has been discussed in detail in a preceding section.

Isolated infundibular stenosis may occur as a fibrous band at the junction of the infundibulum with the body of the right ventricle or may be a fibromuscular obstruction immediately beneath the pulmonary valve. The pathophysiology of these lesions is similar to that of valvar pulmonary stenosis. The natural history is not well documented, but based on

limited data, it appears that there is more rapid progression of the severity of obstruction in patients with infundibular than in patients with valvar stenosis.

The clinical features of isolated infundibular obstruction are, in many respects, similar to those seen with valvar pulmonary stenosis with occasional differences. The signs and symptoms depend on the severity of stenosis. The second heart sound is widely split with a soft pulmonary component. The ejection systolic click is notably absent. A long ejection systolic murmur is heard along the left sternal border at a location slightly lower than that observed with valvar stenosis.

The electrocardiographic findings are similar to valvar stenosis, and the degree of right ventricular hypertrophy is generally proportional to the degree of obstruction. Chest x-ray features are similar to valvar stenosis with notable absence of poststenotic dilatation. Echo-Doppler studies are helpful in distinguishing infundibular from valvar stenosis (140). Instead of doming of pulmonary valve leaflets, as seen in valvar stenosis, systolic fluttering of the pulmonary valve leaflets is seen with isolated infundibular obstruction. Parasternal and subcostal two-dimensional echocardiographic views imaging the right ventricular outflow tract may demonstrate narrowed infundibulum. Two-dimensional and color-flow imaging guided continuous-wave Doppler provides an estimate of the gradient, as discussed above.

Cardiac catheterization demonstrates no gradient across the pulmonary valve and a clearly discernible subvalvar gradient by a pressure pullback with an end-hole catheter. The magnitude of the gradient is proportional to the degree of obstruction. The site and length of infundibular narrowing can be visualized by selective right ventriculography. Poststenotic dilatation of the pulmonary artery is absent.

Treatment of moderate to severe obstruction is surgical resection of obstructing fibrotic and muscle tissue with or without right ventricular outflow tract patch. Balloon dilatation of infundibular pulmonary stenosis has been attempted (141) but was unsuccessful and is not recommended (142).

Double-chamber Right Ventricle

Since its original description by Lucas et al. (143) in 1962, double-chambered right ventricle is recognized as a distinct clinical entity. Obstructive anomalous muscle bundles, consisting of a small ventral and larger dorsal structures, divide the right ventricular cavity into a proximal high-pressure chamber consisting of inflow and sinus portion of the right ventricle and a distal low-pressure chamber consisting of the infundibulum. The anomalous muscle bundles are different from the moderator band and are attached to the interventricular septum below the level of septal leaflet of the tricuspid valve on one side and to the free wall of the right ventricle on the other, crossing the main cavity of the right ventricle. Double-chambered right ventricle is frequently associated with a ventricular septal defect (144).

The pathophysiologic and clinical features are similar to those described for valvar and infundibular pulmonary stenosis as detailed in previous sections of this chapter. The anomalous muscle bundle may be imaged by two-dimensional subcostal views, and Doppler flow velocity indicates the degree of obstruction. Ventricular septal defect with left-to-right shunt may also be seen. Demonstration of intracavity pressure gradient during catheterization and visualization of the anomalous bundle by angiography of the proximal chamber are feasible and are diagnostic. Selective left ventricular angiography to exclude an associated ventricular septal defect is highly desirable.

Double-chamber right ventricle with moderate-to-severe obstruction should undergo surgical resection of the anomalous muscle bundle by right ventriculotomy. The ventricular septal defect, if present, should also be surgically closed.

Because the obstruction is muscular, it is unlikely that balloon dilatation is effective in relieving the obstruction. Chandrashekar et al. (145) performed balloon dilatation in a 21-year-old man with a double-chamber right ventricle and reduced the gradient from 125 to 75 mm Hg. There was improvement in the patient's symptoms, but the residual gradient remained unchanged at follow-up catheterization 1 year later. Although there is no theoretical basis for favorable effect of balloon dilation, severe obstruction with suprasystemic pressure in the proximal chamber may be balloon dilated in an attempt to reduce the gradient, which may make these patients better risk candidates for anesthesia and surgery.

Other Intracavitary Obstructions

Three additional right ventricular outflow tract obstructions are worthy of brief discussion. Hypertrophic cardiomyopathy usually presents as dynamic muscular subaortic stenosis; however, an occasional patient may have severe right ventricular outflow tract obstruction (146–148). The initial management consists of beta-blockade or calcium channel blocker therapy, similar to that used for hypertrophic cardiomyopathy. If there is no good response, surgical resection of obstructing muscle may be necessary.

In congenital corrected transposition of the great arteries (149–151), the atria are normal (i.e., situs solitus of the atria). The finely trabeculated morphologic left ventricle (Fig. 11-17A) is right sided, is connected to the right atrium, and gives rise to a posteriorly located pulmonary artery. The coarsely trabeculated morphologic right ventricle (Fig. 11-17B) is left sided, is connected to the left atrium, and gives rise to an anteriorly located aorta. Thus, atrioventricular and ventriculoarterial discordance (S,L,L) exists. In essence, the ventricles are inverted. However, normal circulatory pattern is preserved: The systemic venous blood is directed into the pulmonary artery, albeit through a right-sided morphologic left ventricle, whereas the pulmonary venous blood is routed into the left-sided morphologic right ventricle and from there into the aorta. The great arteries, by definition, are transposed: The aorta is anterior and the pulmonary artery is posterior, the aorta arises from a morphologic right ventricle, and the pulmonary artery comes off a morphologic left ventricle. Thus, this condition is anatomically a transposition; however, the blood circulation is normal—systemic venous

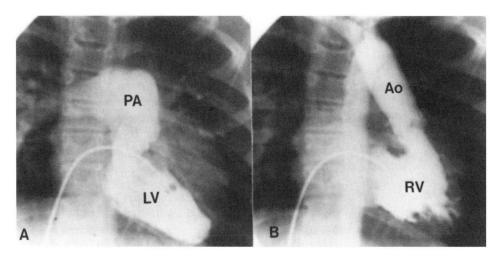

FIG. 11-17. Selective ventricular angiography in a case with congenital corrected transposition of the great arteries. **A:** Angiogram from the right-sided morphologic left ventricle (*LV*) shows a smooth-walled ventricular cavity, with opacification of the pulmonary artery (*PA*). The pulmonary valve is inferior and rightward (also, posterior in the lateral view; not shown). **B:** Cineangiographic frame from the left-sided morphologic right ventricle (*RV*). The catheter has been advanced into the ventricle via a patent foramen ovale and left-sided atrioventricular valve. Note heavily trabeculated ventricle consistent with right ventricular morphology. The aorta (*Ao*) is opacified from this ventricle and is located superiorly and to the left of the pulmonary valve. The aorta is also anterior on the lateral view (not shown). The aorta descends on the left side of the spine and is normal. (From Rao PS. Other tricuspid valve abnormalities. In: Long WA, ed. *Fetal and Neonatal Cardiology*. Philadelphia: WB Saunders, 1990:541–550, with permission.)

blood to the lungs and the pulmonary venous blood to the body. Therefore, the term "congenitally corrected transposition of the great arteries" or "corrected transposition" in short is used to describe this congenital anomaly. Because the aortic valve is to the left of the pulmonary valve (Fig. 11-17) (normally the aortic valve is located to right of the pulmonary valve), it is also referred to as L-transposition. Although patients without any associated defects have been reported (152,153), most patients have other cardiac abnormalities, and these include Ebstein's anomaly of the left-sided morphologic right (tricuspid) atrioventricular valve, heart block, ventricular septal defect, and pulmonary outflow tract obstruction. Discrete subpulmonary membrane (154) and aneurysm of the membranous septum (151) produce subvalvar pulmonary stenosis in patients with corrected transposition, and these are briefed.

The discrete subpulmonary membrane is located in the right-sided morphologic left ventricle of corrected transposition patients. The clinical features are similar to the other subvalvar and valvar pulmonary stenosis described in previous sections. The second heart sound may be single and loud, due to the anteriorly located aorta. Chest x-ray may reveal straightening of the left heart border secondary to abnormal origin and coarse of the ascending aorta. Electrocardiogram may reveal reversed Q waves, that is, Q waves in the right chest leads and no Q waves in the left chest leads. This is due to reversal of septal depolarization that is secondary to inversion of the conduction system associated with ventricular inversion. Echocardiography, apart from revealing corrected transposition, may demonstrate the subpulmonary membrane and increased Doppler flow velocity across the membrane. If the obstruction is moderate to severe (gradient greater than 50 mm Hg), surgical resection of the membrane, a conventional treatment regimen, may be undertaken.

However, Vacek and Goertz (154) were successful in balloon dilating the subvalvar membrane in a 22-year-old woman; the gradient fell from 85 to 34 mm Hg. This gradient remained low at follow-up. Given the success of balloon dilating subaortic membranous stenoses (155–157), it is not surprising that Vacek and Goertz were able to reduce subvalvar obstruction by balloon dilation. If the membrane is thin (less than 2 mm), balloon dilatation should be attempted; otherwise, surgical resection may be required.

Aneurysm of the membranous ventricular septum is one of the mechanisms by which spontaneous closure of ventricular septal defects occurs. In patients with normally related great arteries, higher pressure in the left ventricle favors protrusion of the aneurysm into the right ventricle. Despite this, significant right ventricular outflow obstruction is rare because of the presence of conal septum and crista supraventricularis between the aneurysm and the pulmonary valve (151). By contrast, in patients with inverted ventricles, higher morphologic right ventricular pressure results in protrusion of the aneurysm into the outflow tract of the morphologic left ventricle. Absence of conal septum in the right-sided morphologic left ventricle brings the outflow tract in proximity to the aneurysm and hence can result in obstruction, even with small aneurysms. This type of pulmonary outflow tract obstruction, though rare, is well documented (151,158–162). The clinical features are similar to subpulmonary stenosis described in the preceding section and include increased right ventricular impulse, single second sound, ejection systolic murmur at left upper or mid-sternal borders, and a holosystolic murmur of associated ventricular septal defect at the left lower sternal border. Chest roentgenographic and electrocardiographic features suggestive of corrected transposition may be present. Echocardiogram reveals an echolucent mass in the subpulmonary region with increased Doppler flow velocity across it. Catheterization data reveal peak-to-peak systolic pressure gradient across the subpulmonary region, and selective morphologic left ventriculography (Fig. 11-18) demonstrates

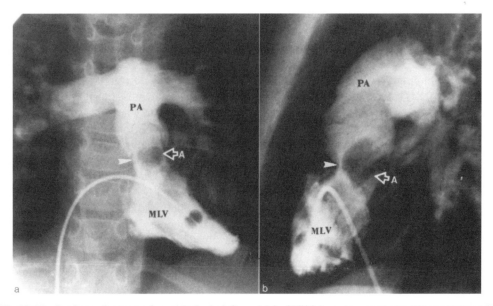

FIG. 11-18. Angiocardiogram of morphologic left ventricle (*MLV*) in anteroposterior **(A)** and lateral **(B)** projections demonstrating smooth trabeculations. A radiolucent structure in the outflow tract, causing obstruction in the subpulmonary region, is seen. *Open arrow,* aneurysm of the membranous septum; *solid arrow,* narrow jet of contrast material. *PA,* pulmonary artery. (From ref. 151, with permission.)

the size of the aneurysm and the extent of obstruction. Treatment consists of surgical resection of the aneurysm along with closure of the ventricular septal defect, if present (151,158–162).

PULMONARY ARTERY STENOSIS

Stenotic lesions of the pulmonary arterial systems may involve the main, left, or right pulmonary arteries; may be single or multiple; and may be discrete or may involve long segments of the pulmonary artery. A variety of classifications has been proposed (163–166) to account for and describe these variations. Pulmonary arterial stenosis may be an isolated defect (nearly one third to one half) or may be associated with other defects, namely, valvar pulmonary stenosis, patent ductus arteriosus, ventricular septal defect, atrial septal defect, or tetralogy of Fallot. Pulmonary artery stenosis may also be associated with rubella syndrome in conjunction with patent ductus arteriosus and/or valvar pulmonary stenosis (167,168); Williams syndrome along with supravalvar aortic stenosis, elfin facies, mental retardation, and infantile hypercalcemia (169,170); and Alagelle syndrome in combination with hepatic ductular hypoplasia, characteristic facies, and vertebral anomalies (171).

Although some studies suggested that the lesions are nonprogressive (172), other observations (173,174) indicate that rapid progression of the degree of obstruction can occur in less than 2 to 4 years.

The clinical features are generally similar to those observed with valvar pulmonary stenosis and generally depend on the degree of obstruction. The second heart sound is split with normal intensity of the pulmonary component. Ejection systolic click is notably absent. An ejection systolic murmur is heard at left upper sternal border and is well transmitted to axillae and the back. If the obstruction is unilateral, it may be heard better in the ipsilateral chest. A small percent of patients may have a continuous murmur secondary to diastolic gradient across the branch pulmonary artery obstruction.

Chest x-ray shows a normal-sized heart unless the obstruction is severe. Main pulmonary artery dilatation is not seen. Unilateral obstructions, if severe, may show ipsilateral decrease in pulmonary vascular markings with increase in the contralateral lung.

Electrocardiogram may be normal in mild cases. Right ventricular hypertrophy may be seen in moderate to severe obstruction. Superiorly oriented mean QRS vector (left-axis deviation) may be present in patients with rubella syndrome (174a) and Noonan's syndrome (23).

Two-dimensional echocardiographic visualization of branch pulmonary arteries is feasible (175), although distal pulmonary arteries may not be seen. Two-dimensional imaging coupled with color-flow mapping provides reasonable visualization of branch stenosis. However, Doppler gradients are inaccurate in estimating the degree of obstruction. Estimation of right ventricular pressure based on tricuspid regurgitant jet velocity may give a good estimate of right ventricular pressure and thereby an estimate of severity of obstruction. Computed tomography and magnetic resonance imaging are useful in demonstrating the branch obstruction but are not routinely used clinically. Pulmonary perfusion scans (Fig. 11-19) are useful in evaluation of relative flow distribution to the lungs and help in decision making regarding intervention (176).

Cardiac catheterization reveals elevated right ventricular pressure, proportional to the degree of obstruction; this is true with main pulmonary artery and bilateral branch pulmonary artery stenosis. In patients with unilateral pulmonary artery stenosis, the right ventricular and main pulmonary artery pressure may be normal or only mildly elevated. However, in long-standing moderate to severe unilateral pulmonary artery stenosis, elevation of the main and contralateral pulmonary artery pressure may be present, and this is secondary to development of increased vascular tone in the contralateral lung. Careful pressure pullback tracing with an end-hole catheter demonstrates a gradient; a peak-to-peak pressure gradient 10 mm Hg or more is considered significant. In unilateral obstructions, quantita-

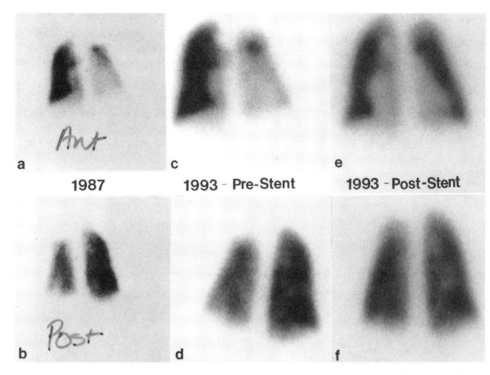

FIG. 11-19. Pulmonary perfusion scan in anterior (*ant*) (**A, C,** and **E**) and posterior (*post*) (**B, D,** and **F**) projections in a teenager with severe residual left pulmonary artery stenosis (see Fig. 11-20) after repair of tetralogy of Fallot. Note markedly decreased perfusion to the left lung (**A** and **B**) in 1987 that remained essentially unchanged (**C** and **D**) before intervention (corresponds to Fig. 11-20A) in 1993. After implantation of a Palmaz-Schatz stent in the left pulmonary artery, the perfusion to left lung (**E** and **F**) increased significantly (corresponds Fig. 11-20B).

tive perfusion scans and angiographic narrowing are better indicators of severity of obstruction than are the pressure gradients. In bilateral obstructions, abnormal contour of the main pulmonary artery pressure trace is present (166,177). The systolic component of the pulmonary arterial pressure trace is similar to that in the right ventricle. The dicrotic notch occurs late and is low, and the diastolic descent of the pressure curve is slow, gradual, and "flat." This results in a wide pulmonary arterial pulse; with increasing severity of obstruction, the pulse pressure becomes increasingly wider.

Selective main pulmonary cineangiogram in a sitting-up view (40 degrees cranial and 15 degrees left anterior oblique) demonstrates location and severity of proximal obstructive lesions (Fig. 11-20A). Distal pulmonary artery stenotic lesions should be demonstrated by selective ipsilateral pulmonary arterial an-

giogram in right anterior oblique or left anterior oblique views, respectively, for right and left pulmonary arteries.

Mild degrees of obstruction do not need treatment. Moderate to severe obstructions should be relieved. Indications for intervention are right ventricular and main pulmonary artery systolic pressures equal to or greater than 50% of aortic systolic pressure along with a peak systolic pressure gradient of at least 20 mm Hg across the stenotic segment and/or decreased ipsilateral perfusion to no more than 30% of total pulmonary flow on a quantitative pulmonary perfusion scan (176). In the past, pericardial or prosthetic patch repair of the stenotic vessel(s) has been attempted (178,179) but has not been uniformly successful. With the advent of balloon angioplasty, because of relatively poor surgical results and surgically inaccessible nature of the lesions, percutaneous

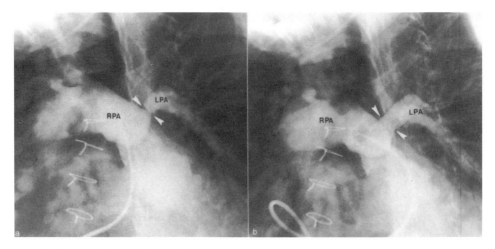

FIG. 11-20. Selected cineangiographic frames from a main pulmonary artery injection in a sitting-up view (15 degrees left anterior oblique and 40 degrees cranial) demonstrating severe narrowing (*solid arrowheads* in **A**) at the origin of left pulmonary artery (*LPA*). After implantation of a stent (**B**), the LPA is wide open. *RPA*, right pulmonary artery.

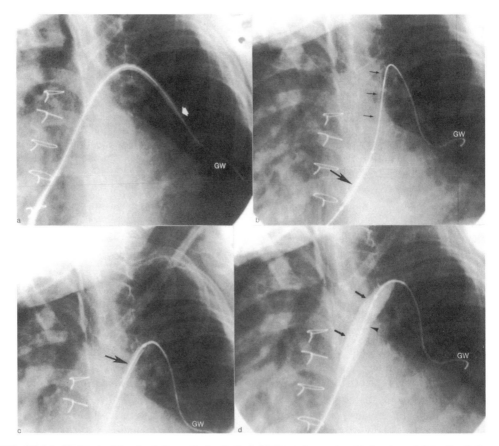

FIG. 11-21. Method of implantation of stent. **A:** Initially, a long sheath is placed into the left pulmonary artery over an already positioned extra-stiff guidewire (GW). **B:** A catheter with the stent mounted on an appropriately sized balloon (*arrow*) is advanced over the GW, but within the sheath. **C:** The stent (*arrow*) is positioned across the stenotic lesion based on other landmarks and the sheath is withdrawn. **D:** The balloon is inflated, thus implanting the stent (*arrow*). Note that the GW is maintained in position throughout the procedure (A–D).

transluminal techniques have been rapidly adopted (180,181). Despite initial enthusiasm and modification of the technique with the use of high-pressure balloon inflation (182), the immediate success rate is low, complication (exsanguination from ruptured pulmonary artery, hemoptysis, pulmonary edema, and pulmonary artery aneurysm) rate is high, and recurrence rate is considerable (183–186). Because of these reasons, intraluminal, balloon-expandable, stainless steel stents, originally described by Palmaz et al. (187), have gained acceptance as a standard mode of therapy (188–190) for the management of branch pulmonary artery stenotic lesions. The procedure of stent implantation (Fig. 11-21) consists of positioning a long 9 to 12F sheath across the stenotic lesion over an extra-stiff Amplatz exchange length wire, positioning a stent mounted on an appropriately sized balloon angioplasty catheter across the stenotic lesion, through the sheath but over the wire, withdrawing the sheath proximally, and inflating the balloon so as to implant the stent across the stenotic lesion. Although the procedure of stent implantation is technically demanding, the results are generally gratifying with improvement of vessel diameter (Fig. 11-20), decrease in pressure gradient and right ventricular pressure, and improved perfusion (Fig. 11-19) to the ipsilateral lung (176,188,190). Restenosis at follow-up has been observed, which appears to be amenable to redilatation (176,189–191).

IDIOPATHIC DILATATION OF THE PULMONARY ARTERY

Idiopathic dilatation of the pulmonary artery is characterized by congenital massive enlargement of the main pulmonary artery and sometimes its primary branches without any discernible causes. Known causes such as pulmonary valve stenosis, severe pulmonary regurgitation, pulmonary vascular obstructive disease (pulmonary hypertension), and syndromes such as Marfan's or Ehlers-Danlos must be excluded.

Clinical presentation is either by the way of an asymptomatic cardiac murmur or detection of an enlarged pulmonary artery on a routine chest x-ray. Whereas the ventricular impulses are normal, visible or palpable impulses of the pulmonary artery in the second left intercostal space may be discerned. No thrills are palpable, although ejection click and pulmonary component of the second sound may be palpable. The first heart sound is normal followed by a late ejection systolic click heard best along the left sternal border. The second heart sound is widely split, with a normal or slightly accentuated pulmonary component. However, the split exhibits normal variation with respiration. The wide split is thought to be related to increased capacitance of the enlarged pulmonary artery with delayed development of recoil to effect pulmonary valve closure (192). A soft, short, mid-systolic murmur of grade I to III/VI may be heard at the left upper sternal border. A low- to medium-frequency early diastolic murmur of pulmonary regurgitation may occasionally be heard.

The electrocardiogram is normal. Chest x-ray shows a normal-sized heart; dilated main pulmonary artery segment, extending sometimes into the left pulmonary artery; and normal pulmonary vascular markings. Echocardiogram reveals normal pulmonary valve leaflets, dilated main pulmonary artery, no transpulmonary valve gradient, and in some cases mild pulmonary regurgitation. Cardiac catheterization is not usually performed, but if performed will reveal no gradient across the pulmonary valve.

The clinical course is benign and the prognosis is excellent, and no treatment other than assurance is necessary.

PULMONARY ATRESIA

Pulmonary atresia with intact ventricular septum is a complex cyanotic congenital cardiac anomaly characterized by complete obstruction of the pulmonary valve, two distinct ventricles, a patent tricuspid valve, and no ventricular septal defect. The right ventricle is usually, but not invariably, small and hypoplastic (Fig. 11-22). This is a rare congenital malformation accounting for approxi-

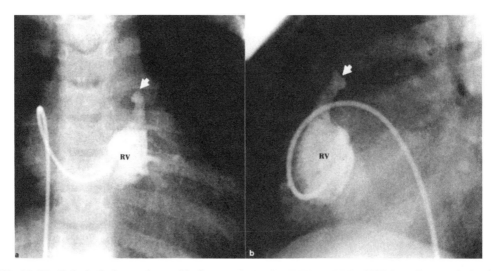

FIG. 11-22. Selected cineangiographic frames from the right ventricle (*RV*) in anteroposterior **(A)** and lateral **(B)** views demonstrating a mid-to-moderately hypoplastic RV. *Arrow*, atretic pulmonary valve.

mately 1% of all congenital cardiac defects and usually presents in the neonatal period. Discussion of this anomaly is beyond the scope of this chapter, and the reader is referred to other publications dealing with the subject (193,194).

Pulmonary atresia can also occur in patients with tetralogy of Fallot and many other complex congenital heart defects such as double-inlet left ventricle, transposition of the great arteries, double-outlet right ventricle, corrected transposition, and tricuspid atresia, and readers are referred to standard textbooks on pediatric cardiology for treatment of these subjects.

SYNDROME OF ABSENT PULMONARY VALVE

The principal features of absent pulmonary valve syndrome are absent or rudimentary pulmonary valve cusps causing pulmonary insufficiency, pulmonary valve ring hypoplasia producing pulmonary stenosis, and massive dilatation of the main and major branch pulmonary arteries resulting in varying degrees of compression of the tracheobronchial tree. This is a rare congenital heart defect and con-

stitutes 3% to 5% of tetralogy of Fallot cases. This syndrome is usually associated with ventricular septal defect and pulmonary stenosis, although it may be occasionally seen as an isolated malformation or with other defects, namely, atrial septal defect, ventricular septal defect, patient ductus arteriosus, endocardial cushion defect, and double-outlet right ventricle.

Two types of clinical presentation are recognized: those who present in early infancy with severe cardiorespiratory distress (because of tracheobronchial compression) and those who present beyond infancy with milder respiratory difficulty. Apart from respiratory difficulty, the infants may have signs of heart failure and are mildly cyanotic. Hyperdynamic cardiac impulses, single second sound, and a to-and-fro murmur of pulmonary stenosis and insufficiency at the left upper sternal border are the other physical findings.

Chest roentgenogram shows mild cardiomegaly, slightly increased pulmonary vascular markings, and, most importantly, prominent right and left pulmonary arteries. Electrocardiogram is suggestive of right ventricular hypertrophy. Echo-Doppler studies demonstrate a large ventricular septal defect, markedly dilated main and branch pulmonary arteries, absent or rudimentary pulmonary valve leaflets, and Doppler evidence for pulmonary stenosis and pulmonary insufficiency. Cardiac catheterization data are suggestive of left-to-right shunt at ventricular level, mild systemic arterial desaturation (secondary to both pulmonary venous desaturation and small interventricular right-to-left shunting), significant peak-to-peak systolic pressure gradient across the pulmonary valve, and an increased ratio of systemic-to-pulmonary flow. Selective cineangiography demonstrates a large subaortic perimembranous ventricular septal defect; moderate-to-severe pulmonary valve ring stenosis; and impressive dilatation of main, right, and left pulmonary arteries (Fig. 11-23A).

Treatment consists of anticongestive measures, chest physiotherapy, and ventilatory support to stabilize the patient followed by total surgical correction (under cardiopulmonary bypass), including closure of the ventricular septal defect, relief of pulmonary stenosis by a transannular pericardial patch as necessary, and partial resection and plastic repair (Fig. 11-23B) of aneurysmally dilated

pulmonary arteries (195). There is some controversy with regard to prosthetic replacement of the pulmonary valve at the time of primary repair (196), but valve replacement may not be necessary at the time of primary repair (195).

PULMONARY REGURGITATION

Pulmonary regurgitation may be caused by a variety of conditions: absent or rudimentary pulmonary valve leaflets (syndrome of absent pulmonary valve is described in the preceding section); congenital abnormality of the pulmonary valve (bicuspid [197] or quadracuspid [198] valves); prolapse of the valve leaflets in an attempt to occlude a high ventricular septal defect (199); idiopathic dilatation of the pulmonary artery (discussed in a preceding section); involvement in carcinoid, rheumatic, or syphilitic disease or endocarditis (all are extremely rare); severe pulmonary hypertension; and, most commonly, iatrogenic, namely, surgical or balloon pulmonary valvotomy/valvuloplasty for pulmonary stenosis or atresia or transannular patch to relieve pulmonary valve ring hypoplasia in patients

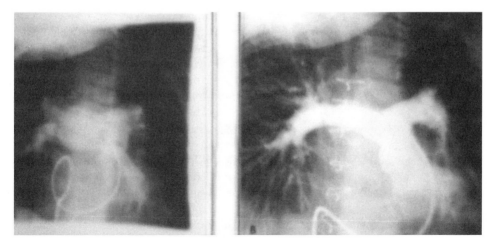

FIG. 11-23. Selected frame from a main pulmonary cineangiogram demonstrating markedly enlarged aneurysmally dilated main, left, and right pulmonary arteries **(A)** in a child with the syndrome of absent pulmonary valves with tetralogy of Fallot. After surgical correction, including partial resection and plastic repair of the pulmonary arteries, repeat pulmonary arteriogram **(B)** reveals near-normal–sized pulmonary arteries. Note pulmonary insufficiency both before and after surgery.

with tetralogy of Fallot or other congenital cardiac defects.

The natural history of pulmonary regurgitation is not well studied. The prognosis of patients with associated defects (e.g., absent pulmonary valve syndrome) and pulmonary vascular obstructive disease (pulmonary hypertension) depends on the primary disease. Based on limited data, isolated pulmonary regurgitation runs a benign course, compatible with an asymptomatic normal lifespan (200–202). However, patients who develop elevated pulmonary artery pressures secondary to lung disease (emphysema), thromboembolism, or left ventricular failure may be subjected to a greater hemodynamic burden with resultant right ventricular failure (197,200, 201,203) and death. Prognosis of patients with pulmonary regurgitation associated with idiopathic dilatation of the pulmonary artery is excellent. Pulmonary regurgitation produced by pulmonary valvotomy for isolated pulmonary stenosis (204) and by total surgical correction of tetralogy of Fallot with or without transannular patch (205,206) is generally well tolerated for years. A small percent of patients may require pulmonary valve replacement to relieve pulmonary regurgitation several years after repair of tetralogy of Fallot (207,208). Finally, pulmonary regurgitation can develop after balloon pulmonary valvuloplasty. However no patient developed severe disease nor required surgical intervention during a follow-up up to 10 years (90). Longer term (15 to 20 years) follow-up may be necessary to confirm the benign nature of the problem.

Isolated pulmonary regurgitation patients come to attention because of a murmur detected on routine examination or because of roentgenographic appearance of a prominent pulmonary artery segment. They usually are asymptomatic. The cardiac impulses are normal, unless the pulmonary regurgitation is severe, in which case hyperdynamic right ventricular impulse may be felt. A prominent impulse may be felt at the left sternal border, indicating a dilated pulsatile pulmonary artery. Thrills are not usually felt. The first heart sound is normal. The second heart sound is normal to widely split, and the pulmonary component may be normal, soft, or inaudible. If the pulmonary artery is significantly dilated, an ejection click may be heard along the left sternal border. An early diastolic decrescendo murmur of grade I to III/VI intensity may be heard best at left upper and mid-sternal border. The murmur is low to medium in pitch in contradistinction to the high-pitched murmur of aortic insufficiency. However, the pulmonary regurgitant murmur associated with pulmonary hypertension is high pitched and is described with an eponym, Graham-Steele murmur. The early diastolic pulmonary regurgitant murmur increases with inspiration. An ejection systolic murmur may also be heard if significant regurgitant volume is present.

The findings in patients with associated defects depend on the features of the associated defects. Postsurgical pulmonary regurgitation patients also exhibit scars of sternotomy.

The electrocardiogram is normal in mild cases. Diastolic overload pattern of QRS complex, manifested by rSR', may be present in moderate to severe pulmonary incompetence. Chest x-ray shows a normal-sized heart with prominent pulmonary artery segment. Cardiomegaly secondary to right ventricular dilatation may be present in severe cases of pulmonary insufficiency. Two-dimensional echocardiography may reveal dilatation of the right ventricle in moderate and severe pulmonary regurgitation cases. The interventricular septal motion may be flat or paradoxical in severe cases. Pulmonary regurgitation can easily be detected by pulsed (Fig. 11-4), continuous-wave (Fig. 11-5), and color Doppler. Color Doppler visualization of pulmonary regurgitation is also observed in normal subjects (up to 40%) and is not necessarily abnormal (209). A short, narrow, nonturbulent, pink jet is characteristic of "normal" pulmonary regurgitation. A combined color Doppler and echocardiographic grading (Table 11-3) has recently been proposed (90) and may be used in quantitation and follow-up evaluation.

TABLE 11-3. *Grading of pulmonary insufficiency by echo-Doppler studies*

None	No pulmonary insufficiency on Doppler study
Grade I	PI jet width[a] ≤ 10% of pulmonary valve annulus diameter in precordial short-axis view No RV volume overload[b]
Grade II	PI jet width between 11% and 25% of pulmonary valve annulus diameter No RV volume overload[b]
Grade III	PI jet width[a] between 26% and 50% of pulmonary valve annulus diameter No volume overload[b] but with or without flat septal motion
Grade IV	PI jet width[a] > 50% of pulmonary valve annulus diameter RV volume overload[b] present

[a]Jet width at the origin of the regurgitation jet rather than jet length was used for grading because the jet width is not influenced by pulmonary artery pressures.

[b]RV volume overload is defined as enlarged RV (greater than 95th percentile) and flat to paradoxical septal motion.

PI, pulmonary insufficiency; RV, right ventricle.

From ref. 90, with permission.

Cardiac catheterization is not necessary in the usual case and may be performed only to exclude any other associated or compounding cardiac abnormality. When performed, the pulmonary arterial pressure trace is abnormal in that there is a wide pulse pressure and, in severe cases, near equilibration of pulmonary artery diastolic and right ventricular end-diastolic pressures (201).

Because of the benign clinical course, no surgical treatment is indicated for isolated pulmonary regurgitation. Bacterial endocarditis prophylaxis and an occasional follow-up is all that is necessary. Appropriate measures to prevent or control secondary pulmonary hypertension may be indicated in selected patients. In postsurgical pulmonary regurgitation cases, a progressive increase in right ventricular volume overload should prompt surgical replacement of the pulmonary valve. Branch pulmonary artery stenosis, if present, should be dealt with, as discussed above.

CONCLUSION

Abnormalities of the pulmonary valve are multiple and varied; valvar stenosis is most common. Careful clinical and noninvasive laboratory evaluation and cardiac catheterization and cineangiography, when indicated, provide accurate diagnosis and assessment of severity. Assurance, clinical follow-up, and/or transcatheter or surgical intervention, as indicated, will generally provide relief of the disease process and augment the prognosis.

REFERENCES

1. Gasul BM, Arcilla RA, Lev M. *Heart Disease in Children: Diagnosis and Treatment*. Philadelphia: JB Lippincott, 1966:763–806.
2. Rao PS. Balloon pulmonary valvuloplasty for isolated pulmonic stenosis. In: Rao PS, ed. *Transcatheter Therapy in Pediatric Cardiology*. New York: Wiley-Liss, 1993:59.
3. Morgagni JB. The seats and causes of diseases investigated by anatomy. *Epistola Anatomico-Medica* 1761;17:435. [Translated from the Latin by Benjamin Alexander, London, Millar, Cadell, Johnson and Payne.]
4. Meckel JR. *Handbuch der menschlichen Anatomie*. Vol. 3. Buchhandlung des Hallischen Waisenhauses, 1817, Berlin.
5. Nadas AS, Fyler DC. *Pediatric Cardiology*, 3rd ed. Philadelphia: WB Saunders, 1972:683.
6. Keith JD, Rowe RD, Vlad P. *Heart Disease in Infancy and Childhood*, 3rd ed. New York: Macmillan, 1978:4–6, 761.
7. Abrahams DG, Wood P. Pulmonary stenosis with normal aortic root. *Br Heart J* 1951;13:519.
8. Campbell M. Simple pulmonary stenosis: pulmonary valvular stenosis with a closed ventricular septum. *Br Heart J* 1954;16:277.
9. Johnson LW, Grossman W, Dalen JE, Dexter L. Pulmonary stenosis in the adult: long-term follow-up results. *N Engl J Med* 1972;287:1159.
10. McCarron WE, Perloff JK. Familial congenital valvar pulmonic stenosis. *Am Heart J* 1974;88:357.
11. Klinger T, Laursen HF. Familial pulmonary stenosis with underdeveloped or normal right ventricle. *Br Heart J* 1975;37:60.
12. Campbell M. Factors in the etiology of pulmonary stenosis. *Br Heart J* 1962;24:625.
13. Nora JJ, Torres FG, Sinha AK, McNamara DG. Characteristic cardiovascular anomalies of XO Turner syn-

drome, XX and XY phenotype and XO/XX Turner mosaic. *Am J Cardiol* 1970;25:639.

14. Nora JJ, Nora AH. Recurrence risk in children having a parent with congenital heart disease. *Circulation* 1976;53:701.

15. Edwards JE. Congenital malformation of the heart and great vessels. In: Gould SE, ed. *Pathology of the Heart.* Springfield, IL: Charles C Thomas, 1953:319.

16. Brock RC. *The Anatomy of the Congenital Pulmonary Stenosis.* New York: Paul B. Hoeber, 1957:1.

17. Gikonyo BM, Lucus RV, Edwards JE. Anatomic features of congenital pulmonary valvar stenosis. *Pediatr Cardiol* 1987;8:109.

18. Roberts WC, Mason DT, Morrow AG, Braunwald E. Calcific pulmonic stenosis. *Circulation* 1968;37:973.

19. Gabriele OF, Scatriff JH. Pulmonary valve calcification. *Am Heart J* 1970;80:299.

20. Koretzky ED, Moller JH, Korns ME, et al. Congenital pulmonary stenosis resulting from dysplasia of the valve. *Circulation* 1969;60:43.

21. Jeffery RF, Moller JH, Amplatz K. The dysplastic pulmonary valve: a new roentgenographic entity. *Am J Roentgenol Ther Radium Nucl Med* 1977;114:322.

22. Linde LM, Turner SW, Sparkes RS. Pulmonary valvular dysplasia: a cardiofacial syndrome. *Br Heart J* 1973;35:301.

23. Noonan JA. Hypertelorism with Turner phenotype: a new syndrome with associated congenital heart disease. *Am J Dis Child* 1968;116:373.

24. Thapar MK, Rao PS. Significance of infundibular obstruction following balloon valvuloplasty for valvar pulmonic stenosis. *Am Heart J* 1989;118:99.

25. Hoffman E. On circumscribed dilatation of an artery immediately distal to a partially occluding band: poststenotic dilatation. *Surgery* 1954;36:3.

26. Rodbard S, Ikeda K, Montes M. Mechanisms of poststenotic dilatation. *Circulation* 1963;28:791.

27. Harnick E, Becker AE, Gittenberger-De Groot AC, et al. The left ventricle in congenital isolated pulmonary stenosis. *Br Heart J* 1977;39:429.

28. Sholler GF, Colan SD, Sanders SP. Effect of isolated right ventricular outflow tract obstruction on left ventricular function in children. *Am J Cardiol* 1988;62: 778.

29. Williams JCP, Barratt-Boyes BG, Lowe JB. Underdeveloped right ventricle and pulmonary stenosis. *Am J Cardiol* 1963;11:458.

30. Nugent EW, Freedom RM, Nora JJ, et al. Clinical course of pulmonic stenosis. *Circulation* 1977;56 [Suppl I]:I.

31. Tinker J, Howitt G, Markman P, et al. The natural history of isolated pulmonary stenosis. *Br Heart J* 1985; 27:151.

32. Moller I, Wennevold A, Lyngborg KE. The natural history of pulmonic stenosis: long-term follow-up with serial heart catheterizations. *Cardiology* 1973;58:193.

33. Mody MR. The natural history of uncomplicated valvar pulmonic stenosis. *Am Heart J* 1975;90:317.

34. Moller JH, Adams P. The natural history of pulmonary valvular stenosis: serial cardiac catheterization in 21 children. *Am J Cardiol* 1965;16:654.

35. Danilowicz D, Hoffman JE, Rudolph AM. Serial studies of pulmonary stenosis in infancy and childhood. *Br Heart J* 1975;37:808.

36. Levine RO, Blumenthal S. Pulmonic stenosis in five congenital cardiac defects. *Circulation* 1985;31-32[Suppl II]:33.

37. Wennevold A, Jacobsen JR. Natural history of valvular pulmonic stenosis in children below the age of two years: long-term follow-up with serial heart catheterizations. *Eur J Cardiol* 1978;8:371.

38. Lueker RD, Vogel JHK, Blount SG, Jr. Regression of valvular pulmonary stenosis. *Br Heart J* 1970;32:779.

39. Hayes CJ, Gersony WM, Driscoll DJ, et al. Second natural history study of congenital heart defects: results of treatment of patients with pulmonary valvar stenosis. *Circulation* 1993;87[Suppl I]:28.

40. Lange PE, Onnasch DGW, Heintzen PH. Valvular pulmonary stenosis: natural history and right ventricular function. In: Doyle EF, et al., eds. *Pediatric Cardiology.* New York: Springer-Verlag, 1986:395–398.

41. Nadas AS. Pulmonary stenosis: indications for surgery in children and adults. *N Engl J Med* 1972;287:1196.

42. Moller JH, Rao S, Lucas RV, Jr. Exercise hemodynamics of pulmonary valvular stenosis: study of 64 children. *Circulation* 1972;46:1018.

43. Krabill KA, Wang Y, Einzid S, Moller JH. Rest and exercise hemodynamics in pulmonary stenosis: comparison of children and adults. *Am J Cardiol* 1985;36:360.

44. Blount SG, Jr, Komesu S, McCord MC. Asymptomatic isolated valvular pulmonary stenosis. *N Engl J Med* 1953;248:5.

45. Wood P. Congenital pulmonary stenosis with left ventricular enlargement associated with atrial septal defect. *Br Heart J* 1942;4:11.

46. Ainworth H, Hunt J, Joseph M. Numerical evaluation of facial pattern in children with isolated pulmonary stenosis. *Arch Dis Child* 1979;54:662.

47. Alday LE, Moreyra E. Calcific pulmonary stenosis. *Br Heart J* 1973;35:887.

48. Vogelpoel L, Schrire V. Auscultatory and phonocardiographic assessment of pulmonary stenosis with intact ventricular septum. *Circulation* 1960;22:55.

49. Rao PS. Evaluation of cardiac murmur in children. *Indian J Pediatr* 1991;58:605.

50. Buckingham WB, Sutton CG, Mezaros WT. Abnormality of the pulmonary artery resembling neoplasms. *Dis Chest* 1961;40:698.

51. Rumbak MJ, Scott M, Walsh FW. Left hilar mass in a 62-year-old man: severe pulmonary valvular stenosis with a poststenotic aneurysm. *South Med J* 1996;89: 824.

52. Diamond EG, Lin TK. The clinical picture of pulmonary stenosis (without ventricular septal defect). *Ann Intern Med* 1954;40:1106.

53. Mehra-Pour M, Whitney A, Liebman J, Borkat G. Quantification of Frank and MacFee-Parunguo orthogonal electrocardiogram in valvar pulmonic stenosis: correlation with hemodynamic measurements. *J Electrocardiol* 1979;12:69.

54. Weyman AE, Dillon JC, Feigenbaum H, Chang S. Echocardiographic patterns of pulmonary valve motion in valvular pulmonary stenosis. *Am J Cardiol* 1974;34:644.

55. LeBlanc MH, Paquet M. Echocardiographic assessment of valvular pulmonary stenosis in children. *Br Heart J* 1981;46:363.

56. Weyman AE, Hurwitz RA, Girod DA. Cross-sectional echocardiographic visualization of the stenotic pulmonary valve. *Circulation* 1977;56:769.

57. Guttgesell HP, et al. Accuracy of two-dimensional echocardiography in the diagnosis of congenital heart disease. *Am J Cardiol* 1985;55:514.

58. Lima CO, Sahn DJ, Valdez-Cruz IM, et al. Noninvasive prediction of transvalvar pressure gradients in patients with pulmonic stenosis by quantitative two-dimensional echocardiographic Doppler studies. *Circulation* 1983;67:866.

59. Johnson GL, et al. Accuracy of combined two-dimensional echocardiography and continuous wave Doppler recordings in the estimation of pressure gradient in right ventricular outlet obstruction. *J Am Coll Cardiol* 1984;3:1013.

60. Currie PJ, et al. Continuous wave Doppler determination of right ventricular pressure: a simultaneous Doppler catheterization study in 127 patients. *J Am Coll Cardiol* 1985;6:750.

61. Rao PS. Doppler ultrasound in the prediction of transvalvar pressure gradients in patients with pulmonic stenosis. *Int J Cardiol* 1987;15:195.

62. Hatle L, Angelsen B. *Doppler Ultrasound in Cardiology: Physical Principles and Clinical Applications.* Philadelphia: Lea & Febiger, 1982.

63. Silove ED, Vogel JHK, Grover RF. The pressure gradient in ventricular outflow obstruction: influence of peripheral resistance. *Cardiovasc Res* 1968;3:234.

64. Rao PS, Linde LM. Pressure and energy in cardiovascular chambers. *Chest* 1974;66:176.

65. Rao PS, Andaya WG, Whisenand HW. Contrast echocardiography in the differential diagnosis of hypoxemia following open heart surgery. *King Faisal Specialist Hosp Med J* 1983;3:121.

66. Gorlin R, Gorlin SG. Hydraulic formula for calculation of the area of the stenotic mitral valve, other valves and central circulatory shunts. *Am Heart J* 1951;41:1.

67. Muster AJ, VanGrandelle A, Paul MH. Unequal pressures in central pulmonary arterial branches in patients with pulmonary stenosis: the influence of blood velocity and anatomy. *Pediatr Cardiol* 1982;2:7.

68. Lewis JM, Montero AG, Kinard SA, Jr, Dennis EQ, Alexander JK. Hemodynamic response to exercise in isolated pulmonic stenosis. *Circulation* 1964;29:854.

69. Howitt G. Haemodynamic effects of exercise in isolated pulmonary stenosis. *Br Heart J* 1966;28:152.

70. Ikkos D, Jonsson B, Linderholm H. Effect of exercise in pulmonary stenosis with intact ventricular septum. *Br Heart J* 1968;28:316.

71. Jonsson B, Lee SJK. Hemodynamic effects of exercise in isolated pulmonary stenosis before and after surgery. *Br Heart J* 1968;39:60.

72. Stone FM, Bessinger FB Jr, Lucas RV Jr, Moller JH. Pre- and postoperative rest and exercise hemodynamics in children with pulmonary stenosis. *Circulation* 1974;49:1102.

73. Neal WA, Lucas RV, Rao S, Moller JH. Comparison of the hemodynamic effects of exercise and isoproterenol infusion in patients with pulmonary valve stenosis. *Circulation* 1974;49:949.

74. Trucone NJ, Steeg CN, Dell R, Gersony WM. Comparison of cardiocirculatory effects of exercise and isoproterenol in children with pulmonary and aortic valve stenosis. *Circulation* 1977;56:79.

75. Moss AJ, Quivers WW. Use of isoproterenol in the evaluation of aortic and pulmonic stenosis. *Am J Cardiol* 1963;11:734.

76. Rao PS, Liebman J, Borkat G. Right ventricular growth in a case of pulmonic stenosis with intact ventricular septum and hypoplastic right ventricle. *Circulation* 1976;53:389.

77. Nakazawa M, Marks RA, Isabel-Jones J, Jarmakani JM. Right and left ventricular volume characteristics in children with pulmonary stenosis with intact ventricular septum. *Circulation* 1976;53:884.

78. Prevention of bacterial endocarditis: recommendation by the American Heart Association by the Committee on Rheumatic Fever, Endocarditis, and Kawasaki Disease. *JAMA* 1997;277:1794.

79. McIntosh HD, Cohen AI. Pulmonary stenosis: the importance of the myocardial factor in determining the clinical course and surgical results. *Am Heart J* 1963; 65:715.

80. Tabatabaei H, Boutin C, Nykanen DC, et al. Morphologic and hemodynamic consequences after percutaneous balloon valvotomy for neonatal pulmonary stenosis: medium-term follow-up. *J Am Coll Cardiol* 1996;27:473.

81. Rao PS. Technique of balloon pulmonary valvuloplasty in the neonate [letter]. *J Am Coll Cardiol* 1994; 23:1735.

82. Rao PS. Balloon valvuloplasty in the neonate with critical pulmonary stenosis [editorial]. *J Am Coll Cardiol* 1996;27:471.

83. Jureidini SB, Rao PS. Critical pulmonary stenosis in the neonate: role of transcatheter management. *J Invasive Cardiol* 1996;8:326.

84. Sellors T. Surgery for pulmonary stenosis: a case in which pulmonary valve is successfully divided. *Lancet* 1948;1:988.

85. Brock RC. Pulmonary valvotomy for relief of congenital stenosis: report of 3 cases. *Br Med J* 1948;1:1121.

86. Mustard WT, Trusler GA. Pulmonic stenosis with normal aortic root. In: Benson CD, Mustard WT, Ravitch MH, Snyder WH Jr, Welch KJ, eds. *Pediatric Surgery.* Vol. I. Chicago: Year Book, 1962;73.

87. Danielson GK, Exarhos ND, Weidman WH, McGoon DC. Pulmonic stenosis with intact ventricular septum: surgical considerations and results of operation. *J Thorac Cardiovasc Surg* 1971;79:464.

88. Bashour T, et al. Pulmonic valvular stenosis: clinical hemodynamic correlation and surgical results. *J Vasc Dis* 1984;35:222.

89. McNamara DG, Latson LA. Long-term follow-up of patients with malformation for which definitive surgical repair has been available for 25 years or more. *Am J Cardiol* 1982;50:560.

90. Rao PS, Galal O, Patnana M, Buck SH, Wilson AD. Three-to-ten-year follow-up results of balloon pulmonary valvuloplasty. *Heart* 1998;80:591.

91. Rubio-Alvarez V, Limon-Lason R, Soni J. Valvulotomias intracardiacas por medio de un cateter. *Arch Inst Cordiol Mex* 1952;23:183.

92. Rubio V, Limon-Lason R. Treatment of pulmonary valvular stenosis and tricuspid stenosis using a modified catheter. 2nd World Congress of Cardiology, Washington, DC, Program Abstract, 1954;II:205.

93. Semb BKH, Tijonneland S, Stake G, et al. "Balloon valvulotomy" of congenital pulmonary valve stenosis with tricuspid valve insufficiency. *Cardiovasc Radiol* 1979;2:239.

94. Kan JS, White RJ Jr, Mitchell SE, Gardner TJ. Percu-

taneous balloon valvuloplasty: a new method for treating congenital pulmonary valve stenosis. *N Engl J Med* 1982;307:540.

95. Dotter CT, Judkins MP. Transluminal treatment of arteriosclerotic obstruction: description of a new technique and a preliminary report of its application. *Circulation* 1967;30:654.

96. Gruntzig AR, Senning A, Siegothaler WE. Non-operative dilatation of coronary artery stenosis: percutaneous transluminal coronary angioplasty. *N Engl J Med* 1979;301:61.

97. Rao PS. Indications for balloon pulmonary valvuloplasty [editorial]. *Am Heart J* 1988;116:1661.

98. Rao PS. Balloon pulmonary valvuloplasty [letter]. *Cathet Cardiovasc Diagn* 1997;40:101.

99. Rao PS. Influence of balloon size on short-term and long-term results of balloon pulmonary valvuloplasty. *Tex Heart Inst J* 1987;14:57.

100. Radtke W, Keane JL, Fellows KE, Lang P, Lock JE. Percutaneous balloon valvotomy of congenital pulmonary stenosis using oversized balloons. *J Am Coll Cardiol* 1986;8:909.

101. Rao PS. Further observations on the effect of balloon size on the short-term and intermediate-term results of balloon dilatation of the pulmonary valve. *Br Heart J* 1988;60:507.

102. Rao PS. Transcatheter treatment of pulmonary outflow tract obstruction: a review. *Progr Cardiovasc Dis* 1995;35:119.

103. Rao PS. Pulmonary valve in children. In: Sigwart U, Bertrand M, Serruys PW, eds. *Handbook of Cardiovascular Interventions.* New York: Churchill Livingstone, 1996:273.

104. Abels JE. Balloon catheters and transluminal dilatation: technical considerations. *AJR Am J Roentgenol* 1980;135:901.

105. Rao PS. Balloon angioplasty and valvuloplasty in infants, children and adolescents. *Curr Probl Cardiol* 1989;14:417.

106. Walls JT, Lababidi Z, Curtis JJ, et al. Assessment of percutaneous balloon pulmonary and aortic valvuloplasty. *J Thorac Cardiovasc Surg* 1984;88:352.

107. Ettedgui JA, Ho SY, Tynan M, et al. The pathology of balloon pulmonary valvuloplasty. *Int J Cardiol* 1987;16:285.

108. Burrows PE, Benson LN, Smallhorn JS, et al. Angiographic features associated with percutaneous balloon valvotomy for pulmonary valve stenosis. *Cardiovasc Intervent Radiol* 1988;11:111.

109. Benson LN, Smallhorn JS, Freedom RM, et al. Pulmonary valve morphology after balloon dilatation of pulmonary valve stenosis. *Cathet Cardiovasc Diagn* 1985;11:161.

110. Rao PS. Right ventricular filling following balloon pulmonary valvuloplasty. *Am Heart J* 1992;123:1084.

111. Rao PS, Thapar MK, Kutayli F. Causes of restenosis following balloon valvuloplasty for valvar pulmonic stenosis. *Am J Cardiol* 1988;62:979.

112. McCrindle BW for VACA Registry. Independent predictors of long-term results after balloon pulmonary valvuloplasty. *Circulation* 1994;89;1751.

113. Rao PS, Galal O, Wilson AD. Feasibility and effectiveness of repeat balloon dilatation of restenosed obstructions following previous balloon valvuloplasty/angioplasty. *Am Heart J* 1996;132:403.

114. Fontes VF, Esteves CA, Eduardo J, et al. Regression of infundibular hypertrophy after pulmonary valvotomy for pulmonic stenosis. *Am J Cardiol* 1988;62:977.

115. Engle ME, Holswade GR, Goldberg HP, Lukas DS, Glenn F. Regression after open valvotomy of infundibular stenosis accompanying severe valvar pulmonary stenosis. *Circulation* 1958;17:862.

116. Johnson AM. Hypertonic infundibular stenosis complicating simple pulmonary valve stenosis. *Br Heart J* 1959;21:429.

117. Gilbert JW, Morrow AG, Talbert JL. The surgical significance of hypertrophic infundibular obstruction accompanying valvular pulmonary stenosis. *J Thorac Cardiovasc Surg* 1963;46:457.

118. Rao PS, Thapar MK. Balloon pulmonary valvuloplasty [letter]. *Am Heart J* 1991;121:1839.

119. Rao PS, Solymar L. Electrocardiographic changes following balloon dilatation of valvar pulmonic stenosis. *J Intervent Cardiol* 1988;1:189.

120. Rao PS. Value of echo-Doppler studies in the evaluation of the results of balloon pulmonary valvuloplasty. *J Cardiovasc Ultrasonogr* 1986;5:309.

121. Rao PS. Balloon dilatation in infants and children with dysplastic pulmonary valves: short-term and intermediate-term results. *Am Heart J* 1988;116:1168.

122. Marantz PM, Huhta JC, Mullins CE, et al. Results of balloon valvuloplasty in atypical and dysplastic pulmonary valve stenosis: Doppler echocardiographic follow-up. *J Am Coll Cardiol* 1988;12:476.

123. Ring JC, Kulik TT, Burke BA, et al. Morphologic changes induced by dilatation of pulmonary valve annulus with overlarge balloons in normal newborn lamb. *Am J Cardiol* 1986;52:210.

124. O'Connor BK, Beekman RH III, Lindaur A, et al. Intermediate-term outcome after balloon pulmonary valvuloplasty: comparison with a matched surgical control. *J Am Coll Cardiol* 1992;20:169.

125. Pepine CJ, Gessner IH, Feldman RI. Percutaneous balloon valvuloplasty for pulmonic valve stenosis in the adult. *Am J Cardiol* 1983;50:1442.

126. Al Kasab S, Ribeiro PA, Al Zaibag M, et al. Percutaneous double balloon pulmonary valvotomy in adults: one-to-two-year follow-up. *Am J Cardiol* 1988;62: 822.

127. Fawzy ME, Mercer EN, Dunn B. Late results of pulmonary balloon valvuloplasty in adults using double balloon technique. *J Intervent Cardiol* 1988;1:35.

128. Silvert H, Kober G, Bussman J, et al. Long-term results of percutaneous pulmonary valvuloplasty in adults. *Eur Heart J* 1989;10:712.

129. Chen CR, Cheng TO, Huang T, et al. Percutaneous valvuloplasty for pulmonic stenosis in adolescents and adults. *N Engl J Med* 1996;335:21.

130. Teupe CHJ, Burger W, Schrader R, Zeiher A. Late (five to nine years) follow-up after balloon dilatation of valvar pulmonary stenosis in adults. *Am J Cardiol* 1997; 80:240.

131. Rao PS. How big a balloon and how many balloons for pulmonary valvuloplasty [editorial]. *Am Heart J* 1989;116:577.

132. Rao PS, Fawzy ME. Double balloon technique for percutaneous balloon pulmonary valvuloplasty: comparison with single balloon technique. *J Intervent Cardiol* 1988;1:257.

133. Lau KW, Jung JS, Wu JJ, et al. Pulmonary valvulo-

plasty in adults using the Inoue balloon catheter. *Cathet Cardiovasc Diagn* 1993;29:99.

134. Bahl VK, Chandra S, Goel A, Goswami KC, Wasir HS. Versatility of Inoue balloon catheter. *Int J Cardiol* 1997;59:75.

135. Gibbs JL, Stanley CP, Dickenson DF. Pulmonary balloon valvuloplasty in late adult life. *Int J Cardiol* 1986;11:237.

136. Cooke JP, Seward JB, Holmes DR Jr. Transluminal balloon valvotomy for pulmonic stenosis in adults. *Mayo Clin Proc* 1987;62:306.

137. Feugelman MY, Lewis BS. Pulmonary balloon valvuloplasty in the seventh decade of life. *Isr J Med Sci* 1988;24:112.

138. Rao PS, Fawzy ME, Solymar L, et al. Long-term results of balloon pulmonary valvuloplasty. *Am Heart J* 1988;115:1291.

139. McCrindle B, Kan J. Long-term results after balloon pulmonary valvuloplasty. *Circulation* 1991;83:1915.

140. Weyman AE, Dillon JC, Feigenbaum H, Chang S. Echocardiographic differentiation of infundibular from valvar pulmonic stenosis. *Am J Cardiol* 1975; 36:21.

141. Mullins CE, Latson LA, Neches WH, Colvin EV, Kan J. Balloon dilatation of miscellaneous lesions: results of Valvuloplasty and Angioplasty of Congenital Anomalies Registry. *Am J Cardiol* 1990;65:802.

142. Rao PS, Thapar MK. Balloon dilatation of other congenital and acquired stenotic lesions of the cardiovascular system. In: Rao PS, ed. *Transcatheter Therapy in Pediatric Cardiology*. New York: Wiley-Liss, 1993: 275.

143. Lucas RV Jr, Varco RL, Lillehei CW, et al. Anomalous muscle bundle of the right ventricle: hemodynamic consequences and surgical considerations. *Circulation* 1962;25:443.

144. Matina D, et al. Subxiphoid two-dimensional echocardiographic diagnosis of double-chambered right ventricle. *Circulation* 1983;67:885.

145. Chandrashekar YS, Anand IS, Wahi PL. Balloon dilatation of double-chamber right ventricle. *Am Heart J* 1990;120:1234.

146. Braunwald E, et al. Idiopathic hypertrophic subaortic stenosis. 1. A description of the disease based on analysis of 64 patients. *Circulation* 1964;29(Suppl IV):3.

147. Morrow AC, Fisher RD, Fogarty TJ. Isolated hypertrophic obstruction to the right ventricular outflow: clinical hemodynamic and angiographic findings before and after operative treatment. *Am Heart J* 1969; 77:814.

148. Dellocchio T, et al. Left ventricular hypertrophy with right ventricular outflow obstruction. *Br Heart J* 1972; 34:754.

149. Anderson RC, Lellehei CW, Lester RG. Corrected transposition of the great vessels of the heart: a review of 17 cases. *Pediatrics* 1957;20:727.

150. Lev M, Rowlatt UF. The pathologic anatomy of mixed levocardia: a review of 13 cases of atrial or ventricular inversion with or without corrected transposition. *Am J Cardiol* 1961;8:216.

151. Reddy SCB, Chopra PS, Rao PS. Aneurysm of the membranous ventricular septum resulting in pulmonary outflow tract obstruction in congenitally corrected transposition of the great arteries. *Am Heart J* 1997;133:112.

152. Rotem CE, Hultgren HN. Corrected transposition of the great vessels without associated defects. *Am Heart J* 1965;70:305.

153. Nagle JP, Cheitlin MD, McCarty RJ. Corrected transposition of the great vessels without associated anomalies: report of a case with congestive heart failure at age 45. *Chest* 1971;60:367.

154. Vacek JL, Goertz KK. Balloon valvuloplasty of a subpulmonary membrane. *Am Heart J* 1990;119:1419.

155. Suarez de Lezo J, Pan M, Sancho M, et al. Percutaneous transluminal balloon dilatation for discrete subaortic stenosis. *Am Heart J* 1986;58:619.

156. Lababidi Z, Weinhaus L, Stoeckle H, Wall JT. Transluminal balloon dilatation for discrete subaortic stenosis. *Am J Cardiol* 1987;59:423.

157. Rao PS, Wilson AD, Chopra PS. Balloon dilatation for discrete subaortic stenosis: immediate and intermediate-term results. *J Invasive Cardiol* 1990;2:65.

158. Summerall CP III, Clowes GHA Jr, Boone JA. Aneurysm of ventricular septum with outflow obstruction of the venous ventricle in corrected transposition of the great vessels. *Am Heart J* 1966;72:525.

159. Falsetti HL, Anderson MN. Aneurysm of the membranous ventricular septum producing right ventricular outflow tract obstruction and left ventricular failure. *Chest* 1971;59:578.

160. Losekoot TG, Andersen RH, Becker AE, et al. Pulmonary stenosis. In: *Modern Pediatric Cardiology: Congenitally Corrected Transposition*. Edinburgh: Churchill Livingstone, 1983:123.

161. Krongard E, Elis K, Steeg CN, et al. Subpulmonary obstruction in congenitally corrected transposition of the great arteries due to ventricular membranous septal aneurysms. *Circulation* 1976;54:679.

162. Ignaszewski AP, Collins-Nakai RL, Gulamhussein SS, et al. Aneurysm of the membranous septum producing subpulmonic outflow tract obstruction. *Can J Cardiol* 1994;10:67.

163. Smith WG. Pulmonary hypertension and a continuous murmur due to multiple peripheral stenosis of the pulmonary arteries. *Thorax* 1958;13:194.

164. Franch RH, Gay BB, Jr. Congenital stenosis of the pulmonary artery branches: a classification, with postmortem findings in two cases. *Am J Cardiol* 1963;35: 512.

165. Gay BB, Franch RH, Shuford WR, Rogers JV. Roentgenographic features of simple and multiple coarctations of the pulmonary artery and branches. *Am J Roentgenol* 1963;90:599.

166. Rowe RD. Pulmonary arterial stenosis. In: Keith JD, Rowe RD, Vlad P, eds. *Heart Disease in Infancy and Childhood*, 3rd ed. New York: Macmillan, 1978:789.

167. Emmanouilides GC, Linde LM, Crittenden IH. Pulmonary artery stenosis associated with ductus arteriosus following maternal rubella. *Circulation* 1964;29: 51.

168. Hastreiter AR, Joorabachi B, Pujatti G, et al. Cardiovascular lesions associated with congenital rubella. *J Pediatr* 1967;71:59.

169. Beuren AJ, Schulze C, Eberle P, et al. The syndrome of supravalvar aortic stenosis, peripheral pulmonary stenosis, mental retardation and similar facial appearance. *Am J Cardiol* 1964;13:471.

170. Roberts N, Moes CAF. Supravalvar pulmonary stenosis. *J Pediatr* 1973;82:838.

171. Allagille D, Odievre M, Gautier M, Dommergues JP. Hepatic ductular hypoplasia associated with characteristic facies, vertebral malformations, retarded physical, mental and sexual development, and cardiac murmur. *J Pediatr* 1975;86:63.

172. Eldregde WJ, Tingelstad JB, Robertsen LW, et al. Observations on the natural history of pulmonary artery coarctations. *Circulation* 1972;45:404.

173. Orell SR, Karnell J, Walhgren F. Malformation and multiple stenoses of the pulmonary arteries with pulmonary hypertension. *Acta Radiol* 1960;54:449.

174. Papadopoulos GG, Folger GM Jr. Progressive pulmonary arterial stenosis. *Am J Cardiol* 1983;51:1662.

174a. Hollaran KH, Sanyal SK, Gardner TH. Superiorly oriented electrocardiographic axis in infants with rubella syndrome. *Am Heart J* 1966;72:600.

175. Tinker DD, Nanda ND, Harris JP, Manning JA. Two-dimensional echocardiographic identification of pulmonary artery branch stenosis. *Am J Cardiol* 1982;50:814.

176. Chandar JS, Wolfe SB, Rao PS. Role of stents in the management of congenital heart defects. *J Invasive Cardiol* 1996;8:314.

177. Augustsson MH, Arcilla RA, Gasul BM, et al. The diagnosis of bilateral stenosis of the primary pulmonary branches based on characteristic pulmonary trunk pressure curves. *Circulation* 1962;26:621.

178. Smith GW, Thompson WM, Muller WH. Surgical treatment of pulmonary hypertension secondary to multiple bilateral pulmonary arterial stenosis. *Circulation* 1964;29[Suppl]:152.

179. McGoon DC, Kincaid OW. Stenosis of branches of the pulmonary artery; surgical repair. *Med Clin North Am* 1964;48:1053.

180. Martin EC, Diamond NG, Casarella WJ. Percutaneous transluminal angioplasty in non-atherosclerotic disease. *Radiology* 1980;135:27.

181. Lock JE, Castaneda-Zuniga WR, Fuhrman BP, Bass JL. Balloon dilatation angioplasty of hypoplastic and stenotic pulmonary arteries. *Circulation* 1983;67:962.

182. Gentles TL, Lock JE, Perry SB. High pressure balloon angioplasty for branch pulmonary artery stenosis: early experience. *J Am Coll Cardiol* 1993;22:867.

183. Rucchani AP, Kveslis D, Dick M, et al. Use of balloon angioplasty to treat peripheral pulmonary stenosis. *Am J Cardiol* 1984;54:1069.

184. Ring JC, Bass JL, Marvin W, et al. Management of congenital stenosis of a branch pulmonary artery with balloon dilatation angioplasty: report of 52 procedures. *J Thorac Cardiovasc Surg* 1985;90:35.

185. Kan JS, Marvin WJ, Bass JL, et al. Balloon angioplasty of branch pulmonary artery stenosis: results of Valvuloplasty and Angioplasty of Congenital Anomalies Registry. *Am J Cardiol* 1990; 65:798.

186. Rothman A, Perry SB, Keane JF, et al. Early results and follow-up of balloon angioplasty for branch pulmonary artery stenosis. *J Am Coll Cardiol* 1990;15:1109.

187. Palmaz JC, Sibbitt RR, Tio FO, et al. Expandable intraluminal vascular graft: a feasibility study. *Surgery* 1986;96:199.

188. O'Laughlin MP, Perry SB, Lock JE, Mullins CE. Use of endovascular stents in congenital heart disease. *Circulation* 1991;83:1923.

189. O'Laughlin MP, Slack MC, Grifka RG, et al. Implantation and intermediate-term follow-up of stents in congenital heart disease. *Circulation* 1993;88:605.

190. Fogelman R, Nykanen D, Smallhorn JF, et al. Endovascular stents in the pulmonary circulation: clinical impact on management and medium-term follow-up. *Circulation* 1995;92:881.

191. Ing FF, Grifka RG, Nihill MR, Mullins CE. Repeat dilatation of intravascular stents in congenital heart defects. *Circulation* 1995;92:893.

192. Schrire V, Vogelpoel L. The role of the dilated pulmonary artery in abnormal splitting of the second heart sound. *Am Heart J* 1962;63:501.

193. Freedom RM. *Pulmonary Atresia with Intact Ventricular Septum.* Mount Kisco, NY: Futura Publishing, 1989:1.

194. Rao PS. Comprehensive management of pulmonary atresia with intact ventricular septum. *Ann Thorac Surg* 1985;40:409.

195. Rao PS, Lawrie GM. Absent pulmonary valve syndrome: surgical correction with pulmonary arterioplasty. *Br Heart J* 1983;50:586.

196. Ilbawi MN, Idriss FS, Muster AJ, et al. Tetralogy of Fallot with absent pulmonary valve: should valve insertion be a part of the intracardiac repair? *J Thorac Cardiovasc Surg* 1981;81:906.

197. Dickens J, Raber CT, Goldberg H. Dynamic pulmonary regurgitation associated with a bicuspid valve. *Ann Intern Med* 1958;48:851.

198. Kissin M. Pulmonary insufficiency with a supernumery cusp in the pulmonary valve: report of a case with review of literature. *Am Heart J* 1936;12:206.

199. Gould I, Lyan AF. Prolapse of the pulmonary valve through a ventricular septal defect. *Am J Cardiol* 1966;18:127.

200. Fish RG, Takaro T, Crymer T. Prognostic consideration in primary isolated insufficiency of the pulmonary valve. *N Engl J Med* 1959;201:739.

201. Hamby RJ, Gulotta SJ. Pulmonary valvar insufficiency: etiology, recognition and management. *Am Heart J* 1967;74:110.

202. Holmes JG, Fowler NO, Kaplan S. Pulmonary valvar insufficiency. *Am J Med* 1968;44:851.

203. Lendrum BL, Shaffer AB. Isolated congenital pulmonic valvar regurgitation. *Am Heart J* 1959;57:298.

204. Hoiser DM, Pitts JL, Taussig HB. Results of valvotomy for valvar pulmonary stenosis with intact ventricular septum: analysis of sixty-nine patients. *Circulation* 1956;14:9.

205. Kay EB, Nogueiru C, Mendelsohn D Jr, Zimmerman HA. Corrective surgery for tetralogy of Fallot: evaluation of results. *Circulation* 1961;24:1342.

206. Finnegan F, Heider R, Patel RG, et al. Results of total correction of tetralogy of Fallot: long-term hemodynamic evaluation at rest and during exercise. *Br Heart J* 1976;38:934.

207. Idriss FS, Markovitz A, Nikaidoh H, et al. Insertion of Hancock valve for pulmonary valve insufficiency in previously repaired tetralogy of Fallot. *Circulation* 1976;54[Suppl II]:100.

208. Miller CS, Rossiter SJ, Stinson EB, et al. Late right heart reconstruction following repair of tetralogy of Fallot. *Ann Thorac Surg* 1979;28:239.

209. Brand A, Dollberg S, Keren A. The prevalence of valvar regurgitation in children with structurally normal hearts: a color Doppler echocardiography study. *Am Heart J* 1992;123:177.

12

Tricuspid Valve Disease

Gordon A. Ewy

Department of Medicine, University of Arizona and Arizona Health Sciences Center,
Tucson, Arizona 85724

Tricuspid valve disease remains a challenge because its malfunction is often difficult to diagnose, its significance often unclear, and therapeutic approaches often unproven. Nevertheless, the clinician should not overlook tricuspid valve disease because it rarely presents as an isolated finding. Its presence should stimulate a search for one of the several potential causes, many of which are treatable.

ANATOMY

The anatomy of the tricuspid valve is complicated and somewhat variable. Tricuspid valve disease can result from malformation or malfunction of any of a number of interrelated structures referred to as the tricuspid valve "complex." An understanding of tricuspid valve disease requires an appreciation of the mitral valve complex. The tricuspid valve complex is composed of several structures whose integrated function is essential for tricuspid valve competence (1–3). For the tricuspid valve to reamin competent, not only the leaflets, but also the chordae, papillary muscles, annulus, and the right atrial and right ventricular myocardium must all be anatomically and physiologically sound.

The normal tricuspid leaflets are delicate translucent structures that have a scalloped appearance when closed. The name of the valve is derived from the presence of three leaflets: anterior, septal, and posterior. The anterior leaflet is the largest, and the septal leaflet the smallest. The posterior leaflet is intermediate in size and is characterized by the presence of from one to three clefts. The clefts in the posterior leaflet can be quite prominent, creating the illusion of multiple tricuspid valve leaflets. The free edges of the three leaflets are longer than the circumference of the annulus, thereby providing a complete and unobstructed opening as the leaflets drop curtainlike into the right ventricle during diastole. When the right heart is opened through the acute margin (Fig. 12-1), the three largest fan-shaped chordae identify the three commissures. Two of the three large fan-shaped chordae arise from the papillary muscles. The anterior papillary muscle supplies fan-shaped chordae to the anterior and posterior leaflets, identifying the anteroposterior commissure. The medial papillary muscle supplies fan-shaped chordae to the posterior and septal leaflets and identifies the posteroseptal commissure. The large fan-shaped chordae to the anterior and the septal leaflets arise from the septal wall (Fig. 12-1).

An average of 25 chordae tendineae attach to the tricuspid valve leaflets. In contrast to mitral chordae, the chordae tendineae to the tricuspid leaflets are quite variable. The scalloped appearance of the tricuspid valve is due to the variability of the chordal attachments. Silver et al. (1) identified five separate types of chordae. In addition to the large fan-shaped

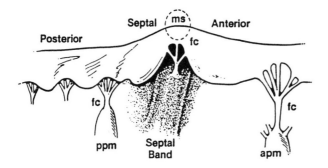

FIG. 12-1. The tricuspid valve as viewed after incision through the acute margin of the right heart. The posterior, septal, and anterior leaflets are identified. The anterior papillary muscle identifies the anteroposterior commissure. *fc,* Fan-shaped chordae; *ms,* membranous septum; *apm,* anterior papillary muscle; *ppm,* posterior papillary muscle. Small fan-shaped chordae identify clefts in the posterior leaflet.

chordae that identify the commissures, there are small fan-shaped chordae to the clefts of the posterior leaflet of the tricuspid valve (Fig. 12-1). Two interesting types of chordae not seen in the mitral apparatus include the "free edge chordae," which are long and attach to the free edge of the leaflets, and the "deep chordae," which are short and attach to the basal portion of each leaflet. Of greatest interest are the short chordae that arise directly from the muscle of the septum and posterior wall and attach to the septal leaflet. This configuration limits the mobility of the septal leaflet and may predispose the tricuspid valve to incompetence. The fixed small septal leaflet allows for little compensation should the free wall of the right ventricle dilate.

The normal circumference of the tricuspid valve annulus in an adult is 11 to 12 cm (2,3). The tricuspid valve leaflets attach to the annulus at different levels. The highest part of the tricuspid valve's attachment occurs at the anteroseptal commissure, which is located near the membranous interventricular septum (Fig. 12-1). As emphasized later, the tricuspid annulus plays an important role in tricuspid valve competence. In addition, the atrial and ventricular myocardium and perhaps the sequence of electrical activation are all important for normal function of the tricuspid valve complex.

Like the mitral valve, the tricuspid valve leaflets consist of three layers: the fibrosa on the ventricular surface, the atrialis on the atrial surface, and the thicker spongiosis layer sandwiched between the atrialis and the fibrosa.

PHYSIOLOGY OF NORMAL TRICUSPID APPARATUS

The right heart is a booster pump that drives blood through the lungs. This requires little work because pulmonary resistance is low, only one eighth of that of the systemic circulation. The normal pulmonary artery pressure is 22/8 mm Hg, with a mean pressure of 13 mm Hg (4). Because the average left atrial mean pressure is about 7 mm Hg, a pressure gradient of 6 mm Hg is adequate to propel the entire blood volume through the lungs. Accordingly, the normal right ventricle is a thinned wall structure. During right ventricular systole, the function of the tricuspid valve is to close, ensuring forward blood flow. During ventricular diastole, the function of the tricuspid valve is to ensure unimpeded forward blood flow from the vena cava and right atrium into the right ventricle.

The human tricuspid valve leaflets and their annular attachments have been studied in detail by two-dimensional echocardiography (5). The size of the human tricuspid annulus was also observed to change dramatically during the cardiac cycle (5). Maximal size occurred just before atrial systole. The major reduction in area occurred with atrial systole and the minimal size was reached in mid-systole. In normal subjects, the annular circumference measured 12 ± 1 cm before atrial contraction and narrowed to 10 ± 1 cm in mid-systole, a 19% reduction in circumference. The annular area was reduced by 33% (5). These findings suggest that a function of atrial contraction is the reduction in size of the tricuspid valve orifice before the onset of systole. With atrial fibrillation, the loss or modification of this sphincterlike motion, especially with annular dilatation, may contribute to tricuspid valvular regurgitation.

ACQUIRED TRICUSPID VALVE DISEASE

Functional (Annular Dilatation)

The most common abnormality of the tricuspid valve is functional tricuspid regurgitation. Even in patients with rheumatic heart disease, functional tricuspid regurgitation is common (6). It is generally accepted that functional tricuspid regurgitation results from annular dilatation. The normal maximal diameter of the tricuspid valve is about 21 mm/m^2 (5). The critical diameter is estimated to be 27 mm/m^2, because above this size, functional tricuspid regurgitation is common (6). Compared with normal, the annular circumference of patients with tricuspid regurgitation is larger (normal 12 ± 1 cm vs. tricuspid regurgitation 14 ± 1 cm) and the percent circumferential reduction from presystole to midsystole is less (normal 19% vs. tricuspid regurgitation 10%) (5). Because the percent reduction of the annulus is less, the minimum systolic tricuspid annular area is almost twice normal (normal 7.6 ± 1.4 cm^2 vs. tricuspid regurgitation 13 ± 1.4 cm^2) (5).

A continued pressure load of the right ventricle from birth usually results in right ventricular hypertrophy with a relatively competent tricuspid valve until heart failure occurs. In contrast, increased afterload applied to the thin-walled right ventricle of an adult is more likely to result in right ventricular failure and annular dilatation. The thin-walled right ventricle handles a volume overload better than a pressure overload.

Functional tricuspid regurgitation due to annular dilatation is common in patients with severe rheumatic mitral stenosis. In the series of 318 consecutive patients from the Massachusetts General Hospital reported by Sagie et al. (7), associated tricuspid regurgitation was severe in 12% and moderate in 19%. In general, the more severe the functional tricuspid regurgitation, the more severe the rheumatic mitral stenosis. Nevertheless, with multivariant analysis, the presence of functional tricuspid valve disease was an independent predictor of poor late outcome. The estimated 4-year event-free (freedom from death, mitral valve surgery, repeat valvuloplasty, and heart failure) survival rate was lower for the group with moderate or severe functional tricuspid regurgitation (7). At 4 years, the event-free survival rate was 68% for mild, 58% for moderate, and 35% for severe functional tricuspid regurgitation (7). At 4 years, the survival rate was 94% for mild, 90% for moderate, and 69% for severe functional tricuspid regurgitation (7). Thus, in patients with mitral stenosis, the presence of moderate or severe tricuspid valve disease may be an indication for surgical repair of the mitral and tricuspid valve rather than only balloon dilatation of the mitral valve. This same group reported that of the patients with significant (moderate or severe) functional tricuspid regurgitation, successful percutaneous valvotomy (valve area at least 1.5 cm^2 or at least 50% increase in valve area) was achieved in only 20 patients (8). In this group of 20 patients, tricuspid regurgitation decreased by one grade in only 4 patients and in none of the patients who did not meet the criteria for valvotomy success (8).

In a study from India, where the patients were younger, Sambasivam et al. (9) reported on 177 patients who underwent percutaneous balloon mitral valvotomy. Of these, 53 had associated functional tricuspid regurgitation. They found that functional tricuspid regurgitation improved only in a subset of younger (age less than 24 years) patients with preoperative cardiomegaly (cardiothoracic ratio greater than 60%) and significant pulmonary hypertension (pulmonary artery systolic greater than 50 mm Hg) (9).

Rheumatic Tricuspid Valve Disease

Rheumatic tricuspid valve stenosis is the result of chronic scarring and fibrosis of the tricuspid valve leaflets with commissural fusion. There is associated fibrosis, thickening, and fusion of the chordae tendineae (10–12). The resultant limitation of leaflet mobility and reduction in tricuspid orifice size may obstruct right ventricular filling. Fibrosis and distortion of leaflet architecture may result in tricuspid regurgitation.

Rheumatic heart disease, and therefore rheumatic involvement of the tricuspid valve, is rare in the Western world but still occurs in areas where rheumatic fever is rampant. Wood (12) concluded that rheumatic involvement of the heart was a pancarditis, involving all parts of the heart. He reasoned that mitral valve disease was the most important long-term sequela because the mitral valve is subject to the greatest pressure, normally having to withstand a systolic pressure of about 120 mm Hg during systole. The aortic valve has to withstand a pressure of 80 mm Hg in diastole. The tricuspid valve has a systolic pressure stress of only 15 to 25 mm Hg. Following this line of reasoning, Wood (12) postulated that rheumatic involvement of the aortic valve was always associated with rheumatic mitral valve disease and that rheumatic tricuspid disease was always associated with rheumatic involvement of the aortic and mitral valves. This postulate proved to be relatively sound. Approximately 15% to 30% of all patients with rheumatic valvular heart disease have evidence at necropsy of rheumatic involvement of the tricuspid valve (13,14). Clinically recognized tricuspid stenosis occurs in approximately 5% of patients with rheumatic heart disease. Rheumatic tricuspid valve disease virtually never occurs in the absence of rheumatic involvement of the mitral valve (15–19). And the natural history of rheumatic tricuspid valve lesions is dictated by the severity of the associated mitral and/or aortic valve lesion (20).

The diagnosis of rheumatic tricuspid stenosis is often difficult, yet important, because residual tricuspid stenosis may preclude clinical improvement despite successful surgical correction of mitral or mitral and aortic valvular lesions (11,15). Echocardiographic investigation of the tricuspid valve is critical in all patients with valvular heart disease.

Significant tricuspid regurgitation is relatively common in patients with chronic rheumatic heart disease. In a series of such patients undergoing diagnostic cardiac catheterization, one third (35 of 99) had angiographic evidence of tricuspid regurgitation (21).

Right Ventricular Infarction

Right ventricular infarction, a condition that occurs almost exclusively with transmural infarction of the left ventricular inferior wall, may result in tricuspid regurgitation (22,23). With right ventricular infarction, tricuspid regurgitation is probably the result of infarction and dysfunction of the papillary muscle and its free wall attachment. The dysfunction may be transient, with normal hemodynamics after recovery, but residual tricuspid regurgitation is common (24). Rupture of a right ventricular papillary muscle after acute myocardial infarction is rare (25).

Endocarditis

Right-sided endocarditis involves the tricuspid valve in 95% of cases (26). Intravenous drug abusers are especially prone to develop right-sided endocarditis, and in these patients the endocarditis frequently develops on a previously normal valve (25). Reports from medical examiners emphasize the frequency of aortic and mitral valve involvement from acute bacterial endocarditis. Reports from large city hospitals, however, emphasize the frequency of tricuspid valve involvement. This apparent discrepancy may be due to the fact that endocarditis of the tricuspid valve does not always result in acute severe hemodynamic embarrassment and rapid deterioration. Infectious endocarditis in drug abusers involves the tricuspid valve alone in about 40% of cases (27).

Patients with infectious endocarditis are often acutely ill with fever, chills, rigors, and pulmonary symptoms. The pulmonary symptoms include cough, hemoptysis, pleuritic chest pain, and dyspnea (28). Chest radiographs have abnormal findings in 70% of patients at initial presentation. Multiple bilateral infiltrates may be noted as a result of septic emboli from the tricuspid valve (29). The characteristic murmur of tricuspid regurgitation is present in only one third of patients at the time of initial presentation (29). The diagnosis is made by echocardiography.

Traumatic Injury

Penetrating and nonpenetrating trauma can result in tricuspid regurgitation from rupture of the leaflets, chordae tendineae, or papillary muscle (30,31). Rarely, traumatic tricuspid insufficiency leads to right atrial enlargement, elevation of mean right atrial pressure, and acquired cyanosis from right to left shunting via a patent foramen ovale (32).

Tricuspid Valve Prolapse

The spectrum of primary tricuspid prolapse is wide, varying from trivial abnormalities of the leaflets or chordae, or both, to severe redundancy of the valvular tissue and marked elongation of the supporting chordae (33–37). The distinguishing pathologic feature of primary tricuspid valve disease is excessive myxomatous tissue in the middle or spongiosis layer of the valve leaflet. Isolated tricuspid valve prolapse is rare (33). In contrast, the combination of tricuspid and mitral valve prolapse is relatively common. The prevalence of concomitant tricuspid valve prolapse in patients with mitral valve prolapse varies widely among reported series, but the combined prevalence of the nine largest series averages 37% (33–37). Because prolapse of the mitral valve is relatively common, affecting almost 4% of the population, tricuspid valve prolapse may be present in 1% to 2% of the population. Patients with combined mitral and tricuspid valve prolapse tend to be older and more symptomatic than patients with isolated mitral valve disease (38–42). Women predominate by a 2:1 ratio in isolated mitral valve prolapse and by a 3:1 ratio in combined atrioventricular prolapse (38).

The clinical features, symptoms, and signs are similar to those of mitral valve prolapse. These include chest pain, dyspnea, palpitations, nonejection systolic clicks, and late systolic murmurs. The identification of tricuspid valve disease is sometimes possible by auscultation. The click is reportedly more prominent at the lower left sternal border. With inspiration, the click occurs later in systole and may merge with the second heart sound. Occasionally, the click is heard along the lower right sternal border. The systolic murmur is also more prominent at the lower left sternal border. With inspiration, the murmur may increase in intensity and may be shorter in duration. Thus, auscultatory changes are thought to be secondary to increased right ventricular volume with inspiration (38,41).

In patients with the mitral valve prolapse syndrome, skeletal abnormalities, including the straight back syndrome, scoliosis, and pectus excavatum, are common. These skeletal abnormalities may be more common in patients with bivalvular involvement (41).

Carcinoid Heart Disease

Carcinoid syndrome is a relatively rare cause of acquired cardiac disease. Patients with the carcinoid heart disease almost always have tricuspid valve involvement (43–45). Cardiac involvement usually occurs in patients who have hepatic metastases from ileocecal tumors (44,45). However, cardiac involvement has also been documented in carcinoid tumors of ovarian and bronchial origin without hepatic metastases (46,47). Although the primary tumors and their metastases tend to have the histologic appearance of malignancy, they often follow an indolent course, thus the name "cancerlike" or "carcinoid." Cardiac failure accounts for significant morbidity and mortality of patients with this syndrome (43,45).

Both the tricuspid and pulmonic valves are commonly involved. Tricuspid regurgitation is the most common clinical abnormality. The pulmonic valve, if involved, is generally stenotic. Tricuspid stenosis with or without tricuspid regurgitation also occurs.

Although the clinical features of tricuspid regurgitation resemble those of other etiologies, the two-dimensional echocardiographic features are relatively characteristic. The tricuspid leaflets are thickened and appear similar to those seen with rheumatic tricuspid stenosis, but the mitral valve is normal, indicating that the right-sided valvular lesions are not due to rheumatic heart disease (48–51). The right atrium is enlarged. In severe cases the valves are virtually immobile with a fixed orifice, resulting in both stenosis and regurgitation (48). In less severely involved valves, the leaflets appear stiff and straightened, moving in a boardlike fashion with diminished total excursion (50). In some there is coaptation of the nodular thickened lesions at the beginning of systole. The leaflets are increasingly pulled apart as right ventricular systole proceeds, due to traction on the leaflets by the thickened chordae tendineae (48). This finding is thought to account for the particularly severe tricuspid regurgitation that is seen in some patients with carcinoid heart disease (48). Occasionally, the leaflets and the right ventricular papillary muscles appear more highly reflective of ultrasound than normal, suggesting endocardial coating by carcinoid-related fibrous plaque (49). Doming of the tricuspid valve has been described in patients with tricuspid stenosis (52,53).

Myxomas

Right atrial myxomas can produce tricuspid stenosis, tricuspid regurgitation, or both. It is easy to imagine how a large myxoma could produce apparent tricuspid stenosis. Tricuspid regurgitation can occur if the myxoma is calcified. In these patients, the myxoma moves in and out of the tricuspid valve orifice, grating and destroying the tricuspid leaflets with the rough calcified areas on its surface.

Atrial myxomas are the most common primary cardiac tumor, and right atrial myxomas account for approximately 25% of cardiac intracavitary myxomas (54–56). This diagnosis should be considered in any patient who has clinical findings of tricuspid valve disease in the absence of aortic and mitral disease. Systemic symptoms of fever, anorexia, and weight loss and changing auscultatory findings suggest either tumor, progressive vasculitis, or endocarditis. The diagnosis of right atrial myxoma can be made with a high degree of accuracy by two-dimensional echocardiography (57). In the rare case of right atrial tumor calcification, the diagnosis is suggested by chest radiograph.

Rare Causes of Acquired Tricuspid Valve Disease

There are a variety of rare causes of tricuspid valve disease that include fibroelastosis (58), endocardial fibrosis (59), fibrolipoma, systemic lupus erythematosus (60), metastatic tumors (61,62), scleroderma (63), hyperthyroidism (64), catheter- or pacemaker-induced thrombus (65), catheter or pacemaker entanglements (66–68), and diseases of the pericardium (69–71). Tricuspid valve regurgitation can occur from iatrogenic causes, such as inadvertent "biopsy" of a chordae during attempted right ventricular biopsy, migration of a Greenfield filter, and radiation injury.

CONGENITAL ABNORMALITIES

Ebstein's Anomaly

Ebstein's malformation is one of the most common congenital abnormalities of the tricuspid valve in adults. Ebstein's anomaly consists of downward displacement of fused malformed portions of tricuspid valvular tissue into the right ventricular cavity (72,73). The leaflets are attached in part to the tricuspid annulus and in part to the right ventricular wall below the annulus (72,73). In general, the anterior leaflet is enlarged at times, forming a large curtain across the right ventricular cavity (74). The posterior leaflet may be rudimentary or entirely absent (75). The right atrium is enlarged. The right ventricular portion that is above the abnormal insertion of the tricuspid valve is said to be "atrialized."

Most patients have either an incompetent or patent foramen ovale or an ostium secundum atrial septal defect (75).

The hemodynamic alterations of Ebstein's anomaly are related to the malformed tricuspid valve and the dysfunction of the right ventricle (76). All gradations of severity exist (73,76), and thus this abnormality may be compatible with a relatively long and active life. When symptoms appear, dyspnea, fatigue, and weakness are most common. Palpitations are usually due to atrial dysrhythmias. Death is due to congestive heart failure, hypoxia, and dysrhythmias (76,77). Cyanosis occurs in 50% to 80% of patients. Perloff (76) emphasized the chronologic sequence of cyanosis as a useful diagnostic feature of the history. Neonatal cyanosis may regress or disappear and then return at a later date. He states, "The functionally inadequate right ventricle copes poorly with the high pulmonary vascular resistance in the newborn. The right atrial pressure rises and a right to left shunt develops through an interatrial communication. When the pulmonary pressure drops to normal, the burden on the right heart is relieved; the right atrial pressure declines, the right to left shunt diminishes or disappears and with it the cyanosis. As time goes on cyanosis may reappear since the inadequate right ventricle, burdened by tricuspid regurgitation, ultimately fails again. Right ventricular end-diastolic pressure rises together with right atrial pressure and a right to left shunt is re-established" (76). The degree of cyanosis does not always coincide with the patient's symptoms (77,78). In fact, a history of relatively good effort tolerance despite cyanosis favors the diagnosis of Ebstein's anomaly (76).

In Ebstein's anomaly, the jugular venous pressure may be normal despite tricuspid incompetence because of the commodious right atrium. On auscultation, the first heart sound is widely split due to the delay in closure of the tricuspid valve. The smaller and poorly contracting right ventricle and the increased excursion of the large anterior leaflet results in a delayed tricuspid component of the first heart sound (79). This early systolic sound is prominent and is due to the large sail-like tricuspid valve reaching the limits of its systolic excursion. Referred to as the "sail sound," this may be the most specific auscultatory finding in Ebstein's anomaly (79). The second heart sound splitting is variable. Systolic murmurs are also quite variable; they may be totally absent or quite prominent. They are best heard along the lower left sternal border. The murmur of tricuspid regurgitation is not necessarily pansystolic. In the absence of pulmonary hypertension, the end-systolic pressure difference between the right ventricle and the V wave of the right atrium is small, and flow is decreased in late systole. In Ebstein's anomaly the murmur of tricuspid regurgitation does not necessarily increase with inspiration. This may be due to the inability of the small right ventricle to increase its stroke volume (76). Early diastolic sounds have been described and are attributed to the "opening snap" of the large anterior tricuspid leaflet or to the rapid filling of a small nondistensible right ventricle. The cadence created by the first heart sound (mitral valve closure), the early systolic sound (tricuspid valve closure), the second heart sound, and the early diastolic sound has been likened to the chugging of a steam locomotive (76).

The electrocardiogram is usually abnormal in the adult with Ebstein's anomaly. The P waves may be prominent and the PR interval prolonged. Preexcitation (Wolff-Parkinson-White) has been described in as many as 20% to 25% of patients with Ebstein's anomaly, and, as would be anticipated, the atrioventricular bypass tracts are usually located on the right (76). Although paroxysmal supraventricular tachycardia occurs from reentry over the bypass tract, other atrial dysrhythmias, such as atrial flutter and fibrillation, are also common because of the enlarged right atrium (76).

The echocardiographic features of Ebstein's anomalies are characteristic. The M-mode recording shows an increased excursion of the tricuspid valve when the echo beam traverses the large anterior leaflet. The most characteristic M-mode feature is delayed closure (50 ms or more) of the tricuspid valve when compared with that of the mitral valve (76). The two-dimensional echocardiogram is also diagnostic. In the apical four-chamber view, the right ventricular displacement of the leaflet and right atrial enlargement can be visualized (76).

Before the advent of echocardiography, the diagnosis of Ebstein's anomaly was made at cardiac catheterization by using a catheter that had an electrode near the opening of the lumen in the pressure-recording catheter. In the right atrium, atrial pressure and an intraatrial electrocardiogram are recorded, but the atrialized portion of the right ventricle generates an intracavitary right ventricular electrogram while registering an atrial pressure pulse. As the catheter tip is advanced across the tricuspid valve, a right ventricular pressure tracing and an intracavitary right ventricular electrogram are recorded (76).

Rare Causes of Congenital Tricuspid Valve Disease

Rare causes of congenital tricuspid valve disease include congenital tricuspid atresia and stenosis (80–83). Tricuspid stenosis is usually associated with an underdeveloped right ventricle. Congenital clefts of the tricuspid valve can be seen as part of the endocardial cushion defects. A straddling tricuspid valve can be part of maldevelopment of the ventricles (single ventricle). The tricuspid valve is the left-sided atrioventricular valve in L-transposition (congenital corrected transposition). In this situation, Ebstein's anomaly is frequent (76). Tricuspid regurgitation has been reported from Ehlers-Danlos syndrome (84).

DIAGNOSIS OF TRICUSPID REGURGITATION

When tricuspid valve disease is severe, the diagnosis is obvious. However, subtle presentations are much more common.

Clinical Findings

Gross tricuspid regurgitation can be diagnosed at the patient's bedside. Lateral head bobbing, large regurgitant CV waves in the jugular veins, and lateral chest wall motion are characteristic. Significant tricuspid regurgitation may result in palpable hepatic pulsations. The method I have found most helpful in feeling hepatic pulsation is to make a fist and place the knuckles and the back side of the metacarpals in the rib interspaces over the liver. Firm pressure facilitates the sensing of rhythmic systolic outward motion of the chest wall. This technique appears to be more sensitive than trying to feel hepatic pulsations below the rib cage with the palmar surface of the fingers.

Subtle presentations are much more common. Attention must be focused on minor alterations of the jugular venous pulse and trivial changes in the frequency or intensity of precordial murmurs with respiration if less severe degrees of tricuspid regurgitation are to be appreciated at the bedside.

Jugular Venous Pulsations

Normal jugular venous pulsation consists of a presystolic A wave, a systolic X descent, a late systolic V wave, and a diastolic Y descent. In normal patients with a slow heart rate, an H wave follows the Y descent and ends with the onset of the next A wave (Fig. 12-2). A C wave may interrupt the early portion of the X descent (Fig. 12-2). In right atrial tracings, the C wave occurs with the bulging of the tricuspid valve into the right atrium at the onset of systole. The larger C waves that are at times present in the neck of some patients are due to impulses transmitted from forceful carotid pulsations. The V wave is the result of continued passive filling of the right atrium during ventricular systole.

Moderate to severe leakage of the tricuspid valve results in a systolic wave that begins with a C wave and peaks at the time of the normal V wave (Fig. 12-2). These regurgitant waves are called CV waves or S waves. Small

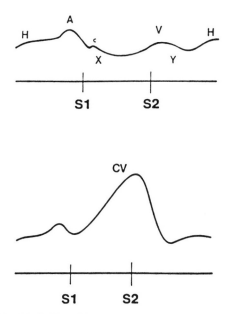

FIG. 12-2. Top: Normal jugular venous pulse illustrating the A and V waves and the X and Y descents. The C wave follows the A wave and interrupts the X descent. The H wave (passive filling of the atrium during diastole) is also shown. **Bottom:** CV wave of tricuspid regurgitation. Note the relationship of the CV wave to the first heart sound (S_1) and the second heart sound (S_2). A small presystolic A wave is shown but is not labeled and is absent in the presence of atrial fibrillation.

CV waves may do little more than obliterate the X descent. As the CV waves become larger, they are easier to recognize as a systolic venous pulse that wells up from the base of the neck. The CV wave should not be confused with the regularly appearing Cannon "A" wave that results from atrial contractions against a closed tricuspid valve. Regular Cannon A waves occur with atrial tachycardia with block or junctional rhythms. Compared with the slow-rising regurgitant CV wave, the Cannon A wave has a quicker rate of rise. Regurgitant CV waves must also be differentiated from large C waves transmitted from forceful carotid pulsations. This differential is easily made if the examining physician applies light pressure with the lateral aspect of his or her hand to the base of the neck just above the clavicle. This maneuver obstructs the internal jugular vein and obliterates regurgitant CV waves but has no effect on carotid pulsations (85).

It is difficult to quantitate the degree of tricuspid regurgitation at the bedside (86,87). The height of the regurgitant CV wave is determined by right atrial size and compliance and by the amount of regurgitation. A large right atrium might absorb a considerable amount of tricuspid regurgitation without altering the venous pulse. Likewise, trivial tricuspid regurgitation may not alter the venous wave form even in patients with a normal-sized right atrium (86,87).

Cardiac Auscultation

The classic auscultatory finding of tricuspid regurgitation is a systolic murmur best heard over the lower sternal area that increases with inspiration. Although the murmur of tricuspid regurgitation is most often heard over the fourth and fifth left intercostal spaces, it may be loudest over the lower right sternal border or over the xiphoid (88). With right ventricular dilatation, the murmur may extend across the entire precordium, mimicking murmurs of ventricular septal defect or mitral regurgitation.

The murmur of tricuspid regurgitation is classically holosystolic, but it can be late systolic or early systolic in timing. At times, holosystolic murmurs of tricuspid regurgitation may be recorded by intracardiac (right atrial) phonocardiography when no or only a mid-systolic murmur can be recorded on the precordium. Rios et al. (89) have emphasized that early systolic murmurs are a feature of tricuspid regurgitation without elevated right ventricular systolic pressures. In this situation, regurgitant flow is thought to decrease in the latter part of systole as the right atrial V wave and the right ventricular systolic pressures tend to equilibrate (89). The intensity and the frequency of the murmur are variable. The intensity of the murmur is not helpful in determining the severity of tricuspid regurgitation. Gross tricuspid regurgitation can be present with little or no murmur. Loud "musical," "honking," or "whooping" murmurs may result from trivial tricuspid regurgitation (33–37). This type of musical murmur is most frequently reported in patients with tricuspid valve prolapse (33–37).

The murmurs resulting from tricuspid and mitral valve regurgitation may be similar in character and have overlapping auscultatory areas. Therefore, emphasis has been placed on inspiratory augmentation of the intensity of tricuspid valve murmurs. Since 1946, when Rivero-Carvallo (90) described this inspiratory increase, this sign has been considered the most important auscultatory feature of tricuspid regurgitation. The inspiratory increase in the intensity of the murmur (Fig. 12-3) is thought to be due to increased venous return (91). The intensity of the murmur can be augmented by applying manual pressure below the liver either before or during inspiration. Occasionally, the murmur may appear only during inspiration while applying manual abdominal pressure (92). Gooch et al. (92) referred to the technique of applying abdominal pressure during inspiration as the "augmented Carvallo sign." The increase in murmur intensity is most marked during early inspiration but is lost if inspiration is held (88). In the presence of right heart failure, right heart output cannot be further increased by inspiration. Thus, the Carvallo sign may be absent in patients with tricuspid regurgitation and right heart failure only to appear after therapy. Occasionally, the murmur of tricuspid regurgitation will appear with the onset of atrial fibrillation and disappear with the return to normal sinus rhythm (88).

Electrocardiogram and Chest Radiograph

The electrocardiogram and chest radiograph are insensitive ways of diagnosing tricuspid valve disease. The electrocardiogram may provide evidence of right atrial enlargement with increased voltage and rightward shift of the P-wave vector. The chest roentgenogram may show rightward displacement of the right heart border (which is formed by the right atrium). The maximal distance of the right heart border of the heart from the midline exceeds the normal value of 4 cm.

Echocardiogram

Echocardiography is used to identify not only the etiology but also the pathologic consequence of tricuspid regurgitation. Echocardiography can be helpful in identifying specific causes of tricuspid regurgitation. Tricuspid valve prolapse, chordal rupture, endocarditis, rheumatic involvement, carcinoid syndrome, and myxomas all have relatively specific echocardiographic appearances (93,94). Echocardiography has also identified the indirect signs of tricuspid regurgitation (i.e., indicators of right ventricular volume overload). With significant tricuspid regurgitation there is an increase in the diameter of the right ventricular chamber or paradoxical

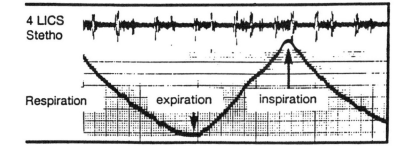

FIG. 12-3. Inspiratory augmentation of the murmur of tricuspid insufficiency from a phonocardiogram recorded at the fourth left intercostal space (*4LICS*)

septal motion, or both. These findings, obviously, are not specific for tricuspid regurgitation because there are other causes of right ventricular volume overload (95).

Doppler Flow Studies

Doppler flow studies enhanced the physician's ability to diagnose abnormalities of the tricuspid valve. By analyzing the returning echoes for a change or shift in the returning sound wave frequency (the Doppler principle), the velocity of blood movement can be estimated (96). Both continuous-wave and single-point Doppler techniques are available (96–99). Color-flow imaging, a technique that provides a real-time two-dimensional image of blood flow superimposed on a real-time two-dimensional anatomic image, results in images that resemble regurgitant flows or stenotic flow jets seen on x-ray cineangiography. The images are color coded to display the direction and relative velocities of the blood flow.

Tricuspid regurgitation results in reverse or disturbed flow in the right atrial chamber and at times in the inferior vena cava or hepatic veins (97–99). Severe tricuspid regurgitation is readily documented by Doppler. However, normal individuals may demonstrate a small systolic flow disturbance in the right atrium. Thus, the sensitivity and specificity of this technique for the diagnosis of mild tricuspid regurgitation are unknown. As the severity of the regurgitation increases, the depth of penetration and the duration and extent of retrograde flow in the right atrium increase. In severe tricuspid regurgitation, the disturbed flow can be detected at the roof of the right atrium. Using this criterion alone, a jet lesion can result in an overestimation of the degree of tricuspid regurgitation.

Hemodynamics and Angiography

Hemodynamic and angiographic diagnosis of tricuspid regurgitation are now of historical interest (100). Intracardiac phonocardiography is another technique no longer used.

DIAGNOSIS OF TRICUSPID STENOSIS

Clinical Findings

Tricuspid stenosis should be suspected in all patients with rheumatic valvular heart disease but especially in those with known mitral and aortic valve involvement who have elevated venous pressure, fatigue, and fluid retention (15). At the bedside, the diagnosis of tricuspid stenosis is made by observing the jugular venous wave form and by auscultation. While the patient is in sinus rhythm, stenosis of the tricuspid valve results in an increase in the height of the A wave of the jugular venous pulse. In the setting of rheumatic heart disease, the presence of a giant A wave in the jugular venous pulse is almost pathognomonic of tricuspid stenosis. In other settings, a large A wave is not diagnostic of tricuspid stenosis because a more common cause is decreased right ventricular compliance. In addition, advanced tricuspid stenosis often results in right atrial enlargement and atrial fibrillation. With the onset of atrial fibrillation, the A wave disappears. Because tricuspid stenosis limits the rapidity with which the right atrium empties, a more specific venous abnormality is the slow Y descent and the absence of the Y trough.

When the patient is in sinus rhythm, a crescendo-decrescendo presystolic murmur is the most important auscultatory sign of tricuspid stenosis. In contrast to the presystolic murmur of mitral stenosis, which is crescendo in configuration, increasing in intensity until truncated by a loud first heart sound, the "atrial systolic" murmur of tricuspid stenosis has a distinct crescendo-decrescendo configuration that ends before right ventricular systole. This murmur parallels the right ventricular right atrial diastolic pressure gradient at the time of the atrial A wave (101). The separation of the presystolic murmur of tricuspid stenosis and the first heart sound is made more distinct by the presence of first-degree heart block, a not uncommon finding in this clinical setting.

The low-frequency diastolic rumble of tricuspid stenosis is best heard along the lower left sternal border. A mid-diastolic murmur is most common in patients with atrial fibrillation. Classically, this rumble increases with inspiration. In general, the configuration of the diastolic murmur (and of the atrial presystolic murmur) parallels the pressure gradient envelope. A low-frequency early diastolic murmur is likewise not diagnostic of tricuspid stenosis, because similar murmurs can be produced by increased flow across a normal tricuspid valve, as seen in patients with a large shunt from an atrial septal defect. The opening snap of tricuspid stenosis is not a helpful diagnostic sign because it is rarely appreciated at the bedside. Occasionally, the tricuspid opening snap can be recorded.

Electrocardiogram and Chest Radiograph

The electrocardiographic findings in patients with tricuspid stenosis include evidence of right atrial or biatrial enlargement or conduction abnormalities in the absence of electrocardiographic evidence of right ventricular hypertrophy (15,102). First-degree heart block and atrial fibrillation are also common. The chest roentgenogram is seldom characteristic but is reported to show a prominent right heart border with a relatively inconspicuous pulmonary artery (15,102).

Echocardiography

The normal tricuspid valve leaflets are seen on two-dimensional echocardiography as two thin, freely moving structures (94). Two-dimensional echocardiography has been found to have a high predictive accuracy for the diagnosis of tricuspid stenosis when the following echocardiographic criteria are used: evidence of rheumatic involvement of the mitral valve; diastolic doming of the anterior tricuspid leaflet (i.e., restriction of leaflet tip motion with greater mobility of the body of the leaflet); reduced excursion of the septal or posterior leaflet, or both; and a reduction in the tricuspid orifice diameter relative to the annular diameter recorded in the same scan plane (94). Thickening and reduced motion of the posterior or septal tricuspid leaflets, or both, with normal anterior leaflet motion may be present with rheumatic involvement but are not considered to represent valvular stenosis (93,94).

Hemodynamics

The hemodynamic diagnosis of tricuspid stenosis often depends on the accurate measurement of a small pressure gradient. Precise simultaneous pressure recordings from the right atrium and right ventricle are required. Pressure recordings are obtained during withdrawal of the catheter tip from the right ventricle. The "pullback" recording technique is limited because atrial fibrillation makes it difficult to superimpose atrial and ventricular pressure curves; tricuspid regurgitation, which frequently accompanies rheumatic tricuspid stenosis, elevates mean right atrial pressure and can create the appearance of a diastolic gradient: and small diastolic gradients, which are typical of tricuspid stenosis, are often overloaded if the pullback technique is used (102,103). Because simultaneous right atrial and right ventricular pressure tracings are not obtained on a routine basis, the diagnosis of tricuspid stenosis is frequently overlooked unless this lesion is suspected from the bedside or noninvasive precatheterization evaluation before catheterization, and the study is designed to specifically determine the presence or absence of tricuspid stenosis (3). Even when simultaneous recording techniques are used, low flow across a stenotic tricuspid valve may result in deceivingly small gradients. Exercise or other methods of increasing the cardiac output may be required for hemodynamic diagnosis.

MANAGEMENT

The management of tricuspid valve disease varies depending on the type (stenosis or regurgitation), etiology, and severity. In most patients with functional tricuspid regurgitation, therapy is initially directed at the contributing abnormality. Examples include treatment of left heart failure, correction of mitral valve disease, thrombolytic therapy of massive pulmonary emboli, or chronic oxygen therapy in patients with cor pulmonale secondary to chronic lung disease and arterial oxygen desaturation. Specific therapy may be necessary: antibiotics and/or surgery for endocarditis and surgery for myxomas, tricuspid stenosis, traumatic rupture of major chordae or heads of the papillary muscle, and so on (104,105).

Because the most common cause of functional tricuspid regurgitation is right heart failure, early therapy of left heart failure is of prime importance. Once severe tricuspid regurgitation is present, diuretics must be used with discretion. Because a large CV wave elevates the mean venous pressure, the physician is tempted to use increasing doses or combinations of diuretics in an effort to lower the venous pressure. Because the CV waves are systolic in timing, the true right ventricular end-diastolic or filling pressure is the pressure at the trough of the venous wave just before its onset. The top of the venous wave is produced by right ventricular systolic pressure. Excessive diuresis may result in an excessively decreased right ventricular filling pressure, decreased cardiac output, and increased fatigue.

Surgery is generally reserved for patients with advanced valvular disease (106–108). It was thought that the tricuspid valve was not necessary for survival because total excision was performed in some patients with endocarditis (109). However, it is now evident that complete removal of the tricuspid valve without replacement eventually results in congestive heart failure (110). Surgical management may require annuloplasty or replacement with a prosthetic valve. Tricuspid annuloplasty should be considered because of its simplicity, safety, and effectiveness. Although tricuspid regurgitation may lessen and disappear in many patients simply as a result of correction of the left-sided valvular disease, this response is not predictable. In patients with severe tricuspid malfunction, valve replacement may be necessary. The mortality of tricuspid valve replacement is high when associated with re-

placement of the aortic and/or mitral valve (106). On the other hand, unrecognized and uncorrected rheumatic tricuspid stenosis can have a deleterious effect on the results of surgery for aortic and mitral valve disease (111,112).

CONCLUSIONS

An appreciation of tricuspid valve disease adds significantly to the physician's clinical acumen. Tricuspid valve disease may be an incidental finding or its presence may provide a clue to otherwise unexplained cardiovascular signs or symptoms. Tricuspid regurgitation is the most commonly seen lesion and when present is most often functional. However, acquired and congenital defects must be excluded. Tricuspid stenosis is seen much less frequently but must be considered in patients with rheumatic heart disease who have involvement of both the mitral and aortic valves, especially if there is failure to improve after corrective surgery.

The clinical diagnosis of severe tricuspid valve disease, particularly tricuspid regurgitation, is usually not difficult. However, clinical signs of mild to moderate disease may be quite subtle and noninvasive techniques such as echo-Doppler are often required to establish the diagnosis. Slight tricuspid regurgitation can be detected by Doppler in many older normal subjects.

Management of tricuspid valve disease is based on the etiology and severity of the disease and is frequently directed at the contributing abnormality. Surgical therapy is usually reserved for patients with advanced valvular disease.

REFERENCES

1. Silver MD, Lam JH, Ranganathan N, et al. Morphology of human tricuspid valve. *Circulation* 1971;43: 333.
2. Wooley CF. Rediscovery of the tricuspid valve. *Curr Probl Cardiol* 1981;6:8.
3. Wooley CF. *The Spectrum of Tricuspid Regurgitation.* Dallas, TX: American Heart Association, 1975.
4. Cournand A. Some aspects of the pulmonary circulation in normal man and in chronic cardiopulmonary diseases. *Circulation* 1952;2:641.
5. Tei C, Pilgrim JP, Shah PM, et al. The tricuspid valve

annulus: study of size and motion in normal subjects and in patients with tricuspid regurgitation. *Circulation* 1982;66:665.

6. Ubango J, Figueroa A, Ochoteco A, et al. Analysis of the amount of tricuspid valve annular dilatation required to produce functional tricuspid regurgitation. *Am J Cardiol* 1983;52:155.

7. Sagie A, Schwammenthal E, Newell JB, et al. Significant tricuspid regurgitation is a marker for adverse outcome in patients undergoing percutaneous balloon mitral valvuloplasty. *J Am Coll Cardiol* 1994;24:696.

8. Sagie A, Schwammenthal E, Palacios IF, et al. Significant tricuspid regurgitation does not resolve after percutaneous balloon mitral valvotomy. *J Thorac Cardiovasc Surg* 1994;108:727.

9. Sambasivam KA, Jose J, Chandy S, Joseph G. Beneficial effect of balloon mitral valvotomy in reducing severity of associated tricuspid regurgitation. *Indian Heart J* 1997;49:271.

10. Hollman A. The anatomical appearance in rheumatic tricuspid valve disease. *Br Heart J* 1957;19:211.

11. Yu PN, Harken DE, Lovejoy FW Jr, et al. Clinical and hemodynamic studies of tricuspid stenosis. *Circulation* 1956;13:680.

12. Wood P. Chronic rheumatic heart disease. In: Wood P, ed. *Diseases of the Heart and Circulation*, 3rd ed. Philadelphia: JB Lippincott, 1968:690–699.

13. Chopra P, Tandon HD. Pathology of chronic rheumatic heart disease with particular reference to tricuspid valve involvement. *Acta Cardiol* 1977;32:423.

14. Edwards WD, Peterson K, Edwards JE. Active valvulitis associated with chronic rheumatic valvular disease and active myocarditis. *Circulation* 1978;57:181.

15. Gibson R, Wood P. The diagnosis of tricuspid stenosis. *Br Heart J* 1955;17:552.

16. Goodwin JF, Rab SM, Sinha AK, et al. Rheumatic tricuspid stenosis. *Br Med J* 1957;2:1383.

17. Kitchin A, Turner R. Diagnosis and treatment of tricuspid stenosis. *Br Heart J* 1964;26:354.

18. Guyer DE, Gillam LD, Foale RA. Comparison of the echocardiographic and hemodynamic diagnosis of rheumatic tricuspid stenosis. *J Am Coll Cardiol* 1984;3:1135.

19. Daniels SJ, Mintz GS, Kotler MN. Rheumatic tricuspid valve disease. Two dimensional echocardiographic. hemodynamic, and angiographic correlations. *Am J Cardiol* 1983;51:492.

20. Gutner RN. Trivalvular rheumatic stenosis: documentation of disease progression by serial cardiac catheterization. *Am J Med Sci* 1980;280:185.

21. Ubago JL, Figueroa A, Colman T, et al. Right ventriculography as a valid method for the diagnosis of tricuspid insufficiency. *Cathet Cardiovasc Diagn* 1981;7:433.

22. McAllister RG, Friesinger GC, Sinclair-Smith BC. Tricuspid regurgitation following inferior myocardial infarction. *Arch Intern Med* 1976;136:96.

23. Zone DD, Botti RE. Right ventricular infarction with tricuspid insufficiency and chronic right heart failure. *Am J Cardiol* 1976;37:445.

24. Bracchetti D, Capucci A. Right ventricular infarction with tricuspid insufficiency. Case report. *Am J Cardiol* 1977;39:133.

25. Eisenberg S, Suyemato J. Rupture of a papillary muscle of the tricuspid valve following acute myocardial infarction. *Circulation* 1964;30:588.

26. Roberts WC. Characteristics and consequences of infective endocarditis (active or healed or both) learned from morphologic studies. In: Rahimtoola SH, ed. *Infective Endocarditis*. New York: Grune & Stratton, 1978.

27. Stimmel B, Dack S. Infective endocarditis in narcotic addicts. In: Rahimtoola SH, ed. *Infective Endocarditis*. New York: Grune & Stratton, 1978;

28. Reid CL, Chandraratua PAN, Rahimtoola SH. Infective endocarditis: improved diagnosis and treatment. In: O'Rourke RH, ed. *Current Problems in Cardiology*. Chicago: Year Book Medical Publishers, 1985.

29. Chambers HF, Koreniowski OM, Sande MA, National Collaborative Endocarditis Study Group. *Staphylococcus aureus* endocarditis: clinical manifestation in addicts and non-addicts. *Medicine (Baltimore)* 1983;63:170.

30. Watanabe T, Katsume H, Matsukubo H, et al. Ruptured chordae tendineae of the tricuspid valve due to nonpenetrating trauma. *Chest* 1981;80:751.

31. Naccarelli GV, Haisty WK, Kahl FR. Left ventricular to right atrial defect and tricuspid insufficiency secondary to nonpenetrating cardiac trauma. *J Trauma* 1980;20:887.

32. Bardy GH, Talano JV, Meyers S, Lesch M. Acquired cyanotic heart disease secondary to traumatic tricuspid regurgitation. *Am J Cardiol* 1979;44:1401.

33. Weinreich DJ, Burke JF, Bharati S, Lev M. Isolated prolapse of the tricuspid valve. *J Am Coll Cardiol* 1985;6:475.

34. Bashour T, Lindsay J Jr. Midsystolic clicks originating from tricuspid valve structures: a sequela of heroin-induced endocarditis. *Chest* 1975;67:620.

35. Sasse L, Froelich CR. Echocardiographic tricuspid prolapse and non-ejection systolic click. *Chest* 1978;73:869.

36. Doi YL, Sugiura T, Bishop RL, et al. High-speed echophonocardiographic detection of tricuspid valve prolapse in mitral valve prolapse with discrepancy in onset of systolic murmur. *Am Heart J* 1982;103:301.

37. Tei C, Shah PM, Tanaka H. Phonographic-echographic documentation of systolic honk in tricuspid prolapse. *Am Heart J* 1982;103:294.

38. Mardelli TJ, Morganroth J, Chen CC, et al. Tricuspid valve prolapse diagnosed by cross-sectional echocardiography. *Chest* 1979;79:201.

39. Ogawa S. Hayashi J, Sasaki H, et al. Evaluation of combined valvular prolapse syndrome by two-dimensional echocardiography. *Circulation* 1982;65:174.

40. Morganroth J, Jones RH, Chen CC, et al. Two-dimensional echocardiography in mitral, aortic and tricuspid valve prolapse: the clinical problem, cardiac nuclear imaging considerations and proposed standard for diagnosis. *Am J Cardiol* 1980;46:1164.

41. Maranhao V, Gooch AS, Yang SS, et al. Prolapse of the tricuspid leaflets in the systolic murmur-click syndrome. *Cathet Cardiovasc Diagn* 1980;1:81.

42. Shrivastava S, Guthrie R, Edwards JE. Prolapse of the mitral valve. *Mod Concepts Cardiovasc Dis* 1977;46:57.

43. Thorson A, Biorck G, Bjorkman G, et al. Malignant carcinoid of the small intestine with metastases to the liver, valvular disease of the right side of the heart (pulmonary stenosis and tricuspid regurgitation without septal defects), peripheral vasomotor symptoms,

bronchoconstriction, and an unusual type of cyanosis. A clinical and pathological syndrome. *Am Heart J* 1954;47:795.

44. Roberts WC, Sjoerdsma A. The cardiac disease associated with the carcinoid syndrome (carcinoid heart disease). *Am J Med* 1964;36:5.

45. Trell E, Ransing A, Ripa J, et al. Carcinoid heart disease: clinicopathologic findings and follow-up in 11 cases. *Am J Med* 1973;54:433.

46. Sworn MJ, Edlin GP, McGill DAF, et al. Tricuspid valve replacement in carcinoid syndrome due to ovarian primary. *Br Med J* 1980;280:85.

47. Erhlichman RT. Carcinoid tumor. *Johns Hopkins Med J* 1979;145:170.

48. Davies MK, Lowry PJ, Littler WA. Cross sectional echocardiographic feature in carcinoid heart disease: a mechanism for tricuspid regurgitation in this syndrome. *Br Heart J* 1984;51:355.

49. Howard RJ, Drobac M, Rider WD, et al. Carcinoid heart disease: diagnosis by two-dimensional echocardiography. *Circulation* 1982;66:1059.

50. Baker BJ, McNee VD, Scovil JA, et al. Tricuspid insufficiency in carcinoid heart disease: an echocardiographic description. *Am Heart J* 1981;10:107.

51. Callahan JA, Wrobleski EM, Reeder GS, et al. Echocardiographic features of carcinoid heart disease. *Am J Cardiol* 1982;50:762.

52. Forman MB, Byrd BF III, Oates JA, et al. Two-dimensional echocardiography in the diagnosis of carcinoid heart disease. *Am Heart J* 1984;107:492.

53. Okada RD, Ewy GA, Copeland JG. Echocardiography and surgery in tricuspid and pulmonary valve stenosis due to carcinoid syndrome. *Cardiovasc Med* 1979;4:871.

54. Zitnik RS, Giuliani ER. Clinical recognition of atrial myxoma. *Am Heart J* 1970;80:689.

55. Bulkley BH, Hutchins GM. Atrial myxomas: a fifty year review. *Am Heart J* 1979;97:639.

56. McAllister HA. Primary tumors and cysts of the heart and pericardium. *Curr Probl Cardiol* 1979;4:1.

57. Giuliani ER, Nasser FN. Two-dimensional echocardiography in acquired heart disease. Part I. *Curr Probl Cardiol* 1981;5:1.

58. Dennis JL, Hansen AE, Corpening TN. Endocardial fibroelastosis. *Pediatrics* 1953;12:130.

59. Davies JNP, Bafl JD. The pathology of endomyocardial fibrosis in Uganda. *Br Heart J* 1955;17:337.

60. Gibson R, Wood P. The diagnosis of tricuspid stenosis. *Br Heart J* 1955;17:552.

61. Thomas JH, Panoussopoulos DG, Jewell WR, et al. Tricuspid stenosis secondary to metastatic melanoma. *Cancer* 1977;39:1732.

62. DeCock KM, Gikonyo DK, Lucas SB, et al. Metastatic tumour of right atrium mimicking constrictive pericarditis and tricuspid stenosis. *Br Med J* 1982;285:1314.

63. Sackner MA, Heinz ER, Steinberg AJ. The heart in scleroderma. *Am J Cardiol* 1966;17:542.

64. Dougherty MJ, Craige E. Apathetic hyperthyroidism presenting as tricuspid regurgitation. *Chest* 1973;63:767.

65. Zager J, Berberich SN, Eslava R, et al. Dynamic tricuspid valve insufficiency produced by a right ventricular thrombus from a pacemaker. *Chest* 1978;74:455.

66. Greco MA, Senesh JD, Aleksic S, et al. Tricuspid

stenosis secondary to entanglement of ventriculoatrial catheter in the valve leaflets. *Surg Neurol* 1982;18:34.

67. Lee ME, Chaux A. Unusual complications of endocardial pacing. *J Thorac Cardiovasc Surg* 1980;80:934.

68. Gibson TC, Davidson RC, DeSilvey DL. Presumptive tricuspid valve malfunction induced by a pacemaker lead: A case report and review of the literature. *Pace* 1980;3:88.

69. Beaver WL, Dillon JC, Jolly W. Pseudo-tricuspid stenosis: A rare entity. *Chest* 1977;71:772.

70. Cintron GB, Snow JA, Fletcher RD, et al. Pericarditis mimicking tricuspid valvular disease. *Chest* 1977;71:770.

71. Wray TM, Prochaska J, Fisher RD, et al. Traumatic pericardial hematoma simulating tricuspid valve obstruction. *Johns Hopkins Med J* 1975;137:147.

72. Ebstein W. On a very rare case of insufficiency of the tricuspid valve caused by severe congenital malformation of the same. *Arch Anat Physiol Wissensch Med Leipz* 1866;238. [Translated by Schiebler GL, Gravenstein JS, Van Mierop LHS. *Am J Cardiol* 1968;22:867.

73. Vacca JB, Bussman DW, Mudd JG. Ebstein's anomaly: complete review of 108 cases. *Am J Cardiol* 1958;2:210.

74. Goodwin JF, Wynn A, Steiner RE. Ebstein's anomaly of the tricuspid valve. *Am Heart J* 1953;45:144.

75. Edwards JE. Pathologic features of Ebstein's malformation of the tricuspid valve. *Proc Staff Meet Mayo Clin* 1953;28:89.

76. Perloff JK. Ebstein's anomaly of the tricuspid valve. In: Perloff JK, ed. *The Clinical Recognition of Congenital Heart Disease*, 2nd ed. Philadelphia: WB Saunders, 1978;184–200.

77. Genton E, Blount SG Jr. The spectrum of Ebstein's anomaly. *Am Heart J* 1967;73:395.

78. Kumar AE, Flyer DC, Miettinsen OS, et al. Ebstein's anomaly: clinical profile and natural history. *Am J Cardiol* 1971;28:84.

79. Fontana ME, Wooley CF. Sail sound in Ebstein's anomaly of the tricuspid valve. *Circulation* 1972;46:155.

80. Mehl SJ, Kaltman AJ, Kronzon I, et al. Combined tricuspid and pulmonic stenosis: clinical, echocardiographic, hemodynamic, surgical, and pathological features. *J Thorac Cardiovasc Surg* 1977;74:55.

81. Cox JN, de Seigneux R, Bolens M, et al. Tricuspid atresia, hypoplastic right ventricle, intact ventricular septum and congenital absence of the pulmonary valve. *Helv Paediatr Acta* 1975;30:389.

82. Greenwood RD. Ossification of the right auriculoventricular opening of the heart. *J Ind State Med Assoc* 1976;69:88.

83. Oeconomos NS, Camilaris DH, Petritis J, et al. Congenital tricuspid valvular stenosis. *J Cardiovasc Surg* 1975;16:100.

84. Leier CV, Call TD, Fulkerson PK, et al. The spectrum of cardiac defects in the Ehlers-Danlos syndrome, types I and III. *Ann Intern Med* 1980;92:171.

85. Ewy GA. Venous and arterial pulsations. In: Horwitz LD, Groves BM, eds. *Signs and Symptoms in Cardiology*. Philadelphia: JB Lippincott, 1985:132.

86. Cairus KB, Kloster FE, Bristow JD, et al. Problems in the hemodynamic diagnosis of tricuspid insufficiency. *Am Heart J* 1968;75:173.

87. Hansing CE, Rowe GG. Tricuspid insufficiency: a

study of hemodynamics and pathogenesis. *Circulation* 1972;45:793.

88. Levine SA, Harvey WP. *Clinical Auscultation of the Heart.* Philadelphia: WB Saunders, 1959:339.

89. Rios JC, Massumi RA, Breesmen WT, et al. Auscultatory features of acute tricuspid regurgitation. *Am J Cardiol* 1969;23:4.

90. Rivero-Carvallo M. Signo para el diagnostico de las insufficiencias tricuspideas. *Arch Inst Cardiol Mex* 1946;16:531.

91. Muller O, Schillingford J. Tricuspid incompetence. *Br Heart J* 1954;16:195.

92. Gooch AS, Maranhao V, Scampardonis G, et al. Prolapse of both mitral and tricuspid leaflets in systolic murmur-click syndrome. *N Engl J Med* 1972;287: 1218.

93. Feigenbaum H. *Echocardiography*, 3rd ed. Philadelphia: Lea & Febiger, 1981:284.

94. Nanna M, Chandraratna PA, Reid C, et al. Value of two-dimensional echocardiography in detecting tricuspid stenosis. *Circulation* 1983;67:221.

95. Seward JB, Tajik AJ, Hagler DJ, et al. Peripheral venous contrast echocardiography. *Am J Cardiol* 1977; 39:202.

96. Hatie L. *Doppler Ultrasound in Cardiology: Physical Principles of Clinical Applications*, 2nd ed. Philadelphia: Lea & Febiger, 1985.

97. Pearlman AS, Stevenson JC. Doppler echocardiography: applications, limitation, and future directions. *Am J Cardiol* 1980;46:1256.

98. Miyatake K, Okamoto M. Evaluation of tricuspid regurgitation by pulsed Doppler and two-dimensional echocardiography. *Circulation* 1982;66:777.

99. Diebold B, Touati R, Blanchard D, et al. Quantitative assessment of tricuspid regurgitation using pulsed Doppler echocardiography. *Br Heart J* 1983;50:443.

100. Cha SD, Gooch A. Diagnosis of tricuspid regurgitation. *Arch Intern Med* 1983;143:1763.

101. Wooley CF, Fontana ME, Kilman JW, Ryan JM. Tricuspid stenosis: atrial systolic murmur, tricuspid open-

ing snap and right atrial pressure pulse. *Am J Med* 1985;78:375.

102. Perloff JK, Harvey WP. Clinical recognition of tricuspid stenosis. *Circulation* 1960;22:346.

103. Sanders CA, Harthome JW, DeSanctis RW, et al. Tricuspid stenosis: a difficult diagnosis in the presence of atrial fibrillation. *Circulation* 1966;33:26.

104. Brandenburg RO, McGoon DC, Campeau L, et al. Traumatic rupture of the chordae tendineae of the tricuspid valve: successful repair twenty-four years later. *Am J Cardiol* 1966;18:911.

105. Tachovsky TJ, Giuliani ER, Ellis FH Jr. Prosthetic valve replacement for traumatic tricuspid insufficiency: report of a case originally diagnosed as Ebstein's malformation. *Am J Cardiol* 1970;26:196.

106. Kochoukos NT, Stephenson LW. Indications for and results of tricuspid valve replacement. *Adv Cardiol* 1976;17:199.

107. Sanfelippo PM, Giuliani ER, Danielson GK, et al. Tricuspid valve prosthetic replacement: early and late results with the Starr-Edwards prosthesis. *J Thorac Cardiovasc Surg* 1976;71:441.

108. Breyer RH, McClenathan JH, Michaelis LL, et al. Tricuspid regurgitation: a comparison of non-operative management, tricuspid annuloplasty, and tricuspid valve replacement. *J Thorac Cardiovasc Surg* 1976;72: 867.

109. Arbulu A, Thoms NW, Wilson RF. Valvulectomy without prosthetic replacement: a lifesaving operation for tricuspid pseudomonas endocarditis. *J Thorac Cardiovasc Surg* 1972;64:103.

110. Robin E, Belamaric J, Thoms NW, et al. Consequences to total tricuspid valvulectomy without prosthetic replacement in treatment of pseudomonas endocarditis. *J Thorac Cardiovasc Surg* 1974;68:461.

111. Sheikhzadeh A, Tarbiat S, Paydar D, Shakibi J. Rheumatic tricuspid stenosis: a clinical overview. *Acta Cardiol* 1978;33:431.

112. Watson H, Lowe K. Severe tricuspid stenosis revealed after aortic valvotomy. *Br Heart J* 1962;24:241.

13

Prosthetic Heart Valves

Hoang M. Thai and Joel M. Gore

Section of Cardiology, University of Arizona College of Medicine, Veteran's Administration Medical Center, Tucson, Arizona 85724; Division of Cardiovascular Medicine, University of Massachusetts Medical School and Memorial Health Care, Worcester, Massachusetts 01655

In 1960, a major advance in the management of valvular heart disease occurred when diseased cardiac valves were replaced by mechanical prosthetic valves. Harken et al. (1) in Boston and Starr and Edward (2) in Oregon used ball-and-cage mechanical prostheses in the aortic and mitral positions. Today, valve replacement is the most common operation for adults with symptomatic valvular heart disease. During the past 25 years, operative mortality has declined significantly, and the long-term outlook for patients undergoing valve replacement has continually improved. Since 1960, hundreds of thousands of valves have been implanted throughout the world; in the United States alone, greater than 60,000 are implanted annually (3).

Despite substantial improvements in design and characteristics, the ideal valve substitute does not yet exist nor have we met the criteria of the perfect valve outlined by Harken et al. in 1962 (4). The optimal prosthetic valve, according to Harken et al., should have "lasting physical geometric features and be capable of permanent fixation in the normal anatomic site. It should be chemically inert, nonthrombogenic, harmless to blood elements and must not annoy the patient. It must open and close promptly during the appropriate phase of the cardiac cycle and should offer no resistance to physiological blood flow."

All currently available prosthetic valves fall short of these standards, and the search for the ideal valve continues (5). Physicians caring for patients with valvular heart disease need to be aware of the advantages and disadvantages of the various types of prosthetic valves (6). In addition, familiarity with the proper care and follow-up of patients with prosthetic valves is necessary. At present, there are more than 80 different varieties of prosthetic valves available (3,7). To make a rational decision as to which valve is best for a particular patient, several variables important to consider include long-term complication rates, need for anticoagulation, age of patient, coexistent disease, patient lifestyle, anatomic and hemodynamic factors, and the surgeon's experience. No particular valve substitute is clearly superior, and operative mortality does not appear to be related to valve selection but rather to the patient's general condition and the degree of myocardial dysfunction. Individualization of valve selection is important; a valve ideal for one patient may be disastrous for another. The size of the patient and his or her heart are extremely important variables that must be considered if the correct prosthetic valve is to be chosen.

Prosthetic heart valves are available as either totally mechanical devices or as bioprosthetic (tissue) valves (Tables 13-1 and

TABLE 13-1. *Prosthetic heart valves*

Design	Valve name	Comments
Mechanical		
Caged ball	Starr-Edwards	Cloth and non–cloth-covered models of this valve identified by four-digit code
	Braunwald-Cutter	Discontinued
	Smeloff-Cutter	
	DeBakey-Surgitool	
Low profile		
Disc valves	Starr-Edwards	Series 6500, 6520
	Kay-Shiley	
	Beall	
	Harken	Discontinued
	Cooley-Bloodwell-Cutter	
Hinged-leaflet	Gott-Daggett	Discontinued
Central flow, eccentric	Lillehei-Kaster	
monocusp valves	Bjork-Shiley	
	St. Jude	
Tissue		
Bovine pericardium	Ionescu-Shiley	
Porcine heterograft	Hancock	
	Carpentier-Edwards	
	Angell-Shiley	

TABLE 13-2. *Features of commonly used prosthetic valves*

Valve type	Durability	Advantages	Disadvantages
Starr-Edwards	Good	Longest record of reliability and durability	Anticoagulation mandatory, hemolysis, poor hemodynamics in small sizes
Bjork-Shiley	Good	Durability, good hemodynamics even in small sizes	Anticoagulation mandatory, high potential for thrombotic occlusion
St. Jude	Uncertain	Low profile, good hemodynamics even in small sizes	Anticoagulation mandatory, thrombotic occlusion (?)
Porcine	Uncertain	Anticoagulation not mandatory, little hemolysis	Uncertain long-term durability, small sizes have poor hemodynamics, calcification in young patients

13-2). The mechanical substitutes are made of metal and/or synthetic materials such as Dacron, Teflon, pyrolytic carbon, silicone rubber, graphite, chromium cobalt, nickel, and stainless steel. The mechanical valve has a cufflike sewing ring of cloth, used to attach the prosthesis to the valve annulus. The sewing ring presents both inflow and outflow surfaces to blood and has an outer rim that forms the peripheral margin of the prosthesis and an inner ring that defines the valve orifice. Caged-ball prosthetic valves have struts that project from the inner ring on the outflow surface to form a cage that limits movement of the occluder.

TYPES OF PROSTHETIC VALVES

Caged-Ball Valves

Caged-ball valves have been used longer and more extensively than any other type of valve (8). The caged-ball devices are designed with a central ball occluder and a cage made with three or four struts that project from the inner ring on the outflow surface to form a cage that limits movement of the ball (Fig. 13-1). The struts may or may not be joined at their apex. In the closed position, the ball, made of cured silicone rubber, sits on a cloth-covered ring; in the open position the ball is restrained by the cage struts. Several modifications in this type of

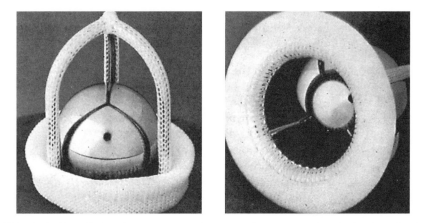

FIG. 13-1. Starr-Edwards aortic valve **(left)** and Starr-Edwards mitral valve **(right)**.

valve have been made, including using a metallic ball and covering the struts with cloth. These modifications were made in an attempt to improve durability and decrease thromboembolism; however, they presented other complications, and these two modifications are no longer used. The currently available caged-ball valve has unclothed struts and a silicone ball. The most common valve-related cause of death has been thromboembolism. It is clear that thrombogenic potential depends on valve type and location. Patients with caged-ball prostheses have the highest thrombogenicity, followed by those with single tilting-disk prostheses. Patients with bileaflet tilting disks have the lowest thrombogenic potential (9). Chronic anticoagulant therapy is required in all patients with mechanical prosthetic valves.

Disc Valves

Disc valves were introduced in the mid-1960s for mitral valve replacement on the assumption that they would be less likely to obstruct the aortic outflow tract or irritate the interventricular septum than ball valves in the mitral position. These valves are often referred to as low-profile valves. There have been many modifications in the tilting-disc valves since they were first introduced. The design principle of these valves is the incorporation of an occluder that pivots on its central axis in the open position to allow for the free flow of blood. Disc valves come in several different configurations. The oscillatory disc (e.g., Starr-Edwards, Kay-Shiley) is composed of a central metal disc that in the closed position sits on a ring and moves directly away from the ring in the open position and is restrained by open or closed metal struts. The mechanism of action of this valve is similar in concept to the caged-ball type, but the occluder is a flat disc rather than a ball, allowing for a smaller cage. These oscillating disc valves are infrequently used because they have little if any advantage over caged-ball valves. Caged-disc valves have a greater risk of thrombotic occlusion than caged-ball valves.

The tilting-disc valves (e.g., Bjork-Shiley) have an eccentric free-floating occluder (Fig. 13-2). The occluder pivots into the open position, providing a major and a minor orifice for blood flow. The tilting-disc valves open to varying angles, resulting in different flow patterns through the major and minor orifices: the wider the opening angle, the smaller the flow differences. These valves permit central laminar flow. The durability of the Bjork-Shiley pyrolytic-carbon prosthesis has been excellent to date (10). The major reservation regarding this valve is the possibility of sudden catastrophic valve thrombosis. The latest disc design is the bileaflet St. Jude valve that opens to provide two lateral major flow orifices and a minor central orifice (11) (Fig. 13-3).

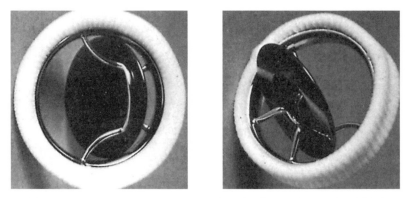

FIG. 13-2. Bjork-Shiley valve **(left)** and Bjork-Shiley mitral valve **(right)**.

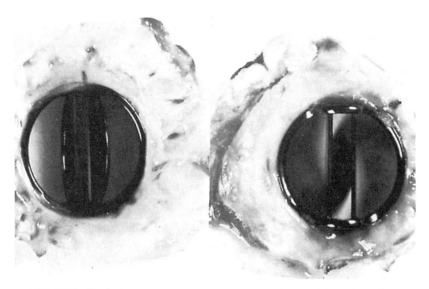

FIG. 13-3. St. Jude prosthetic valves. **Left:** top view; **right:** bottom view.

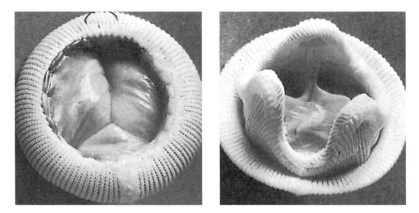

FIG. 13-4. Porcine bioprosthetic valves. **Left:** ventricular side (bottom); **right:** aortic root side (top).

Bioprosthetic (Tissue) Valves

Tissue valves are derived from human homografts or from bovine or porcine tissue. Tissue valves have three cusps that open and close like a normal human aortic valve. Before insertion, the valve is usually treated with glutaraldehyde to sterilize the valve and to reduce tissue antigenicity and stabilize proteins. The cusps of tissue valves may be unsupported but more often are mounted on a frame (Fig. 13-4). This includes a sewing ring that facilitates insertion and cloth-covered struts that provide a stent.

Despite the success of bioprosthetic valves, novel surgical techniques are on the horizon. Valve reconstruction from bovine or autologous pericardial tissue has recently been demonstrated to be a promising alternative to bioprosthetic valve replacement (12).

HEMODYNAMIC FEATURES OF PROSTHETIC VALVES

Design of the currently available prosthetic valves is such that there is minimal if any regurgitant flow; however, they all are "stenotic" because the effective *in vivo* valve area is less than the normal aortic or mitral valve area (13). After implantation, the effective *in vivo* valve area may diminish secondary to tissue ingrowth and endothelialization. In some instances, the resting transvalvular gradient may not be hemodynamically significant at rest; however, with exercise, significant gradients may develop. The Starr-Edwards caged-ball valve is intrinsically stenotic because of its design with blood flowing around the occluder. The resting transvalvular gradient is 6 to 20 mm Hg in the aortic position and 3 to 8 mm Hg in the mitral position (14). When the cloth covering was extended onto the struts, the gradient increased. The tilting-disc valves have smaller gradients as a result of their central flow design. In the larger disc valves (aortic 23 to 27 mm and mitral 29 to 33 mm), the resting transvalvular gradient in the aortic position is

5 to 15 mm Hg and 3 to 7 mm Hg in the mitral position (14). With smaller valves, larger gradients are found; however, the gradients are less than with similar-sized caged-ball devices. The St. Jude valve has transvalvular gradients in both the aortic and mitral position of less than 5 mm Hg when large valves are used. Measurement of gradients across the St. Jude valve is variable and dependent on the technique used. Because of the phenomenon of downstream pressure recovery, Doppler ultrasound measurements often overestimate the pressure gradient compared with catheter measurements (15). With smaller St. Jude valves, the gradient is no different than with similarly sized Bjork-Shiley valves (16). The porcine bioprosthetic valves have transvalvular gradients that have been reported from 6 to 23 mm Hg in the aortic area and in the mitral position from 2 to 8 mm Hg (17,18). There is a significant increase in transvalvular gradients when smaller valves are used.

OPERATIVE MORTALITY AND RESULTS

In the early years of valve replacement, the operative mortality approached 25%. Technical improvements have reduced the current risk to 2% to 10% for aortic or mitral valve replacement and 5% to 10% for multiple valve operations (19,20). In most cases, symptomatic improvement accompanies valve replacement. Valve replacement is highly likely to prolong the survival of patients with symptomatic aortic stenosis and mitral stenosis (21). It has been more difficult to show, however, improved survival in patients having valve replacement because of regurgitant lesions. The replacement of a diseased valve for whatever reason is not a cure, and the 10-year survival for operative survivors who received aortic and mitral Starr-Edwards valves is 60%, with most deaths being cardiac related (22,23). The major abnormalities that contribute to morbidity and mortality in patients with prosthetic heart valves relate to myocardial disease, other cardiac lesions, and/or prosthesis related problems (24,25).

Left ventricular function has an extremely important impact on the long-term results of prosthetic valve surgery. Myocardium may be damaged by long-standing pressure or volume overload with resultant hypertrophy and fibrosis. Improvement in ventricular function is more commonly seen after correction of stenotic lesions rather than regurgitant ones. However, clinical data now indicate that left ventricular function is preserved in patients with regurgitant lesions if valve repair is done instead of valve replacement (26). Myocardial dysfunction may occur as a result of the surgery itself. Necrosis and fibrosis may result from ischemia during surgery, further compromising ventricular function. Myocardial protection during valve replacement must be accomplished. New techniques of myocardial protection, such as cold cardioplegia and retrograde delivery, have decreased myocardial damage during surgery.

Other cardiac abnormalities may coexist with valvular heart disease. Alterations in the conduction system, coronary arteries, pulmonary vasculature, and other heart valves may influence the postoperative results.

DURABILITY OF PROSTHETIC VALVES

The durability of prosthetic heart valves remains a major problem (27). Ideally, a substitute cardiac valve should last a patient's lifetime. To date, mechanical valves have a much better record for reliable long-term performance than bioprosthetic valves. Long-term follow-up studies have shown that mechanical valves last well into the second and even the third decade after implantation. This is in contrast to the bioprostheses, which can have a 10% to 30% failure rate after 10 years (28,29). Durability of the early types of caged-ball valves may be compromised by ball variance: Valve malfunction is caused by chemical and physical alterations in the oc-

cluder. An increased or decreased diameter, grooving, cracking, fragmentation, and formation of fluid lakes in the core of the occluder all affect valve durability. Ball variance rarely occurs with the currently used ball valves.

Disc-valve durability may be compromised by disc variance. The discs move up and down in a fixed axis. This movement results in an uneven distribution of stress on contacting parts. If the disc wears to such an extent that it cannot cover the primary orifice, valvular regurgitation results.

The long-term durability and biologic fate of bioprosthetic valves are uncertain. The glutaraldehyde-preserved porcine valves have produced excellent results with minimal complications, although present evidence suggests degeneration may develop after 5 to 7 years (20,30–35). Bioprosthetic valves are contraindicated in patients with abnormal calcium metabolism, such as patients with severe kidney disease and in young patients (less than age 35) because of early valve calcification (36,37).

FOLLOW-UP OF PATIENTS WITH PROSTHETIC HEART VALVES

The follow-up of patients with prosthetic heart valves requires careful attention. All patients require regular follow-up. Patients with mechanical valves require life-long chronic anticoagulation. This is accomplished by dosing oral coumadin to a desired international normalized ratio. The intensity of anticoagulation should be determined by the age of the patient, the type and number of valves, and the position of the valve (3). Those with porcine valves usually need to be anticoagulated for the first 3 months after surgery but not after that unless they are in atrial fibrillation, have a history of systemic embolism, or had an intracardiac clot at the time of operation. Each time the patient is seen, the physician should assess the overall medical status and seek evidence of prosthetic valve complications.

Auscultatory Findings

Each type of prosthetic heart valve is associated with distinct auscultatory findings caused by the altered flow characteristics of the valve itself (38) (Table 13-3). Auscultation can provide the earliest clues to prosthetic valve malfunction (Table 13-4). Caged-ball valves have easily audible opening and closing sounds corresponding to the maximal excursion and seating of the ball. In the mitral position, there is a very prominent opening click, which one can usually detect 0.1 seconds after the aortic second sound (A_2). Shortening or prolongation of this A_2 opening click interval suggests prosthetic obstruction or interference with excursion of the ball. Systolic murmurs due to turbulence of flow around the prosthesis are common, but a diastolic murmur indicates prosthetic dysfunction or obstruction. In the aortic position, the ball valve produces a loud opening click that is clearly separated from S_1. A softer closing sound is also audible. A systolic ejection murmur is usually present, which at times may be quite harsh, but a diastolic murmur should not be present.

In contrast with caged-ball valves, tilting and caged-disc valves produce faint opening sounds; however, they do have distinct closing sounds that tend to be high pitched or clicking in quality. In the mitral position, there is a prominent closing sound at the apex. The systolic ejection murmur, which is usually heard, is thought to be due to the turbulent flow around the mitral valve apparatus lying in the left ventricular outflow tract. A diastolic murmur may be heard and is thought to result from turbulent flow across the valve. Disc valves in the aortic position also produce dis-

TABLE 13-3. *Normal auscultatory findings in patients with prosthetic heart valves*

Valve	Caged-ball	Disc	Bioprosthetic
Aortic	Sharp opening sound after S_1 Sharp closing sound at S_1 "Rattling" of ball during systole Systolic ejection murmur	Soft opening sound after S_1 Sharp closing sound at S_2 Systolic ejection murmur	Systolic ejection murmur
Mitral	Sharp opening sound after S_2 Sharp closing sound at S_1 "Rattling" of ball during diastole Systolic ejection murmur	Soft opening sound after S_2 Sharp closing sound at S_1	"Diastolic rumble" (may represent obstruction) Systolic ejection murmur Opening snap

TABLE 13-4. *Auscultatory findings suggesting prosthetic valve dysfunction*

Valve	Caged-ball	Disc	Bioprosthetic
Aortic	Diastolic murmur	Diastolic murmur (may hear faint diastolic murmur because disc does not contact the ring)	Diastolic murmur
	Diminished opening sound (ball variance)	Absent closing sound	
Mitral	Prolonged S_2-OS interval (prosthetic obstruction, severe mitral regurgitation) Shortened S_2-OS interval (interference with ball excursion) Loss of previously audible opening and closing prosthetic clicks Systolic murmur louder than grade 2/6 Diastolic murmur (prosthetic dysfunction/obstruction)	Absent closing sound Systolic murmur louder than grade 2/6	Increasing systolic murmur New or changing diastolic murmur

OS, opening snap.

tinct closing sounds. A systolic murmur is common because of turbulent flow across the valve, but the presence of a diastolic murmur indicates valve dysfunction.

The most common tissue valves in use today are glutaraldehyde-stabilized porcine valves (7). They produce opening and closing sounds that are much less prominent than those of the mechanical valves. In the mitral position, some patients have an audible opening snap at the apex—most have a closing sound audible at the left lower sternal border that is like the normal mitral closing sound. In the aortic position, tissue valves also produce closing and, occasionally, opening sounds. Frequently, there is a systolic flow murmur, but a diastolic murmur is abnormal.

Chest X-Ray Findings

The chest x-ray can provide useful information in patients with prosthetic heart valves (39). It may be helpful in diagnosing extremely uncommon but life-threatening complications such as ball or disc dislodgement. The chest x-ray may also be helpful in identifying the type of prosthetic valve the patient has had implanted (Table 13-5). Chest fluoroscopy can reveal abnormal rocking of a dehiscing prosthesis or limitation of the occluder, if the latter is opaque (40). Cineradiographic imaging has been used successfully to detect single-leg separations in the Bjork-Shiley convexo-concavo valves. Failure of these struts can lead to disk embolization and catastrophic valvular incompetence (41).

Echocardiography

Echocardiography provides useful information regarding prosthetic valve function or dysfunction (42–44). Two-dimensional (2D) and Doppler echocardiography are the most reliable techniques for the noninvasive evaluation of prosthetic heart valves (45). By examining the opening and closing motion of the poppet and its excursion within the cage, gross abnormalities of poppet mobility due to ball variance or thrombus formation can sometimes be detected. The echocardiographic appearance of tilting-disc valves can be extremely variable because the tilting disc opens in an arc and the orientation of the arc depends on the orientation of the valve within the heart. Echocardiography for tilting-disc valves is usually limited to the detection of gross motion abnormalities of the disc. Phonocardiography of the time interval between aortic closure and the opening click of a mechanical mitral poppet can be helpful in identifying prosthetic dysfunction in the absence of atrial fibrillation: Prolongation or marked variability of this interval may indicate mechanical interference with poppet motion.

Schapira et al. (46) found that M-mode echocardiography provided a 67% diagnostic accuracy rate in patients evaluated for bioprosthetic valve dysfunction, and 2D echocardiography was significantly better with a 97% diagnostic accuracy. Useful echocardiographic features include diastolic fluttering of the mitral leaflets, which suggests prosthetic aortic insufficiency; normal septal motion, which

---

TABLE 13-5. *Radiologic appearance of prosthetic heart valves*

Type of valve	Valve name	Identifying factors
Caged-ball valves	Starr-Edwards 6000	Four struts joined at apex, radiolucent poppet
	Braunwald Cutter	Open-ended cage, radiolucent poppet
Low-profile disc	Starr-Edwards	Low-profile cage, cross struts, radioopaque poppet, concave perforations
	Kay-Shiley	Single or double muscle guard, two parallel struts, radiolucent poppet
Central flow, eccentric monocusp	Lillehei-Kaster	Two teardrop-shaped pivots, two lateral disc guide-shields, radiolucent poppet
	Bjork-Shiley	Two eccentrically located support struts, radiolucent poppet
Bioprosthesis		Radiolucent stents

suggests prosthetic regurgitation because the septum usually moves paradoxically for up to 5 years after implantation; and visualization of normal thin bioprosthetic cusps without fluttering, which helps to exclude the possibility of bioprosthetic stenosis, endocarditis, or regurgitation secondary to flail cusps.

COMPLICATIONS OF PROSTHETIC VALVES

Although most patients with prosthetic heart valves do well, they are subject to a variety of complications (Table 13-6) (47–51). All patients require close follow-up to permit early detection of complications if they occur. History and physical examination, including careful auscultation, provide clues to the presence of complications in most patients. Fluoroscopy, 2D echocardiography, nuclear scans, or even cardiac catheterization may be needed in some cases.

Thromboembolism

Although the precise incidence is uncertain (it is believed to range from 0.1% to 5.7% per patient-year), thromboembolism continues to be the most common complication of prosthetic heart valves, especially for patients with mechanical valves (52–55). Strokes and other disabling thromboembolic complications are estimated to occur at a rate of 1% to 5% per year (this includes bioprosthetic valves without anticoagulation therapy and other valves with adequate anticoagulation) (56). Patients requiring anticoagulation are subjected to an additional risk of hemorrhagic

complications, estimated to be 1% per year for life-threatening hemorrhages and up to 20% per year for other hemorrhagic complications (57). Accurate comparison of the frequency that various prosthetic valves develop thromboembolic complications is difficult because of lack of standardized reporting of thromboembolic complications, variable anticoagulation compliance and monitoring, and unrecognized embolic complications.

Thrombosis and embolism may occur for several reasons: The prosthetic valve may cause turbulence, shearing stress, stagnation, eddy currents that may damage cellular elements, and release factors that evoke the normal clotting reaction. The valve materials themselves may encourage thrombosis. Furthermore, the presence of atrial fibrillation may lead to left atrial thrombosis with resultant systemic embolism in patients with any type of mechanical or bioprosthetic valve.

When comparing different mechanical valves in the aortic position, thromboembolic events per 100 patient-years have been reported as follows: 3.4 for non–cloth-covered Starr-Edwards, 1.8 for the Bjork-Shiley, 1.4 for the Lillehei-Kaster, and 0.7 for the St. Jude (53). Early reports with the St. Jude valve reveal incidences of thromboembolism not significantly different from those of bioprosthetic valves in the mitral position. Bioprostheses are inherently less thrombogenic than mechanical valves. This is particularly true in the aortic position. In the presence of atrial fibrillation, however, thrombi may form in the left atrium.

All patients with mechanical valves require anticoagulation for life. The incidence of

---

TABLE 13-6. *Potential complications in patients with prosthetic heart valves*

Hemorrhagic complications of anticoagulation
Systemic embolism
Endocarditis
Hemolytic anemia
Mechanical dysfunction
    Obstruction—thrombotic persistent stenosis due to patient-prosthetic mismatch
    Insufficiency—disruption of tissue leaflets, valve sticking in open position
Parabasilar leak
Other—ball variance, ball wear, sturt fracture, dehiscence

thromboembolism remains fairly constant over time. Patients with bioprosthetic valves have a low incidence of thromboembolism unless one or more of four risk factors is present: atrial fibrillation, a large left atrium, a clot in the left atrium at the time of operation, or a history of prior systemic embolism. The incidence of embolism depends directly on the number of risk factors present. Because the incidence of thromboembolism for bioprostheses appears to be highest in the first 3 months after implantation, patients are frequently maintained on anticoagulants for 3 months after valve replacement (24). Withholding anticoagulants during surgical procedures or other interventions is less risky in patients with bioprosthetic valves than for those with mechanical valves. Sudden interruption of anticoagulants should be avoided unless absolutely necessary. A 20% to 25% rate of embolization in the first year after withdrawal of anticoagulants has been reported in patients with Bjork-Shiley valves (24). When discontinuation of anticoagulation is required because of elective surgery, warfarin should be stopped 3 to 4 days before surgery and restarted as soon as possible postoperatively. Many physicians admit patients with prosthetic heart valves to the hospital when warfarin is stopped and begin intravenous heparin therapy. The heparin may be discontinued 4 to 6 hours before the procedure and restarted postoperatively. A patient with a mechanical valve in the aortic position can probably have anticoagulants withheld for 3 to 5 days without incuring added risk of thrombosis or embolism. The risk of acute thrombosis with a mitral prosthetic valve, however, increases significantly after the first 24 hours, especially with the Bjork-Shiley valve. Management of anticoagulation is difficult, and unfortunately there is no uniformly accepted approach (see Chapter 15). Surgery is the current therapy of choice for patients with acute prosthetic valve thrombosis. Thrombolytic therapy is recommended for patients who are at high surgical risk. A high rate of cerebral thromboembolism is seen in these individuals (58).

The use of antiplatelet agents without warfarin has not been adequate in the prevention of thrombosis and embolism in patients with mechanical prosthetic valves. The addition of dipyridamole and/or aspirin to warfarin has not been shown to be more effective than warfarin alone despite one initially favorable report (59,60). If a patient develops recurrent emboli with a mechanical prosthesis despite adequate anticoagulation, replacement with a bioprosthetic valve may be required.

Infective Endocarditis

Endocarditis involving prosthetic heart valves is a life-threatening complication (61–64). Patients with prosthetic heart valves demonstrate increased vulnerability to endocarditis, and once infection has developed, eradication is difficult. The documented incidence of infection ranges from 3% to 6% of patients (65). Prosthetic endocarditis can be divided into that which occurs early after surgical implantation and that which occurs late. Within 60 days of the operation, infection usually results from contamination during the surgical procedure or an infection occurring in the immediate postoperative period. The incidence of early endocarditis is low, approximately 2% (66,67). The infecting organism is most commonly staphylococcus (either *S. aureus* or *S. epidermidis*) but may be a fungus or a gram-negative bacterium. These organisms tend not to respond to antibiotics, and the overall mortality is in excess of 75% (68). Antibiotic prophylaxis is recommended immediately before implantation of a valve substitute and for a few days afterward (69).

Prosthetic endocarditis occurring late after surgery is more likely to resemble typical subacute bacterial endocarditis. The incidence of endocarditis on prosthetic valves is approximately 1% per patient-year (68). Streptococcal strains are the usual causative agents. Staphylococci are less common, and fungal and gram-negative organisms are rare. The mortality for late prosthetic endocarditis is approximately 25% (70). This lower rate probably reflects less virulent organisms or ones that are more sensitive to antibiotics. Patients with late endocarditis usually present with fever, fatigue, malaise, lethargy, or anorexia. Onset is usually gradual but occasionally can be abrupt. Physical examination may reveal new murmurs of regurgitation and evidence of systemic embolization.

Medical therapy is effective in only one third of patients with endocarditis involving a prosthetic valve (71). It is more likely to be effective if there are no new regurgitant murmurs and the organism is of low virulence and high antibiotic sensitivity. When medical therapy is of no avail (uncontrolled infection) or if systemic embolism or left ventricular failure occurs, the physician must recognize this promptly and plan for immediate reoperation.

Because all prosthetic heart valves can become infected, every patient should receive endocarditis prophylaxis whenever the potential for bacteremia exists. Chapter 14 reviews the recommended antibiotic prophylaxis for patients with prosthetic heart valves. The recommended antibiotic prophylaxis is broader for prosthetic heart valves than for native diseased valves because of the higher incidence of infection with virulent organisms in the former. Inadequate antibiotic prophylaxis places the patient with a prosthetic heart valve at high risk for endocarditis.

Hemolysis

The incidence and degree of hemolysis relate to the type of cardiac prosthesis implanted; it is highest in patients with non–cloth-covered Starr-Edwards aortic valves. In general, hemolytic anemia occurs more commonly with prosthetic valves in the aortic than in the mitral position, and hemolysis is more common with caged-ball mechanical prostheses than with tilting-disc valves (72,73). This is a result of several factors, including less central and more turbulent blood flow with ball valves. In addition, red cell compression by the ball when it comes into contact with the seating ring can lead to red blood cell trauma and hemolysis. Hemolysis tends to be greatest when the orifice

through which the red cells travel is small, as in slitlike perivalvular leaks or stenotic valves. Hemolysis may eventually cause iron deficiency, which increases the fragility of the red cells and leads to a vicious cycle with increased hemolysis. Also, anemia increases cardiac output and flow across the valve, further increasing red cell lysis. Hallmarks of significant prosthetic valve hemolysis are hemosiderinuria, schistocytosis, reticulocytosis, absent serum haptoglobin, and elevated serum lactate dehydrogenase. Treatment is achieved with supplemental iron and folate and blood transfusions if the hematocrit becomes too low. Patients with symptomatic refractory anemia should be closely evaluated for signs of prosthetic dysfunction, especially perivalvular leak. Replacement of the valve is indicated only if the anemia is refractory to therapy and causes high output failure or if the hemolysis is due to significant valve dysfunction. Specific echo-Doppler findings have been demonstrated in patients with hemolysis thought to be secondary to a prosthetic valve. In particular, patterns of flow associated with high shear stress seem to be of significance (74).

Left Ventricular Failure Due to Malfunction of Prosthetic Valves

The occurrence of left ventricular failure in a patient with a prosthetic mitral or aortic valve is ominous. Heart failure may be unrelated to the prosthetic valve and may be due to coronary artery or myocardial disease resulting from the long-standing effects of the valvular lesion before correction. Associated uncorrected valvular disease may also cause heart failure. For a significant number of patients, however, left ventricular failure is due to mechanical failure of the prosthetic valve. Endocarditis of the prosthesis can also present as heart failure.

Careful evaluation is necessary to uncover the cause of heart failure. Blood cultures should be obtained, and noninvasive testing should be performed. 2D echocardiography of the suspected failing prosthesis can yield valuable information. Radionuclide ventriculography is also useful. Normal or near-normal left ventricular function suggests prosthetic valve dysfunction as the cause of left ventricular failure. Fluoroscopy of the prosthetic valve may detect abnormal rocking of the valve or altered motion of a mechanical component of the valve. Finally, cardiac catheterization and angiography may be required. The diagnosis of myocardial disease due to chronic effects of valvular heart disease should not be made until all correctable causes of left ventricular failure are excluded.

Valve failure has been reported with all types of prosthetic valves (Table 13-7). It is generally gradual in onset, but occasionally it occurs suddenly with fatal outcome. Modes of valve failure include valvular or parabasilar regurgitation, disruption of tissue leaflets, thrombotic obstruction, ball variance (which can cause the ball to stick in the open position), fracture of supporting struts, or dislodging of the ball or disc. The tilting-disc prosthesis has a very low mechanical failure rate but is quite sensitive to thrombotic occlusion in either the aortic or mitral position. This results in disc immobility with obstruction and severe regurgitation, causing rapid deterioration of the patient. Ball variance can be caused by swelling, fissuring, fracture, or fragmentation of the prosthetic poppet, which results in impaction, dislodgement, or embolization (23,75,76). Other rare causes of mechanical failure include incorporation of the cage into the left ventricle and cocking of the disc (47). The most important potential disadvantage of porcine valves is that with time they are at increased risk of fibrocalcific degeneration. This process is accelerated in children and young adults. When a patient with a prosthetic valve develops new or unstable angina, syncope or near syncope, dyspnea, increasing hemolysis, or transient ischemic attacks, valve failure should be suspected.

All prosthetic valves have effective *in vivo* orifices that are smaller than the normal native valve. Thus, the prosthetic valve is stenotic compared with the normal valve. This is a particular problem in cases of patient-prosthesis mismatch that occurs in those individuals in whom a small prosthetic valve has been implanted because of a small aortic or mitral anulus. These patients are left with residual obstruction across the prosthetic valve. If the prosthesis is in the mitral position, one can expect symptoms of pulmonary venous hypertension when valve flow is significantly increased, as with exertion (77).

Unrecognized or untreated valvular lesions may cause significant impairment of prosthetic valve function. The regurgitant jet of associated but uncorrected aortic insufficiency in a patient with a mitral prosthesis may impede the proper function of the prosthesis and even cause damage to the mitral disc with resultant mitral regurgitation (78). With an aortic prosthesis, if concomitant subvalvular left ventricular outflow obstruction is not identified, little or no clinical improvement occurs after aortic valve replacement. In this circumstance, clinical failure may be incorrectly attributed to the prosthesis or to myocardial disease.

Pregnancy in patients with prosthetic heart valves presents a difficult problem (79,80). In women with bioprosthetic valves who do not require anticoagulation and who have a good

TABLE 13-7. Structural failure of prosthetic heart valves

Caged-ball	Disc	Bioprosthetic
Strut fracture	Sewing ring dehiscence (secondary to endocarditis)	Spontaneous tissue degeneration
Ball variance (rare)	Thrombosis interfering with proper disc motion	Leaflet perforation
Sewing ring dehiscence	Eccentric wearing of disc	Leaflet calcification (leading to stenosis or regurgitation)

hemodynamic result, pregnancy carries a low risk for both mother and fetus. In these women, the use of prophylactic aspirin has been suggested. In one series, aspirin resulted in no maternal mortality or morbidity from thromboembolism or hemorrhages nor any apparent adverse effect to the fetus (80). In women with mechanical valves or in those with bioprostheses who require warfarin, a dilemma exists. Unfortunately, warfarin is teratogenic and cannot be used during the first trimester. At term, warfarin may cause lethal cerebral hemorrhage in the fetus. The teratogenic effect of warfarin may already have occurred before the pregnancy is recognized. The efficacy of fixed low-dose heparin administered subcutaneously as thromboembolic prophylaxis has been studied (79). Although the regimen was well tolerated, it did not provide adequate thromboembolic prophylaxis in patients with prosthetic heart valves during pregnancy. These risks of anticoagulation make the decision of valve type a difficult one in women of childbearing age. If a woman wishes to have subsequent pregnancies, a strong argument is present for a bioprosthetic valve; however, the questionable durability of the bioprostheses raises the probability of future reoperation.

Examination of currently available data reveals advantages and disadvantages of each of the available prosthetic valves. The surgeon together with the cardiologist should choose the best type of valve substitute for a particular patient (81).

REFERENCES

1. Harken DE, et al. Partial and complete prostheses in aortic insufficiency. *J Thorac Cardiovasc Surg* 1960;40: 744.
2. Starr A, Edward ML. Mitral replacement: clinical experience with a ball-valve prosthesis. *Ann Surg* 1961;154: 726.
3. Teply JF, et al. The ultimate prognosis after valve replacement: an assessment at twenty years. *Ann Thorac Surg* 1981;32:11.
4. Harken DE, Taylor SJ, Lafemine AA. Aortic valve replacement with a caged ball. *Am J Cardiol* 1962;9:292.
5. Carpentier A, et al. Continuing improvements in valvular bioprostheses. *J Thorac Cardiovasc Surg* 1982;83: 27.
6. Bonchek LJ. Current status of cardiac valve replace-ment: selection of a prosthesis and indications for operation. *Am Heart J* 1981;101:96.
7. Silverman NA, Levitsky S. Current choices for prosthetic valve replacement. *Mod Concepts Cardiovasc Dis* 1983;52:35.
8. Bonchek LJ, Starr A. Ball valve prostheses: current appraisal of late results. *Am J Cardiol* 1975;35:843.
9. Cannegieter SC, Rosendaal FR. Thromboembolic and bleeding complications in patients with heart valve prostheses. *Circulation* 1994;89:635.
10. Bjork VO, Heinze A. Ten year experience with the Bjork-Shiley tilting disc valve. *J Thorac Cardiovasc Surg* 1979;78:331.
11. Emery RW, Mettler E, Nicoloff DM. A new cardiac prosthesis: the St. Jude medical cardiac valve. *Circulation* 1979;60[Suppl]:148.
12. Bjornstad K, Duran RM, Nassau K, Gometza B, Hatle LK, Duran CM. Clinical and echocardiographic followup after aortic valve reconstruction with bovine or autologous pericardium. *Am Heart J* 1996;132:1173.
13. Horskotte D, et al. Central hemodynamics at rest and during exercise after mitral valve replacement with different prostheses. *Circulation* 1983;68[Suppl 11]:161.
14. Pyle RB, et al. Hemodynamic evaluation of Lillehei-Kaster and Starr-Edwards prostheses. *Ann Thorac Surg* 1978;26:336.
15. Vandervoort PM, Greenberg NL, Pu M, Powell KA, Cosgrove DM, Thomas JD. Pressure recovery in bileaflet heart valve prostheses. *Circulation* 1995;92:3464.
16. Nicoloff DM, et al. Clinical and hemodynamic results with the St. Jude medical cardiac valve prosthesis. *J Thorac Cardiovasc Surg* 1981;82:674.
17. Levine FH, Carter JE, Buckley MJ. Hemodynamic evaluation of Hancock and Carpentier-Edwards bioprosthesis. *Circulation* 1981;64[Suppl]:192.
18. Chaitman BR, Bronan R, Lepage G. Hemodynamic evaluation of the Carpentier-Edwards porcine xenograft. *Circulation* 1976;60:1170.
19. West PN, Ferguson TB, Clar RE. Multiple valve replacement: changing status. *Ann Thorac Surg* 1978;26: 32.
20. [Removed]
21. Selzer A. Present status of prosthetic cardiac valves. *Arch Intern Med* 1983;143:1965.
22. McGoon MD, et al. Aortic and mitral valve incompetence: long-term follow-up (10 to 19 years) of patients treated with Starr-Edwards prosthesis. *J Am Coll Cardiol* 1984;3:930.
23. Lefrak EA, Starr A. *Cardiac Valve Prostheses.* New York: Appleton-Century-Crofts, 1979.
24. Morton MT, Rahimtoola SH. How to follow patients with prosthetic heart valves. *J Cardiovasc Med* 1980;5:475.
25. St John Sutton MG, et al. Valve replacement without preoperative cardiac catheterization. *N Engl J Med* 1981;305:1233.
26. Ren JF, Aksut S, Lighty GW, et al. Mitral repair is superior to vavle replacement for the early preservation of cardiac function: relation of ventricular geometry to function. *Am Heart J* 1996;131:974.
27. McGoon DC. Long term effects of prosthetic materials. *Am J Cardiol* 1982;50:621.
28. Schoevaerdts JC, Buche M, el Gariani A, et al. Twenty years experience with the model 6120 Starr-Edwards valve in the mitral position. *J Thorac Cardiovasc Surg* 1987;94:375.

29. O'Brien MF, Stafford EG, Gardner MAF, et al. Allograft aortic valve replacement: long term follow-up. *Ann Thorac Surg* 1995;60:S65.

30. Goffin YA, et al. Normally and abnormally functioning left sided porcine bioprosthetic valves after long term implantation in patients: distinct spectra of histologic and histochemical changes. *J Am Coll Cardiol* 1984;4:324.

31. Magillan DJ, et al. Spontaneous degeneration of porcine bioprosthetic valves. *Ann Thorac Surg* 1980;30:259.

32. Oyer PE, et al. Clinical durability of the Hancock porcine bioprosthetic valve. *J Thorac Cardiovasc Surg* 1980;80:824.

33. Cohn LH, et al. Five to eight year follow up of patients undergoing porcine heart valve replacement. *N Engl J Med* 1981;304:257.

34. Lakier JB, et al. Porcine xenograft valves. *Circulation* 1980;62:313.

35. Gallo J, et al. Degeneration in porcine bioprosthetic cardiac valves: incidence of primary tissue failures among 938 bioprostheses at risk. *Am J Cardiol* 1984;53:1061.

36. Sanders SP, et al. Use of Hancock porcine xenografts in children and adolescents. *Am J Cardiol* 1980;46:429.

37. Dunn JM. Porcine valve durability in children. *Ann Thorac Surg* 1981;32:357.

38. Smith ND, Raizada V, Abrams J. Auscultation of the normally functioning prosthetic valve. *Ann Intern Med* 1981;95:594.

39. Chun PKC, Nelson WP. Common cardiac prosthetic valves. *JAMA* 1977;238:401.

40. Sands MJ, et al. Diagnostic value of cinefluoroscopy in the evaluation of prosthetic heart valve dysfunction. *Am Heart J* 1982;104:622.

41. O'Neill WW, Chandler JG, et al. Radiographic detection of strut separation in Bjork-Shiley convexo-concavo mitral valves. *N Engl J Med* 1995;333:414.

42. Kotler MN, et al. Noninvasive evaluation of normal and abnormal prosthetic valve function. *J Am Coll Cardiol* 1983;2:151.

43. Johnson ML, Paton BC, Holmes JH. Ultrasonic evaluation of prosthetic valve motion. *Circulation* 1970;41 [Suppl II]:3.

44. Grenadier E, et al. Detection of deterioration or infection of homograft and porcine xenograft bioprosthetic valves in mitral and aortic positions by two dimensional echocardiographic examination. *J Am Coll Cardiol* 1983;2:452.

45. Williams GA, Labovitz AJ. Doppler hemodynamic evaluation of prosthetic and bioprosthetic cardiac valves. *Am J Cardiol* 1985;56:325.

46. Schapira JN, et al. Two dimensional echocardiographic assessment of patients with bioprosthetic valves. *Am J Cardiol* 1979;43:511.

47. Roberts WC. Complications of cardiac valve replacement: characteristic abnormalities of prostheses pertaining to any or specific site. *Am Heart J* 1982;103:113.

48. Gore JM, Dalen JE. Complications of prosthetic heart valves. *J Cardiovasc Med* 1983;8:1153.

49. Horstkottle D, et al. Late complications in patients with Bjork-Shiley and St. Jude mechanical heart valve replacement. *Circulation* 1983;68[Suppl II]:175.

50. Giuliani ER. Cardiac prostheses: a twentieth century problem. *Int J Cardiol* 1983;3:203.

51. Schoen EJ, Titus JL, Lawne GM. Autopsy determined causes of death after cardiac valve replacement. *JAMA* 1983;249:899.

52. Kontos GJ, Schaff HV. Thrombotic occlusion of a prosthetic heart valve: diagnosis and management. *Mayo Clin Proc* 1985;60:118.

53. Edmunds LH. Thromboembolic complications of current cardiac valvular prostheses. *Ann Thorac Surg* 1982; 34:96.

54. Pumphrey CW, Fuster V, Cheseboro JH. Systemic thromboembolism in valvular heart disease and prosthetic heart valves. *Mod Concepts Cardiovasc Dis* 1982;51:131.

55. Metzdorff MT, et al. Thrombosis of mechanical cardiac valves: a qualitative comparison of the silastic ball valve and the tilting disc valve. *J Am Coll Cardiol* 1983;4:50.

56. Edmunds LH. Thromboembolic complications of current cardiac valvular prostheses. *Ann Thorac Surg* 1982;34:96.

57. Lieberman A, et al. Intracranial hemorrhage and infarction in anticoagulated patients with prosthetic heart valves. *Stroke* 1978;9:18.

58. Lengyel M, Fuster V, et al. Guidelines for management of left-sided prosthetic valve thrombosis: a role for thrombolytic therapy. *J Am Coll Cardiol* 1997;30:1521.

59. Cheseboro JH, et al. Trial of combined warfarin plus dipyridamole or aspirin therapy in prosthetic heart valve replacement. *Am J Cardiol* 1983;51:1537.

60. Altman R, Boollan F, Rouvier J. Aspirin and prophylaxis of thromboembolic complications in patients with substitute heart valves. *J Thorac Cardiovasc Surg* 1976;72:127.

61. Dismikes WE. Prosthetic valve endocarditis: factors influencing outcome and recommendations for therapy. In: Bisno AI, ed. *Treatment of Infective Endocarditis.* New York: Grune & Stratton, 1981.

62. Calderwood S, et al. Risk factors for development of prosthetic valve endocarditis. *Circulation* 1985;72:31.

63. Murphy ES, Kloster FC. Late results of valve replacement surgery: complications of prosthetic heart valves. *Mod Concepts Cardiovasc Dis* 1979;48:59.

64. Wilson WR, Jaumin P, Danielson GK. Prosthetic valve endocarditis. *Ann Intern Med* 1975;82:751.

65. Threlkeld MG, Cobbs CG. Infectious disorders of prosthetic valves and intravascular devices. In: Mandell GL, Bennette JE, Dolin R, eds. *Mandell, Douglas, and Bennette's principles and practice of infectious diseases, 4th edition.* Vol. 1. New York: Churchill Livingstone, 1995.

66. Calderwood SB, Swinski LA, Waternaux CM. Risk factors for the development of prosthetic valve endocarditis. *Circulation* 1985;72:31.

67. Saffle JR, et al. Prosthetic valve endocarditis: the case for prompt valve replacement. *J Thorac Cardiovasc Surg* 1977;73:416.

68. Murphy ES, Kloster FC. Late results of valve replacement surgery. II. Complications of prosthetic heart valves. *Mod Concepts Cardiovasc Dis* 1979;48:59.

69. Goldmann DA, et al. Cephalothin prophylaxis in cardiac valve surgery: a prospective, double-blind comparison of two-day and six-day regimens. *J Thorac Cardiovasc Surg* 1977;73:470.

70. Shemin RJ, et al. Prosthetic aortic valves indications for and results of reoperation. *Arch Surg* 1979;114:63.

71. Rodewald G, et al. The risk of reoperation in acquired valvular heart disease. *J Thorac Cardiovasc Surg* 1980; 28:77.

72. Santinga JT, Kirsh MM. Hemolytic anemia in series 2300 and 2310 Starr-Edwards prosthetic valves. *Ann Thorac Surg* 1972;14:539.

73. Austen WG. Heart valve substitutes. In: Johnson RA, Haber E, Austen WG, eds. *The Practice of Cardiology.* Boston: Little, Brown, 1980.

74. Yeo TC, Freeman WK, Schaff HV, Orszulak TA. Mechanisms of hemolysis after mitral valve repair: assessment by serial echocardiography. *J Am Coll Cardiol* 1998;32:717.

75. Hylen JC. Mechanical malfunction and thrombosis of prosthetic heart valves. *Am J Cardiol* 1972;30:396.

76. Krosnick A. Death due to migration of the ball from an aortic-valve prosthesis. *JAMA* 1965;191:1083.

77. Dalen JE, Alpert JJ, eds. *Valvular Heart Diseases.* Boston: Little, Brown, 1981:79–81.

78. Carlson CJ. Mitral regurgitation due to intermittent prosthetic valvular dysfunction. *Chest* 1971;71:90.

79. Wang RY, et al. Efficacy of low dose, subcutaneously administered heparin in treatment of pregnant women with artificial heart valves. *Med J Aust* 1983;2:126.

80. Nunez L, et al. Pregnancy in 20 patients with bioprosthetic valve replacement. *Chest* 1983;84:26.

81. Cooley DA. Current status of surgical treatment of acquired valvular heart disease. *Tex Med* 1983;79:41.

14

Antimicrobial Prophylaxis of Bacterial Endocarditis and Acute Rheumatic Fever

Kathryn A. Taubert

Department of Science and Medicine, American Heart Association; Department of Physiology,
University of Texas Southwestern Medical School, Dallas, Texas 75231

Bacterial infections can cause serious cardiac disease. Two examples are endocarditis and rheumatic fever. The American Heart Association (AHA) states that in 1994, total hospital discharges with the diagnosis of bacterial endocarditis (International Classification of Diseases, 9th edition [ICD/9] code 421.0) was about 22,000. For that same year, total hospital discharges for rheumatic fever/rheumatic heart disease (ICD/9 codes 390–398) was about 17,000 (1). Primary prevention of both of these potentially devastating conditions can often be accomplished by antimicrobial prophylaxis. Antibiotic prophylaxis given before certain surgical or dental procedures can decrease the likelihood of endocarditis in individuals at risk. Likewise, antibiotics can prevent rheumatic fever by eradicating group A streptococci from the throat. In individuals who have already had rheumatic fever, secondary prevention is accomplished by long-term administration of antibiotics.

ENDOCARDITIS

Bacterial endocarditis occurs when certain bloodborne bacteria lodge on damaged endocardial (endothelial) surfaces of the heart, usually an abnormal or prosthetic valve or an anatomic cardiac defect. In the preantibiotic era, mortality was virtually 100%. Although advances in antimicrobial therapy and the development of better diagnostic and surgical techniques have reduced the morbidity and mortality, it remains a potentially life-threatening disease. Therefore, primary prevention is very important.

Rationale

The rationale for endocarditis prophylaxis was succinctly defined by Durack (2). He stated that endocarditis usually follows bacteremia, certain health care procedures cause bacteremia with organisms that can cause endocarditis, and these bacteria are usually sensitive to antibiotics; therefore, antibiotics should be given to patients with predisposing heart disease before procedures that may cause bacteremia. Although no clinical trials or prospective studies have been conducted, recommendations for prevention of endocarditis are based on experimental animal data, *in vitro* studies, and clinical experiences (3–6).

It is not always possible to predict which patients will develop endocarditis or which particular procedure will be responsible. In fact, most cases of endocarditis are not attributable to a given invasive procedure (2). In spite of this, certain bacteria are known to be associated with endocarditis in at-risk individuals. Therefore, antibiotic recommendations for prevention of bacterial endocarditis have been issued by various organizations. Those most widely used in the United States are written by the AHA (3) and serve as a point of reference for the discussion below. These recommendations were developed in collaboration with the American Dental Association and American Society for Gastrointestinal Endoscopy. They were designed to assist practitioners in appropriate use of prophylaxis and take into account both the risk of the patient's underlying cardiac condition and the risk of an endocarditis-producing bacteremia during the surgical/dental procedure. Underuse of prophylaxis could lead to possible cases of endocarditis, whereas overuse promotes the development of resistant microorganisms and leads to risk of adverse drug reactions. No one set of guidelines can be used for all patients in all situations. Clinicians should use their own judgment when making recommendations for which patient to treat, which antibiotic to use, or the number of doses to be administered. Furthermore, endocarditis may occur despite the use of an appropriate antimicrobial regimen. Therefore, practitioners should maintain a high index of suspicion regarding any unexplained clinical event such as fever, night chills, back pain, stiff neck, weakness, myalgia, arthralgia, lethargy, or malaise after procedures in which prophylaxis was administered.

Cardiac Conditions

It is known that certain cardiac conditions are more frequently associated with endocarditis than others (7). When endocarditis does occur, it can be associated with higher morbidity and mortality in some groups of individuals than others. This has led to a stratification of patients by the AHA (3). They have listed cardiac condition categories of high, moderate, and negligible risk (Table 14-1). Patients in the high- and moderate-risk categories are those for whom prophylaxis is recommended. The negligible-risk category represents those individuals for whom the risk of endocarditis is no greater than the general population.

High-risk Category

Patients in the high-risk category include individuals who have prosthetic heart valves, a previous history of endocarditis (even in the

---

TABLE 14-1. Cardiac conditions

Endocarditis prophylaxis recommended
  High-risk category
    Prosthetic cardiac valves, including bioprosthetic and homograft valves
    Previous bacterial endocarditis
    Complex cyanotic congenital heart disease (e.g., single ventricle states, transposition of the great arteries, tetralogy of Fallot)
    Surgically constructed systemic-pulmonary shunts or conduits
  Moderate-risk category
    Most other congenital cardiac malformations (other than above and below)
    Acquired valvular dysfunction (e.g., rheumatic heart disease)
    Hypertrophic cardiomyopathy
    Mitral valve prolapse with valvular regurgitation and/or thickened leaflets
Endocarditis prophylaxis not recommended
  Negligible-risk category (no greater risk than the general population)
    Isolated secundum atrial septal defect
    Surgical repair of atrial septal defect, ventricular septal defect, or patent ductus arteriosus (without residua beyond 6 months)
    Previous coronary artery bypass graft surgery
    Mitral valve prolapse without valvular regurgitation
    Physiologic, functional, or innocent heart murmurs
    Previous Kawasaki disease without valvular dysfunction
    Previous rheumatic fever without valvular dysfunction
    Cardiac pacemakers (intravascular and epicardial) and implanted defibrillators

From ref. 3, with permission.

absence of other cardiac disease), complex cyanotic congenital heart disease, or surgically constructed systemic shunts or conduits (3,7,8). When these individuals contract endocarditis, it is associated with a higher morbidity and mortality than in individuals in the lower risk categories.

Moderate-risk Category

The moderate-risk category includes most uncorrected congenital cardiac defects (other than those listed above or below) and various other cardiac conditions such as acquired valvular dysfunction from previous rheumatic fever, collagen vascular disease, or other causes. Hypertrophic cardiomyopathy is also in the moderate-risk category. It is recognized that not all conditions in this category pose the same risk for endocarditis; they all have a risk higher than the general population, however. Patients with mitral valve prolapse (MVP) are among the most problematic for whom to choose prophylaxis. Estimates of the number of individuals in the United States who have MVP varies but probably is somewhere between 2% and 6% (9). For those with no mur-

mur, the incidence of endocarditis is no greater than the general population, whereas one study has shown that for patients with a mitral regurgitant murmur, the incidence of endocarditis is about tenfold greater (10). The AHA has given a detailed description of the spectrum of MVP and has produced an algorithm (Fig. 14-1) for the approach to the patient with suspected MVP (3). Further discussion of MVP can be found in Chapter 6.

Negligible-risk Category

The negligible-risk category lists cardiac conditions that are not associated with a risk for the development of endocarditis that is any greater than that of the general population. This category includes isolated secundum atrial septal defects and surgically repaired (without residua beyond 6 months) atrial septal defect, ventricular septal defect, and patent ductus arteriosus. If closure of these defects results in any form of residual shunting, continued antibiotic prophylaxis is indicated as in the preprocedure state. There is no evidence that previous coronary artery bypass graft surgery carries any risk for subsequent endo-

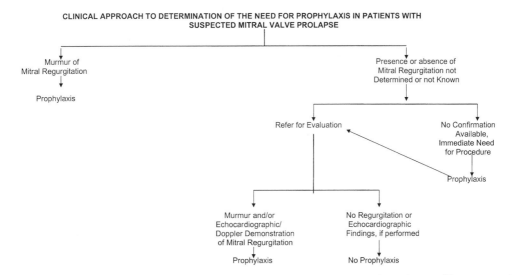

FIG. 14-1. Clinical approach to determination of the need for prophylaxis in patients with suspected mitral valve prolapse.

carditis. Other cardiac conditions in the negligible-risk category are listed in Table 14-1.

Endocarditis with No Underlying Heart Disease

Clearly, individuals with no underlying heart disease contract endocarditis. This is often the case in young children, intravenous drug abusers, and in individuals with nosocomial endocarditis. In infants (particularly premature newborns) and young children, endocarditis is often associated with indwelling arterial and central venous catheters (8,11–13). It has been estimated that 50% to 70% of cases of endocarditis in children under the age of 2 years occur in structurally normal hearts (14). Over one half of intravenous drug abusers who contract endocarditis have structurally normal hearts (14). This group of individuals develop endocarditis (usually right sided) at a rate higher than the general population and even higher than that of patients with rheumatic heart disease or with prosthetic cardiac valves (15,16). Between 14% and 40% of cases of nosocomially acquired endocarditis occur in hearts with no underlying cardiac defect (17,18).

Bacteremia

Invasion of the circulation by microorganisms is the initiating event in bacterial endocarditis. The sites of origin of the bacteria are typically the oropharynx, the gastrointestinal tract, and the genitourinary tract (19). Transient bacteremias occur commonly (20,21). They may occur spontaneously, such as with tooth brushing, food or gum chewing, or eating hard candy. Antibiotic prophylaxis is impractical for preventing a transient bacteremia secondary to these common daily activities; however, maintenance of good oral hygiene decreases the amount of gum disease, which is a key determinant of the frequency of a transient bacteremia after any dental manipulation. Bacteremias can also be the result of a local infection (e.g., poor dental hygiene, periodontal/periapical infection, urinary tract infection, pneumonia, or cellulitis) or can be procedure related. Bacteremia is common after many invasive procedures, but it is important to remember that only certain bacteria usually cause endocarditis. The largest number of cases of endocarditis is attributed to streptococci, with other organisms including staphylococci, enterococci, and gram-negative bacteria (22). Invasive procedures performed through surgically scrubbed skin (such as at the site of insertion of a catheter during cardiac catheterization) are not likely to produce such bacteremias. Certain dental and surgical procedures, especially those involving mucosal surfaces or contaminated tissue, can cause transient bacteremia with those bacteria associated with endocarditis. This bloodborne bacteremia usually lasts for only a few minutes (generally less than 15 minutes), and quantitative blood cultures usually show that the number of organisms is usually less than ten per milliliter of blood (20,23,24). These bacteria may lodge on the endothelial surface of damaged or abnormal heart valves or other cardiac defects, however, resulting in bacterial endocarditis or endarteritis.

The oral cavity and upper respiratory tract harbor multiple organisms, especially viridans streptococci (α-hemolytic streptococci). Therefore, prophylactic regimens for dental, oral, respiratory tract, or esophageal procedures are specifically directed against these organisms. Studies have shown that dental extraction is associated with positive blood cultures in up to 85% of patients (19,20). Bacterial endocarditis that occurs after gastrointestinal tract or genitourinary tract procedures is most often due to organisms of the *Enterococcus* genus (25). Enterococci are normal inhabitants of the gastrointestinal tract and cause genitourinary tract infection. Thus, prophylaxis in these circumstances is directed primarily against the enterococci.

Bacteremia-producing Procedures

Dental and Oral Procedures

Poor dental hygiene and periodontal disease can produce a bacteremia even in the absence

TABLE 14-2. Dental procedures

Endocarditis prophylaxis recommended[a]
    Dental extractions
    Periodontal procedures including surgery, scaling and root planing, probing, recall maintenance
    Dental implant placement and reimplantation of avulsed teeth
    Endodontic (root canal) instrumentation or surgery only beyond the apex
    Subgingival placement of antibiotic fibers/strips
    Initial placement of orthodontic bands but not brackets
    Intraligamentary local anesthetic injections
    Prophylactic cleaning of teeth or implants where bleeding is anticipated
Endocarditis prophylaxis not recommended
    Restorative dentistry[b] (operative and prosthodontic) with/without retraction cord[c]
    Local anesthetic injections (nonintraligamentary)
    Intracanal endodontic treatment; postplacement and buildup
    Placement of rubber dams
    Postoperative suture removal
    Placement of removable prosthodontic/orthodontic appliances
    Taking of oral impressions
    Fluoride treatments
    Taking of oral radiographs
    Orthodontic appliance adjustment
    Shedding of primary teeth

---

[a]Prophylaxis is recommended for patients with high- and moderate-risk cardiac conditions.
[b]This includes restoration of decayed teeth (filling cavities) and replacement of missing teeth.
[c]Clinical judgment may indicate antibiotic use in selected circumstances that may create significant bleeding.
From ref. 3, with permission.

of specific dental procedures. In fact, both the frequency and magnitude of bacteremias have been shown to be proportional to the degree of oral inflammation and infection (26,27). Therefore, the maintenance of optimal oral health through professional dental care and home care, which reduces possible sources of bacterial seeding, may be an even more important preventive measure than procedure-focused antibiotic prophylaxis (21,26,28). Procedure-related dental and oral procedures for which endocarditis prophylaxis is or is not recommended are listed in Table 14-2. Not all procedures need prophylaxis. In general, prophylaxis is recommended for those procedures that are associated with bacteremias—significant bleeding from hard or soft tissues, dental extractions, periodontal operations, scaling, and professional teeth cleaning (3). If a series of dental procedures is planned, the AHA recommends observance of an interval 9 to 14 days between procedures to minimize the potential for the emergence of resistant strains and to allow repopulation of the mouth with antibiotic-susceptible flora (3).

Respiratory, Gastrointestinal, and Genitourinary Tract Procedures

The most recent AHA recommendations (3) have given greater flexibility concerning which patients and which procedures involving respiratory, gastrointestinal, and genitourinary tract procedures need antimicrobial prophylaxis (Table 14-3). For gastrointestinal procedures listed under endocarditis prophylaxis recommended (upper half of Table 14-3), they state that prophylaxis is recommended for the high-risk patient and is optional for the medium-risk patient. For certain procedures involving respiratory, gastrointestinal, and genitourinary tract procedures listed under endocarditis prophylaxis not recommended (lower half of Table 14-3), the practitioner may choose to administer prophylactic antibiotics to patients in the high-risk category.

Certain procedures involving the oropharynx and respiratory tract may result in bacteremia, including tonsillectomy, surgical operations that involve the respiratory mu-

CHAPTER 14

TABLE 14-3. Other procedures

Endocarditis prophylaxis recommended
   Respiratory tract
      Tonsillectomy and/or adenoidectomy
      Surgical operations that involve respiratory mucosa
      Bronchoscopy with a rigid bronchoscope
   Gastrointestinal tract[a]
      Sclerotherapy for esophageal varices
      Esophageal stricture dilation
      Endoscopic retrograde cholangiography with biliary obstruction
      Biliary tract surgery
      Surgical operations that involve intestinal mucosa
   Genitourinary tract
      Prostatic surgery
      Cystoscopy
      Urethral dilation
Endocarditis prophylaxis not recommended
   Respiratory tract
      Endotracheal intubation
      Bronchoscopy with a flexible bronchoscope, with or without biopsy[b]
      Tympanostomy tube insertion
   Gastrointestinal tract
      Transesophageal echocardiography[b]
      Endoscopy with or without gastrointestinal biopsy[b]
   Genitourinary tract
      Vaginal hysterectomy[b]
      Vaginal delivery[b]
      Cesarean section
      In uninfected tissue
         Urethral catheterization
         Uterine dilatation and curettage
         Therapeutic abortion
         Sterilization procedures
         Insertion or removal of intrauterine devices
   Other
      Cardiac catheterization, including balloon angioplasty
      Implanted cardiac pacemakers, implanted defibrillators, and coronary stents
      Incision or biopsy of surgically scrubbed skin
      Circumcision

[a]Prophylaxis is recommended for high-risk patients; optional for medium-risk patients.
[b]Prophylaxis is optional for high-risk patients.
From ref. 3, with permission.

cosa, and rigid-tube bronchoscopy (which causes mucosal damage) (19). Positive blood cultures, however, rarely occur in association with flexible fiberoptic bronchoscopy and lung biopsy (29). This contrasts with a rate of bacteremia of 15.4% associated with the use of a rigid bronchoscope (20).

Various procedures involving the gastrointestinal tract are associated with bacteremia (3). Sclerotherapy of esophageal varices is associated with a bacteremia rate of approximately 31%, and esophageal stricture dilation is associated with bacteremia rates as high as 45% (30). The bacteremia rates for endo-scopic retrograde cholangiography in the absence of ductal obstruction are approximately equal to most other endoscopic procedures. An obstructed biliary tree, however, may be colonized with a variety of organisms; therefore, chemoprophylaxis is recommended for endoscopic retrograde cholangiography with biliary obstruction. In surgery that involves the intestinal mucosa or biliary tract, there is a potential for bacteremia with organisms known to cause endocarditis (predominantly enterococci). Therefore, prophylaxis is recommended, especially for patients in the high-risk category.

Transient bacteremia and endocarditis can occur after urinary tract, obstetric, and gynëcologic instrumentation or surgical or diagnostic procedures (2,19,20,31). Although the risk that any particular patient will develop endocarditis is low, the genitourinary tract is second only to the oral cavity as a portal of entry for organisms that cause endocarditis (3). Genitourinary tract procedures for which endocarditis prophylaxis is recommended for all high- and moderate-risk category patients (Table 14-3) include prostatic surgery, cystoscopy, and urethral dilation. A study in 300 patients undergoing various urologic procedures found that transient bacteremia occurred in 8% of patients undergoing urethral catheterization, 24% of those undergoing urethral dilation, 17% of those having cystoscopy, and 31% of those having transurethral prosthetic resection (32). The frequency of positive blood cultures increases severalfold in patients with infection at the instrumented site (32). One example of such an infection is that of the urinary tract. Sterilization of the urinary tract with antimicrobial therapy in patients with bacteriuria should be attempted before elective procedures, including lithotripsy. Preprocedure culture of the urine will allow the practitioner to choose antibiotics appropriate to the recovered organisms.

Transient bacteremia after uncomplicated vaginal delivery is infrequent—only 1% to 5% of procedures (2)—and well-documented cases of endocarditis after normal vaginal delivery are uncommon (33,34). Therefore, antibiotic prophylaxis for normal vaginal delivery is not recommended. If an unanticipated bacteremia is suspected during vaginal delivery, intravenous antibiotics can be administered at that time. Chemoprophylaxis is optional for high-risk patients for both vaginal delivery and vaginal hysterectomy. Bacteremias have not been detected in studies after cervical biopsy or manipulation of an intrauterine device in the absence of obvious infections (2,35) Infected intrauterine devices have been associated with endocarditis (36). Bacteremia after removal of an infected intrauterine device is unresolved (37) but would seem possible and therefore should warrant prophylaxis. Other genitourinary procedures performed in the presence of infection should also warrant prophylaxis.

Prophylactic Regimens

Chemoprophylaxis is most effective when serum antibiotic levels during and after the procedure are adequate to inhibit the bacteremia expected from that procedure. It is also important to use the antibiotics only during the perioperative procedure to minimize the emergence of resistance.

Dental, Oral, Respiratory Tract, or Esophageal Procedures

Amoxicillin is a standard antibiotic prophylaxis for dental, oral, respiratory tract, and esophageal procedures directed against viridans streptococci (Table 14-4). All patients in the high- and moderate-risk categories are eligible for this regimen unless they are allergic to penicillins or cannot take oral medications. Oral prophylaxis for high-risk patients has been a part of the recommendations from the AHA since 1990 (3,38), and an increased incidence of prophylaxis failures has not been reported. The most current recommendations have lowered the preprocedure adult dose of amoxicillin from 3.0 to 2.0 g and eliminated the follow-up dose. A comparative study of 2.0- and 3.0-g dosing regimens showed that a 2.0-g dose resulted in adequate serum levels for several hours and was associated with fewer gastrointestinal side effects (39). Alternatives to the amoxicillin regimen are listed in Table 14-4. The AHA no longer includes erythromycin because of the complicated pharmacokinetics of the various formulations and its propensity for gastrointestinal upset. Practitioners who have successfully used erythromycin in individual patients in the past and wish to continue using this antibiotic in these patients can use the dosing regimen given by the AHA in their 1990 recommendations (38).

TABLE 14-4. Prophylactic regimens for dental, oral, respiratory tract, or esophageal procedures

Situation	Agent	Regimen[a]
Standard general prophylaxis	Amoxicillin	Adults: 2.0 g Children: 50 mg/kg p.o. 1 h before procedure
Unable to take oral medications	Ampicillin	Adults: 2.0 g i.m. or i.v. Children: 50 mg/kg i.m. or i.v. within 30 min before procedure
Allergic to penicillin	Clindamycin	Adults: 600 mg Children: 20 mg/kg p.o. 1 h before procedure
	OR Cephalexin[b] or cefadroxil[b]	Adults: 2.0 g Children: 50 mg/kg p.o. 1 h before procedure
	OR Azithromycin or clarithromycin	Adults: 500 mg Children: 15 mg/kg p.o. 1 h before procedure
Allergic to penicillin and unable to take oral medications	Clindamycin	Adults: 600 mg Children: 20 mg/kg i.v. within 30 min before procedure
	OR Cefazolin[b]	Adults: 1.0 g Children: 25 mg/kg i.m. or i.v. within 30 min before procedure

[a]Total children's dose should not exceed adult dose.
[b]Cephalosporins should not be used in individuals with immediate hypersensitivity reaction (urticaria, angioedema, or anaphylaxis) to penicillins.
From ref. 3, with permission.

Genitourinary and Nonesophageal Gastrointestinal Procedures

Prophylaxis recommendations for patients undergoing genitourinary and nonesophageal gastrointestinal tract procedures are directed against enterococci and generally require intravenous or intramuscular antibiotic administration (Table 14-5). In moderate-risk patients not allergic to penicillins, there is a choice of an oral or a parenteral regimen. A physician may choose to administer prophylactic antibiotics to patients in the high-risk category undergoing procedures in which prophylaxis is not normally recommended.

Special Situations in Patients Needing Endocarditis Prophylaxis

Patients Already Receiving Antibiotics

If a patient is currently taking, or has recently completed, a course of an antibiotic normally used for endocarditis, the practitioner should select a drug from a different class rather than increase the dose of the current antibiotic. This includes those patients on oral penicillin for secondary prevention of rheumatic fever or for other purposes. They may have penicillin-resistant viridans streptococci in their oral cavity. In this situation, one of the alternate regimens listed in Table 14-4 should be used. Cephalosporins, however, should be avoided because of their possible cross-resistance. Alternatively, the practitioner could delay the procedure for at least 9 days after completion of the antibiotic to allow repopulation of the oral cavity with the usual antibiotic susceptible flora.

Patients on Anticoagulation Drugs

In these patients, one should avoid intramuscular antibiotic administration, especially if the anticoagulant is heparin. The use of

TABLE 14-5. *Prophylactic regimens for genitourinary and gastrointestinal (excluding esophageal) procedures*

Situation	Agent(s)[a]	Regimen[b]
High-risk patients	Ampicillin plus gentamicin	Adults: ampicillin 2.0 g i.m./i.v. plus gentamicin 1.5 mg/kg (not to exceed 120 mg) within 30 min of starting the procedure. Six hours later, ampicillin 1.0 g i.m./i.v. or amoxicillin 1 g p.o. Children: ampicillin 50 mg/kg i.m. or i.v. (not to exceed 2.0 g) plus gentamicin 1.5 mg/kg within 30 min of starting the procedure. Six hours later, ampicillin 25 mg/kg i.m./i.v. or amoxicillin 25 mg/kg p.o.
High-risk patients allergic to ampicillin/ amoxicillin	Vancomycin plus gentamicin	Adults: vancomycin 1.0 g i.v. over 1–2 h plus gentamicin 1.5 mg/kg i.v./i.m. (not to exceed 120 mg). Complete injection/infusion within 30 min of starting procedure. Children: vancomycin 20 mg/kg i.v. over 1–2 h plus gentamicin 1.5 mg/kg i.v./i.m.. Complete injection/infusion within 30 min of starting the procedure.
Moderate-risk patients	Amoxicillin or ampicillin	Adults: amoxicillin 2.0 g p.o. 1 h before procedure, OR ampicillin 2.0 g i.m./i.v. within 30 min of starting the procedure. Children: amoxicillin 50 mg/kg p.o. 1 h before procedure, OR ampicillin 50 mg/kg i.m./i.v. within 30 min of starting the procedure.
Moderate-risk patients allergic to ampicillin/ amoxicillin	Vancomycin	Adults: vancomycin 1.0 g i.v. over 1–2 h. Complete infusion within 30 min of starting the procedure. Children: vancomycin 20 mg/kg i.v. over 1–2 h. Complete infusion within 30 min of starting the procedure.

[a]No second dose of vancomycin or gentamicin is recommended.
[b]Total children's dose should not exceed adult dose.
From ref. 3, with permission.

warfarin is a relative contraindication to intramuscular injections.

Patients Who Have Procedures Involving Infected Tissue

If an individual at high or moderate risk for developing endocarditis has a procedure involving incision and/or drainage of infected tissue, the ensuing bacteremia may cause endocarditis. Therefore, prophylactic antibiotics should be given before the procedure. The choice of antibiotic should be directed at the pathogen causing the infection.

Patients Undergoing Cardiac Surgery

If a patient in the high- or moderate-risk category undergoes open heart surgery, they are at risk for developing bacterial endocarditis. Similarly, patients who are undergoing surgery for implantation of a prosthetic heart valve are also at risk for developing endocarditis. Because of the serious consequences if infection occurs, perioperative antibiotic prophylaxis is recommended by the AHA (3), is used essentially universally by cardiac surgeons, and has influenced the incidence of prosthetic valve endocarditis (40). *Staphylococcus aureus*, coagulase-negative staphylococci, or diphtheroids most often cause endocarditis associated with open heart surgery and early-onset prosthetic valve endocarditis. Prophylaxis at the time of cardiac surgery, therefore, is directed against staphylococci. First-generation cephalosporins (such as cefazolin) are most often used, although the choice of an antibiotic should be influenced by the antibiotic susceptibility patterns at each hospital (41). Prophylaxis should be of short duration—beginning immediately before the operative procedure, repeating during prolonged procedures, and continuing for no more than 24 hours postoperatively to minimize emergence of resistant microorganisms.

Patients Who Have Had Heart Transplants

The AHA makes no specific recommendations for these patients. They do point out that these individuals are at risk for acquired valvular dysfunction, especially during rejection episodes. Additionally, there is immunosuppression use in this group of patients. One survey of transplant centers conducted by the AHA and published in abstract form indicated that 97% of these centers recommend routine prophylaxis before dental, oral, or respiratory tract procedures in the months and years after the transplant (42).

RHEUMATIC FEVER

Prevention of an initial attack of rheumatic fever depends on the proper diagnosis and control of the antecedent group A streptococcal tonsillopharyngitis (strep throat). "Primary prevention" of rheumatic fever refers to treatment and eradication of group A streptococci from the throat and thus prevention of an initial attack of rheumatic fever. "Secondary prevention" refers to prevention of recurrent attacks of rheumatic fever. An individual who has had one attack of rheumatic fever is inordinately susceptible to a second attack and therefore needs continuous prophylaxis, usually with penicillin, to prevent a recurrence. The AHA published guidelines for primary and secondary prevention of rheumatic fever in 1995; these guidelines are the basis for the recommendations given here (43).

The proper diagnosis of an initial attack of acute rheumatic fever must be made for secondary prevention to be initiated. The Jones' criteria are the guidelines most often used for the diagnosis of rheumatic fever. They were initially written by T. Duckett Jones in 1944 (44) and were most recently updated by the AHA in 1992 (45).

Primary Prevention

Penicillin is recommended for primary prevention of rheumatic fever (Table 14-6). This can either be accomplished by one injection of benzathine penicillin G or by 10 days of oral penicillin V. Erythromycin is the drug of choice for penicillin-allergic individuals. Azithromycin (approved by the Food and Drug Administration as a second-line therapy in individuals 16 years of age or older) and oral cephalosporins are also acceptable, although they are more expensive than penicillin or erythromycin.

Secondary Prevention

The likelihood of a recurrent attack of rheumatic fever is influenced by several factors: the interval since the most recent attack, the number of previous attacks, and whether the individual is in an environment where he or she is often exposed to streptococcal infections (e.g., children, parents of young children, teachers, health care personnel in contact with children, military recruits). Regimens for secondary prevention are listed in Table 14-7. Penicillin or sulfadiazine is considered the

TABLE 14-6. *Primary prevention of rheumatic fever (treatment of streptococcal tonsillopharyngitis)*

Agent	Dose	Mode	Duration
Benzathine penicillin G	600,000 units for patients ≤ 27 kg 1,200,000 units for patients > 27 kg OR	i.m.	Once
Penicillin V (phenoxymethyl penicillin)	Children: 250 mg 2–3 times daily Adolescents and Adults: 500 mg 2–3 times daily	p.o.	10 days
For individuals allergic to penicillin Erythromycin			
Estolate	20–40 mg/kg/day 2–4 times daily (maximum 1 g/day) OR	p.o.	10 days
Ethylsuccinate	40 mg/kg/day 2–4 times daily (maximum 1 g/day)	p.o.	10 days

Other acceptable alternatives listed in text. The following are not acceptable: sulfonamides, trimethoprim, tetracyclines, and chloramphenicol.
From ref. 43, with permission.

TABLE 14-7. *Secondary prevention of rheumatic fever (prevention of recurrent attacks)*

Agent	Dose	Mode
Benzathine penicillin G	1,200,000 units every 4 wk[a]	i.m.
	OR	
Penicillin V	250 mg twice daily	p.o.
	OR	
Sulfadiazine	0.5 g once daily for patients ≤ 27 kg (60 lb)	
	1.0 g once daily for patients > 27 kg (60 lb)	p.o.
For individuals allergic to penicillin and sulfadiazine		
Erythromycin	250 mg twice daily	p.o.

[a]In high-risk situations, administration every 3 weeks is justified and recommended.
From ref. 43, with permission.

first-line agent. The presence or absence of carditis and valvular disease primarily determines the duration of secondary prophylaxis. Individuals who have had rheumatic carditis, even without valvular disease, are at high risk for recurrences of carditis in subsequent attacks of rheumatic fever, and each recurrence incurs increasingly severe cardiac involvement (46–48). The duration of secondary prevention prophylaxis in patients who have had rheumatic fever without carditis is 5 years, or until age 21, whichever is longer (43,49). For patients who have had rheumatic fever with carditis but without clinical or echocardiographic evidence of valvular disease, prophylaxis should continue for 10 years or well into adulthood, whichever is longer (43). Finally, for those patients who have had rheumatic fever with carditis and clinical or echocardiographic evidence of persistent valvular disease, the duration of prophylaxis is at least 10 years since the last episode and at least until age 40; sometimes, lifelong prophylaxis is warranted (43).

REFERENCES

1. American Heart Association. *1997 Heart and Stroke Statistical Update.* Dallas, TX: American Heart Association, 1997:17–18.
2. Durack DT. Prevention of infective endocarditis. *N Engl J Med* 1995;332:38–44.
3. Dajani AS, Taubert KA, Wilson W, et al. Prevention of bacterial endocarditis. *JAMA* 1997;277:1794–1801.
4. Leport C, Horstkotte D, Burckhardt D, Group of Experts of the International Society of Chemotherapy. Antibiotic prophylaxis for infective endocarditis from an international group of experts towards a European consensus. *Eur Heart J* 1995;16:126–131.
5. Hay DR, Chambers ST, Ellis-Pegler RB, et al. Prevention of infective endocarditis associated with dental treatment and other medical interventions. *N Z Med J* 1992;105:192–197.
6. Simmons NA, Ball AP, Cawson RA, et al. Antibiotic practice and infective endocarditis. *Lancet* 1992;339:1292–1293.
7. Steckelberg JM, Wilson WR. Risk factors for infective endocarditis. *Infect Dis Clin North Am* 1993;7:9–19.
8. Saiman L, Prince A, Gersony WM. Pediatric infective endocarditis in the modern era. *J Pediatr* 1993;122:847–853.
9. Bonow RO, Carabello B, de Leon AC, et al. ACC/AHA guidelines for the management of patients with valvular heart disease. *J Am Coll Cardiol* 1998;32:1486–1588.
10. MacMahon SW, Roberts JK, Kramer-Fox R, et al. Mitral valve prolapse and infective endocarditis. *Am Heart J* 1987;113:1291–1298.
11. Baltimore RS. Infective endocarditis in children. *Pediatr Infect Dis J* 1992;11:907–912.
12. Noel GJ, O'Loughlin JE, Edelson PJ. Neonatal staphylococcus epidermidis right-sided endocarditis: description of five catheterized infants. *Pediatrics* 1988;82:234.
13. Millard DD, Shulman ST. The changing spectrum of neonatal endocarditis. *Clin Perinatol* 1988;15:587–608.
14. Harris SL. Definitions and demographic characteristics. In: Kaye D, ed. *Infective Endocarditis*, 2nd ed. New York: Raven Press, 1992:1–18.
15. Sande MA, Lee BL, Mills J, Chambers HF. Endocarditis in intravenous drug users. In: Kaye D, ed. *Infective Endocarditis*, 2nd ed. New York: Raven Press, 1992:345–359.
16. Levine DP, Crane LR, Zervos MJ. Bacteremia in narcotic addicts at the Detroit Medical Center. II. Infectious endocarditis: a prospective comparative study. *Rev Infect Dis* 1986;8:374–396.
17. Friedland G, Von Reyn CF, Levy B, Arbeit R, Dasse P, Crumpacker C. Nosocomial endocarditis. *Infect Control* 1984;5:284–288.
18. Terpenning MS, Buggy BP, Kauffman CA. Hospital-acquired infective endocarditis. *Arch Intern Med* 1988;148:1601–1603.
19. Livornese LL, Korzeniowski OM. Pathogenesis of infective endocarditis. In: Kaye D, ed. *Infective Endocarditis*, 2nd ed. New York: Raven Press, 1992:19–35.
20. Everett ED, Hirschmann JV. Transient bacteremia and endocarditis prophylaxis: a review. *Medicine (Baltimore)* 1977;56:61–77.

21. Guntheroth WG. How important are dental procedures as a cause of infective endocarditis? *Am J Cardiol* 1984; 54:797–801.

22. Tunkel AR, Mandell GL. Infecting organisms. In: Kaye D, ed. *Infective Endocarditis*, 2nd ed. New York: Raven Press, 1992:85–97.

23. LeFrock JL, Ellis CA, Klainer A, Weinstein L. Transient bacteremia associated with barium enema. *Arch Intern Med* 1975;135:835–837.

24. LeFrock JL, Ellis CA, Turchik JB, Weinstein L. Transient bacteremia associated with sigmoidoscopy. *N Engl J Med* 1973;289:467–469.

25. Rice LB, Calderwood SB, Eliopoulos GM, Farber BF, Karchmer AW. Enterococcal endocarditis: a comparison of prosthetic and native valve disease. *Rev Infect Dis* 1991;13:1–7.

26. Pallasch TJ, Slots J. Antibiotic prophylaxis and the medically compromised patient. *Periodontol 2000* 1996;10: 107–138.

27. Bender IB, Naidorf IJ, Garvey GJ. Bacterial endocarditis: a consideration for physicians and dentists. *J Am Dent Asso* 1984;109:415–420.

28. Van der Meer JTM, Thompson J, Valkenburg HA, Michel MF. Epidemiology of bacterial endocarditis in the Netherlands. II. Antecedent procedures and use of prophylaxis. *Arch Intern Med* 1992;152:1869–1873.

29. Alexander WJ, Baker GL, Hunker FD. Bacteremia and meningitis following fiberoptic bronchoscopy. *Arch Intern Med* 1979;139:580–583.

30. Botoman V, Surawicz C. Bacteremia with gastrointestinal endoscopic procedures. *Gastrointest Endosc* 1986; 32:342–346.

31. Vosti KL. Special problems in prophylaxis of endocarditis following genitourinary tract and obstetrical and gynecological procedures. In: Kaplan EL, Taranta AV, eds. *Infective Endocarditis*. American Heart Association Monograph 52. Dallas, TX: American Heart Association, 1977:75–79.

32. Sullivan N, Sutter V, Mims M, Marsh V, Finegold S. Clinical aspects of bacteremia after manipulation of the genitourinary tract. *J Infect Dis* 1973;127:49–55.

33. Sugrue D, Blake S, Troy P, MacDonald D. Antibiotic prophylaxis against infective endocarditis after normal delivery—is it necessary? *Br Heart J* 1980;44:499–502.

34. Seaworth BJ, Durack DT. Infective endocarditis in obstetric and gynecologic practice. *Am J Obstet Gynecol* 1986;154:180–188.

35. Ritvo R, Monroe P, Andriole VT. Transient bacteremia due to suction abortion: implications for SBE prophylaxis. *Yale J Biol Med* 1977;50:471–479.

36. Cobbs CG. IUD and endocarditis. *Ann Intern Med* 1973;78:451.

37. Child JS. Risks for and prevention of infective endocarditis. *Cardiol Clin* 1996;14:327–343.

38. Dajani AS, Bisno AL, Chung KJ, et al. Prevention of bacterial endocarditis. *JAMA* 1990;264:2919–2922.

39. Dajani AS, Bawdon RE, Berry MC. Oral amoxicillin as prophylaxis for endocarditis: what is the optimal dose? *Clin Infect Dis* 1994;18:157–160.

40. Douglas JL, Cobbs CG. Prosthetic valve endocarditis. In: Kaye D, ed. *Infective Endocarditis*, 2nd ed. New York: Raven Press, 1992:375–396.

41. Bayer AS, Nelson RJ, Slama TG. Current concepts in prevention of prosthetic valve endocarditis. *Chest* 1990; 97:1203–1207.

42. Taubert KA, Dajani AS. Usual practice patterns for endocarditis prophylaxis in cardiac transplant patients [abstract 125]. Abstracts of the 3rd International Symposium on Modern Concepts in Endocarditis. Boston, MA, July 1995.

43. Dajani A, Taubert K, Ferrieri P, Peter G, Shulman S. Treatment of acute streptococcal pharyngitis and prevention of rheumatic fever. *Pediatrics* 1995;96: 758–764.

44. Jones TD. Diagnosis of rheumatic fever. *JAMA* 1944; 126:481–484.

45. Dajani AS, Ayoub E, Bierman F, et al. Guidelines for the diagnosis of rheumatic fever (Jones criteria, updated 1992). *JAMA* 1992;268:2069–2073.

46. Majeed HA, Yousof AM, Khuffash FA, Yusuf AR, Farwana S, Khan N. The natural history of acute rheumatic fever in Kuwait: a prospective six year follow-up report. *J Chronic Dis* 1986;39:361–369.

47. Taranta A, Kleinberg E, Feinstein AR, Wood HF, Tursky E, Simpson R. Rheumatic fever in children and adolescents: a long-term epidemiologic study of subsequent prophylaxis, streptococcal infections, and clinical sequelae. V. Relation of the rheumatic fever recurrence rate per streptococcal infection to pre-existing clinical features of the patients. *Ann Intern Med* 1964;60 [Suppl]:58–67.

48. Kuttner AG, Mayer FE. Carditis during second attacks of rheumatic fever—its incidence in patients without clinical evidence of cardiac involvement in their initial rheumatic episode. *N Engl J Med* 1963;268: 1259–1261.

49. Berrios X, del Campo E, Guzman B, Bisno AL. Discontinuing rheumatic fever prophylaxis in selected adolescents and young adults. *Ann Intern Med* 1993;118: 401–406.

15

Endocarditis: An Enduring Challenge

Karam C. Mounzer, Antonio J. Chamoun, and Mark J. DiNubile

*Department of Internal Medicine, University of Medicine and Dentistry of New Jersey/
Robert Wood Johnson Medical School, Camden, New Jersey 08103; Division of Cardiology,
University of Texas Medical Branch at Galveston, Galveston, Texas 77555*

Over three centuries ago, Riviere described a patient dying of infective endocarditis (1); later Sir William Osler referred to this condition as malignant endocarditis (2). Endocarditis was almost invariably fatal in the preantibiotic era. However, with the discovery of penicillin, cure of infective endocarditis became possible. Unfortunately, the hope for universal cure has been tempered by the realization that not all pathogens can be eradicated quickly enough to prevent life-threatening hemodynamic changes or emboli. In addition, antimicrobial resistance has kept ahead of the enlarging armamentarium of powerful antibiotics. In the mid-1960s, the role of valve replacement emerged as a salvage intervention for patients failing medical therapy and further improved outcome. But, even now, despite the broad spectrum of available antimicrobial agents, advances in diagnostic modalities and surgical treatment, and sophisticated supportive care, infective endocarditis still remains a life-threatening entity and continues to challenge the diagnostic acumen and therapeutic judgment of physicians. Currently, the overall mortality rate remains over 10% (3).

In this chapter, we focus primarily on the pathogenesis, microbiology, clinical presentations, and complications of infective endocarditis. The diagnostic role and prognostic implications of echocardiography in infective endocarditis and the timing of surgical intervention are also stressed. Our intent is not to provide a comprehensive summary of all aspects of endocarditis (which can be readily found in standard textbooks of medicine, cardiology, and infectious diseases) but to frame the areas of change and controversy.

PATHOGENESIS AND MICROBIOLOGY

Endocarditis technically refers to inflammation of the endocardium. Although the heart valves are most often involved, the process can affect and can even be confined to mural endocardium. Furthermore, not all causes of endocarditis are microbial in origin. Nevertheless, most cases of endocarditis represent bacterial infections of the valve leaflets.

Native valve infective endocarditis has traditionally been classified into "subacute" and "acute" forms. Subacute infective endocarditis by definition presents as an indolent disease, but if left untreated is uniformly fatal within the ensuing several months. In stark contradistinction, the less common acute endocarditis is an aggressive and rapidly progressive illness that can lead to death in a few days from sepsis, intractable heart failure due to valvular incompetence, and/or major central nervous system (CNS) events.

Infections with *Staphylococcus aureus* cause most acute infections, often involving previously normal heart valves (4). *S. aureus* may also be the cause of subacute disease. However, subacute endocarditis typically results from hematogenous seeding of already damaged heart valves with oral flora of low virulence, as illustrated by the viridans (i.e., "green" or α-hemolytic) streptococci (5). These species encompass *Streptococcus mitis, S. sanguis,* and *S. salivarius.* Bacteremia with viridans streptococci often follows dental procedures associated with bleeding, especially when intense gingivitis is present; however, most cases of streptococcal endocarditis are not associated with discrete dental manipulations. This observation limits the utility of endocarditis prophylaxis before procedures (5a).

Many organisms cause endocarditis only under specific and definable circumstances (Fig. 15-1) Gram-negative bacilli are rare causes of native valve endocarditis except in populations injecting recreational drugs. The specific bacteria involved vary by geographic region, but *Pseudomonas aeruginosa* is a widespread gram-negative pathogen among parenteral drug users (6). *Candida* species also infrequently cause community-acquired native valve endocarditis, and again such cases occur almost exclusively in injection drug users (7). However, the most important pathogen in the drug-using population remains *S. aureus,* regardless of geography. Right-sided involvement, typically affecting the tricuspid valve, is characteristically a consequence of injecting drug use.

Other examples of pathogens causing endocarditis that need to be considered in certain restricted contexts include *Coxiella burnetti* (Q fever) after visiting a farm or exposure to par-

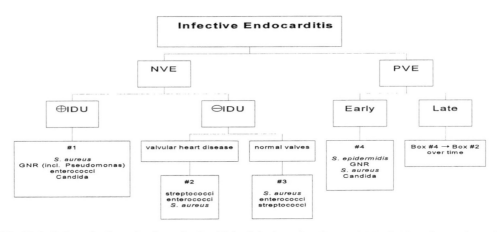

FIG. 15-1. Categorization of selected microbial etiologies of native and prosthetic valve endocarditis. NVE, native valve endocarditis; PVE, prosthetic valve endocarditis; IDU, injecting drug use; GNR, gram-negative rods.

1. All *S. epidermidis* are coagulase-negative staphylococci, but all coagulase-negative staphylococci are not *S. epidermidis*; if you encounter a "Staph" species with an unfamiliar name, it is a species of coagulase-negative staphylococci, e.g., *S. hemolyticus, S. saprophyticus,* etc. *S. lugdunesis* has been peculiarly associated with community-acquired native valve endocarditis.

2. "Strep. viridans" is not a true species but refers to α-hemolytic (viridans = "green") streptococci. If the name is not familiar, e.g., *S. mitis, S. sanguis, S. salivarius,* etc., the streptococci are probably from the viridans group.

3. Enterococci are no longer included among the "group D streptococci" and are now considered a separate genus distinct from the streptococci. *E. facium* is less common but more resistant than *E. faecalis. S. bovis* is a highly penicillin-sensitive group D streptococcus that often causes endocarditis in patients with gastrointestinal (predominantly colonic) lesions (often, but not always malignant).

4. Late PVE increasingly over time resembles NVE occurring on abnormal heart valves, but infections with enteric GNR remain an additional concern indefinitely. After the first postoperative year, *S. epidermidis* is a rare cause of PVE.

turient cats and *Bartonella quintana* in homeless alcoholics (8). A diagnostic evaluation for one of these organisms would be pursued in patients suspected of having endocarditis in the appropriate epidemiologic setting when routine blood cultures are unrevealing. *Brucella* and the HACEK group of gram-negative coccobacilli (*Hemophillus, Actinobacillus, Cardiobacterium, Eikenella*, and *Kingella* species) also cause culture-negative endocarditis but can be cultivated using special media or prolonged incubation periods, respectively (9). *Actinobacillus actinomycetescomitans* should be specifically sought in patients with culture-negative endocarditis after dental procedures. The causative agents in infective endocarditis that will not be recovered from routine blood cultures also include *Legionella* species, atypical mycobacteria, endemic yeast and opportunistic molds, and the Whipple bacillus (*Tropheryma whippelii*). But, in the end, recent prior antibiotic therapy, not unusual or fastidious organisms, is the most frequent cause of culture-negative endocarditis.

Gastrointestinal lesions predispose to endocarditis with streptococcus (*S.*) *bovis* and enterococci; these lesions are usually colonic and often malignant (10). Enterococcal endocarditis is also associated with urinary tract infections and manipulations. Line infections can result in endocarditis due to staphylococci and *Candida*; nosocomial endocarditis secondary to line-related bacteremia is predominantly due to *S. aureus* (11).

Cardiac lesions that predispose to endocarditis are those that result in high-velocity turbulent flow leading to eddy currents and/or denudement of the endocardial endothelium. Rheumatic valvular disease and most congenital heart malformations set the stage for the deposition of platelets and fibrin, leading to the formation of a sterile thrombus referred to as "nonbacterial thrombotic endocarditis." This nidus is susceptible to infection through hematogenous seeding. The risk of seeding a prolapsed mitral valve during bacteremia is much smaller, but mitral valve prolapse remains an important predisposing factor for endocarditis because of its high prevalence in the general population (12). Particulate material injected by parenteral drug users may damage the tricuspid and pulmonic valves, predisposing to right-sided infection. When septicemia of sufficient magnitude and duration due to microorganisms with valvular tropism supervenes occurs, the fibrin platelet thrombus formed at the site of valvular dysfunction can serve as a hospitable nidus, which then shelters proliferating bacteria or fungi in its interstices from phagocytic cells. The histopathologic hallmark of endocarditis is the vegetation, an amorphous clot typically harboring abundant microorganisms but scant inflammatory cells. The observation that organisms buried in the vegetative lesion are protected from host defenses perhaps explains why long courses of bactericidal antibiotics are needed for reliable cures of endocarditis.

Over the last few decades, there has been a shift in the frequency of cardiac conditions predisposing to infective endocarditis. Rheumatic heart disease, still problematic in developing countries, has become relatively less important in the industrial world with the widespread availability of antibiotics. In addition, congenital heart disease, traditionally an underlying condition in children, has become an increasingly relevant substrate in adults with the successes in surgical repair of complex congenital heart diseases. On the other hand, with the growing elderly population, degenerative valve diseases have emerged as a leading predisposing factor in those older than 60 years of age. In this group, enterococci and *S. aureus* are the major pathogens.

In a few cases, infective endocarditis develops on presumably normal valves. *S. aureus* is particularly virulent in attacking undamaged tissues (13). Hence, prevention strategies focused on persons with underlying valvular heart disease can at best prevent 50% to 70% of infections (5a). Nevertheless, because the prevalence of organic valvular disease in the American population is relatively low, it is clear that preexistent valve disease increases the risk of endocarditis after streptococcal bacteremia by several orders of magnitude.

The pathogenesis and microbiology of prosthetic valve endocarditis are related to the time of onset after valve replacement. The prosthesis epitomizes the most extreme form of a damaged valve. Mechanical valve infection differs from infection on native valves because the lesion in the former case routinely involves the valve ring and periannular tissue. Endocarditis on bioprosthetic valves shares pathologic features of both native and mechanical valve infection.

Mechanical and bioprosthetic valves seem to have a similar cumulative risk of infection (400-fold more than normal native valves), although some centers report higher infection rates in mechanical valves compared with bioprostheses during the first postoperative year (14,15). In early infections (manifested less than 2 months after valve replacement), the valve is seeded intra- or perhaps perioperatively; the causative organisms are common skin contaminants, like *Staphylococcus epidermidis* and diptheroids, and nosocomial flora, including *S. aureus*, gram-negative rods, and even yeasts (16). In contrast, in late prosthetic valve endocarditis (more than 6 months after surgery), the infection is typically acquired outside the hospital in a manner very similar to subacute native valve endocarditis. Nevertheless, nosocomial or community-acquired bacteremia with enteric gram-native bacilli, which rarely adhere to even severely damaged native valves, may stick to prostheses at any time and thus are well-recognized causative agents of late prosthetic valve endocarditis. The period ranging from 2 to 6 months after valve replacement encompasses a hybrid of early and late pathogens. *S. epidermidis* remains the most common etiologic agent in this time frame, but the usual etiologies of native valve endocarditis are increasingly encountered over time (Table 15-1).

Not all cases of endocarditis result from infection. Endocardial changes, varying from inflammatory to fibrotic, can be seen in diseases as diverse as malignancy (marantic endocarditis) (17), systemic lupus (Libman-Sacks endocarditis), Loeffler's eosinophilic endocarditis, and carcinoid. Even drugs may occasionally cause endocardial damage.

CLINICAL PRESENTATIONS AND COMPLICATIONS

Manifestations of infective endocarditis can appear in any organ system. Symptoms can result from direct invasion of the myocardium by the expanding vegetation, the sustained bacteremia that is a distinguishing feature of this infection, septic embolization to distant sites, and/or the immune complex-mediated phenomena associated with this process. The most common complaints reported by patients are fever, anorexia, and malaise. In the acute form of endocarditis, the abrupt onset of fever, shaking chills, and a toxic appearance is common, but in the more frequent subacute presentation, fever may be low grade and systemic toxicity absent. Subacute endocarditis can often be a nondescript illness, with an indolent course, sometimes mistaken for a nagging viral syndrome or even the early manifestations of a collagen vascular disease or lymphoma. Patients sometimes receive multiple short courses of antibiotics with transient improvement during therapy, but ultimately they relapse. This vague presentation explains why subacute endocarditis is a major cause of classic "fever of unknown origin." Arthralgia and myalgia, mostly localized to the low back, are frequent presenting complaints, and these false localizing signs may further delay diagnosis (18).

Most patients with endocarditis have heart murmurs, although it is not always clear whether the valvular dysfunction predisposed to the infection or resulted from it. Innocent flow murmurs in febrile patients further confound the association of fever and murmur. In a small fraction of patients, the murmur can be documented as new or significantly changed. The development of organic valvular involvement, resulting in a new diastolic or holosystolic murmur, in the setting of a febrile illness is essentially pathognomic of endocarditis. In less than 10% of patients with endocarditis, murmurs are not recognized. These patients include those without significant underlying valvular disease and those with extravalvular infection.

Perivalvular intramyocardial abscesses can lead to conduction abnormalities translated clinically into dizziness, dyspnea, and syncope. Most significant abscesses are complications of aortic valve infection, typically associated with at least moderate regurgitation. Electrocardiographic evidence of new and persistent heart block involving the bundle of His, the bundle branches, and left anterior fasciculus has been correlated with perivalvular abscesses in patients with aortic or prosthetic valve endocarditis (18a). Congestive heart failure is usually present in invasive infection and accounts for most deaths in infective endocarditis. Purulent pericarditis is an unusual but catastrophic complication of a valve ring abscess erupting into the pericardial space.

Systemic emboli occur in nearly a third of cases, especially when the mitral valve is involved. An embolic event may be the presenting symptom; the clinical manifestations depend on the targeted organ(s). Emboli to visceral organs result in infarction or abscess formation. Almost half of the patients with systemic emboli also have CNS involvement (19). Embolization to the CNS may result in ischemic or hemorrhagic strokes, seizures, and/or psychiatric disturbances. Microemboli to the vasa vasorum lead to the formation of mycotic aneurysms, which may expand and sometimes rupture to cause potentially fatal complications. Hematogenous meningitis and macroscopic brain abscess are rare complications, almost always encountered with *S. aureus* endocarditis.

Splenomegaly is found in half of the patients with subacute endocarditis. Back pain from vertebral osteomyelitis and/or epidural abscesses occasionally dominates the clinical picture and needs to be differentiated from the much more commonly encountered nonspecific lumbar myalgias. Localized spinal tenderness, especially with neurologic findings in the appropriate distribution, is a cause for concern in this regard.

Approximately 25% of patients with native valve endocarditis develop some type of pe-

ripheral mucocutaneous signs during their illness. The most frequently observed lesions are petechiae and hemorrhages, involving the conjunctivae, the nails (splinter hemorrhages), the palms and soles (Janeway lesions), and the pulps of the distal digits (Osler's nodes). Fundoscopic examination may reveal retinal lesions; those with a central pale area surrounded by a hemorrhagic rim are designated Roth spots (20).

Right-sided endocarditis caused by *S. aureus* is a frequent complication of injection drug use. Isolated tricuspid valve involvement is the rule in the absence of preexisting valvular heart disease (21). In general, isolated right-sided endocarditis is a less aggressive infection than left-sided endocarditis. This prognostic difference can be partially explained by the greater hemodynamic significance of left-sided as opposed to right-sided valves. Most studies indicate a mortality rate below 5% for staphylococcal tricuspid valve endocarditis, and surgical intervention (with or without valve replacement) is only rarely necessary (21,22). Injecting drug users who present with pneumonia may harbor occult right-sided endocarditis. In these patients, endocarditis should be suspected when pleuritic chest pain and/or hemoptysis are presenting complaints. Multifocal pulmonary infiltrates, often nodular, are often seen as a result of multiple septic pulmonary emboli. On the other hand, pyophlebitis at the site of injection may exactly mimic the syndrome of right-sided endocarditis.

DIAGNOSIS

The diagnosis of infective endocarditis must be suspected and investigated when patients with fever present with one or more of the following cardinal elements: a predisposing cardiac lesion, a high-risk epidemiologic context (e.g., intravenous drug use, recent dental procedure), bacteremia without an obvious source, an embolic event (often to the CNS, especially in a young person), and/or direct evidence of an active endocardial process (particularly a new or changing organic heart murmur). As simple as it sounds, and despite the large body of information concerning pathophysiology, clinicians still often fail to suspect endocarditis or to confirm the diagnosis once suspected. A firm diagnosis is warranted, because treatment regimens are long and potentially toxic. In 1994, Durack et al. amended the older Von Reyn criteria (Beth Israel) for the diagnosis of infective endocarditis (22a). These diagnostic criteria, now quoted as the Duke criteria, incorporate echocardiographic evidence of endocarditis. The Duke criteria appear to be highly specific and more sensitive than the Beth Israel criteria for the diagnosis of infective endocarditis (23,24,25).

Blood cultures remain the cornerstone of the diagnosis of infective endocarditis. They are positive in over 90% of cases when drawn before any antibiotic administration (26). Blood cultures not only serve to identify the causative organism but can demonstrate sustained bacteremia that characterizes the infection as endovascular. In acute endocarditis, two to three sets of blood cultures should be obtained over a short period of time, dictated by the urgency of the clinical picture. The volume of blood drawn is critical to optimizing the diagnostic yield, but the exact amount depends on the culture system used. In subacute endocarditis, three sets of blood cultures can be spaced over at least several hours. In patients who have been ill for several weeks or even months, making the diagnosis of endocarditis by blood culture in a few hours is not often necessary. If antibiotic use in the recent past is documented or suspected, more blood cultures spaced over longer time intervals are worthwhile when the patient's status allows delay in the institution of therapy.

In strongly suspected cases of endocarditis where routine blood cultures fail to grow, the microbiology laboratory should be notified to incubate the cultures for 2 or more weeks. Sometimes special media or handling are needed to establish a microbiologic diagnosis. Occasionally, serologic tests are required to make an etiologic diagnosis for endocarditis caused by *Brucella, Legionella, Bartonella, Coxiella burnetti*, or *Chlamydia*. If the patient experiences peripheral emboli leading to embolectomy, the embolus should be sent for histologic examination and culture. The polymerase chain reaction technique has been used on excised heart valves and other tissue removed at surgery to make the diagnosis in some culture-negative cases (26a).

The most common hematologic abnormality in patients with subacute endocarditis is a normochronic normocytic anemia of chronic disease, reflecting the chronic inflammatory nature of the process. Moderate leukocytosis is a common but variable finding. The erythrocyte sedimentation rate and the C-reactive protein levels are almost always elevated at presentation; although these tests have been used as a crude estimate of the response to treatment, their lack of specificity renders them essentially useless in diagnosis and management. Circulating immune complexes are frequently detectable in subacute endocarditis. These can deposit in glomeruli, leading to acute glomerulonephritis, associated with low complement levels in 85% of cases (27). Hematuria may also result from embolization to the renal arteries. A positive rheumatoid factor is encountered in nearly half of subacute cases (28).

ECHOCARDIOGRAPHY

Echocardiography potentially can help the clinician in three different but related aspects of the care of patients with suspected endocarditis: by confirming the diagnosis through imaging of valvular vegetations; by identifying the hemodynamic and other intracardiac complications that affect the prognosis of the disease; and by dictating specific interventions, such as length of the antibiotic treatment and the need for surgical intervention. Since the initial description by Dillon et al. in 1973 (29), debate has continued over the exact indications for echocardiography in patients with suspected endocarditis and the implications of specific findings on prognosis and management.

The sensitivity and specificity of echocardiography in the detection of vegetations or specific complications (e.g., valve ring abscess) depend on several variables, most importantly the ultrasonographic technique (two-dimensional transthoracic echocardiography [TTE] versus transesophageal echocardiography [TEE]). The predictive values of positive and negative studies are also a function of the pretest probability of endocarditis and the degree of suspicion for a complication. Echocardiographic vegetations should be classified into two subcategories: a definite vegetation recognized as a distinct oscillating mass attached to an incompetent valvular apparatus or a possible vegetation suspected because of a fixed or ill-defined mass on a thickened or calcified leaflet (30).

The old M-mode imaging technique is the least sensitive (<50%) and specific. With the advance of two-dimensional echocardiography, a better spatial definition of the vegetation, its dimensions, and extensions as it relates to intracardiac structures became possible. Studies suggest an incremental likelihood of vegetation detection with increasing size (31). Using TEE as the comparative standard, Erbel et al. (32) found that TTE identified only 25% of vegetations less than 5 mm, 69% of vegetations between 6 and 10 mm, and all those larger than 10 mm. The overall sensitivity of TTE for vegetations is approximately 60%, but it has a specificity exceeding 90% in skilled hands. TTE views may be inadequate in 20% of adult patients because of obesity, chronic obstructive pulmonary disease, or chest wall deformities (33).

Many patients with native valve endocarditis involving the aortic and mitral valves can be adequately imaged by TTE. However, higher resolution images are provided by TEE. Both TTE and TEE can be enhanced by continuous, pulsed, or color Doppler techniques (34). In comparative studies, TEE is both more sensitive and probably more specific in detecting vegetations and other structural abnormalities than TTE (35). Because of the location of the TEE transducer in the esophagus in physical proximity to the aortic root and basal septum, TEE is superior to TTE in detecting valvular and perivalvular compli-

cations and visualizing prosthetic valves, particularly in the mitral position (36). A negative TEE does not totally exclude infective endocarditis, especially early in the course of infection. A repeat TEE a week later may be positive when the initial study had been interpreted as negative or indeterminate. Monoplanar TEE has a reported sensitivity of 85% on initial examination. Using biplanar TEE, Lowry et al. (37) demonstrated nearly 100% sensitivity for native valve endocarditis and 90% for prosthetic valve endocarditis on a single examination; however, this study was confounded by using a clinical diagnosis of endocarditis, which incorporated the echocardiographic findings as their gold standard.

Many, but not all, studies looking at the complication rates associated with detectable vegetations on echocardiography suggest an increased risk of adverse outcomes, including embolic events, congestive heart failure, and need for surgery, when vegetations are visible on TTE (38,39). Several small series using TTE have reported an increased incidence of embolic events with vegetations greater than 1 cm (38,40). However, other studies have failed to reveal any significant correlation between the risk of embolic events and the size of the vegetation (41,42). The mobility of vegetations is apparently not an independent risk factor for embolic complications, perhaps in part because highly mobile vegetations tend to be large.

The relative risk of embolization appears to be microorganism dependent, with an increased frequency seen in patients with *S. aureus* endocarditis (41). With this virulent pathogen, the risk of emboli may not be greatly affected by the presence or size of a vegetation. However, in a recent publication, visualization of vegetations by TTE in patients with *S. aureus* endocarditis was associated with a higher risk of embolization and death compared with those patients who had their vegetations seen only on TEE (11,43). In contrast, the risk of emboli in patients with endocarditis caused by viridans streptococci increases directly and dramatically with vegetation size (41).

The natural history of vegetation size during therapy is variable. In patients without embolic complications, emboli become increasingly unlikely after the first week of effective antimicrobial therapy (41,44,45). Using TEE, Rohmann et al. (46) followed 83 patients with either aortic or mitral valve vegetations whose initial vegetation averaged 8 ± 1 mm for a mean of 74 weeks. Near the conclusion of antibiotic therapy, the patients were divided into two groups based on whether the vegetation had enlarged or shrunk: group A, where the mean vegetation size had increased to 11 mm (and *S. aureus* was the most common etiology), and group B, where the vegetation size decreased to 5 mm (and streptococci predominated). In both groups, vegetations subsequently decreased in size over months. However, even after 30 weeks, vegetations remained detectable in 75% of group A and 43% of group B. Following the size of the vegetation is not clinically useful. Occasionally, embolization may occur long after microbiologic cure.

Echocardiography is not a useful screening test for the diagnosis of infective endocarditis in low-risk settings. Moreover, in patients with a high pretest clinical suspicion, echocardiography is often unnecessary for the diagnosis when more traditional parameters (i.e., history, physical findings, and blood cultures results) confirm the diagnosis. In selected patients where the clinical and microbiologic data are suggestive but inconclusive, an echocardiographic study may provide useful diagnostic information. Whether the cost-to-benefit analysis favors going directly to a TEE, which is more invasive but would have a higher negative predictive value, or starting with a TTE and completing the workup with a TEE, if the TTE is nondiagnostic, has still not been clearly determined.

Despite recent trends, including the wide acceptance of the Duke criteria, we do not routinely recommend echocardiography in uncomplicated patients with a firm diagnosis of endocarditis unless there are open issues of therapeutic importance that may be clarified by imaging. If complications occur later, echocardiography can promptly be performed at that time. To the best of our knowledge, there is no convincing evidence to suggest that stable patients with endocarditis in the absence of complications will benefit from routine echocardiography if they are followed closely by careful clinical examinations. In fact, the excessive use of TEE, which has operationally redefined perivalvular abscess in patients with endocarditis, has motivated unnecessary operative interventions. For example, patients with streptococcal endocarditis on a native mitral valve and an uncomplicated clinical course, in whom a perivalvular abscess is detected solely by TEE, do not routinely require surgery. As new techniques gain popularity among echocardiographers, such as second harmonic and three-dimensional imaging, carefully designed management-outcome studies will be needed to determine how to incorporate more detailed information into clinical practice.

MEDICAL AND SURGICAL TREATMENT

The successful treatment of infective endocarditis has two major goals: to eradicate the infecting microorganism and to correct or at least limit the cardiac and extracardiac complications caused by this infection. Reliably successful antibiotic regimens have almost universally contained a bactericidal cell wall-active agent. Unfortunately, medical treatment of endocarditis alone may not always be sufficient to fulfill these objectives, and cardiac surgery sometimes must be performed for complete eradication of the organism, hemodynamic stabilization of the patient, and prevention of extracardiac sequelae. The emergence of antimicrobial resistance in bacteria that commonly cause endocarditis raises novel challenges to medical therapy and perhaps presents another impetus for operative intervention. In this respect, it appears that we are moving back toward the preantibiotic era. For standard treatment recommendations, one should refer to the comprehensive guidelines published by the American Heart Association (47) and summarized for staphylococcal and streptococcal native valve endocarditis in Table 15-1. We briefly discuss some areas presently in flux.

TABLE 15-1. *A summary of therapeutic options for left-sided native valve endocarditis caused by gram-positive cocci*

	PEN × 4 wk[a] + AG × 2 wk	PEN × 2 wk[a] + AG × 2 wk	PEN × 4 wk[a]	PEN × 4 wk + AG × 4 wk
Streptococci				
MIC of penicillin				
MIC < 0.1	++	+++	+++	+
0.1 < MIC < 0.5	+++	+	+	+
MIC > 0.5	+	±	±	+++
Enterococci[b]	−	−	−	+++
	Naf or cefazolin × 4–6 wk ± AG × < 1 wk	Vanco × 4–6 wk ± AG × < 1 wk		Vanco + Rif × 6 wk + AG × 2 wk
Staphylococci				
MSSA	+++	+		±
MRSA	−	+++		+

MIC, minimum inhibitory concentration; PEN, penicillin; AG, aminoglycoside; Naf, nafcillin; Vanco, vancomycin; Rif, rifampin; MSSA, MRSA, methicillin-sensitive and methicillin-resistant *S. aureus*, respectively; +++, preferred regimen; ++ or +, more or less acceptable regimen in selected patients; ±, controversial regimen under these circumstances; -, unacceptable regimen.

[a]Ceftriaxone can be substituted for penicillin in a once-daily (potentially outpatient) treatment regimen for stable uncomplicated patients.

[b]Ampicillin can be substituted for penicillin in the therapy of enterococcal endocarditis. None of the cephalosporin antibiotics cover enterococci; in severely penicillin-allergic patients with enterococcal endocarditis, patients must either be desensitized to penicillin or treated with vancomycin (in combination with an AG). Tobramycin must *not* be substituted for streptomycin or gentamicin in patients infected with *E. faecium*.

Antibiotic Therapy for Exclusively Right-sided Endocarditis Caused by *S. aureus*

The most common type of endocarditis in injection drug users is due to *S. aureus* confined strictly to the right-sided heart valves. In view of its good prognosis, the high cost and toxicity of prolonged parenteral antibiotic therapy, and the frequent reluctance of drug users to stay in the hospital after they feel better, selected patients with staphylococcal tricuspid valve endocarditis can be treated with a 2-week course of antibiotics under certain conditions (48). Short-course treatment should be considered only in the absence of evidence of hemodynamic compromise, systemic embolic complications, or metastatic infection. Although the prognostic implications of large vegetations are still unclear, patients with echocardiographic vegetations greater than 2 cm are often excluded from short-course therapy. Usually, short-course therapy is accomplished with a combination of a penicillinase-resistant penicillin and an aminoglycoside antibiotic (49,50). However,

there is one study that suggests the use of a penicillinase-resistant penicillin alone for 2 weeks in the treatment of these patients may itself be sufficient (51). Vancomycin and even cefazolin may afford less-effective anti-staphylococcal treatment than nafcillin or oxacillin. Patients should be repeatedly evaluated for complications at the start, during the course, and at the potential conclusion of treatment. Candidates who do not respond clinically and bacteriologically within 96 hours after the initiation of therapy and those with intolerance to penicillins or aminoglycosides should be excluded from short-course therapy. In counterdistinction, septic pulmonary emboli occurring during the initial few days of treatment are not a contraindication to the shorter regimen.

The expense and inconvenience of even 2 weeks of parenteral antibiotic therapy for endocarditis are considerable. Now with the advent of potent oral agents with excellent bioavailability and long half-lives, oral therapy consisting of ciprofloxacin and rifampin for 4 weeks may offer a viable alternative to intravenous treatment for patients with un-complicated right-sided endocarditis due to susceptible *S. aureus* (52). The absorption of quinolone antibiotics is reduced by the con-comitant ingestion of cations because of chelation in the stomach; therefore, coadmin-istration of antacids, iron, calcium, magne-sium, and sulcrafate must be separated by at least 2 hours from the quinolone. The patient population eligible for oral therapy is similar to those who might be selected for a 2-week course of intravenous combination treatment, as discussed previously. The potential role of oral antibiotics in uncomplicated cases of gram-negative and left-sided endocarditis de-serves further studies but is still unresolved.

Antibiotic Therapy for Enterococcal Endocarditis

The treatment of enterococcal endocarditis is complicated because these bacteria are gen-erally resistant to the bactericidal action of cell wall-active antibiotics like penicillin and vancomycin when used as monotherapy. Killing, as opposed to merely inhibition, of enterococci can be achieved by the addition of an aminoglycoside (appropriate to the partic-ular species), unless the organism exhibits high-level resistance to that aminoglycoside. Minimum inhibitory concentrations greater than or equal to 2,000 µg/mL of streptomycin and 500 to 2,000 µg/mL of gentamicin are considered the critical values in predicting whether penicillin and the aminoglycoside agent will synergistically kill enterococci (53). Tobramycin cannot be routinely substi-tuted for streptomycin or gentamicin because tobramycin does not provide synergistic killing of *E. faecium* even in the absence of high-level resistance (54). If endocarditis is caused by enterococci that exhibit high-level resistance to gentamicin, synergy cannot be obtained with any other aminoglycoside ex-cept possibly streptomicin. Enterococci with high-level resistance to gentamicin and strep-tomicin pose a difficult therapeutic problem; prolonged monotherapy (8 to 12 weeks) with high-dose ampicillin, optimally administered by continuous infusion, may cure half of the patients.

Patients with a life-threatening allergy to penicillin can be treated with vancomycin and an aminoglycoside or undergo desensitization to penicillin. The incidence of vancomycin re-sistance in enterococcus, mainly *E. faecium*, has continued to increase during the past 5 years; such strains may also be resistant to penicillin (minimum inhibitory concentration > 100 µg/mL) and all aminoglycoside antibi-otics. Treatment with quinupristine/dalfopris-tine (Synercid) or minocycline ± rifampin, perhaps in conjunction with valve replace-ment, has been advocated in these cases (55).

Continued Fever Despite Appropriate Antibiotic Therapy

Persistent fever during endocarditis is usu-ally defined as fever lasting for more than 10 to 14 days after institution of appropriate treatment. It represents a serious diagnostic challenge and should be differentiated from recurrent fever in a patient who initially had responded to therapy. Cardiac complications (e.g., refractory valvular and perivalvular in-fection, sometimes with the formation of a frank myocardial abscess) remain a major rea-son for persistent fever; other important causes include abscesses in distant organs, such as the spleen and other intraabdominal or retroperitoneal viscera (56). Multiple metastatic foci of infection are particularly common in patients after *S. aureus* bac-teremia. Intercurrent nosocomial infections, phlebitis, and drug-induced fever are more of-ten associated with relapsing as opposed to unabated fever. Repetitive emboli causing er-ratic fevers may continue for weeks despite effective antimicrobial therapy, especially in patients with right-sided endocarditis.

Cardiac and Neurovascular Surgery in Active Native Valve Endocarditis

It must be remembered that patients with in-fective endocarditis who do well without valve replacement are spared both the immediate operative morbidity and multiple additional life-long risks associated with prosthetic valves. However, surgery has assumed an increasingly important role in the optimal treatment of selected patients with infective endocarditis. The procedures can range from mitral valve repair to complete tricuspid valvulectomy to aortic root reconstruction necessitating reimplantation of the coronary arteries (57). Ideally, surgical intervention would be performed before the onset of hemodynamic instability and CNS emboli. Such prophylactic intervention can prevent serious complications, thus improving prognosis significantly. However, predicting these complications in individual cases is fraught with imprecision and uncertainty given the currently available clinical, microbiologic, and echocardiographic tools. Thus, in most cases, operative intervention is precipitated by a complication but can hopefully be performed before irreversible damage develops or another complication ensues (58,59) (Table 15-2).

Heart failure secondary to left-sided valvular incompetence is the most common and widely accepted indication for valve replacement. A 10-year comparative analysis from the University of Alabama revealed that early surgical intervention decreases the mortality rate in patients with native valve endocarditis and moderate or severe heart failure. In those patients with *S. aureus* native valve endocarditis, regardless of their hemodynamic status, early valve replacement appeared to improve the overall outcome (60). In this analysis, the benefit of surgery was apparent during the hospitalization and for 2 years after discharge. A prospective study looking at immediate and long-term survival after emergent valve replacement, compared with patients who were treated only with antimicrobials, also revealed a better short- and long-term outcome in the former group of patients (61). Emergent operation was not significantly associated with an increased operative mortality compared with elective surgery, as long as the intervention preceded the onset of severe heart failure and the spread of infection beyond the valve annulus (61).

TABLE 15-2. *Criteria for operative intervention during active endocarditis*

Major indications for prompt operation	Major indications for surgery if findings persist or progress after 1 week of optimal medical therapy	Indications for operation if at least three minor indications coexist
Severe heart failure due to valvular insufficiency or obstruction	Progressive heart failure despite medical therapy	Heart failure resolved on medical therapy
Endocarditis due to highly resistant pathogens[a]	Persistent bacteremia despite appropriate antibiotics	Single macroembolic event
Prosthetic valve dehiscence or malfunction	*New* conduction disturbances in the setting of *aortic* valve endocarditis (not caused by drugs or noninfectious cardiac disease)	Definite left-sided vegetations visualized by TTE
Multiple major embolic events (unless recent cerebral event mandates delaying valve replacement)	Microbiologic relapse of prosthetic valve endocarditis during or after an appropriate course of therapy	Prosthetic valve endocarditis caused by other than exquisitely penicillin-sensitive viridans streptococci
Purulent pericarditis (secondary to direct extension of valvular infection)		Persistent fever without another suspected etiology except unresponsive intracardiac infection
		Lack of bactericidal antibiotic options

[a]Fungal endocarditis has traditionally been considered a firm indication for prompt surgery, although recent data suggest that indefinite "suppressive" azole therapy might be considered in some patients who are poor operative candidates. Left-sided or prosthetic valve endocarditis due to *S. aureus* or *P. aeruginosa* are believed by some authors to be independent indications for valve replacement.

TTE, transthoracic echocardiography.

Hemodynamic status at the time of cardiac surgery is the major determinant of operative mortality; in fact, the mortality rate increases in direct proportion to the degree of hemodynamic disability (62). It has been repeatedly observed that adverse outcomes occur more frequently when operative intervention is delayed in a hemodynamically unstable patient to allow a longer duration of antibiotic therapy to be administered preoperatively.

Surgery should be performed promptly in patients with active endocarditis when severe or progressive heart failure ensues. The only relative contraindication to this approach is the presence of a fresh cerebral infarct. When cardiac function permits, surgery is best delayed for patients suffering from a recent cerebral insult. Preoperative risk factors for exacerbation of neurologic deficits include the severity of the stoke, the presence of an intracranial bleed, and the time interval between the event and the surgical procedure. In the case of an embolic infarct, surgery should be postponed, if possible, until 1 to 2 weeks have elapsed since the stroke; longer delays are often recommended when hemorrhage is present (63).

Angiography is the only test that can reliably exclude mycotic aneurysms, with a sensitivity of approximately 90%. An angiogram should be performed shortly before cardiothoracic surgery for patients who have experienced strokes or bothersome headaches during the course of endocarditis (64). Although mycotic aneurysms may develop in up to 5% of patients with bacterial endocarditis, only 10% of these aneurysms will rupture (65). Unfortunately, hemorrhage may be the first manifestation without any premonitory symptoms. In these cases, the mycotic aneurysm should be urgently resected and any cardiac surgery delayed for 2 or more weeks (63). Aneurysms that have not leaked will stabilize or regress with antimicrobial therapy alone in most cases. Under these circumstances, serial angiograms are used to follow the size of the aneurysm (64). Large, expanding, and/or leaking aneurysms are indications for prompt

neurosurgical intervention. Patients with mycotic aneurysms are at high risk of bleeding when anticoagulated, as may be required during and after valve replacement. It reasonably follows then that a lower threshold for aneurysm repair is appropriate for patients likely to require valve replacement, especially when subsequent anticoagulation is unavoidable. Although persistent stable aneurysms may rupture after completion of standard antibiotic treatment, the risk for late rupture cannot be precisely estimated, and recommendations for delayed surgical repair are made on an individual basis. If possible, drainage of extracardiac sites of active infection should be performed before valve replacement. Attention to dental issues is advised in all patient with endocarditis for at least two reasons: if they go on to valve replacement, subsequent circumstances may not permit a delay to address dental disease, and once a left-sided heart valve is infected, the risk of reinfection is increased.

Management of Prosthetic Valve Endocarditis

Prosthetic valve endocarditis occurs in 1.4% to 3.1% of patients within the first postoperative year and in 3.2% to 5.7% within 5 years of valve replacement surgery (66). Despite increasingly sophisticated diagnostic and treatment modalities, the overall mortality rate remains as high as 23% to 48%. The mortality rate in early prosthetic valve endocarditis (less than 60 days after surgery) is higher than for late prosthetic valve endocarditis (67–69). Continued but carefully monitored anticoagulation is usually advocated for patients with prosthetic valve endocarditis when otherwise required by the valve type and position. Anticoagulation must be immediately reversed in cases of intracerebral bleeding. It should be used very cautiously, if at all, in the immediate aftermath of nonhemorrhagic cerebral infarctions. Heparin, because of its shorter effects, is preferred to warfarin during the period of active infection;

whether the newer low-molecular-weight heparins offer any advantages under these circumstances has not been systematically studied.

"Complicated" prosthetic valve endocarditis has been defined by the presence of heart failure, a murmur reflective of prosthesis malfunction, new electrocardiographic conduction abnormalities, unexplained fevers beyond 10 days of appropriate antibiotic therapy, or relapsed infection. Prosthetic aortic valve endocarditis due to *S. aureus* is often anticipated as a complicated infection. Complicated cases, which disproportionately occur among early cases, have a sixfold higher mortality rate than uncomplicated infections. Most of these patients are best treated with a combined medical-surgical approach. The optimal timing of cardiac surgery is almost exclusively determined by the hemodynamic and neurologic status of the patient and should be individualized on a case by case basis.

ACKNOWLEDGMENT

We are deeply indebted to Deanne Schufreider-Conners and Cindy Harker for their tireless efforts in patching together this manuscript.

REFERENCES

1. Major RH. Notes on the history of endocarditis. *Bull Hist Med* 1945;17:351.
2. Osler W. The Gulstonian lectures on malignant endocarditis. *BMJ* 1885;1:467, 522, 577.
3. Watanakunakorn C, Burkert T. Infective endocarditis at a large community teaching hospital. A review of 210 episodes. *Medicine (Baltimore)* 1993;72:90.
4. Mortara AM, Bayer AS. Staphylococcus aureus bacteremia and endocarditis. New diagnostic and therapeutic concepts. *Infect Dis Clin North Am* 1993;7: 53–68.
5. Fulton MN, Levines A. Subacute bacterial endocarditis with special reference to the valvular lesions and previous history. *Am J Med Sci* 1938;183:60.
5a. Strom BL, et al. Dental and cardiac risk factors for infective endocarditis. A population-based, case-control study. *Ann Intern Med* 1998;129:761.
6. Wieland M, et al. Left-sided endocarditis due to

Pseudomonas aeruginosa: a report of 10 cases and a review of the literature. *Medicine (Baltimore)* 1986; 65:180.
7. Rubinstein E, Lang R. Fungal endocarditis. *Eur Heart J* 1995;16[Suppl B]:84.
8. Drancourt M, et al. Bartonella quintana endocarditis in three homeless men. *N Engl J Med* 1995;332:419.
9. Geraci JE, Wilson WR. Symposium on infective endocarditis. III. Endocarditis due to gram negative bacteria, report of 56 cases. *Mayo Clin Proc* 1982;57:145.
10. Ruoff KL, et al. Bacteremia with *Streptococcus bovis* and *Streptococcus salivarius*: clinical correlates of more accurate identification of isolates. *J Clin Microbiol* 1989;27:305.
11. Fowler GV, et al. Infective endocarditis due to *Staphylococcus aureus*: 59 prospectively identified cases with follow-up. *Clin Infect Dis* 1999;28:106.
12. Nishimura RA, et al. Echocardiographically documented mitral valve prolapse. Long term follow-up of 237 patients. *N Engl J Med* 1985;313:1305.
13. Johnson CM. Adherence events in the pathogenesis of infective endocarditis. *Infect Dis Clin North Am* 1993; 7:21.
14. Ivert TSA, et al. Prosthetic valve endocarditis. *Circulation* 1984;69:223.
15. Bortolotti UG, et al. Pathological study of infective endocarditis on Hancock porcine bioprostheses. *J Thorac Cardiovasc Surg* 1981;81:934.
16. Karchmer AW, Gibbons WG. Infections of prosthetic heart valves and grafts. In: Biano AL, Walvogel AF, ed. *Infections Associated with Indwelling Medical Devices*, 2nd ed. American Society for Microbiology, Washington; 1994:213.
17. Chino F, et al. Non-bacterial thrombotic endocarditis in a Japanese autopsy sample. A review of 80 cases. *Am Heart J* 1975;90:190.
18. Churchill MA Jr, Goraci JE, Hunder GG. Musculoskeletal manifestations of bacterial endocarditis. *Ann Intern Med* 1977;87:754.
18a. DiNubile MJ, et al. Cardiac conduction abnormalities complicating native valve active infective endocarditis. *Am J Cardiol* 1986;58:1213.
19. Greenle GE, Mandell GL. Neurological manifestations of infective endocarditis: a review. *Stroke* 1973; 4:958.
20. Rabinovich I, et al. A long term view of bacterial endocarditis. 337 cases 1924 to 1963. *Ann Intern Med* 1965;63:185.
21. Bayer AS, Norman DC. Valve site-specific pathogenic differences between right-sided and left-sided bacterial endocarditis. *Chest* 1990;98:200.
22. Robins MJ, et al. Right-sided valvular endocarditis: etiology, diagnosis, and an approach to 1990.therapy. *Am Heart J* 1986;11:128.
22a. Durack DT, Lukas AS, Bright DK. The duke endocarditis service. New critieria for diagnosis of infective endocarditits. *Am J Med* 1994;96:200.
23. Bayer AS, et al. Evaluation of new clinical criteria for the diagnosis of infective endocarditis. *Am J Med* 1994;96:211.
24. Hoen B, et al. The Duke criteria for diagnosing infective endocarditis are specific: analysis of 100 patients with acute fever of unknown origin. *Clin Infect Dis* 1996;23:298.

25. Gagliardi JP, et al. Native valve infective endocarditis in elderly and younger adult patients: comparison of clinical features and outcomes with use of the Duke criteria and the Duke endocarditis database. *Clin Infect Dis* 1998;26:1165.

26. Werner AS, et al. Studies on the bacteremias of bacterial endocarditis. *JAMA* 1967;202:199.

26a. Kostman JR, et al. Detection of the etiologic agents of culture-negative endocarditis by polymerase chain reaction. Abstracts of the 34th ICAAC. Orlando, FL, abstract D7, 1998.

27. Bayer AS, et al. Circulating immune complexes in infective endocarditis. *N Engl J Med* 1976;295:1500.

28. Williams RC Jr, Kunkel HG. Rheumatoid factor, complement, and conglutinin aberrations in patients with subacute bacterial endocarditis. *J Clin Invest* 1962;41: 666.

29. Dillon JC, et al. Endocardiographic manifestation of valvular vegetation. *Am Heart J* 1973;86:698.

30. Roy P, et al. Spectrum of echocardiographic findings in bacterial endocarditis. *Circulation* 1976;53:474.

31. Stafford WJ, et al. Vegetations in infective endocarditis: clinical relevance and diagnosis by cross sectional echocardiography. *Br Heart J* 1985;53:310.

32. Erbel R, et al. Improved diagnostic value of echocardiography in patients with infective endocarditis by transesophageal approach. A prospective study. *Eur Heart J* 1988;9:43.

33. Murphy GJ, Foster-Smith K. Management of complications of infective endocarditis with emphasis on echocardiographic findings. *Infect Dis Clin North Am* 1993;7:153.

34. Shapiro SM, et al. Transesophageal echocardiography in diagnosis of infective endocarditis. *Chest* 1994;105: 377.

35. Daniel WG, et al. Improvement in the diagnosis of abscesses associated with endocarditis by transesophageal echocardiography. *N Engl J Med* 1991; 324:795.

36. Karalis DG, et al. Transesophageal echocardiographic recognition of subaortic complications in aortic valve endocarditis, clinical and surgical implications. *Circulation* 1992;86:353.

37. Lowry RW, et al. Clinical impact of transesophageal echocardiography in the diagnosis and management of infective endocarditis. *Am J Cardiol* 1994;73:1089.

38. Stewart JA, et al. Echocardiographic documentation of vegetative lesions in infective endocarditis: clinical implications. *Circulation* 1980;61:374.

39. Mugge A, et al. Echocardiography in infective endocarditis: reassessment of prognostic implications of vegetation size determined by the transthoracic and transesophageal approach. *J Am Coll Cardiol* 1989;14:631.

40. Wann LS, et al. Comparison of M-mode and cross-sectional echocardiography in infective endocarditis. *Circulation* 1979;60:728.

41. Steckelberg JM, et al. Emboli in infective endocarditis: the prognostic value of echocardiography. *Ann Intern Med* 1991;114:635.

42. Buda AJ, et al. Prognostic significance of vegetations detected by two-dimensional echocardiography in infective endocarditis. *Am Heart J* 1986;112:1291.

43. Karchmer AW. Staphylococcal endocarditis. In: Kaye D, eds. *Infective Endocarditis,* 2nd ed. New York: Raven Press, 1992:225.

44. Bayer AS, et al. Diagnosis and management of infective endocarditis and its complication. *Circulation* 1998;98:2936.

45. Garvey GJ, Neu HC. Infective endocarditis: an evolving disease. A review of endocarditis at the Columbia-Presbyterian Medical Center. *Medicine (Baltimore)* 1978;57:105.

46. Rohmann S, et al. Clinical relevance of vegetation localization by transesophageal echocardiography in infective endocarditis. *Eur Heart J* 1992;13:446.

47. Wilson WR, et al. Antibiotic treatment of adults with infective endocarditis due to streptococci, enterococci, staphylococci, and HACEK microorganisms. *JAMA* 1995;274:1706.

48. DiNubile MJ. Short-course antibiotic therapy for right-sided endocarditis caused by *Staphylococcus aureus* in injection drug users. *Ann Intern Med* 1994;121:873.

49. Chambers HF, et al. Right-sided *Staphylococcus aureus* endocarditis in intravenous drug abusers: two-week combination therapy. *Ann Intern Med* 1988;109:619.

50. Torres-Tortosa M, et al. Indications and therapeutic results of an antibiotic regime lasting two weeks in intravenous drug users with right-sided S. aureus infective endocarditis: a multicentre study of 139 consecutive cases. *Eur J Clin Microbiol Infec Dis* 1994;13:533.

51. Ribera E, et al. Effectiveness of cloxacillin with and without gentamicin in short-term therapy for right-sided *Staphylococcus aureus* endocarditis. A randomized, controlled trial. *Ann Intern Med* 1996;125:969.

52. Heldman AW, et al. Oral antibiotic treatment of right-sided staphylococcal endocarditis in injection drug users: prospective randomized comparison with parenteral therapy. *Am J Med* 1996;101:68.

53. Eliopoulos GM. Enterococcal endocarditis. In: Kaye D, ed. *Infective Endocarditis*, 2nd ed. New York: Raven Press, 1992:209.

54. Eliopoulos GM. Aminoglycoside resistant enterococcal endocarditis. *Med Clin North Am* 1993;17:117.

55. Finch RG. Antimicrobial activity of quinupristin-dalfopristin. *Drugs* 1997;51:31.

56. Blumberg EA, et al. Persistent fever in association with infective endocarditis. *Clin Infect Dis* 1992;15:933.

57. Pagano D, Allen SM, Boner RS. Homograft aortic valve and root replacement for severe destructive native and prosthetic endocarditis. *Eur J Cardiothorac Surg* 1994;8:173.

58. David TE, et al. Heart valve operations in patients with active infective endocarditis. *Ann Thorac Surg* 1990; 49:701–705.

59. DiNubile MJ. Surgery in active endocarditis. *Ann Intern Med* 1982;96:650.

60. Alsip SG, et al. Indications for cardiac surgery in patients with active infective endocarditis. *Am J Med* 1985;78[Suppl 6B]:138.

61. Reinhartz O, et al. Timing of surgery in patients with acute infective endocarditis. *J Cardiovasc Surg* 1996; 37:397.

62. Gillinov AM, et al. Valve replacement in patients with endocarditis and acute neurologic deficit. *Ann Thorac Surg* 1996;61:1125.

63. Eishi K, et al. Surgical management of infective endocarditis associated with cerebral complications. Multicenter retrospective study in Japan. *J Thorac Cardiovasc Surg* 1995;110:1745.

64. Matsushita K, et al. Hemorrhagic and ischemic cere-

brovascular complications of active infective endocarditis of native valve. *Eur Neurol* 1993;33:267.

65. Brust CMJ, et al. The diagnosis and treatment of cerebral mycotic aneurysms. *Ann Neurol* 1990;27:238.

66. Calderwood SB, et al. Risk factors for the development of prosthetic valve endocarditis. *Circulation* 1985;72:31.

67. Yu VL, et al. Prosthetic valve endocarditis: superiority of surgical valve replacement versus medical therapy only. *Ann Thorac Surg* 1994;58:1073.

68. Calderwood SB, et al. Prosthetic valve endocarditis: analysis of factors affecting outcome of therapy. *J Thorac Cardiovasc Surg* 1986;92:776.

69. Malcolm DV, et al. *Staphylococcus aureus* prosthetic valve endocarditis: optimal management and risk factors for death. *Clin Infect Dis* 1998;26:1302.

16

Management of Antithrombotic Therapy in Patients with Prosthetic Heart Valves

Paul D. Stein

Henry Ford Heart and Vascular Institute, Detroit, Michigan 48202

MECHANICAL PROSTHETIC HEART VALVES

All patients with mechanical prosthetic heart valves require some form of prophylaxis. Experience in patients without antithrombotic prophylaxis has been devastating. The prevalence of thromboemboli among patients with St. Jude aortic valves (1), St. Jude mitral valves (1), and with Bjork-Shiley spherical disc aortic valves (2) is shown in Fig. 16-1.

The prevalence of thromboemboli depends on the type of mechanical prosthetic heart valve. The prevalence of thromboemboli is lower with modern valves than with first-generation valves. Among patients treated with anticoagulants at an international normalized ratio (INR) of 2.0 to 4.9, the prevalence of thromboemboli among patients treated with oral anticoagulants was 0.5%/yr with bileaflet valves, 0.7%/yr with tilting-disc valves, and 2.5%/yr with caged-ball and caged-disc valves (Fig. 16-2) (3). Trends in patients with caged-ball or caged-disc valves showed the lowest incidence of adverse effects at an INR of 4.0 to 4.9, although at this level of the INR, there is a considerable risk of bleeding (3).

The prevalence of thromboemboli is greater in patients with valves in the mitral position than in the aortic position, and the prevalence of thromboemboli is highest in patients with two prosthetic valves. A higher prevalence of thromboemboli has been shown with valves in the mitral position compared with the aortic position among patients with the St. Jude bileaflet valve (4), the Bjork-Shiley spherical disc valve (5), the Bjork-Shiley convexo-concave valve (6), and with the Medtronic Hall valve (7) (Fig. 16-3). These data and data from several other studies have been reviewed (8). Cannegieter et al. (3) showed an incidence of thromboembolism of 0.5%/yr with a prosthetic aortic valve, 0.9%/yr with a prosthetic mitral valve, and 1.2%/yr with both aortic and mitral valves. The reason for a higher prevalence of thromboembolic complications with valves in the mitral position is probably due to atrial fibrillation, but it has been speculated that left atrial enlargement, and perhaps endocardial damage from rheumatic mitral valve disease, may contribute (4).

Trends suggested that an INR of 4.0 to 4.9 might show fewer adverse effects in patients with two mechanical prosthetic valves (3), but a high percentage of patients with such levels of the INR have bleeding (8,9).

For any particular valve in a specific position (aortic or mitral), it seems that there may be an INR above which small if any reduction of thromboemboli occur. However, the data are sparse and conflicting. With the St. Jude valve in the aortic position, combined data from sev-

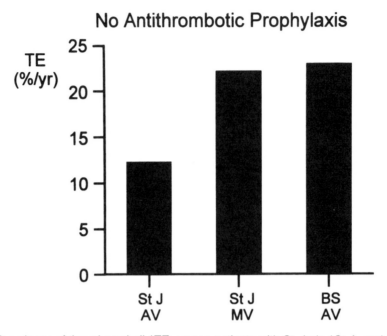

FIG. 16-1. Prevalence of thromboemboli (*TE*) among patients with St. Jude (*St J*), and Bjork-Shiley (*BS*) valves. *AV*, aortic valves; *MV*, mitral valves (1,2).

eral investigators showed that the prevalence of thromboembolism was not diminished by increasing the level of the INR above 2.0 to 3.0 (Fig. 16-4) (4,10,11). Individual investigators, however, showed differing results. Horstkotte et al. (4) showed fewer thromboemboli with higher levels of the INR in patients with St. Jude aortic valves. Acar et al. (10) showed comparable prevalences of thromboemboli with levels of the INR of 2.0 to 3.0 and 3.0 to

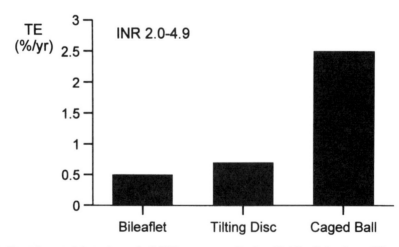

FIG. 16-2. Prevalence of thromboemboli (*TE*) among patients with bileaflet valves, tilting-disc valves, and caged-ball or caged-disc valves (3).

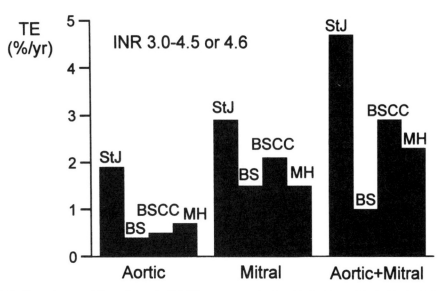

FIG. 16-3. Prevalence of thromboemboli (*TE*) among patients with St. Jude (*St J*), Bjork-Shiley (*BS*), Bjork-Shiley convexo-concave (*BSCC*), and Medtronic Hall (*MH*) valves. Thromboemboli were more frequent among patients with prosthetic mitral valves than aortic valves, and TE were most frequent among patients with two prosthetic valves (4,6,7).

4.5 in patients with aortic prosthetic valves, 96% of which were St. Jude.

Among patients with St. Jude valves in the mitral position, combined data showed that the prevalence of thromboemboli did not di-minish with levels of the INR above 2.8 to 4.3 (Fig. 16-5) (4,11). Horstkotte et al. (4), how-ever, showed fewer thromboemboli with higher levels of the INR in patients with St. Jude mitral valves.

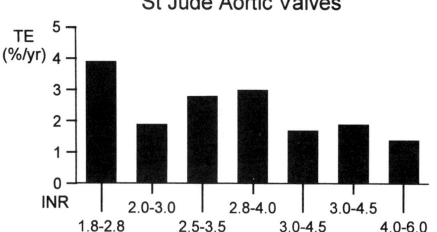

FIG. 16-4. Prevalence of thromboemboli among patients with St. Jude aortic valves. A comparable frequency of thromboemboli with an INR of 2.0 to 3.0 or higher is seen (4,10,11).

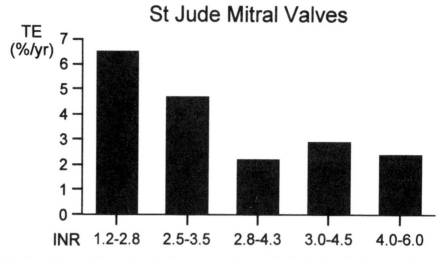

FIG. 16-5. Prevalence of thromboemboli among patients with St. Jude mitral valves. A comparable frequency of thromboemboli with an INR of 2.8 to 4.3 or higher is seen (4,11).

Regarding patients with two St. Jude valves, the prevalence of thromboemboli did not diminish with levels of the INR higher than 2.5 to 3.5 (Fig. 16-6) (4).

Regarding mechanical prosthetic valves of various types, patients with an INR of 7.4 to 10.8 had no fewer thromboemboli than patients with an INR of 1.9 to 3.6 (Fig. 16-7) (12). Major hemorrhage, however, was twice as high in the group treated with the higher INR.

Regarding the relation of the INR to major hemorrhagic events, an association was shown by Wilson et al. (13) based on the North American prothrombin time. A direct relation of the level of the INR to the frequency of bleeding was also shown by Horstkotte et al. among patients with St. Jude valves. van der Meer et al. (14) observed 42% more major bleeding for every one point increase in INR. Comparison of data from sev-

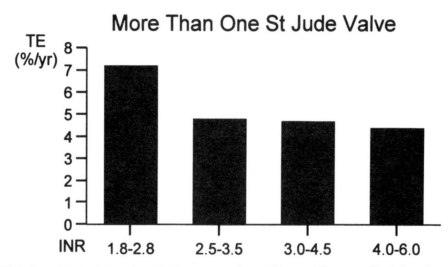

FIG. 16-6. Prevalence of thromboemboli among patients with more than one St. Jude valve. A comparable frequency of thromboemboli occurred with an INR of 2.5 to 3.5 or higher (4).

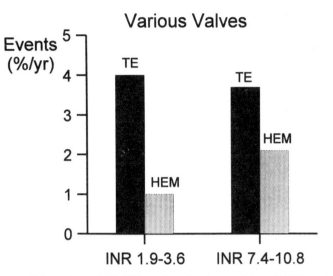

FIG. 16-7. Prevalence of thromboemboli (*TE*) and major hemorrhage (*HEM*) among patients with various types of mechanical prosthetic valves. A comparable frequency of thromboemboli occurred with an INR of 1.9 to 3.6 and an INR of 7.4 to 10.8. Major hemorrhage was more frequent at the higher INR (12).

eral individual reports suggested a relation of the frequency of hemorrhagic events to the level of the INR, but there was considerable variability (Fig. 16-8) (4,5,7,10–12,15–17). Major bleeding occurred more frequently in patients 70 years of age or older than in younger patients (3).

There appears to be an optimal level for individual valves inserted in specific locations at which the event rate (thromboemboli and major hemorrhage) is lowest. Beyond a given level of the INR, for a particular valve in a particular position, there is little if any reduction of the prevalence of thromboemboli, but the

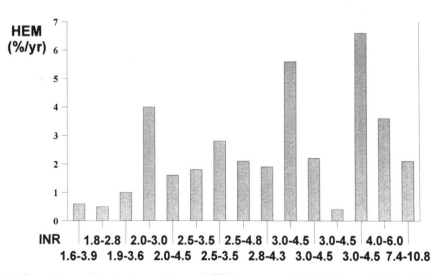

FIG. 16-8. Prevalence of major hemorrhage (*HEM*) among patients with prosthetic valves treated with various levels of the INR. In general, major hemorrhage was more frequent at higher levels of the INR (4,5,7,10–12,15–17).

prevalence of major bleeding increases. An optimal level of the INR exists, therefore, at which the combined rates of thromboemboli and major bleeding is lowest. This has been shown for bileaflet and tilting-disc valves (18). For tilting-disc valves and bileaflet mechanical valves, when the estimated INR was no lower than 2.5 or 3.0 (minimal INR), there was a low thromboembolic rate with an acceptable hemorrhagic event rate (18). If the lower range of the INR was 1.6 or 1.9, then the thromboembolic rate increased considerably, whereas the hemorrhagic event rate decreased only somewhat. Regarding the upper end of the therapeutic range (maximal INR), the thromboembolic rate with a maximal level of the INR of 2.5 or 3.6 was not different from the thromboembolic rate with a maximal level of the INR of 3.9 or 4.8. Increasing the maximal value of the INR to 8.2 caused no further reduction of the thromboembolic rate, but the hemorrhagic rate increased. An INR in the range of 2.5 to 3.6, therefore, was effective in reducing the risk of thromboembolic events and in minimizing the risk of major bleeding

in patients, most of whom had tilting-disc or bileaflet mechanical heart valves (18). Cannegieter et al. (3), among patients with various valves, most of which were tilting disc, but some were caged-ball or caged-disc and some were bileaflet, showed the fewest adverse events at an INR that ranged between 2.5 to 2.9 and 4.5 to 4.9.

Aspirin in Combination with Oral Anticoagulants May Be Effective and Safe

Turpie et al. (17) reintroduced the concept that aspirin in combination with oral anticoagulants might reduce the prevalence of thromboemboli without greatly increasing the risk of major bleeding. Low doses of aspirin (100 mg/day) were administered in combination with oral anticoagulants at an INR of 3.0 to 4.5. This resulted in a reduced frequency of thromboemboli with only a trend toward increased major bleeding, although there was an increased frequency of minor bleeding (Fig. 16-9) (17). Meschengieser et al. (19) showed in patients with various types of mechanical

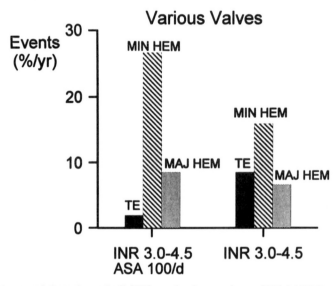

FIG. 16-9. Prevalence of thromboemboli (*TE*), major hemorrhage (*MAJ HEM*), and minor hemorrhage (*MIN HEM*) among patients with various types of mechanical prosthetic valves. Patients treated with oral anticoagulants at an INR of 3.0 to 4.5 in combination with aspirin (*ASA*) 100 mg/day showed fewer thromboemboli and a comparable frequency of major hemorrhage as those treated with oral anticoagulants alone at the same INR. Minor bleeding was more frequent among patients treated with oral anticoagulants in combination with ASA (17).

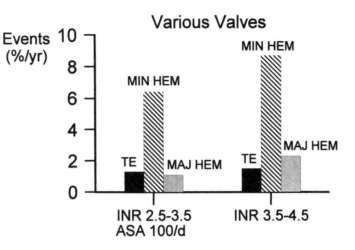

FIG. 16-10. Prevalence of thromboemboli (*TE*), major hemorrhage (*MAJ HEM*), and minor hemor-rhage (*MIN HEM*) among patients with various types of mechanical prosthetic valves. Patients treated with oral anticoagulants at an INR of 2.5 to 3.5 in combination with aspirin (*ASA*) 100 mg/day showed a comparable frequency of thromboemboli but somewhat less frequent major and minor hemorrhage in comparison with those treated with oral anticoagulants alone at an INR of 3.5 to 4.5 (19).

prosthetic valves that the use of anticoagu-lants at an INR of 2.5 to 3.5 combined with aspirin 100 mg/day was as effective as an INR of 3.5 to 4.5 and the likelihood of major and minor bleeding tended to be lower in the as-pirin group (Fig. 16-10). With a low INR of 2.0 to 3.0, a high dose of aspirin plus dipyri-damole was effective and safe (20). Available evidence, based on several investigations, is shown in Fig. 16-11 (17,19–22). The data

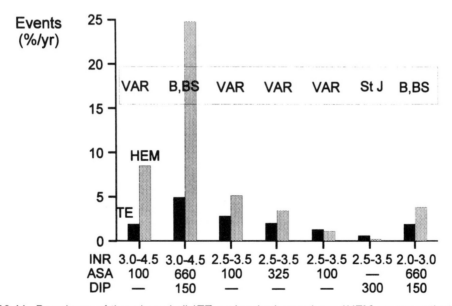

FIG. 16-11. Prevalence of thromboemboli (*TE*) and major hemorrhage (*HEM*) among patients with various types of mechanical prosthetic valves (*VAR*), Bicor valves (*B*), Bjork-Shiley (*BS*) valves, and St. Jude (*St J*) valves who were treated with oral anticoagulants and antiplatelet agents in combina-tion. The level of INR, daily dose of aspirin (*ASA*), and dipyridamole (*DIP*) are shown (17,19–22).

suggest both a low frequency of thromboemboli and low frequency of major hemorrhage
are accomplished with oral anticoagulants in
combination with aspirin if the level of the
INR is low (Fig. 16-11). High levels of both
the INR and of aspirin cause more bleeding
but do not reduce the frequency of thromboemboli (Fig. 16-11).

The combination of oral anticoagulants and
aspirin may be particularly useful in patients
with coronary artery disease or stroke (19).
Mortality from other vascular causes was
lower among patients treated with aspirin in
combination with oral anticoagulants (17).

Dipyridamole in Combination with Oral Anticoagulants

In regard to dipyridamole in addition to
oral anticoagulants, a few investigations were
performed on first-generation valves between
1969 and 1983. Some showed an additive
benefit (23,24), one showed no benefit (25),
and some showed only a trend (26–28). The
intensity of oral anticoagulants in these investigations, based on the INR, is not known.

Meta-analysis based on the investigations that
were randomized showed that oral anticoagulants in combination with dipyridamole reduced the frequency of thromboembolism
when compared with anticoagulants alone
(29). There was no difference between treatment groups with respect to hemorrhagic
events.

Prophylaxis with Antiplatelet Agents Alone or in Combination with Fixed Low Doses of Oral Anticoagulants

Most data related to antithrombotic prophylaxis are based on treatment with oral anticoagulants adjusted to a certain level of the
prothrombin time ratio or, more recently, the
INR. Other approaches to prophylaxis have
been attempted, however. The use of a fixed
low dose of warfarin (2.5 mg/day) in combination with aspirin and dipyridamole showed
good results in patients with St. Jude bileaflet
valves (Fig. 16-12) (30). Antiplatelet agents
alone also have been shown by some to offer
satisfactory protection in adults in sinus
rhythm with St. Jude valves in the aortic posi-

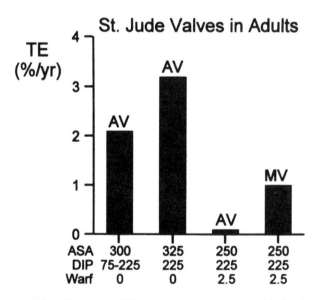

FIG. 16-12. Prevalence of thromboemboli (*TE*) among adult patients with St. Jude aortic valves (*AV*)
and mitral valves (*MV*) who were treated with antiplatelet agents alone or in combination with fixed low
doses of warfarin (*Warf*). The daily dose of aspirin (*ASA*) and dipyridamole (*DIP*) is shown (30–32).

tion (31,32) (Fig. 16-12). Antiplatelet agents alone in patients with the Bjork-Shiley spherical disc valve showed unsatisfactory results (2).

Elderly Patients

Among patients with various types of mechanical heart valves, most thromboemboli occurred in patients 50 years of age or older (Fig. 16-13) (3). Major hemorrhage was also more frequent in patients 50 years of age or older, and the highest frequency of bleeding was in elderly patients (70 years of age or older) (Fig. 16-13) (3). Among elderly patients with St. Jude valves in the aortic position, an INR of 1.8 to 2.8 was effective and major hemorrhage was infrequent (33). The INR was unknown among some of the elderly patients in this study who were treated before the INR was in use (33).

Antithrombotic Therapy in Children

Attempts have been made to entirely avoid antithrombotic treatment in children with various types of prosthetic valves. The results were sometimes (34) but not always (35) disastrous. Some investigators attempted pro-

phylaxis with antiplatelet agents alone. These results were variable and sometimes tragic (36,37), although some investigators showed borderline (38) or good results (34,39–42). Antithrombotic therapy in children has been reviewed (43).

WARFARIN

International Normalized Ratio

The prothrombin time ratio and the prothrombin time depend on the thromboplastin reagent (9). An INR based on a World Health Organization standard thromboplastin was defined that permits reporting of the prothrombin time ratio in a standardized fashion. This permits comparison of the anticoagulant effect, irrespective of the local thromboplastin reagent that was used for measurement of the prothrombin time.

The INR is calculated as follows:

$$INR = (prothrombin\ time\ ratio)^{ISI}$$

where ISI is international sensitivity index of the thromboplastin reagent used for measurement of the prothrombin time. The prothrombin time ratio (the ratio of patient prothrombin time to control prothrombin time) is measured in the local laboratory. The ISI is a

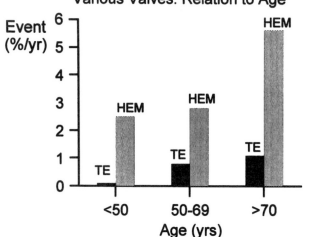

FIG. 16-13. Prevalence of thromboemboli (*TE*) and major hemorrhage (*HEM*) in relation to age among patients with various types of mechanical prosthetic valves (*VAR*) (3).

measure of the responsiveness of a given thromboplastin to a reduction of the vitamin K-dependent coagulation factor, compared with the international reference preparation (9). The value of the ISI for commercial thromboplastins is now indicated by many manufacturers on the reagent packages and therefore is easily reported by the laboratory. The INR is calculated simply by raising the prothrombin time ratio to the ISI power. For example, if the patient prothrombin time is 18 seconds and the control prothrombin time is 12 seconds, the prothrombin time ratio is 1.5. If the ISI is 2, then INR = $1.5^2 = 2.25$.

The ISI of commercial thromboplastin reagents varies according to manufacturer and from batch to batch. Most thromboplastins used in the United States vary from 1.8 to 2.8 (44). Most thromboplastins used in the United Kingdom, and in many parts of Scandinavia and the Netherlands, have ISI values of 1.0 to 1.1 (9).

Administration of Warfarin

The prothrombin time may become prolonged before a full anticoagulant effect is reached. This is a result of a rapid reduction of factor VII, which has a half-life of 6 to 7 hours (45). Full anticoagulant activity is delayed 72 to 96 hours after the administration of warfarin because the half-lives of factors II, IX, and X are considerably longer than the half-life of factor VII (46). Protein C and protein S are vitamin K-dependent natural anticoagulants that are also affected by warfarin. There is a potential for the early anticoagulant effect of warfarin to be counteracted by a reduction of protein C because the half-life is short, similar to factor VII (9,47). Warfarin-induced skin necrosis has been attributed to this reduction in protein C (9). It is recommended to begin warfarin therapy with an appropriate maintenance dose of about 5 mg/day (9). Loading doses are not recommended (9).

Anticoagulant Clinics

Regarding the management of anticoagulant therapy in patients with mechanical prosthetic heart valves, the risk of thromboemboli and the risk of major hemorrhagic events were both significantly lower when patients attended an anticoagulation clinic than when the same patients were followed by their physicians (48).

Recommendations of American College of Chest Physicians Conference on Antithrombotic Therapy

In 1998, based on extensive review of the literature, the American College of Chest Physicians Consensus Conference on Antithrombotic Therapy concluded the following for patients with mechanical prosthetic heart valves (8):

1. Permanent therapy with oral anticoagulants is strongly recommended.
2. An INR 2.0 to 3.0 is recommended for patients with bileaflet aortic valves provided there is a sinus rhythm, a normal left atrium and normal ejection fraction.
3. An INR of 2.5 to 3.5 is recommended for patients with tilting disc valves, bileaflet mitral valves or bileaflet aortic valves with atrial fibrillation. An alternative recommendation in such patients is an INR of 2.0 to 3.0 in combination with aspirin 80 to 100 mg/day.
4. An INR of 2.5 to 3.5 in combination with aspirin 80 to 100 mg/day is recommended for patients with caged ball or caged disk valves, patients with additional risk factors, and patients who suffered a systemic embolism despite adequate prophylaxis with oral anticoagulants.

Whether low doses of aspirin in combination with oral anticoagulants should be recommended in all patients with mechanical prosthetic valves is uncertain. It seems reasonable to consider low-dose aspirin in combination with oral anticoagulants for patients at a higher risk of thromboembolism. Higher risk patients are those with a prior thromboembolism, atrial fibrillation, large left atrium, left atrial thrombus, ball valve, and more than one mechanical prosthetic valve. Patients with a mechanical prosthetic mitral valve are at higher risk than patients with a mechanical aortic valve.

Anticoagulants During Pregnancy

There is a considerable difference of opinion on the management of anticoagulants during pregnancy. It was recommended by some that warfarin during the first trimester of pregnancy should be avoided because of the risk of embryopathy or fetal bleeding (9,49,50). Hirsh et al. (9) recommended that, if possible, oral anticoagulants should be avoided throughout pregnancy and heparin should be used instead.

Some investigations suggest that warfarin may be used throughout pregnancy. Among pregnant patients with mechanical prosthetic valves, the frequency of thromboemboli was high in those treated with subcutaneous un-fractionated heparin compared with those who received oral anticoagulants (51,52), and fetal outcome was not improved (52). According to literature reviewed by Oakley (51), the incidence of embryopathy among women who took oral anticoagulants throughout pregnancy or during the first trimester was 4% to 7.9%. Women who required 5 mg/day or less of warfarin had little risk of embryopathy (53). In addition, some reported a high frequency of abortion (37.5%) among women who took heparin during the 6th to 12th weeks of gestation (52). The European Society of Cardiology therefore suggested that oral anticoagulant therapy throughout pregnancy is preferred (54). Full discussion with the patient and her partner about the risks and benefits were recommended (54). The manufacturer's package insert states that warfarin is contraindicated during pregnancy. This statement has medicolegal implications (50).

Delivery presents an additional problem about which there is not uniform opinion. A planned cesarian section at 38 weeks of gestation has been recommended by some (53), but greater safety for this approach has not been validated (54). If vaginal delivery is preferred, it is recommended that heparin is administered intravenously in the hospital during the last 2 or 3 weeks of pregnancy (54). Heparin should be withdrawn at the onset of labor and resumed 6 to 12 hours after delivery (54).

Regarding the postpartum period, warfarin in nursing mothers appears not to induce an anticoagulant effect in the breast-fed infant (55,56).

Interruption of Anticoagulant Therapy

Major Surgery

Some circumstances, such as noncardiac surgery, may necessitate the interruption of oral anticoagulant therapy. Experience with a few patients showed significant perioperative bleeding with various noncardiac operations when anticoagulation was maintained (57). Others, however, during cholecystectomy or gastric resection showed no difference in blood loss between patients who were anticoagulated versus those who were not (58).

Tinker and Tarhan (59), in patients with first-generation aortic or mitral valves, showed no difference in thromboembolism between patients who discontinued oral anticoagulants 1 to 3 days before operation and did not receive heparin versus those who continued oral anticoagulants at therapeutic levels. Katholi et al. (57), however, also in patients with first-generation valves, showed a high rate of postoperative thromboembolism in patients with prosthetic valves in the mitral position when oral anticoagulants were discontinued 3 to 5 days before operation and heparin was not administered. Thromboemboli were not observed in patients with prosthetic valves in the aortic position when oral anticoagulants were discontinued (57,60).

After a risk-to-benefit assessment is made, one can elect to do one of the following: discontinue oral anticoagulants several days before the procedure to allow the INR to return to nearly normal and reinstitute therapy shortly after operation (59,61–63), reduce the dose of oral anticoagulants to maintain a lower or subtherapeutic INR during the procedure, or discontinue oral anticoagulants and institute intravenous heparin therapy (57).

The safest approach would be to discontinue oral anticoagulants 3 to 5 days before operation and maintain the patient on heparin. Intravenous heparin is recommended in doses sufficient to prolong the activated partial thromboplastin time to at least twice the control level. In these latter patients, heparin is discontinued 2 to 4 hours before operation and reinstituted when considered safe after operation. Thereafter, oral anticoagulation is reinstituted. The last of these three options provides the shortest interval totally free of anticoagulation but usually requires hospitalization for heparin therapy before surgery. The cost effectiveness of this practice, as applied to all patients, has been questioned (64). Low molecular weight heparin is a potential alternative (9). Some recommend that only those patients with the most thrombogenic prostheses are treated with perioperative heparin, unless such therapy can be given within the confines of the hospitalization required for the procedure (64).

Minor Surgery

Bleeding was no greater among patients who underwent dental extractions while receiving oral anticoagulants than among patients who were not receiving anticoagulants (65). For patients who require minimal invasive procedures (dental extractions, superficial biopsies), the American College of Chest Physicians Consensus Conference on Antithrombotic Therapy recommended briefly reducing the INR to the low or subtherapeutic range and resuming the normal dose of oral anticoagulants immediately after the procedure (9). Tranexamic acid or epsilon amino caproic acid mouthwash has been used successfully without interrupting anticoagulant therapy (9).

Management of Patients with Mechanical Prosthetic Valves Who Suffer Bleeding

If reversal of oral anticoagulation needs to be achieved rapidly, small parenteral doses of vitamin K_1 are recommended (0.5 to 1 mg i.v.) (66). With normal liver function, such therapy should significantly reduce the INR in 12 to 24 hours without creating a state of relative resistance to oral anticoagulants when anticoagulant therapy is resumed, as might occur with larger doses of vitamin K_1. If the INR is above the therapeutic range but below 6.0 and there is no bleeding, vitamin K_1 does not need to be administered (9).

For long-term anticoagulant therapy in patients who suffered a bleeding episode, every effort should be made to reverse the cause of the bleeding (9). Recognizing that the risk of bleeding is related to the level of the INR, it has been suggested that an INR of 2.0 to 2.5 might be reasonable for patients with mechanical prosthetic valves (9). Perhaps even a lower INR combined with aspirin 80 mg/day might be considered, but there is no evidence to support such an approach (9).

Bioprosthetic Valves

First 3 Months After Valve Insertion

Thromboemboli have been reported to be high in the first 3 months after bioprosthetic valve insertion among patients not receiving antithrombotic therapy, particularly among patients with bioprosthetic valves in the mitral position. Some investigators reported that 67% to 80% of patients had thromboemboli during the first 3 months (67–69). Heras et al. (70) reported thromboembolic rates during the first 10 days after operation of 41%/yr for the aortic valve and 55%/yr for the mitral valve (70). Other investigators, however, did not observe this high rate of thromboemboli (71). Among patients who received only subcutaneous heparin 22,500 IU/day and aspirin 100 mg/day for the first 14 to 22 days after aortic valve replacement, the frequency of thromboemboli was 3.5%/yr (72).

During the first 3 months after bioprosthetic valve insertion, oral anticoagulants appear to diminish the prevalence of thromboemboli, but thromboemboli are not eliminated (73). Among patients with either aortic or mitral bioprosthetic valves, 1.9% of patients with an INR of 2.5 to 4.5 had thromboemboli during the first 3 months, and 2.0% of patients with an INR of 2.0 to 2.3 had thromboemboli during that period (73).

Prophylaxis at an INR of 2.0 to 2.3 was associated with fewer bleeding complications. None with prosthetic valves in the aortic position had thromboemboli, but 5.0% and 5.1% with valves in the mitral position had thromboemboli. These patients also had atrial fibrillation. This is equivalent to a prevalence of thromboemboli in patients with mitral prosthetic valves of 20.0%/yr with the higher INR and a 20.4% with the lower INR (73). These patients also received heparin 5,000 units 12 hourly for venous prophylaxis.

Heras et al. (70) also reported that oral anticoagulants (estimated INR 3.0 to 4.5) in patients with bioprosthetic valves in the mitral position decreased the frequency of thromboemboli a statistically significant amount. However, the frequency remained high (48%/yr) during the first 10 postoperative days. This may have been due to delay in achieving therapeutic levels and variable and unstable levels of the INR. It was suggested that the early administration of heparin might explain why some groups observed lower rates of thromboemboli in patients who received short-term oral anticoagulants (70). In view of these observations, The American College of Chest Physicians Consensus Conference on Antithrombotic Therapy recommended that all patients with bioprosthetic valves in the mitral position should be for the first 3 months after valve insertion with oral anticoagulants at an INR of 2.0 to 3.0 (8). Anticoagulant therapy in patients with bioprosthetic valves in the aortic position who are in sinus rhythm was considered optional during the first 3 months after insertion.

Long-term Results

The normal aortic valve is covered with a surface of endothelial cells (Fig. 16-14). Glu-

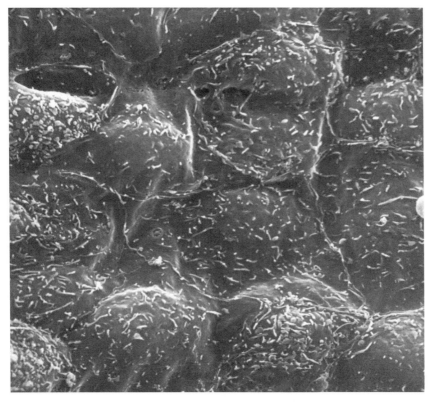

FIG. 16-14. Electron micrograph of normal aortic valve from a dog. The endothelial cells are intact and cover the entire surface of the valve.

taraldehyde processing of porcine bioprosthetic valves results in extensive denudation
of the endothelial surface with exposure of
the basement membrane and subendothelial
fibers (Fig. 16-15) (74). Adherent reversible
and irreversible platelet aggregates were frequently observed by scanning electron mi-
croscopy on the surface of degenerated
porcine bioprosthetic valves (Fig. 16-16) (74).
Regarding bioprosthetic valves in the aortic
position in patients in sinus rhythm, the frequency of thromboemboli among patients
who did not receive long-term antithrombotic
therapy was 0.2% to 2.9%/yr (75–77). This was
comparable with the frequency of thromboemboli in patients with mechanical prosthetic valves who received oral anticoagulants. There is therefore some risk of
thromboemboli, even in patients with bioprosthetic valves in the aortic position. The
frequency of thromboemboli in patients with
bioprosthetic valves in the mitral position
who were in sinus rhythm and did not receive
long-term antithrombotic therapy unless they
had a giant left atrium or prior history of
thromboembolism was 0.4% to 1.9%/yr
(78,79). Among a few untreated patients with
bioprosthetic valves in the mitral position
who were in sinus rhythm and had no risk factors for thromboembolism, including enlarged left atrium, preoperative thromboembolism, or thrombi in the left atrium, no
thromboemboli occurred during 6 years of
follow-up (80).

Among patients with bioprosthetic valves
in the mitral or mitral plus aortic position who

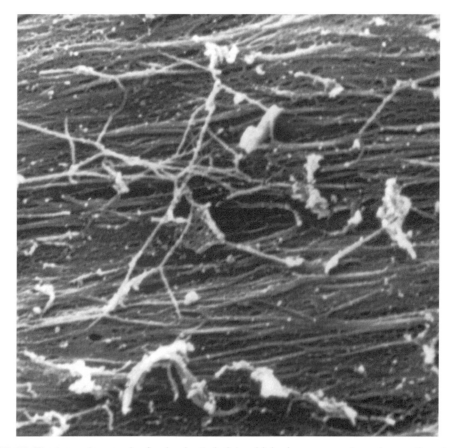

FIG. 16-15. Electron micrograph of unimplanted glutaraldehyde-processed porcine aortic valve. The endothelial cells are completely denuded. The subendothelial surface is shown.

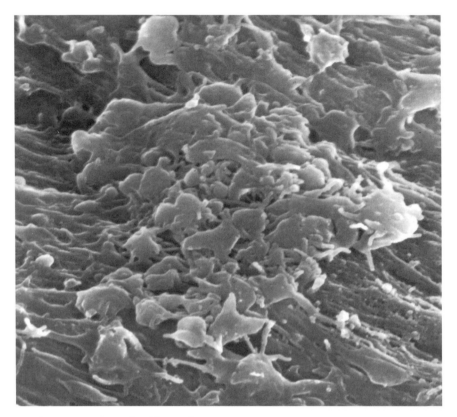

FIG. 16-16. Degenerated porcine bioprosthetic valve removed at surgery. The endothelial surface is denuded. Subendothelial fibers are shown. An aggregate of platelets is deposited on the surface of the valve.

were treated with long-term aspirin, no thromboemboli occurred in those with sinus rhythm followed an average of 32 months (81). Also, no thromboemboli occurred in 31 patients with a giant left atrium (81). In view of these observations, The American College of Chest Physicians Consensus Conference on Antithrombotic Therapy recommended that long-term therapy with aspirin, 162 mg/day, may offer protection against thromboembolism and may be considered optional in patients with bioprosthetic valves who are in sinus rhythm (8).

Thromboemboli in patients with bioprosthetic valves who are in atrial fibrillation presumably relate to both the bioprosthetic valve and to the atrial fibrillation. The occurrence of thromboemboli in these patients was reported to be as high as 16% at 31 to 36 months (82,83). Most investigations in patients with atrial fibrillation who did not have prosthetic valves showed that long-term oral anticoagulants are effective, more effective than aspirin (84).

The American College of Chest Physicians Consensus Conference recommended that patients with bioprosthetic valves who have atrial fibrillation should be treated with long-term oral anticoagulants with a dose sufficient to prolong the INR to 2.0 to 3.0. This recommendation was based on evidence for treatment of patients with atrial fibrillation who did not have prosthetic heart valves (8). Long-term anticoagulants (INR 2.0 to 3.0) were also recommended for patients with bioprosthetic valves who have a left atrial thrombus at surgery and for patients who have a history of systemic embolism (8). Data to support these recommendations, the level of INR, and the duration of therapy, are sparse or nonexistent.

REFERENCES

1. Baudet EM, Oca CC, Roques XF, et al. A 5 1/2 year experience with the St. Jude Medical cardiac valve prosthesis: early and late results of 737 valve replacements in 671 patients. *J Thorac Cardiovasc Surg* 1985;90: 137–144.
2. Björk VO, Henze A. Management of thrombo-embolism after aortic valve replacement with the Björk-Shiley tilting disc valve: medicamental prevention with dicumarol in comparison with dipyridamole-acetylsalicylic acid. Surgical treatment of prosthetic thrombosis. *Scand J Thorac Cardiovasc Surg* 1975; 9:183–191.
3. Cannegieter SC, Rosendaal FR, Wintzen AR, Van Der Meer FJM, Vandenbroucke JP, Breit E. Optimal oral anticoagulant therapy in patients with mechanical heart valves. *N Eng J Med* 1995;333:11–17.
4. Horstkotte D, Schulte HD, Bircks W, et al. Lower intensity anticoagulation therapy results in lower complication rates with the St. Jude Medical prosthesis. *J Thorac Cardiovasc Surg* 1994;107:1136–1145.
5. Bloomfield P, Wheatley DJ, Prescott RJ, et al. Twelve-year comparison of a Bjork-Shiley mechanical heart valve with porcine bioprostheses. *N Engl J Med* 1991; 324:573–579.
6. Sethia B, Turner MA, Lewis S, Rodger RA, Bain WH. Fourteen years' experience with the Björk-Shiley tilting disc prosthesis. *J Thorac Cardiovasc Surg* 1986;91: 350–361.
7. Vallejo JL, Gonzalez-Santos JM, Albertos J, et al. Eight years' experience with the Medtronic-Hall valve prosthesis. *Ann Thorac Surg* 1990;50:429–436.
8. Stein PD, Alpert JS, Dalen JE. Antithrombotic therapy in patients with mechanical and biological prosthetic heart valves. *Chest* 1998;114[Suppl]:602S–610S.
9. Hirsh J, Dalen JE, Anderson D, et al. Oral anticoagulants: Mechanism of action, clinical effectiveness, and optimal therapeutic range. *Chest* 1992;102[Suppl]: 1998;114[Suppl]:445S–469S.
10. Acar J, Iung B, Boissel JP, et al. AREVA: multicenter randomized comparison of low-dose versus standard dose anticoagulation in patients with mechanical prosthetic heart valves. *Circulation* 1996;94:2107–2112.
11. Vogt S, Hoffmann A, Roth J, et al. Heart valve replacement with the Björk-Shiley and St. Jude Medical prostheses: A randomized comparison in 178 patients. *Eur Heart J* 1990;11:583–591.
12. Saour JN, Sieck JO, Mamo LAR, Gallus AS. Trial of different intensities of anticoagulation in patients with prosthetic heart valves. *N Engl J Med* 1990;322: 428–432.
13. Wilson DB, Dunn MI, Hassanein K. Low-intensity anticoagulation in mechanical cardiac prosthetic valves. *Chest* 1991;100:1553–1557.
14. van der Meer FJM, Rosendaal FR, Vandenbroucke JP, et al. Bleeding complications in oral anticoagulant therapy. An analysis of risk factors. *Arch Intern Med* 1993; 153:1557–1562.
15. Butchart EG, Lewis PA, Grunkemeier GL, Kulatilake N, Breckenridge IM. Low risk of thrombosis and serious embolic events despite low-intensity anticoagulation. *Circulation* 1988;78[Suppl I]:I-66–I-77.
16. Gossinger H, Neissner H, Grubeck B, et al. Thromboembolism in patients with prosthetic heart valves. An adequately controlled intense anticoagulant therapy and its influence on the occurrence of thromboembolism in relation to valve type. *Thorac Cardiovasc Surg* 1986;34: 283–286.
17. Turpie AGG, Gent M, Laupacis A, et al. Comparison of aspirin with placebo in patients treated with warfarin after heart-valve replacement. *N Engl J Med* 1993;329: 524–529.
18. Stein PD, Grandison D, Hua TA, et al. Therapeutic levels of oral anticoagulation with warfarin in patients with mechanical prosthetic heart valves: review of literature and recommendations based on international normalized ratio. *Postgrad Med J* 1994;70[Suppl 1]:S72–S83.
19. Meschengieser SS, Carlos GF, Santarelli MT, et al. Low-intensity oral anticoagulation plus low-dose aspirin versus high-intensity oral anticoagulation alone: a randomized trial in patients with mechanical prosthetic heart valves. *J Thorac Cardiovasc Surg* 1997;113: 910–916.
20. Altman R, Rouvier J, Gurfinkel E, et al. Comparison of two levels of anticoagulant therapy in patients with substitute heart valves. *J Thorac Cardiovasc Surg* 1991;101:427–431.
21. Skudicky D, Essop MR, Wisenbaugh T, et al. Frequency of prosthetic valve complications with very low level warfarin anticoagulation combined with dipyridamole after valve replacement using St Jude Medical prostheses. *Am J Cardiol* 1994;74:1137–1141.
22. Albertal J, Sutton M, Pereyra D, et al. Experience with moderate intensity anticoagulation and aspirin after mechanical valve replacement. A retrospective, non-randomized study. *J Heart Valve Dis* 1993;2:302–307.
23. Sullivan JM, Harken DE, Gorlin R. Effect of dipyridamole on the incidence of arterial emboli after cardiac valve replacement. *Circulation* 1969;39–40[Suppl 1]:I-149–I-153.
24. Kasahara T. Clinical effect of dipyridamole ingestion after prosthetic heart valve replacement: especially on the blood coagulation system. *J Jpn Assoc Thorac Surg* 1977;25:1007–1021.
25. Groupe de recherche P.A.C.T.E. Prevention des accidents thrombo-emboliques systemiques chez les porteurs de protheses valvulaires artificielles. *Coeur* 1978; 9:915–969.
26. Chesebro JH, Fuster V, Elveback LR, et al. Trial of combined warfarin plus dipyridamole or aspirin therapy in prosthetic heart valve replacement: danger of aspirin compared with dipyridamole. *Am J Cardiol* 1983;51: 1537–1541.
27. Bran M, Capel P, Messin R. Reduction of platelet activity in patients with prosthetic heart valves. *Rev Med Brux* 1980;1:71–75.
28. Starkman C, Estampes B, Vernant P, et al. Prevention de des accidents thrombo-emboliques systemiques chez les patients porteurs de protheses valvulaires artificielles: essai prospectif de l'association anti-vitamines-K-dipyridamole. *Arch Mal Coeur* 1982;75:85–88.
29. Pouleur H, Buyse M. Effects of dipyridamole in combination with anticoagulant therapy on survival and

thromboembolic events in patients with prosthetic heart valves. A meta-analysis of the randomized trials. *J Thorac Cardiovasc Surg* 1995;110:463–472.

30. Yamak B, Karagoz HY, Zorlutuna Y, et al. Low-dose anticoagulant management of patients with St. Jude Medical mechanical valve prostheses. *Thorac Cardiovasc Surg* 1993;41:38–42.

31. Hartz RS, LoCicero J III, Kucich V, et al. Comparative study of warfarin versus antiplatelet therapy in patients with a St. Jude medical valve the aortic position. *J Thorac Cardiovasc Surg* 1986;92:684–690.

32. Ribeiro PA, Al Zaibag MA, Idris M, et al. Antiplatelet drugs and the incidence of thromboembolic complications of the St. Jude medical aortic prosthesis in patients with rheumatic heart disease. *J Thorac Cardiovasc Surg* 1986;91:92–98.

33. Arom KV, Emery RW, Nicoloff DM, et al. Anticoagulant related complications in elderly patients with St. Jude mechanical valve prostheses. *J Heart Valve Dis* 1996;5:505–510.

34. Rao PS, Solymar L, Mardini MK, et al. Anticoagulant therapy in children with prosthetic valves. *Ann Thorac Surg* 1989;47:589–592.

35. Sade RM, Crawford FA Jr, Fyfe DA, et al. Valve prostheses in children: a reassessment of anticoagulation. *J Thorac Cardiovasc Surg* 1988;95:533–561.

36. Serra AJS, McNicholas KW, Olivier HG Jr, et al. The choice of anticoagulation in pediatric patients with the St. Jude Medical valve prostheses. *J Cardiovasc Surg* 1987;28:588–591.

37. McGrath LB, Gonzalez-Lavin L, Eldredge WJ, et al. Thromboembolic and other events following valve replacement in a pediatric population treated with antiplatelet agents. *Ann Thorac Surg* 1987;43:285–287.

38. Bradley LM, Midgley FM, Watson DC, et al. Anticoagulation therapy in children with mechanical prosthetic cardiac valves. *Am J Cardiol* 1985;56:533–535.

39. El Makhlouf A, Friedi B, Oberhansli I, et al. Prosthetic heart valve replacement in children. *J Thorac Cardiovasc Surg* 1987;93:80–85.

40. Solymar L, Rao PS, Mardini MK, et al. Prosthetic valves in children and adolescents. *Am Heart J* 1991; 121:557–568.

41. Borkon AM, Soule L, Reitz BA, et al. Five year follow-up after replacement with the St. Jude medical valve in infants and children. *Circulation* 1986;74[Suppl]: I110–I115.

42. LeBlanc JG, Sett SS, Vince DJ, et al. Antiplatelet therapy in children with left-sided mechanical prostheses. *Eur J Cardiothorac Surg* 1993;7:211–215.

43. Michelson AD, Boville E, Andrew M. Antithrombotic therapy in children. *Chest* 1995;108[Suppl]:506S–520S.

44. Bussey HI, Force RW, Bianco TM, Leonard AD. Reliance on prothrombin time ratios causes significant errors in anticoagulation therapy. *Arch Intern Med* 1992; 152:278–282.

45. O'Reilly RA, Aggeler PM. Determinants of the response to oral anticoagulant drug in man. *Pharmacol Rev* 1970;22:35–96.

46. Hellemans J, Vorlat M, Verstraete M. Survival time of prothrombin and factors VII, IX, and X after complete synthesis blocking doses of coumarin derivatives. *Br J Haematol* 1963;9:506–512.

47. Vigano S, Mannucci PM, Solinas S, Bottasso B, Mariani G. Decrease in protein C antigen and formation of

an abnormal protein soon after starting oral anticoagulant therapy. *Br J Haematol* 1984;57:213–220.

48. Cortelazzo S, Finazzi G, Viero P, et al. Thrombotic and hemorrhagic complications in patients with mechanical heart valve prosthesis attending an anticoagulation clinic. *Thromb Haemost* 1993;69:316–320.

49. Hall JAG, Pauli RM, Wilson KM. Maternal and fetal sequelae of anticoagulation during pregnancy. *Am J Med* 1980;68:122–140.

50. Ginsberg JS, Hirsh J. Use of antithrombotic agents during pregnancy. *Chest* 1995;108[Suppl]:305S–311S.

51. Oakley CM. Anticoagulants in pregnancy. *Br Heart J* 1995;75:107–111.

52. Salazar E, Izaguirre R, Verdejo J, et al. Failure of adjusted doses of subcutaneous heparin to prevent thromboembolic phenomena in pregnant patients with mechanical cardiac valve prostheses. *J Am Coll Cardiol* 1996;27:1698–1703.

53. Cotrufo M, de Luca TSL, Calabro R, et al. Coumarin anticoagulation during pregnancy in patients with mechanical valve prostheses. *Eur J Cardiovasc Surg* 1991:5:300–305.

54. Study Group of the Working Group on Valvular Heart Disease of the European Society of Cardiology. Guidelines for prevention of thromboembolic events in valvular heart diseases. *Eur Heart J* 1995;16: 1320–1330.

55. McKenna R, Cale ER, Vasan U. Is warfarin sodium contraindicated in the lactating mother? *J Pediatr* 1983; 103:325–327.

56. Lao TT, DeSwiet M, Letsky SE, Walters BN. Prophylaxis of thromboembolism in pregnancy: an alternative. *Br J Obstet Gynaecol* 1985;92:202–206.

57. Katholi RE, Nolan SP, McGuire LB. Living with prosthetic heart valves: subsequent noncardiac operations and the risk of thromboembolism or hemorrhage. *Am Heart J* 1976;92:162–167.

58. Rustad H, Myhre E. Surgery during anticoagulant treatment. *Acta Med Scand* 1963;173:115–119.

59. Tinker JH, Tarhan S. Discontinuing anticoagulant therapy in surgical patients with cardiac valve prostheses. *JAMA* 1978;239:738–739.

60. Katholi RE, Nolan SP, McGuire LB. The management of anticoagulation during noncardiac operations in patients with prosthetic heart valves. *Am Heart J* 1978;96: 163–165.

61. Grady RF. Noncardiac surgery in the elderly patient with heart disease. *Mt Sinai J Med* 1985;52:634–642.

62. Chesebro JH, Adams PC, Fuster V. Antithrombotic therapy in patients with valvular heart disease and prosthetic heart valves. *J Am Coll Cardiol* 1986;8[Suppl]: 41B–56B.

63. Bodnar AG, Hutter AM. Anticoagulation in valvular heart disease preoperatively and postoperatively. *Cardiovasc Clin* 1984;14:247–264.

64. Eckman MH, Beshansky JR, Durand-Zaleski I, et al. Anticoagulation for noncardiac procedures in patients with prosthetic heart valves. *JAMA* 1990;263: 1513–1521.

65. McIntyre H. Management, during dental surgery, of patients on anticoagulants. *Lancet* 1966;2:99–100.

66. Shetty HGM, Backhouse G, Bentley DP, et al. Effective reversal of warfarin-induced excessive anticoagulation with low dose vitamin K_1. *Thromb Haemost* 1992;67: 13–15.

67. Hetzer R, Topalidis T, Borst HG. Thromboembolism and anticoagulation after isolated mitral valve replacement with porcine heterografts. In: Cohn LH, Gallucci V, eds. *Proceedings, Second International Symposium on Cardiac Bioprostheses.* New York: Yorke Medical Books, 1982:170–172.

68. Oyer PE, Stinson EB, Griepp RB, et al. Valve replacement with the Starr-Edwards and Hancock prostheses: comparative analysis of late morbidity and mortality. *Ann Surg* 1977;186:301–309.

69. Ionescu MI, Smith DR, Hasan SS, et al. Clinical durability of the pericardial xenograft valve: ten years experience with mitral replacement. *Ann Thorac Surg* 1982; 34:265–277.

70. Heras M, Chesebro JH, Fuster V, et al. High risk of early thromboemboli after bioprosthetic cardiac valve replacement. *J Am Coll Cardiol* 1995;25:1111–1119.

71. Magilligan DJ Jr, Lewis JW Jr, Tilley B, et al. The porcine bioprosthetic valve—twelve years later. *J Thorac Cardiovasc Surg* 1985;89:499–507.

72. Babin-Ebell J, Schmidt W, Eigel P, et al. Aortic bioprosthesis without early anticoagulation—risk of thromboembolism. *Thorac Cardiovasc Surg* 1995;43: 212–214.

73. Turpie AGG, Gunstensen J, Hirsh J, et al. Randomised comparison of two intensities of oral anticoagulant therapy after tissue heart valve replacement. *Lancet* 1988;1: 1242–1245.

74. Riddle JM, Magilligan DJ Jr, Stein PD. Surface morphology of degenerated porcine bioprosthetic valves four to seven years following implantation. *J Thorac Cardiovasc Surg* 1981;81:279–287.

75. Cohn LH, Allred EN, DiSesa VJ, et al. Early and late risk of aortic valve replacement: a 12-year concomitant comparison of the porcine bioprosthetic and tilting disc prosthetic aortic valves. *J Thorac Cardiovasc Surg* 1984;88:695–705.

76. Bolooki H, Kaiser GA, Mallon SM, et al. Comparison of long-term results of Carpentier-Edwards and Hancock bioprosthetic valves. *Ann Thorac Surg* 1986;42: 494–499.

77. Bloomfield P, Kitchin AH, Wheatley DJ, et al. A prospective evaluation of the Bjork-Shiley, Hancock, and Carpentier-Edwards heart valve prostheses. *Circulation* 1986;73:1213–1222.

78. Cohn LH, Allred EN, Cohn LA, et al. Early and late risk of mitral valve replacement. *J Thorac Cardiovasc Surg* 1985;90:872–881.

79. Louagie YA, Jamart J, Eucher P, et al. Mitral valve Carpentier-Edwards bioprosthetic replacement, thromboembolism, and anticoagulants. *Ann Thorac Surg* 1993;56:931–937.

80. Gonzalez-Lavin L, Chi S, Blair TC, et al. Thromboembolism and bleeding after mitral valve replacement with porcine valves: influence of thromboembolic risk factors. *J Surg Res* 1984;36:508–515.

81. Nunez L, Aguado GM, Larrea JL, et al. Prevention of thromboembolism using aspirin after mitral valve replacement with porcine bioprosthesis. *Ann Thorac Surg* 1984;37:84–87.

82. Williams JB, Karp RB, Kirklin JW, et al. Considerations in selection and management of patients undergoing valve replacement with glutaraldehyde-fixed porcine bioprostheses. *Ann Thorac Surg* 1980;30:247–258.

83. Gonzalez-Lavin L, Tandon AP, Chi S, et al. The risk of thromboembolism and hemorrhage following mitral valve replacement. *J Thorac Cardiovasc Surg* 1984;87:340–351.

84. Laupacis A, Albers GW, Dalen JE, et al. Antithrombotic therapy in atrial fibrillation. *Chest* 1995;108[Suppl]: 352S–359S.

Anticoagulation for the Patient with Valvular Heart Disease and Atrial Fibrillation

Kodangudi B. Ramanathan and Howard R. Horn

Department of Medicine/Cardiology, University of Tennessee 38163;
VA Medical Center, Memphis, Tennessee 38104; Department of Medicine,
University of Tennessee Memphis Health Center; U.T. Bowld Hospital, Memphis, Tennessee 38163

The association between valvular heart disease and thrombosis has been recognized for over 150 years. In 1814, Wood (1) described the occurrence of a spherical ball thrombus in the left atrium of a 15-year-old girl with mitral stenosis at autopsy. This was long before the recognition of atrial fibrillation by Vulpian in 1874 (2), who described the replacement of the normal systole by an uncoordinated fluttering of the atrial tissue in dogs. The electrocardiographic recognition had to await the work of Sir Thomas Lewis (3) and Rothberger and Winterberg in 1909 (4). Yet among arrhythmias, atrial fibrillation is considered the grandfather of cardiac arrhythmias (5,6). Although the association between atrial fibrillation and stroke has been known for many years, routine use of anticoagulants to prevent such complications had to await the latter part of the 20th century, especially for those with nonvalvular heart disease (7). The delay was not irrational because anticoagulant therapy is not devoid of complications. Use of anticoagulants is one of the most common causes of iatrogenic complications in patients, and it is only in the last few years that international standardization has been achieved for their use (8,9).

Although atrial fibrillation complicates all forms of heart disease, its association with rheumatic mitral valve disease has been most notable. In the Framingham study, rheumatic heart disease, especially in women, provided the highest age-adjusted risk for the occurrence of atrial fibrillation (10). Whereas the presence of valvular heart disease alone increases the risk of thromboembolism, the development of atrial fibrillation multiplies the risk many times, especially in rheumatic mitral valve disease (11). Although the occurrence of atrial fibrillation and thromboembolism in rheumatic mitral valvular disease is related to left atrial hypertension, the pathologic changes induced by the rheumatic heart disease may indeed have some role in the pathogenesis (12).

Besides systemic embolism with its attendant disability such as stroke, atrial fibrillation associated with valvular heart disease also increases the mortality significantly. Gajewski and Singer (13) in their analysis of 3,099 life insurance applicants found that chronic atrial fibrillation associated with mitral stenosis increased mortality 17.4-fold. Even paroxysmal atrial fibrillation in those with mitral stenosis increased mortality 12.9-fold (13).

The focus of this chapter is limited to the use of anticoagulants in valvular heart disease complicated by atrial fibrillation. Valvular heart disease is divided into rheumatic and nonrheumatic. Although rheumatic heart disease can affect all the valves in the heart, the two valves commonly involved are the mitral and aortic. Both mitral and aortic valves can also be affected by nonrheumatic disease states.

With the gradual disappearance of rheumatic heart disease in the developed world, one of the emerging causes of nonrheumatic mitral regurgitation is mitral valve prolapse (14). Both mitral valve stenosis and insufficiency can also result from congenital involvement, and ischemic involvement of the papillary muscles can result in acute or subacute mitral insufficiency. Mitral insufficiency due to involvement of the anterior leaflet of the mitral valve is part of the syndrome of hypertrophic obstructive cardiomyopahty. All these nonrheumatic mitral valvular disease states have the potential to develop atrial fibrillation with embolic sequelae. Finally, mitral annular calcification with or without valvular insufficiency also has been associated with atrial fibrillation and thromboemboli, and bacterial endocarditis with valvular involvement with or without atrial fibrillation also has embolic potential of a different kind.

The aortic valve can also be involved in rheumatic and nonrheumatic disease states, but the embolic potential of isolated aortic valvular disease either due to stenosis or insufficiency is minimal. Unlike mitral valve disease where the rheumatic etiology greatly increases the thromboembolic potential, the etiology of aortic valve disease has minimal bearing on embolic potential unless associated with concomitant mitral valve disease and atrial fibrillation.

MITRAL VALVE DISEASE

Rheumatic Mitral Valve Disease

Both rheumatic mitral stenosis and insufficiency are associated with marked increase in the propensity for systemic embolism. The occurrence of systemic embolism is greater than most other disease states, especially in the presence of atrial fibrillation. Of the 642 autopsied patients with history of atrial fibril-

lation, Aberg (15) noted systemic emboli in 54% with mitral valve disease or coronary artery disease. Among those with other forms of organic heart disease, only 42% had emboli (15). Hinton et al. (16), in a similar autopsy study of 333 patients with atrial fibrillation, noted an incidence of systemic emboli of 41% among those with mitral valve disease, 35% among those with coronary artery disease, and only 7% among those with idiopathic atrial fibrillation.

Although several autopsy studies dating from 1933 described the association of systemic emboli with mitral valve disease complicated by atrial fibrillation, Paul Dudley White and his colleagues were among the earliest to critically study patients in their clinical practice with rheumatic heart disease and systemic embolism; they also subsequently studied some of them at autopsy (17,18). They noted a considerable discrepancy between clinical recognition of thromboembolic episodes and pathologic demonstration of emboli that far exceeded clinical recognition.

In clinical studies, Wood (19) noted a prevalence of 9% to 14% of systemic emboli in patients with mitral stenosis. Ellis and Harken in 1961 (20) reported that 27% of 1,500 patients undergoing mitral valvuloplasty had a history of systemic embolization. Szekely (11), in his review of 754 patients followed for many years, observed an incidence of 1.5% of systemic emboli per patient year. Dervall et al. (21) in their search of literature in 1968 noted the incidence to vary between 1.5% and 4.7% per year.

In both mitral stenosis and mitral regurgitation, the incidence of systemic embolization is greatly enhanced by the development of atrial fibrillation. Szekely (11) reported a seven fold greater risk for systemic embolism for patients with mitral valve disease and atrial fibrillation compared with those in normal sinus rhythm. Similarly, Coulshed et al. (22) noted systemic emboli in 8% of patients with mitral stenosis in sinus rhythm, whereas 31.5% had embolization among those in atrial fibrillation. In mitral regurgitation, the incidence of systemic embolization increased to

22% for those in atrial fibrillation compared with 7% for those in normal sinus rhythm.

In rheumatic mitral valve disease, the incidence of thromboemboli increases with increasing age. Between the ages of 10 and 39 years, the incidence is 18%, between 40 and 49 years it increases to 39%, and between the ages of 50 and 79 years it is as high as 47% (23). In a similar study, Daley et al. (17) noted an incidence of less than 5% for patients below 30 years of age, and this increased by 1.5% per year such that it reached almost 40% by the time the patient reached 70. Besides atrial fibrillation and increasing age, other factors that may increase the embolic potential have been decrease in left ventricular function and increase in left atrial size. The data on left atrial size are controversial. Madden (24) first proposed that increase in left atrial size might be associated with an augmented risk for systemic embolization. This was supported by Sommerville and Chambers (25), who reported a threefold increase in embolism in patients with mitral stenosis who had enlarged left atrial appendage on the chest x-ray compared with those who did not. This observation was not supported by subsequent studies, including a multifactorial study by Peterson et al. (26). However, in nonvalvular atrial fibrillation, a recent study for stroke prevention found left atrial size and left ventricular dysfunction to be the strongest independent predictors for systemic thromboembolism (27).

The severity of mitral valve disease as denoted by clinical classification or mitral valve area does not correlate with the risk of future thromboemboli. In fact, in 12.5% of patients with rheumatic mitral valve disease, systemic embolization is the initial manifestation of the disease (19). Recurrent embolization is frequent and occurs in 30% to 65% of cases, most episodes occurring within the first 6 months (28,29).

The incidence of rheumatic heart disease has decreased significantly in the developed world. Even among the small number of patients with rheumatic mitral valve disease, the incidence of systemic emboli may have decreased due to increased use of anticoagulation. However, surgical correction of the valvular disease has not diminished the propensity for embolization. Mitral valvuloplasty does not decrease the incidence and therefore requires continued anticoagulation (21). Similarly, valve replacement by prosthetic devices confers its own need for anticoagulation and is discussed in a separate chapter. Even the use of tissue valves does not obviate the need for anticoagulation, especially if atrial fibrillation persists.

The use of long-term anticoagulation with warfarin has become accepted in patients with rheumatic mitral valvular heart disease for many years. However, such use has never been subjected to the scrutiny of a large-scale randomized trial. Szekely (11) was an early advocate for the use of anticoagulation in rheumatic mitral valvular heart disease, and he demonstrated an incidence of recurrent embolism of 3.4% per year for those who received warfarin as compared with 9.6% per year for those who did not. In another observational study, Adams et al. (30) followed 84 patients with mitral stenosis for about 20 years in two different decades. The first half who were followed between the years 1949 and 1959 did not receive anticoagulants, whereas the second half, followed between the years 1959 and 1969, received warfarin. There were 13 deaths among those who did not receive anticoagulants as opposed to only 4 deaths among those treated with warfarin. Fleming and Bailey (31) in another observational study found a 25% incidence of emboli among 500 patients not treated with anticoagulants, whereas among the 217 patients treated with warfarin, there were only five embolic episodes over a period of 9.5 years. Roy et al. (32), in a retrospective study of 254 patients with atrial fibrillation, noted an embolic rate of 5.46% per patient year among those not anticoagulated and 0.7% per patient year for those given warfarin.

Although none of these retrospective and observational studies will stand the scrutiny of modern epidemiologists and statisticians, the overwhelming message that anticoagulants prevent systemic emboli in patients with atrial fibrillation and rheumatic mitral valve disease would discourage most institutional review boards from approving randomized trials. Thus, the confirmation that anticoagulants do prevent systemic embolization has been derived from the many recently randomized multicenter trials in nonvalvular atrial fibrillation where the incidence of thromboembolism is lower and use of anticoagulants less accepted by the practicing physician. The conclusion from all these trials has been that long-term anticoagulation prevents stroke in nonvalvular atrial fibrillation (33–37).

Thus, as stated by the guidelines of the American College of Chest Physicians (ACCP) in 1992, long-term warfarin therapy sufficient to prolong the international normalized ratio to 2.0 to 3.0 is strongly recommended for patients with mitral valvular heart disease who have either a history of systemic embolism or have chronic or paroxysmal atrial fibrillation. The ACCP guidelines also recommend the use of long-term anticoagulation for patients with rheumatic mitral valvular disease but in sinus rhythm who had left atrial enlargement greater than 5.5 cm. This recommendation is based on the belief that such patients may be at a higher risk for the development of atrial fibrillation (38).

Exceptions to the use of long-term anticoagulation with warfarin exist, especially in conditions such as pregnancy, higher risk for bleeding due to concomitant disease, contact sports, trauma, or inability to control the prothrombin time. In pregnancy, especially in a patient with noncritical rheumatic mitral valve disease and atrial fibrillation, it may be wise to switch the patient to low-molecular-weight heparin. Heparin does not cross the placental barrier, and use of heparin is not associated with fetal malformation. In other situations, individual risk stratification should choose between the risk of anticoagulation and the risk of systemic embolization.

Mitral balloon valvuloplasty has been shown to be as effective as closed or open mitral valvuloplasty, but the procedure of passing the balloon across the left atrium might increase the possibility of dislodging a clot. It is therefore recommended that these patients are treated with anticoagulants for at least 3 weeks before the procedure (38). Also, as stated previously, valvuloplasty does not remove the embolic potential postprocedure, and anticoagulation needs to be continued, especially if atrial fibrillation persists.

Nonrheumatic Mitral Valve Disease

As stated before, nonrheumatic causes of mitral insufficiency have become more common than rheumatic valvular disease in the developed world. Although 75% of patients with rheumatic mitral insufficiency have atrial fibrillation, in nonrheumatic mitral insufficiency either due to ischemic or congenital etiology, the occurrence of atrial fibrillation is decreased to 40% (39). The propensity for systemic embolization is greater in mitral stenosis than in mitral insufficiency even among the rheumatic population. Wood (19) noted that systemic emboli occurred 1.5 times more frequently in rheumatic mitral stenosis than mitral regurgitation. More recently it was noted that in nonrheumatic valvular disease, the development of mitral insufficiency may protect against the development of thrombus formation (40). However, whether the protection offered by the development of mitral insufficiency is of sufficient magnitude to offset the embolic potential in patients with atrial fibrillation is unclear.

Mitral Valve Prolapse

Mitral valve prolapse is the most common cause of valvular heart disease in the Western world. During the past two decades, there have been numerous reports of patients with cerebral ischemia in whom no cause other than mitral valve prolapse has been demonstrated. Barnett et al. (42) in their study of 60 patients younger than 45 years with partial stroke demonstrated mitral valve prolapse in 40%, whereas in the other 60 age-matched control patients, the incidence of mitral valve prolapse was only 6.8% ($p < 0.001$). The pathologic basis for the development of thromboembolism is speculative. These include the presence of fibrinous endocarditis, endothelial denudation with fibrin deposition on the denuded surface of mitral valve, and mural thrombus deposition on the prolapsed mitral leaflet. However, the ubiquitous occurrence of mitral valve prolapse in the population coupled with the rarity of embolic events makes routine use of anticoagulants unwarranted. Unfortunately, there are currently no reliable ways to recognize a subset with a greater risk for thromboemboli. The severity of mitral valve prolapse, or mitral valve thickening, or laboratory studies demonstrating shortened platelet survival in mitral valve prolapse have not been helpful. The indication for long-term anticoagulation with warfarin is limited to those with documented systemic embolism or those with chronic atrial fibrillation complicating mitral valve prolapse (39).

Mitral Annular Calcification

In the Framingham study, the incidence of atrial fibrillation was 12 times higher among those demonstrating mitral annular calcification than in those without such calcification (10). Fulkerson et al. (40) noted a 29% incidence of atrial fibrillation among the patients they studied with mitral annular calcification. Mitral annular calcification is a clinical syndrome that may be associated with mitral stenosis or insufficiency, calcific aortic stenosis, conduction disturbances, atrial fibrillation, systemic emboli, and even endocarditis. The disease state has a strong female preponderance, and the mean age of the patient is 73 to 75 years. Thus, the disease affects the older age group, and systemic emboli occur more frequently among these patients with or without atrial fibrillation. Although thrombi have been demonstrated on the heavily calcified annular tissue, it is unclear whether the embolic potential is due solely to thrombi or dislodgment of calcified spicules from the ulcerated calcified annulus. In the latter instance, anticoagulation will be of no avail. Given the greater chance of drug-induced mishap among these older patients, long-term anticoagulation should be limited to those in whom it can be clearly demonstrated that systemic emboli are not due to dislodgment of calcified spicules or to those in whom the presence of chronic atrial fibrillation in itself justifies long-term warfarin (38).

Hypertrophic Obstructive Cardiomyopathy

Mitral regurgitation occurs commonly in patients with hypertrophic cardiomyopathy. This is possibly related to the approximation of the anterior leaflet of the mitral valve to the outflow tract during systole that is characteristic of hypertrophic obstructive cardiomyopathy. Atrial fibrillation complicates about 15% of patients with this syndrome and can lead to clinical deterioration and systemic emboli. However, the occurrence of atrial fibrillation does not correlate with the degree of mitral valvular insufficiency (43). Prompt anticoagulation with heparin and subsequently with warfarin is essential to prevent thromboembolic complications.

AORTIC VALVE DISEASE

The isolated occurrence of aortic valve disease is rather uncommon in patients with rheumatic heart disease. Daley et al. (17) in their study of 194 patients with rheumatic valvular disease and systemic emboli found only six patients with isolated aortic valve disease. All six of them were in atrial fibrillation. Thus, the risk for systemic emboli in patients with aortic valvular disease often resides in its association with mitral valvular disease complicated by atrial fibrillation. In the absence of mitral valve disease, isolated aortic valve disease is rarely complicated by atrial fibrillation. Myler and Sanders (44) found only one patient with atrial fibrillation in their study of 122 consecutive patients with isolated aortic valve disease. Thus, in the absence of concomitant mitral valve disease, atrial fibrillation, or previous thromboemboli, anticoagulation with warfarin is not indicated.

Even if there is a history of a previous embolic episode, it is often unclear whether such an event is due to a thromboembolus or calcific microemboli from the heavily calcified aortic valve. Obviously, long-term anticoagulant therapy is unlikely to benefit calcific emboli. There is considerable discrepancy between clinical and pathologic studies in patients with severe calcific aortic valve disease. Stein et al. (45) in a pathologic study demonstrated microthrombi on 10 of 19 calcific aortic valves. In an autopsy study of 165 patients, Holley et al. (46) noted systemic emboli in 19% of patients. However, on neither of these two series was there clinical evidence of systemic embolism.

INFECTIVE ENDOCARDITIS

Both aortic valve and mitral valve can be affected by infective endocarditis. This leads to formation of vegetations on the valve leaflets with propensity for subsequent embolization. With the advent of effective antibiotic therapy, the incidence of systemic embolization has decreased. Transesophageal echocardiography has made detection of vegetations easier so that the diagnosis of bacterial endocarditis is in doubt in the absence of demonstrable vegetations (47). However, there is little correlation between the presence of vegetations and the frequency of systemic emboli. The primary treatment for endocarditis is prolonged, and appropriate antibiotic therapy and the use of anticoagulants in native valve endocarditis has shown little benefit. Except for situations such as recent onset atrial fibrillation in someone with mitral valve disease complicated by endocarditis, routine use of anticoagulants is contraindicated. It is unclear if the infected embolic material responds to anticoagulant therapy, and there appears to be a greater likelihood of developing intracranial hemorrhage with their use in endocarditis (38). Bacterial endocarditis superimposed on prosthetic and tissue valves poses yet another special situation, discussed in Chapter 16.

NONBACTERIAL THROMBOTIC ENDOCARDITIS

This syndrome occurs in a variety of malignant neoplasms, chronic debilitating disease states, acute septicemia, burns, and in association with any condition that leads to disseminated intravascular coagulation (48). This disease is associated with fibrin thrombi commonly located on the aortic and mitral valves with a very high embolic potential. Unlike bacterial endocarditis, evidence of infection is lacking and the small vegetations are not usually detected by echocardiography. Nor are there clinical manifestations such as new onset heart murmurs as noted in bacterial endocarditis. Similar to bacterial endocarditis, treatment should be directed toward the primary disease, and anticoagulant therapy with warfarin is not indicated or useful. However, use of intravenous heparin is beneficial in the presence of disseminated intravascular coagulation and especially in those with treatable forms of cancer. Even among those with chronic debilitating diseases and lingering forms of cancer, subcutaneous heparin is indicated in the presence of demonstrable aseptic vegetations on echocardiography. The latter recommendation is primarily to improve the quality of life in these chronically sick patients (38).

USE OF ANTIPLATELET AGENTS

Anticoagulation with warfarin requires frequent determination of prothrombin times to maintain the international normalized ratio at a therapeutic level. Numerous drugs interact with warfarin, and a constant vigil is needed to stay between the Scylla of thromboembolism and Charybdis of excessive bleeding. Even alterations in diet can affect prothrombin time, and it is a difficult exercise for both patients and physicians alike. Patients would much prefer to use a simple agent such as aspirin to prevent embolic complications without having to undergo periodic blood tests.

The use of antiplatelet agents for the prevention of thromboembolism has been proposed because numerous studies have indicated that systemic embolism occurs more frequently in patients with valvular heart disease with shortened platelet survival time (49,50). Although shortened platelet survival time has been shown to be a sensitive index of past thromboembolism in rheumatic valvular disease, the test has very poor specificity (51). Numerous antiplatelet agents have been tried, but none has been found to be a useful primary agent to prevent thromboemboli in rheumatic mitral valve disease. Both sulfinpyrazone and dipyridamole have been shown to normalize platelet survival times, and their addition to warfarin has been shown to reduce thromboembolic complications compared with warfarin alone (52). In prosthetic valves, aspirin similarly has been shown to prevent thromboemboli when combined with warfarin (53).

Recently, numerous large-scale multicenter trials have been undertaken among patients with nonvalvular atrial fibrillation comparing placebo, aspirin, and warfarin (33–37). Whereas all the trials showed warfarin to be superior to aspirin, in some of the trials, use of aspirin did show some benefit. In the Danish trial, a modest reduction of stroke incidence was noted among patients randomized to aspirin. However, the 18% reduction did not reach statistical significance (33). In the SPAF-1 trial a significant 44% reduction in stroke rate was noted among those taking aspirin alone (34). A reduction of this magnitude was not duplicated by other trials that were equally well conducted. The SPAF investigators did a second trial, and in SPAF-2, aspirin was useful in reducing thromboembolic risk among younger patients without significant risk factors for stroke such as hypertension, heart failure, or previous history of thromboembolism (54).

With regard to valvular heart disease, it is most unlikely that such trials will ever be undertaken. However, in situations where use of warfarin is contraindicated, aspirin might offer some benefit. In young patients with an active life and asymptomatic mitral valve disease in sinus rhythm, aspirin might be useful. More importantly, in patients with thromboembolic episodes in spite of warfarin, addition of as-

pirin should be undertaken. In mitral valve prolapse with history of transient ischemic attacks, use of aspirin is strongly recommended (38).

More recently, trials are being undertaken to study low-dose combinations of warfarin and aspirin such that blood tests are unnecessary. In SPAF-3, the combination of low-dose warfarin and aspirin was compared with adjusted-dose warfarin in high-risk patients with nonvalvular atrial fibrillation. The trial was stopped prematurely because the low-dose warfarin–aspirin combination had a much higher incidence of systemic embolism than adjusted-dose warfarin (55). If the low-dose combination did not succeed in nonvalvular atrial fibrillation, the chances that such a combination will prevent systemic embolism in valvular heart disease where the risk is much higher is unlikely.

Two new groups of antiplatlet agents have been introduced lately. Ticlopidine works differently from aspirin and has been shown to be an effective antiplatelet agent. This drug has been used extensively to prevent coronary stent occlusions (56). Another antiplatelet agent, clipodregel, has been recently introduced with good credentials in coronary disease (57). Whether these drugs will ever replace anticoagulation for atrial fibrillation in valvular heart disease remains to be seen. Ticlopidine has been advocated for use in mitral valve prolapse patients in sinus rhythm who suffer from transient ischemic attacks despite aspirin intake (38).

Finally, platelet glycoprotein IIb-IIIa antagonists have been shown to be useful in unstable angina and to prevent thrombotic occlusion after percutaneous transluminal coronary angioplasty. It is likely that oral agents will soon be available and may offer an effective alternative to anticoagulation even in rheumatic valvular disease (58,59).

COMPARISON OF VALVULAR AND NONVALVULAR HEART DISEASE WITH ATRIAL FIBRILLATION

It has been recognized for many years that patients with rheumatic mitral valvular heart disease complicated by atrial fibrillation have a greater risk for systemic embolization. A patient with such disease has a one in five chance of having a clinical episode of systemic embolization during the course of the disease. The recognition that patients with nonvalvular heart disease complicated by atrial fibrillation also have an increased risk for systemic embolization has occurred only recently. The reason for the delay is related to the greatly increased risk for systemic emboli in patients with rheumatic heart disease. As shown in the Framingham study, the risk of stroke is 4% to 5% annually among patients with nonvalvular atrial fibrillation. The risk is increased 17-fold when the etiology is rheumatic heart disease (10).

Nonvalvular atrial fibrillation is a disease of old age. The mean age of patients in all the nonvalvular atrial fibrillation trials is greater than 65 years (33–37). However, both in nonvalvular and valvular heart disease with atrial fibrillation, the incidence of embolic complications increases with advancing age. In rheumatic heart disease, anticoagulation with warfarin was established based on observational studies, but nonvalvular atrial fibrillation patients have been subjected to many multicenter clinical trials. In both disease states, however, warfarin remains the effective anticoagulant. Use of aspirin has been shown in some of the trials to be effective in preventing stroke in nonvalvular atrial fibrillation. This may not be true in rheumatic heart disease with atrial fibrillation.

Besides age, multiple risk factors such as hypertension, diabetes, coronary artery disease, and congestive heart failure play a dominant role in the development of thromboemboli in nonvalvular atrial fibrillation (Table 17-1) (33–37). In rheumatic heart disease, on the other hand, these factors do not have a major role, as the severity of valvular heart disease, if untreated, often determines the patient's ultimate outcome.

ANTICOAGULATION FOR CARDIOVERSION IN PATIENTS WITH ATRIAL FIBRILLATION AND VALVULAR HEART DISEASE

Because the development of atrial fibrillation is not always related to the severity of underlying valvular disease, it is often justified to attempt cardioversion in those instances where the valvular involvement is considered minimal. This is especially true if the rhythm abnormality is of recent onset or indicated for hemodynamic stability.

The general rules are the same with valvular disease as in nonvalvular atrial fibrillation. Anticoagulation with warfarin is given for at least 3 weeks before cardioversion and continued for 4 weeks after. An alternative approach is to use transesophageal echocardiography. The patients are heparinized to therapeutic levels before transesophageal echocardiography, and cardioversion is carried out if there are no thrombi seen in the left atrium. After cardioversion, the patients have to be anticoagulated for 4 weeks with warfarin (60,61).

There is a general consensus in nonvalvular atrial fibrillation that anticoagulation is not required if the duration of atrial fibrillation is less than 48 hours. However, in rheumatic valvular disease complicated by atrial fibrillation, it may be wise to use intravenous heparin and subsequent anticoagulation by warfarin for 3 weeks before cardioversion because

TABLE 17-1. *Comparison of valvular and nonvalvular heart disease with atrial fibrillation*

	Nonvalvular	Valvular
Incidence	Increasing	Decreasing
Mean age	>65 yr	Younger
Use of aspirin	Useful in some subsets	Not useful
Stroke incidence	4–5%/yr	17-fold higher
Risk factors to systemic emboli	Age, left atrial size, and left ventricular function	Age, hypertension, diabetes mellitus, and coronary artery disease

thrombi are often present in the left atrium in these cases (62,63).

REFERENCES

1. Wood W. Letter enclosing the history and dissection of a case in which a foreign body was found within the heart. *Edinb Surg J* 1814;10:50–54.
2. Vulpian A. Note sur les effets de faradisation directe des ventricules du coeur chez le chien. *Arch Physiol* 1874; 1:976.
3. Lewis T. Auricular fibrillation: a common clinical condition. *Br Med J* 1909;2:1528.
4. Rothberger CJ, Winterberg H. Vorhofflimmern und arrhythmia perpetua. *Wien Klin Wochenschr* 1909;22:839.
5. Selzer A. Atrial fibrillation revisited. *N Engl J Med* 1982;306:1044–1045.
6. Lie JT. Atrial fibrillation and left atrial thrombus: an insufferable odd couple. *Am Heart J* 1988;116: 1374–1377.
7. Albers GW. Atrial fibrillation and stroke. Three new studies, three remaining questions. *Arch Intern Med* 1994;154:1443–1448.
8. Landefeld CS, Beyth RJ. Anticoagulant-related bleeding: clinical epidemiology, prediction, and prevention. *Am J Med* 1993;95:315–328.
9. Hirsh J, Poller L. The international normalized ratio: a guide to understanding and correcting its problems. *Arch Intern Med* 1994;154:282–288.
10. Kannel WB, Abbott RD, Savage DD, McNamara PM. Epidemiologic features of chronic atrial fibrillation. *N Engl J Med* 1982;306:1018.
11. Szekely P. Systemic embolism and anticoagulant prophylaxis in rheumatic heart disease. *BMJ* 1964;1: 209–212.
12. Martin D, Mendelsohn ME, John RM, Loscalzo J. *Atrial Fibrillation*. Boston: Blackwell Scientific Publications, 1994:60–67.
13. Gajewski J, Singer RB. Mortality in an insured population with atrial fibrillation. *JAMA* 1981;245:1540.
14. Jeresaty RM. *Mitral Valve Prolapse*. New York: Raven Press, 1979.
15. Aberg H. Atrial fibrillation—necropsy analysis of emboli. *Acta Med Scand* 1969;185:373.
16. Hinton RC, Kistler JP, Fallon JT, Friedlich AL, Fisher CM. Influence of etiology of atrial fibrillation on incidence of systemic embolism. *Am J Cardiol* 1977;40: 509.
17. Daley R, Mattingley TW, Holt CL, Bland EF, White PD. Systemic arterial embolism in rheumatic heart disease. *Am Heart J* 1951;42:566–581.
18. Graham GK, Taylor JA, Ellis LB, Greenberg DJ, Robbins SL. Studies in mitral stenosis: a correlation of postmortem findings with the clinical course in the disease in one hundred and one cases. *Arch Intern Med* 1951; 88:532–547.
19. Wood P. *Diseases of the Heart and Circulation*. Philadelphia: JB Lippincott, 1956.
20. Ellis LB, Harken DE. Arterial embolization in relation to mitral valvuloplasty. *Am Heart J* 1961;62:611–620.
21. Dervall PB, Olley PM, Smith DR, et al. Incidence of stenosis embolism before and after mitral valvotomy. *Thorax* 1968;23:530–540.
22. Coulshed N, Epstein EJ, McKendrick CS, et al. Systemic embolism in mitral valve disease. *Br Heart J* 1970;32:26–34.
23. Garvin CF. Mural thrombi in the heart. *Am Heart J* 1941;21:713.
24. Madden JL. Resection of the left auricular appendage—aprophylaxis for recurrent arterial emboli. *JAMA* 1949;140:769.
25. Somerville W, Chambers RJ. Systemic embolism in mitral stenosis-relation to the size of the left atrial appendix. *Br Med J* 1964;2:1167.
26. Peterson P, Kastrup J, Helweg-Larsen S, Boysen G, Gotfredsen J. Risk for thromboembolic complications in chronic atrial fibrillation. *Arch Intern Med* 1990;150: 819.
27. The Stroke Prevention in Atrial Fibrillation Investigators. Predictors of thromboembolism in atrial fibrillation. V. Clinical features of patients at rest. *Ann Intern Med* 1992;116:1a.
28. Levine HJ. Which atrial fibrillation patients should be on chronic anticoagulation? *Cardiovasc Med* 1981;6: 483–487.
29. Carter AB. Prognosis of cerebral embolism. *Lancet* 1965;2:514–519.
30. Adams GF, Merrett JD, Hutchinson WM, et al. Cerebral embolism and mitral stenosis: survival with and without anticoagulants. *J Neurol Neurosurg Psychiatry* 1974; 37:378–383.
31. Fleming HA, Bailey SM. Mitral valve disease, systemic embolism and anticoagulants. *Postgrad Med J* 1971;47: 599–604.
32. Roy D, Marchand E, Gagne P, et al. Usefulness of anticoagulant therapy in the prevention of embolic complications of atrial fibrillation. *Am Heart J* 1986;112: 1039–1043.
33. The Stroke Prevention in Atrial Fibrillation Investigators. The stroke prevention in atrial fibrillation study: final results. *Circulation* 1991;84:527–539.
34. Peterson P, Godtfredson J, Boysen G, et al. Placebo controlled, randomized trial of warfarin and aspirin for prevention of thromboembolic complications in chronic atrial fibrillation: the Copenhagen AFASAK Study. *Lancet* 1985;1:175–179.
35. The Boston Area Anticoagulation Trial for Atrial Fibrillation Investigators. The effect of low dose warfarin on the risk of stroke in patients with nonrheumatic atrial fibrillation. *N Engl J Med* 1990;323: 1505–1511.
36. Connolly S, Laupacis A, Gent M. Canadian atrial fibrillation anticoagulation (CAFA) study. *J Am Coll Cardiol* 1991;18:349–355.
37. Ezekowitz M, Bridgers S, James K, et al. VA cooperative study of warfarin in the prevention of stroke associated with nonrheumatic atrial fibrillation. *N Engl J Med* 1992;327:1406–1412.
38. Levine RJ, Pauker, SG, Salzman EW, Eckman MH. Antithrombotic therapy in valvular heart disease. *Chest* 1992;102:434S–444S.
39. Probst P, Goldschlager N, Selzer A. Left atrial size and atrial fibrillation in mitral stenosis: factors influencing their relationship. *Circulation* 1973;48:1282–1287.
40. Fulkerson PK, Beaver BM, Auseon J, et al. Calcification of the mitral annulus: etiology, clinical associations, complications and therapy. *Am J Med* 1979;66: 967–977.
41. Fukazawa H, Yamamoto K, Ikeda U, Shimada K. Effect

of mitral regurgitation on coagulation activity in atrial fibrillation. *Am J Cardiol* 1998;81:93–96.

42. Barnett HJM, Jones ME, Boughner DR, et al. Cerebral ischemic events associated with prolapsing mitral valve. *Arch Neurol* 1976;33:777–782.

43. Glancy DL, O'Brien KP, Gold HK, Epstein SE. Atrial fibrillation in patients with idiopathic hypertrophic subaortic stenosis. *Br Heart J* 1970;15:1279.

44. Myler RK, Sanders CA. Aortic valve disease and atrial fibrillation: report of 122 patients with electrocardiographic, radiographic and hemodynamic observations. *Arch Intern Med* 1968;121:530.

45. Stein P, Sabbath H, Apitha J. Continuing disease process of calcific aortic stenosis. *Am J Cardiol* 1977;39:159–163.

46. Holley KE, Bahn RC, McGoon DC, et al. Spontaneous calcification associated with calcific aortic stenosis. *Circulation* 1963;27:197–202.

47. Popp RL. Echocardiography. *N Engl J Med* 1990;323:165–172.

48. Lopez JA, Ross RS, Fishbeim MC, et al. Non-bacterial thrombotic endocarditis: a review. *Am Heart J* 1987;113:773–784.

49. Harker LA, Slichter SJ. Platelet and fibrinogen consumption in man. *N Engl J Med* 1972;287:999–1005.

50. Steele PP, Weily HS, Davis H, et al. Platelet survival in patients with rheumatic heart disease. *N Engl J Med* 1974;290:537–539.

51. Steele P, Rainwater J. Favorable effect of sulfinpyrazone in thromboembolism in patients with rheumatic heart disease. *Circulation* 1980;62:462–465.

52. Sullivan JM, Harken DE, Gorlin R. Pharmacologic control of thromboembolic complications of cardiac-valve replacement. *N Engl J Med* 1971;284:1391–1394.

53. Turpie AGG, Gent M, Laupacis A, et al. A comparison of aspirin with placebo in patients treated with warfarin after heart valve replacement. *N Engl J Med* 1993;329:524–529.

54. The Stroke Prevention in Atrial Fibrillation Investigators. Warfarin versus aspirin for prevention of thromboembolism in atrial fibrillation: stroke prevention in atrial fibrillation II study. *Lancet* 1996;343:687–691.

55. The Stroke Prevention in Atrial Fibrillation Investigators. Adjusted dose of warfarin versus low intensity, fixed dose warfarin plus aspirin for high risk patients with atrial fibrillation: stroke prevention in atrial fibrillation III randomized clinical trial. *Lancet* 1996;348:633–638.

56. Schomig A, Neumann FJ, Kastrati A, et al. A randomized comparison of antiplatelet and anticoagulant therapy after the placement of coronary artery stents. *N Engl J Med* 1996;344:1084–1089.

57. The CAPRIE Steering Committee. A randomized, blinded, trial of clopidogrel versus aspirin in patients at risk of ischaemic events. *Lancet* 1996;348:1329–1339.

58. The EPIC Investigators. Use of a monoclonal antibody directed against the platelet glycoprotein IIb/IIIa receptor in high risk coronary angioplasty. *N Engl J Med* 1994;330:956–964.

59. Chesebro JH, Badimon JJ. Platelet glycoprotein IIB/IIIa receptor blockade in unstable coronary disease. *N Engl J Med* 1998;338:1539–1541.

60. Laupacis A, Albers G, Dalen J, Dunn M, Feinberg W, Jacobson A. Antithrombotic therapy in atrial fibrillation. *Chest* 1995;108:3525–3595.

61. Klein AL, Grimm RA, Black IW, et al. Cardioversion guided by transesophageal echocardiography: the ACUTE pilot study. *Ann Intern Med* 1997;126:200–209.

62. Stoddard MF, Dawkins PR, Prince CR, Ammash NM. Left atrial appendage thrombus is not uncommon in patients with acute atrial fibrillation and a recent embolic event: a transesophageal echocardiographic study. *J Am Coll Cardiol* 1995;25:452–459.

63. Prystowsky EN, Benson DW, Fuster V, et al. Management of patients with atrial fibrillation. A statement for healthcare professionals from the subcommittee on electrocardiography and electrophysiology, American Heart Association. *Circulation* 1996;93:1262–1277.

Subject Index

Page numbers followed by f refer to figures; page numbers followed by t refer to tables.